1 MONTH OF
FREE
READING

at

www.ForgottenBooks.com

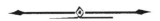

By purchasing this book you are eligible for one month membership to ForgottenBooks.com, giving you unlimited access to our entire collection of over 1,000,000 titles via our web site and mobile apps.

To claim your free month visit:
www.forgottenbooks.com/free789933

ISBN 978-0-483-58716-8
PIBN 10789933

This book is a reproduction of an important historical work. Forgotten Books uses
state-of-the-art technology to digitally reconstruct the work, preserving the original format
whilst repairing imperfections present in the aged copy. In rare cases, an imperfection in
the original, such as a blemish or missing page, may be replicated in our edition. We do,
however, repair the vast majority of imperfections successfully; any imperfections that
remain are intentionally left to preserve the state of such historical works.

INTERNATIONAL DENTAL JOURNAL

A MONTHLY PERIODICAL

DEVOTED TO

DENTAL AND ORAL SCIENCE

EDITED BY

JAMES TRUMAN, D.D.S.

VOL. XXV

PHILADELPHIA
INTERNATIONAL DENTAL PUBLICATION COMPANY
1904

LIST OF CONTRIBUTORS TO VOLUME XXV.

AINSWORTH, GEORGE C., D.D.S.
ALLEN, FREEMAN, M.D.
ANDREWS, R. R., A.M., D.D.S.
ANEMA, R., D.D.S.
ARRINGTON, B. F., D.D.S.
BAKER, H. A., D.D.S.
BAKER, LAWRENCE W., D.M.D.
BALDWIN, A. E., M.D., D.D.S., LL.B.
BOUTWELL, LESLIE BARNES, D.M.D.
CAUSH, DOUGLAS E., L.D.S.
CHADDOCK, CHARLES GILBERT, M.D.
CHITTENDEN, CHARLES C., D.D.S.
CRANDALL, G. C., B.S., M.D.
CRYER, M. H., M.D., D.D.S.
CUMSTON, CHARLES GREENE, M.D.
CURTIS, G. LEROY, M.D., D.D.S.
DAWBARN, R. H. M., M.D.
DECKER, WALTER E., D.D.S.
EAMES, GEORGE F., M.D., D.D.S.
ENDELMAN, JULIO, D.D.S.
FINE, WM. MIDDLETON, D.D.S.
FITZHARDINGE, H. C., D.D.S.
FLETCHER, M. H., M.D., D.D.S.
FRANKLIN, MILTON, M.D.
GIBLIN, THOMAS J., D.M.D.

GILLETT, HENRY W., D.M.D.
GILMER, THOMAS L., M.D., D.D.S.
GRANT, GEORGE F., D.M.D.
GREEN, LEO, A.B., D.M.D.
HALES, LEONARD C., D.D.S.
HICKMAN, H. B., D.D.S.
HOGUE, F. WILSON, D.M.D.
JANLUSZ, HENRY J., D.D.S.
KIRK, EDWARD C., D.D.S., SC.D.
KYLE, D. BRADEN, M.D.
LATHAM, V. A., M.D., D.D.S., F.R.M.S.
McCULLOUGH, P. B., D.D.S.
MARSHALL, JOHN S., M.D., M.S.
MAYER, FRANK R., D.D.S.
MOFFATT, R. T., D.M.D.
MORGENSTERN, MICHAEL.
OTTOLENGUI, RODRIGUES, M.D.S.
PEIRCE, C. N., D.D.S.
PIKE, CHARLES C., D.M.D.
POTTER, WILLIAM L., D.M.D.
READE, ROBERT J., M.D., D.D.S.
RHEIN, M. L., M.D., D.D.S.
SANGER, R. M., D.D.S.
SMITH, D. D., M.D., D.D.S.
SMITH, EUGENE H., D.M.D.

iii

SMITH, F. MILTON, D.D.S.

SOUTHWELL, CHARLES, D.D.S.

STANLEY, NED A., D.M.D.

STOREY, J. E., D.D.S.

TALBOT, EUGENE S., M.D., D.D.S.

TOUSEY, SINCLAIR, A.M., M.D.

TRUEMAN, W. H., D.D.S.

WALKER, WILLIAM ERNEST, M.D., D.D.S.

WEDELSTAEDT, E. H., D.D.S.

WHEELER, H. L., D.D.S.

WHITNEY, J. M., M.D., D.D.S.

WORMAN, J H.

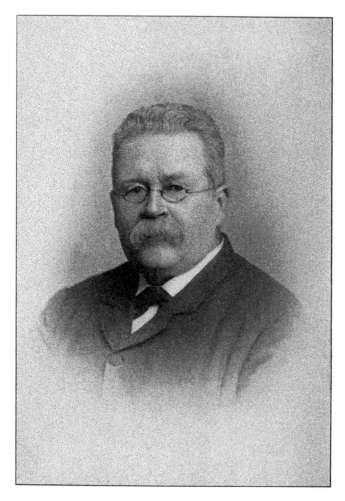

DR. J. FOSTER FLAGG.

THE

International Dental Journal.

| VOL. XXV. | JANUARY, 1904. | No. 1 |

Original Communications.[1]

THE ART OF CARVING AND BAKING PORCELAIN TEETH AND CROWNS.[2]

BY R. T. MOFFATT, D.M.D., BOSTON, MASS.

THE carving of teeth by dentists as a part of their every-day practice is not at all common, and, in fact, I doubt if there are to-day more than fifteen or twenty men in the dental profession in the entire United States who really know anything about it. The carving of teeth, and the preparation of the bodies and enamels wherewith to do it, is so old that to the present generation it is entirely new. It is, in fact, nearly a lost art. This class of work is not taught in the dental schools, though to my mind it should be, if for no other reason than for the education of the eye and hand. Neither is it treated of in the text-books, except those published away back in the '50's. The reason for this lack of appreciation of a useful, practical, and really desirable art is somewhat difficult for me to explain. Those who have been fortunate enough

---

[1] The editor and publishers are not responsible for the views of authors of papers published in this department, nor for any claim to novelty, or otherwise, that may be made by them. No papers will be received for this department that have appeared in any other journal published in the country.

[2] Read before The New York Institute of Stomatology, October 6, 1903.

to acquire the art could not by any possibility do without it, unless sacrificing their artistic ideals of prosthetic work. It seems to me that the "commercial bug" has affected modern dentists to such a degree that in their desire to get rich quickly, they prefer methods that will enable them to turn out artificial teeth in quantity, rather than of a quality that would satisfy an artistic sense. There is as much difference beween a well-carved tooth and a "store" or moulded tooth as between an ordinary cheap photograph of a person and an oil portrait that is a speaking likeness of the subject.

Carving teeth is a delicate art, requiring skill, experience, and artistic taste. As any simple object needs skill and training in its imitation, the beginner must not expect to be able to produce the forms of natural teeth in porcelain without many failures and much perseverance. It will be necessary to study the shapes of many different types of teeth, those belonging to all the different temperaments, in order that the results for each case may not seem as if made from the same hand, or reproduced by means of a mould that is merely mechanically perfect. However, if one will persevere, more or less success may attend his efforts. It has been suggested that an art student, preferably a young lady, might be taught to carve and bake teeth for dentists with satisfaction to the latter and profit to herself. It is possible that this would work well, but it has not my approval, for this reason: for really artistic work that will imitate nature, I think none would be able to do it so well as a dentist, who, with practised eye and fingers, is constantly working over, examining, and repairing the natural teeth, and he best of all knows exactly what he wants as to color, form, and characteristics.

Porcelain teeth were first introduced to this country by a Frenchman, who brought some to Philadelphia about 1820. According to the "American System of Prosthetic Dentistry," Charles W. Peale, in 1822, and Samuel W. Stockton, in 1825, were the next after the Frenchman to manufacture porcelain teeth. They were soon followed by many others, and by 1838 mineral, porcelain, or incorruptible teeth, as they were variously called, had come into general use. Apparently those above mentioned did not carve teeth for individual cases, but they manufactured them from moulds so that they could make them in quantities.

In 1838 there appeared in the *Boston Annual Advertiser and Directory* the following advertisement. This was the only advertisement of the kind in the *Boston Directory* between 1825 and 1860.

IMPROVEMENT IN DENTAL SURGERY.

WHITE TEETH.

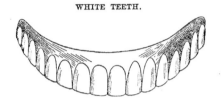

Removal to Granite Building, No. 14 Howard St.

Dr. B. T. Prescott, would inform his friends and the public generally, that he has removed from his old stand, Hanover, corner of Portland St. to the Granite Building, No. 14 Howard St., directly opposite Pemberton House (formerly Holland's Coffee House), where he continues to perform all the necessary operations on the teeth, both for their beauty and preservation. Particular attention paid to cleansing and filling carious teeth with gold, thereby arresting the progress of decay and rendering them useful for many years. Mineral teeth of superior quality inserted on the most reasonable terms.

Dr. Prescott, having obtained the latest and highly approved method of inserting the mineral or incorruptible teeth on gold plates, so recently introduced in Paris, feels assured that he cannot fail to give a general and acknowledged satisfaction to all who may favor him with their call.

Persons requiring operations on the teeth will please call and see specimens at his office, Stone Building, No. 14 Howard St., a few doors West of Concert Hall, Boston.

N.B.—Dentists supplied with mineral or incorruptible teeth, European and American, Wholesale and Retail, on the most reasonable terms. Orders from the country promptly answered.

As far as I have been able to determine, Boston seems to be unique in having fostered a taste for something better than manufactured teeth, turned out of moulds in quantities, entirely lacking in character and individuality. At the time of which I speak conditions in dentistry were much different from what they are to-day, as one would suppose, and these conditions should be understood before I proceed further with my paper. The principal usefulness of dentists at this time was in the extraction of teeth and the manufacture of artificial teeth, so that what we call laboratory work played a prominent part. Plates were then made entirely with metal and the teeth themselves were prepared in secret.

Among the most notable dentists of Boston in their time were

4   *Original Communications.*

the following, with date at which they commenced practice in Boston:

1826. W. P. Greenwood (a famous character), Nathan Cooley Keep (principal witness in Webster-Parkman murder case), Samuel O. Bemis, Thomas Barnes, Moses F. Randall, Richard R. Smith.

1828. Josiah F. Flagg, Thomas W. Parsons (afterwards the great Latin scholar).

1830. Daniel Harwood.

1836. Joshua Tucker.

1842. Elisha Tucker (brother to above).

1846. David Jordan, E. G. Leach.

1848. D. M. Parker, W. T. G. Morton (who needs no introduction).

1849. Willard W. and Benjamin Codman (the latter afterwards founding the firm of Codman & Shurtleff), A. F. Preston.

1851. Jacob L. Williams.

1853. E. T. Wilson.

1855. I. A. Salmon, A. L. Snow (inventors of an automatic mallet), H. D. Osgood (who was constantly in practice until his death last August).

1856. C. E. Dearborn (who is still alive, aged eighty-three).

1857. George T. Moffatt (afterwards Professor of Operative Dentistry, Harvard Dental School).

1858. I. J. Wetherbee (afterwards Dean of Boston Dental School).

1859. Henry Jordan.

1860. Samuel F. Ham, W. E. Woodman.

1862. Thomas B. Hitchcock.

1864. Thomas H. Chandler (afterwards Dean of Harvard Dental School), Nathaniel W. Hawes (afterwards Adjunct Professor of Operative Dentistry, Harvard Dental School), Aaron H. Parker.

1865. Thomas Cogswell, E. N. Harris.

1867. John T. Codman.

1868. R. R. Andrews, Peter Burchaell, L. D. Shepard, John T. Stetson, F. F. Gage.

1870. Charles S. Bartlett.

1872. E. P. Bradbury, D. M. Clapp, D. D. Dickinson, T. O. Loveland.

Out of the above, those whom I have found to have been carvers of teeth were the following: N. C. Keep, Daniel Harwood, Joshua

Tucker, C. E. Dearborn, W. E. Woodman, George T. Moffatt, Henry Jordan, Thomas H. Chandler, S. F. Ham, Aaron H. Parker, Peter Burchaell, F. F. Gage, and Charles S. Bartlett, truly not a large number for a period of forty-six years, from 1826 to 1872.

Nathan Cooley Keep was probably the first carver of teeth in Boston. His work was celebrated for its artistic merit and its individuality. It was by his identifying some teeth which he had carved, and which fitted some models that he had saved, that Professor Parkman was hanged for the murder of Dr. Webster. The porcelain of which Dr. Keep made his bodies and enamels was considered very beautiful, and was noted for the lifelike appearance that it gave his teeth. In those days knowledge in dentistry was kept secret by those who possessed any, and consequently posterity has no authentic formula of Dr. Keep's, as it was said that he kept them in his head, and his secrets died with him.

Next to Dr. Keep was Daniel Harwood. It was related of him that in 1838 he went to Philadelphia, and finding a broken saucer that seemed to be made of material suitable for artificial teeth, he got the receipt for its composition and then constructed some porcelain for incorruptible teeth. He was an artistic carver of teeth and a very busy man. I was told recently by Dr. A. H. Parker that Dr. Harwood had told the latter that many a time he (Harwood) had sat up nearly all night carving teeth, while his wife held a lamp for him to see by. In these days under discussion it was the custom for a dentist with a large practice to take under his training and tuition some promising young man, treating him like an apprentice. These apprentices would pay one thousand dollars for the privilege of being with a man like Dr. Harwood. Dr. Harwood had in all sixteen of these young men or apprentices, four of whom were David M. Parker, C. E. Dearborn, A. H. Parker, and Wilbur Parker, the two latter being brothers. David Parker never carved teeth, but the others did. I commenced my dental career under Dr. A. H. Parker, entering as a laboratory boy, at the age of sixteen, and after four years with him, entered the Harvard Dental School. After graduation I was associated with him for two years. I commenced to carve teeth before I really had studied dentistry, and while with Dr. Parker I had the valuable experience of running the old-fashioned coal and coke furnaces, helping in the manufacture of the improved gas furnaces, grinding and preparing titanium, silex, felspar, and clay, mixing the bodies, enamels, etc. I afterwards received some valuable information from my father on these same subjects and as he studied with Dr. Joshua Tucker, and A. H. Parker studied with Dr. Daniel Harwood, and Drs. Harwood and Tucker were at one time associated, I feel that I am rightfully descended, by the "carving genealogical tree," from the pioneer workers in porcelain dental art.

C. E. Dearborn's teeth had a sameness of expression that suggested a mechanical treatment. W. E. Woodman, I have understood, carved beautiful and artistic teeth. He left a son, who is now the tooth-carver for the Boston Dental Laboratory. Of the work of Henry Jordan, T. H. Chandler, and S. F. Ham I can say little, as I have never seen the work of either of them. - I will give you later, however, some formulas of Dr. Chandler's and Dr. Ham's.

Porcelain for carving teeth is an entirely different material in every way from the material at present on the market that is used for porcelain inlays and restorations. Porcelain teeth are composed of two parts, the body representing the dentine of natural teeth, and the enamel representing what its name implies. The body is made of silex (pure quartz), felspar, and kaolin, or clay, and an oxide of a metal for the coloring. Enamel is made of felspar and a small proportion of silex, and the coloring pigment.

The qualities of a good body are a natural, "bony, lifelike appearance, density sufficient to withstand the strains of mastication, power to withstand the heat of the blow-pipe, a not undue amount of shrinkage during baking, and sufficient plasticity when unbaked to permit of easy handling during carving. The enamel should melt at a temperature slightly below that of the body, for if too fusible it will melt into, rather than upon the latter. Porcelain undergoes a notable diminution of volume during baking, varying from one-eighth to one-fifth according to the formula and amount of moisture, but the same mixture, if moistened always to the same consistency, will contract an amount that is always constant, and which can be properly allowed for. The density is increased with the contraction.

Bodies are best kept in a moist state, as they undergo a process of mouldering, owing to a fermentation of organic matter. This process seems to make the bodies smoother, more homogeneous, and more plastic. It is said that the Chinese have handed down the moistened clay, used for their porcelain wares, through their families for several generations before it is used for its ultimate purpose. If kept too wet the suspended particles will settle into a cake at the bottom of the vessel and the water rise to the top. This settling can be overcome by the addition of acetic acid, which increases the density of the water, but it has the disadvantage of making a rather nauseating odor.

As a consideration of the physical qualities of the constituents of bodies and enamels may not be amiss, I will briefly mention them.

Silex, or quartz, is the main constituent of body, as it gives density and stability and maintains the shape of the tooth during the fusing process; it is practically infusible. It varies much in quality, that from some localities being better than that from others, most of the best coming from Pennsylvania. As the method for reducing silex to a degree of fineness suitable for the purpose under consideration is well described in the "American Text-Book of Prosthetic Dentistry," pages 226, 227, I will omit it here and refer you to that. Coarse silex is used on the planche or tray as a bed for the teeth and to prevent the fusion of the latter to the tray.

Felspar, when finely ground, is a white powder that looks so much like finely ground silex that care must be used not to get them mixed until you are prepared to do so. Felspar, commonly spoken of as spar, is the flux which binds the particles of silex and clay together in the baked tooth. It is the main constituent of the enamel, and it gives the glaze to the tooth.

Kaolin, or clay, should be of the very finest, free from sand and mica or any traces of iron. I have seen blue clay and yellow clay of vastly different appearance in large lumps, but when properly prepared and mixed in the body there was no appreciable difference. Clay gives plasticity to body and assists in making an opaque, bony look. All clays are not plastic, however, nor are they always pure. When perfectly pure, clay is infusible even at the highest heats, but it will soften and become lustrous.

The coloring pigments are oxides of various metals, those of titanium, cobalt, chromium, and nickel being most used, and giving respectively the colors yellow, blue, green, and dark brown. Platinum "sponge" gives a grayish-blue color, and purple of Cassius, a preparation of gold, is used to give red and pink tints for the gum. The preparation of this pigment is a matter of great nicety, and sometimes the most experienced fail to get the desired results. The oxide of titanium can be made to give many shades of yellow, from a good warm orange-color to a pale canary yellow, according to its purity, the fineness to which it is ground, and to the presence or absence of iron. If coarsely ground a warm orange yellow will obtain, while fine grinding will give a lemon yellow. The presence of iron will make it look muddy and brownish. Some titanium containing iron, which I use, will give the black necessary to imitate tobacco stains. The art of tinting porcelains depends upon a knowledge of the management of the vitrifiable pigments. Like all other pigments they may be so mixed as to produce a great variety of tone and tints, but, unlike common coloring matters, chemical changes and reactions take place among them at the high heat to which they are necessarily exposed, so that this latter factor should also be taken into account in the preparation and use of the colors.

Frit is a mixture of a metallic oxide and felspar. By this means a greater subdivision of the pigment is secured, and hence a more thorough permeation of the mass to be colored. Dr. Parker does not frit his titanium, but he does his chromium and the other oxides.

Floating is a process of preparing porcelain materials so as to do away with much of the laborious grinding. The silex, spar, clay, or titanium is mixed with a large quantity of water, stirred, and the heavier particles allowed to settle from one-quarter to one-half hour. The water containing the suspended material is then drawn off and allowed to settle from twenty-four to forty-eight hours, when the water is again drawn off and the material at the bottom dried, and it is then ready for use. If allowed to settle too long, the material will be too fine to be of use for tooth body or enamel. Some felspar that Dr. Parker allowed to settle for four days was too fine, and was useless on account of excessive shrinkage.

We now come to the practical manipulation of the body and enamel in order to make a tooth. First, the instruments. These are few and can be made by any dentist. A " carving-knife," with a small blade about an inch long, three-sixteenths of an inch wide at its widest part, and about 26 gauge; it should have a wooden handle to secure lightness, and be about the size of an ordinary lead-pencil and four inches long. A similar knife with a very thin blade, say 36 gauge, and only about five-eighths of an inch long and one-fourth of an inch wide for separating the teeth. Formerly a bow of whalebone with a fine cotton thread was used for this purpose, but it is not so good or so handy. A little drill for making holes for the pins. A small, flat separating file. A small pair of tweezers with the points grooved for holding a pin, and having a snap catch, so that you can hold a tooth by the pins while enamelling it. A few small camel's-hair brushes for applying the enamel. In addition, you should have handy a small dish or cup full of *clean* water, a little bottle of olive oil with a brush, and a spirit lamp, or a small Bunsen burner with a clean flame. The blade of the carving-knife should be highly polished and the edges dulled and smooth rather than sharp.

The actual carving of a single tooth is a very easy matter, provided one is skilled with his fingers and has an artistic taste. As the description of the carving of a single crown will illustrate the method as well as for a whole set, I will take the simplest form which comes to us, and endeavor to make plain the making of a crown for an upper central incisor. We will suppose that the natural crown of an upper right central incisor has been broken off, leaving a good solid root, and that the other front teeth are all present and in good shape. After preparing the end of the root as you consider proper (and here let me state that you can give it almost any shape you wish, leaving the end practically as you find it, with the exception of removing decay), you fit your platinum post in the canal, giving it whatever direction you desire. Now take a plaster impression of the pin in the root, the end of the root, and at least two teeth on either side of the space to be supplied with the artificial substitute. Any other kind of impression material will not do; plaster *must* be used if you would have an artistic and accurate result. If you are to make a lateral, you should be sure to get an accurate impression of the other lateral, in order that you may have a guide that will enable you to imitate any natural characteristic peculiar to that particular patient's teeth. The same thing applies to cuspid and bicuspid teeth. Make sure that your impression is correct and that the pin has come away in the right place. If the impression breaks, fit the pieces together and wax them so that they will not fall off; then shellac and oil the impression, taking care not to use too much oil; then melt a very thin film of yellow wax on the part of the pin that projects from the impression and that was up in the root-canal.

Now plaster into your impression, and when sufficiently hard cut away the impression carefully, and you should have an accurate model of the patient's teeth, with the end of the root and the pin in place exactly as in the mouth. As soon as you have taken the impression of the teeth, after allowing the patient to rinse the mouth of stray bits of plaster, you should seal the root-canal with temporary gutta-percha. Now take a bit of yellow wax about the size of a walnut and warm and soften it, then press it into the space of the lost crown, and, pressing it firmly into place, let the excess of wax take an impression of the adjoining teeth and then let the patient bite into it, keeping the teeth closed for about two minutes, or until the wax hardens. Carefully remove the wax, taking great care not to distort it, and you will have an accurate occlusion of the lower teeth. Now, with your sample colors select the correct shade, and you can dismiss the patient. All the above should not take more than forty-five to fifty minutes. Now take your model with the pin still in it, and, turning it over in your hand so that the bottom or reverse side presents, make a hole of half an inch diameter in the direction of the apical end of the pin. As soon as you come upon the end of the pin, stop. Now take a fine pointed instrument and gently push the pin out from the impression, if necessary, first gently warming the pin to soften the film of wax before mentioned. Now properly shellac and oil the model, first making grooves or depressions that will guide the " bite half" always to its proper position; then take your little wax impression and bite and set it in its proper place upon the model. Now cast the bite in plaster, and when the latter is hard enough soften the wax in warm water and separate.

You now have an accurate and correct working model. Shellac the bite half and the entire model outside, where your hands or the tooth body would come in contact with it, the object of this being to keep the plaster from getting into the body and to show any scars or marks made upon the model. Next oil the model with olive oil at any part where the body will be placed. Now take an amount of the body sufficient to fill the space, and have it moistened with clean water to the consistency of putty; mix it in the palm of your hand with an ivory, bone, or celluloid spatula (the flat handle of an old tooth-brush will do nicely) until it is entirely free from air bubbles. Then put your pin back in place on the model, pack the body around it, and fill in the entire space, then close the bite half of the model. Next, pat it gently in with the finger in order to make the body as dense and solid as possible; it is even better to squeeze it into position. Now, with the carving-knife you can trim off the surplus body and gradually work it into the shape desired; you can cut, or scrape, or model with the flat of the knife as seems to be required. If you cut off too much, dip the knife-blade in the clean water and touch a drop to the body, then add a little more to give the contour desired; you will find there will be no difficulty in this patching. The tooth should be carved about one-fifth larger than you wished the finished tooth to be, to allow for shrinkage. Sometimes a little smoothing with a moistened camel's-hair brush will make the tooth look more as you wish. If this were a tooth for a plate instead of a crown that we are carving, you could put the platinum pins in now, using head or looped pins for rubber work or headless pins for gold plate work. Dip your drill in water, drill your hole wherever you desire the pin to be, then dip the pin in water, carry it to place, and insert in the hole, and then pat the body down around it to make it solid. Care must be used not to confine an air-bubble at the end of the pin, or you will weaken the tooth, or have a miniature balloon when the tooth is baked. Gently dry the tooth over a spirit lamp and remove from the model. Place some clean coarse silex on your tray or planche and lay the tooth upon this. Dry it out slowly over a Bunsen burner and then bake to a biscuit bake. Partially baking a tooth so that it has about the consistency of a piece of chalk is called biscuiting, or cruzing. The object is to make the tooth more easy to handle, and this final shaping should now be given the tooth. This is also the best time, in my opinion, to put the pins in, although it can be done when the body is soft. In the Parker gas furnace the biscuiting takes three minutes; in the Hammond No. 2 Electric, if you start with a cold furnace you can do the drying out in ten minutes on the first notch, and then heating up for one minute on each consecutive notch, give it four minutes on the sixth notch and then shut off current and cool down. On a biscuit bake you can take the cruzed tooth out at once without danger of cracking it. The biscuited tooth can now be handled with comparatively little danger of injury, and any smoothing up or finishing touches can be given

now. Some prefer to put in the pins at this time. Burs in the
engine can be used to drill the holes for the pins, and if in making
a crown you desire one with a hole through it for the post, in
preference to baking the post in, you can put it in now. Sand-
paper disks in the engine can be used to cut or trim the tooth
should you have cruzed it too hard.

ENAMELLING.

After the tooth has been biscuited it is ready for enamelling.
The tooth or crown should be held with tweezers, having a catch
which will lock it firmly. The tooth should be held in a horizontal position, with the cutting edge towards you. The enamel
should be in a small dish or saucer, such as is used by artists for
water-color paints, and conveniently placed within reach. The
enamel should be moistened with clean water to the consistency
of thick cream. The enamel is applied with a small camel's-hair
brush, the brush sopping up sufficient enamel to have it flow readily
from the point of the brush on touching the tooth. It is better
to have the tooth slightly warm, as the moment the enamel touches
the tooth it is absorbed and dried at once upon its surface. The
enamelling should commence at the cutting edge of the tooth. A
ridge of the enamel should then be made along the cutting edge
of the tooth, then from this a line of enamel should be made upon
the centre of the tooth, parallel with its long axis, so that it
makes a guiding line to show to what thickness the enamel should
be applied over the remaining surface of the crown. The enamel
should be applied in just the same manner as the natural enamel
is found upon the tooth; in other words, quite thick on the cutting
edge and tapering off to nothing at the neck. Care should be used
to lay the enamel on without bubbles, or without getting frothi-
ness. After the crown surface is enamelled about as you think
it should be, little strokes with a moist brush, or with a small
carving-knife, will enable you to put on artistic touches or characteristics which you wish to bring out in the finished tooth. If
you wish to stain the tooth to imitate a tobacco stain or green
stain, now is the time to apply it. This stain is applied on top of
the enamel previously put on. When this is accomplished to your
satisfaction, the tooth should be dried in the flame of a spirit-
lamp. The tooth is now ready for baking.

Dr. Parker's directions for enamelling are to " wet the enamel with water to the consistency of thin cream, and lay or paint it on with a camel's-hair brush, in thickness and contour exactly like the natural enamel. A good effect can be produced, if desired, by too heavily enamelling a tooth, then, when baked, grinding off to match, and polishing in lathe with a buff-wheel or reglazing the surface in the furnace. In this way a greasy, dull surface is made, which has a more natural appearance than the highly glazed, crockery-like surface which is so much the characteristic of artificial teeth. If the color is not deep enough, a second coating of enamel can be brushed on and the tooth rebaked. A second bake always deepens the color, and makes the tooth more transparent. Another desirable effect is secured by levelling the enamel surface with a carving-knife after it has been laid on with the brush and while it is still wet and plastic; characteristic elevations and depressions can now be made. To a beginner a good, practical view of the enamel can be had from a section of a superior central incisor. Gum enamel is applied with a carving-knife."

FURNACES.

The early and common form of furnace was made of fire clay, bound and secured with wrought iron bands and hoops. (See illustration.) It was cylindrical in shape and made in three parts. The total height was about three and a half feet, and the diameter eighteen inches. The lower part contained the grate and ash-pit, the middle section contained a fire-clay muffle placed horizontally with external communication by a door, and the dome-shaped top section had two openings, one directly on top, in the centre, for the smoke-pipe, the other on the front side for the introduction of the fuel, usually coal. The muffle had to be securely luted so as to make it impervious to the gases from the coal, which would have " gassed" and spoiled the work. The external opening to the muffle was closed by a fire-clay door, which was perforated with a hole of about an inch diameter. Through this hole was arranged a clay stopper carrying a platinum wire, on the free end of which was placed a small quantity of body and enamel with each baking, so that the progress of the fusion could be determined from time to time. These furnaces made a lot of dirt. The time of baking varied according to the draft, but it was practically an all-day piece of work, including the gradual cooling off, and the muffles would sag and sometimes break and drop the work into the fire.

About 1870 Dr. A. H. Parker, of Boston, constructed a furnace on this principle, but of much smaller dimensions, it being

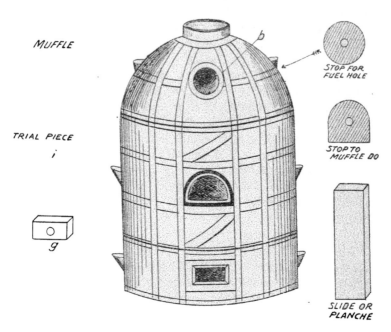

MUFFLE

TRIAL PIECE

g

b

STOP FOR FUEL HOLE

STOP TO MUFFLE DO

SLIDE OR PLANCHE

about the size of a man's silk hat. In this furnace he used coke,
which gave a fire more easily managed, and which reduced the
dirt, time, and labor to about one-half. In 1889 he invented what
came to be known as the Parker Improved Gas Furnace, a little
cylindrical fire-clay furnace four and one-half inches in diameter,
set in a wrought-iron case and covered by a clay dome, the whole
being about six inches high. To the bottom of the iron case was
attached a burner, by which a mixture of gas and air was carried
to the centre of the furnace, where it was ignited. At the lower
end of this burner tube entered two small tubes, through one of
which gas was supplied, the other being used to conduct an air-
blast from the bellows. On the clay bottom of the furnace inside are three little supports for the clay planche, or tray, on
which the teeth are placed for the baking. This planche and the
teeth are protected from the flame and blast by a small clay

cover. The teeth could not be laid directly upon a planche, for they would stick to it when fused, so they are put upon some coarse clean silex. With this furnace the time of baking was reduced to twelve minutes, and the dirt problem was entirely eliminated.

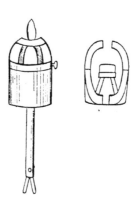

The air blast was maintained by means of a bellows worked by the foot, or connected to a one-fourth horse-power motor and operated by electricity. This form of furnace I have used constantly with success and profit until within a year, when I adopted the Hammond furnace with the No. 2 muffle. As this furnace is well known to all of you, I will not describe it except to say that the time required to bake the porcelain that I use requires ten or twelve minutes to heat and seventeen minutes to bake; in all, I count on about one-half hour. My preference for an electric furnace is on account of the fact that I can have it in my operating-room, and, being noiseless and odorless, I can have baking going on while attending to a patient in the chair. I am also saved the trouble of going up and down two flights of stairs to my laboratory. Its capacity is somewhat limited, which is an objection. Were I in my laboratory nearly all the time, I would still prefer the gas furnace.

BAKING.

Baking with the gas furnace, when the tooth is thoroughly dried, put the tray containing it upon the supports in the bottom of the furnace, cover with the little clay cover, turn on the gas, light it, and then turn on the air-blast (either foot bellows or mechanical pump). Gradually increase the flow of both gas and

air, and when both are on full force put the top of the furnace
in position and continue the baking from ten to fourteen minutes. Shut off gas and air together and allow to cool gradually.
If you wish a rapid cooling, take the furnace top off and remove
tray and cover together, with appropriate tongs, and place in a
large fire-clay muffle. Porcelain can be cooled comparatively
quickly without accident, providing it is cooled equally and evenly.
If, however, the top part cools more rapidly than the part which
is in contact with the silex on the bottom, and which of course
holds the heat longer, you will be sure to find your work cracked.
I would never try to cool a thin gum section rapidly. With a gas
furnace you must carefully regulate the gas supply at the stop-
cock so that the flame visible at the orifice at the top of furnace
is straw-color, thus showing perfect combustion and preventing
" gassing." A blue flame will " gas" the baking. The baking may
be examined by removing the top, but after a little experience
one can bake by " time."

With the Hammond electric furnace No. 2 I use a little platinum planche and cover (gauge 34) on which to put my work.
Start with cold furnace, heat ten minutes on first stop, two minutes each on the second, third, fourth, and fifth stops, and about
fifteen minutes on the sixth stop. Total, thirty-three minutes from
start to finish. Cool slowly, and do not remove the teeth from
the furnace until it has cooled so that you can bear your hand
upon the outside of the muffle dome.

In concluding this brief sketch of the history and art of carving
teeth, I wish to say that I consider that the advantages of this
sort of work over the ready-made teeth are, better colors, a more
natural and lifelike appearance, the possibility of taking conditions in the mouth exactly as you find them, especially concerning crowns and partial dentures, the fact that you can put the pins
exactly where needed for greatest strength, and lastly, a result
which enables art to conceal art, pleases your patient, and satisfies
your own inner consciousness.

FORMULAS FOR BODIES AND ENAMELS.

Thomas H. Chandler's body:

> Silex, 1 oz.;
> Felspar, 2 oz.;
> Kaolin, 2 dwts.;
> Yellow frit, 3 grs. and upward.

YELLOW FRIT.

Spar, 45 dwts.;
Ox. titanium, 5 dwts.;
Ox. chromium, 3 to 10 grs.

Drs. C. P. Wilson and G. T. Moffatt say that the old Harwood and Tucker body was:

Spar, 12 dwts.;
Silex, 8 dwts.;
Clay, 20 grs.;
Color frit.

Dr. A. H. Parker says that the above should be:

Spar, 4 oz.;
Silex, 3 oz.;
Clay, 1 dwt.;

which is what he uses, and as he learned tooth carving of Dr. Harwood, and was with him many years, it is to be presumed he would know. My father and Dr. Wilson's father, Dr. E. T. Wilson, were both with Dr. Tucker, and they obtained the former formula from him.

Dr. S. F. Ham's formula:

BODY.

Spar, 45 dwts.;
Silex, 15 dwts.;
Clay, 2 dwts.;
Color frit.

ENAMEL.

Spar, 10 parts;
Silex, 1 part;
Color frit.

YELLOW FRIT FOR BODY.

Spar, 40 dwts.;
Titanium, 5 dwts.;
Ox. chromium, 2 to 10 grs.

For dark bodies double the amount of chromium in the frit.

GRAY FRIT.

Felspar, 15 dwts.;
Ammoniated muriate of platina, 1 dwt.

Grind the above dry, then wet sufficiently to form into a cake, fuse on a tile, and plunge into cold water while red hot. Grind and float off.

Dr. John D. Dickinson uses for body:

> Spar, 2 oz.;
> Silex, 1 oz.;
> Clay, 2 dwts.;
> Coloring.

ENAMEL.

> Spar, 18 parts;
> Silex, 2 parts;
> Coloring.

Dr. A. H. Parker's enamel is:

> Spar, 6 parts;
> Silex, 1 part;

BLUE FRIT FOR ENAMELS.

> Spar, 15 dwts.;
> Platina sponge, 1 dwt.

YELLOW FRIT.

> Spar, 45 dwts.;
> Titanium, 5 dwts.

BROWN FRIT.

> Spar, 40 dwts.;
> Titanium, 5 dwts.
> Ox. chromium, 10 grs.

GRAYISH FRIT.

> Spar, 10 dwts.;
> Titanium, 2 dwts.;
> Manganese, 12 grs.

BLUE BODY FRIT.

> Felspar, 19 dwts.;
> Oxide cobalt, 1 dwt.

A CARD SYSTEM FOR KEEPING DENTAL RECORDS AND ACCOUNTS.[1]

BY WALTER E. DECKER, BOSTON, MASS.

SYSTEM is an assemblage of objects in regular arrangement. Index is that which guides, points out, informs, or manifests. An index system, therefore, as applied in our present subject, is a regular arrangement of cards that clearly point out or inform.

The value of careful records and accounts cannot be too greatly emphasized.

The conditions that exist during the treatment of a tooth at one time may very materially affect the course pursued later. The observation of different methods and materials under known conditions is a teacher that no successful man can possibly do without.

A systematic record requires very little time, frequently, not more than one minute for each operation.

A dentist's time is his capital, and he can ill afford to waste valuable minutes when they can easily be saved. Furthermore, the loss of energy must be considered. Thought is energy expended, and anything that can be done with little thought and effort conserves energy. A search through several books and over many pages for a particular record is not only a waste of time and energy, but a sore aggravation. Record ledgers, if used as much as they should be, soon wear out and must be rebound and new indices written, or a new book added to the list.

For these reasons a card system is particularly adapted to dentists. The principal arguments in its favor can be clearly stated under the following heads: Adaptability, Contractibility, Expansibilty, and Accessibility.

Its adaptability to dentists is its most conspicuous feature. In few callings are there occasions to refer to past records as frequently as in our profession, and at such times there are few men whose minutes are as valuable.

With books it is necessary to refer, first, to the index, then to the page, or, likely, to several pages, and, finally, to the record. Then, too, it is not convenient to have the books at the chair during an examination, for instance, while the cards may lie upon the

---

[1] Read before the Massachusetts Dental Society, June 3 and 4, 1903.

tray and the record be referred to without even taking the mirror from the patient's mouth. As I have said, this sort of observation and comparison is a most valuable teacher. Our methods change from time to time, likewise our materials. If we may know by a glance the method or material employed at a previous sitting, it may be of great value in choosing and eliminating.

A card system has contractibility,—no useless matter need be retained. In the book old matter which has ceased to be of use continues to occupy valuable space, and there is no way of weeding it out except by rewriting. In the card index active and dead matter may be separated and yet one class referred to as readily as the other. The card containing the dead matter may be removed without interfering with the remaining cards in any way. As a result the card list is always an accurate up-to-date source of information.

The expansibility of a card system is limitless.

Additions can be made by the insertion of new cards without disturbing the former occupants.

It is far less expensive than keeping books. One outfit answering the purpose of any number of new ledgers. The original outlay is only once. After that one only buys the leaves, as it were.

It also has accessibility,—always " get-at-able." For convenience of reference nothing can equal the card index. The record cards are arranged under certain heads and subdivided under alphabetical guides in such manner that from the patient's name his card can be turned to instantly and, as I will show you later, when the card is in one's hand the record stands out clear and distinct.

Not only do I advise the casting aside of record books, but also other books, papers, etc., whose matter can be systematically recorded in the same cabinet. For instance, a cash account, a directory, prescriptions under certain heads, various filling-materials and medicaments, legal and other matters of whatever nature can be indexed in very convenient forms.

With a record pertaining to the practice, four divisions, each with alphabetical guides, is the most convenient arrangement. One for " Unfinished Operations," one for " Outstanding Accounts," one for " Settled Accounts," and one for " Old Charts for Reference." During a series of sittings for a patient the card is kept under " Unfinished Operations." When the mouth has been placed in order at the last sitting the card is placed under " Outstanding

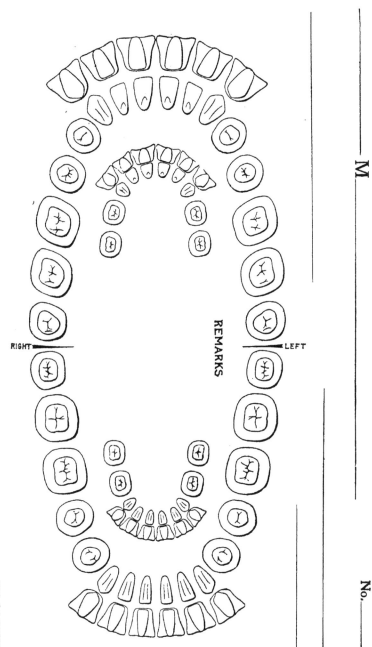

M.

REMARKS

RIGHT

LEFT

No.

Accounts." This second section, only, has to be gone through when sending out bills. This is a great advantage over books where the outstanding accounts are scattered and the whole book, or books, must be gone over.

It is said of dentists that they are poor collectors. Possibly the books are to blame for a part of this, as the due accounts are not in a conspicuous place and the bills may not go when they should.

When an account is paid the card is so credited and placed under " Settled Accounts." When the account is reopened the card starts on the same routine again and continues until it is filled, when it is given a number and then placed under the fourth head, or, " Old Charts for Reference."

The simplicity of this arrangement enables one to find at once anything that has been done in the mouth.

There are a great many charts on the market, but, to me, all are defective in some important feature.

Some are too extensive, requiring a compound filling to be marked in several different places. Others are so small it is impossible to tell from a marking which of several fillings in the same tooth a description refers to.

The vast majority do not show all the approximal sides of the
The only original feature, however, displays the approximal surfaces, this is an annoying defect.

In this chart we have endeavored to overcome the failings of others.

The only original feature, however, displays the approximal surfaces of the twelve anterior teeth.

The relative sizes and shapes of the teeth on this chart are nearer normal than any other. The sulci, also, are the most constant found.

Of course, in a measure, it is diagrammatic, and yet a complete and comprehensive record can easily be drawn upon it.

The chart shows two drawings of the twelve anterior teeth. The inner cuts representing the inner, or palatal and lingual aspects. The outer ones display the labial and approximal surfaces.

The masticating surfaces of the posterior teeth are represented by the inner circles along the sides of the card, the outer circles representing the gum margins. The same description applies to the smaller arch, which represents the temporary teeth.

If desired, after marking each operation the date and material used. can be written opposite, and only the charge placed upon the back of the card. The better way, however, is to give each operation a number, which is also written on the back of the card with the record and account.

The back is ruled in such a manner that the date, operation, and charge can be recorded thereon. As there are fifty lines, one card will last a long time.

These cards can be obtained of the Eugene Smith Company, 108 Pemberton Building, Makers of Special Card Index Systems for Physicians and Dentists. Mr. Smith has kindly consented to keep this card in stock and arrange outfits in any style and for almost any price.

The popular outfit costs seven dollars, and contains cards enough to last from six to ten years.

REPORT OF THE DEMONSTRATOR OF OPERATIVE DENTISTRY OF THE G. V. BLACK DENTAL CLUB (INC.), OF ST. PAUL, FOR THE OCTOBER, 1903, MEETING.

BY E. K. WEDELSTAEDT, DEMONSTRATOR.

MR. PRESIDENT AND GENTLEMEN,—For a number of years you have elected me to the office of demonstrator of operative dentistry. Each month during this long period of time a report has been made you regarding the current dental literature of the day and some special features of our operations. There has also been a large number of discussions of the ideas and methods advanced by others. On many occasions we have wondered at some of the things printed in the journals, and many times we have been unable to understand how it was possible for men to display such a limited comprehension of our operations.

In my dealings with you the changes which have taken place in your ideas regarding our methods and operations have perhaps been of more satisfaction to me than anybody knows. This continual advance is as it should be. You know that intelligent men who are interested in their different vocations do more or less reading, as well as have a constant interchange of ideas with others

in their special calling. By following such a course, we change our
ideas, our methods, our operations, etc.   In the fewest possible
words, we broaden our views and look at things generally in a
much more comprehensive way. A man who does not do any reading cares nothing for an interchange of opinion with others, is
perfectly satisfied with himself and his methods, is not, in fact,
interested in what he himself or others are doing; he becomes
more and more narrow, until at last his ideas may not be broader
than the edge of a razor. It is from the men who are in the last-
named class that we hear so much about the beauty of following
the obsolete methods. As a rule, these men are unwilling to
progress, and, worse still, are unwilling to permit others or the
profession to advance beyond their own ideals or standards. Imagine for a moment the situation, if other professions were handicapped in a similar manner. Suppose the medical journals were
continually filled with many essays which should advocate the
necessity for bleeding all people who had fevers. Or suppose, at
the regular meetings of physicians, there was a constant discussion
regarding the efficacy of following the hot-water treatment of
Dr. Ferrara, so beautifully depicted in Gil Blas, what advance in
their calling would physicians make? To speak plainly, we have
altogether too many writers who are forever dwelling on the past
history of our profession and who are forever giving entirely too
little consideration to the present and future welfare of our calling.
No man, I do not care who he is, honors the memory of Townsend,
Varney, Webb, Cushing, McKellops, and all others who were in-
strumental in assisting to raise the standard of our profession,
more than I do, nor does any man place a higher value upon their
efforts in doing good. But I also try to make use of the knowledge
which has been developed since the time of these men, instead of
continually dwelling on the beauty of the ideas that were promulgated twenty or thirty years ago. It is hardly necessary for me
to say to you, that unless I could assist in raising the standard
to a higher plane, try to interest you in progressive dentistry, try
to interest you in being of greater worth to humanity, both my
pen and voice would be forever silent, and I would not, month
after month, come to you as I have requesting that you make
greater use of and give more consideration to the knowledge as it
has been developed. An honest dentist is the noblest work of God,
and an honest dentist dwells rather with the present than with the

past. He takes the best out of the old and applies it to the new. He is a radical, but he is the king of conservatives. Intelligent men so recognize him and the position which he has taken, but ignorant men are apt to call him an extremist. Few persons seem to know that the term " extremist" is equally applicable to ignorant as well as to intelligent people. You know also that the greater the departure from our own personal standard or ideals the more we are inclined to think it extreme.

But all this preface has been for the purpose of leading up to other things.

On many occasions we have all wondered how long it would be before some little ray of light would begin to break in on others, and when they would look at conditions from our point of vantage. The light has at last reached one of my friends. In the INTERNATIONAL DENTAL JOURNAL for September is an essay from the pen of Dr. M. L. Rhein, of New York. The subject chosen is, " The Technique of Approximal Restorations with Gold in Posterior Teeth." The essay, being published, is public property, and I have a right to discuss the ideas which it contains. The essay has been read by me a number of times, and I shall try to discuss it in a perfectly fair and impartial manner. To discuss it in this way, however, is a somewhat difficult thing to do, for the reason that there are so many unknown terms used with which I am not familiar. Neither can I quite understand the use of a number of words for which there is no authority and which, so to speak, do not quite fill the bill. Besides, Dr. Rhein's interpretation of the fundamental principles is very different from our own, he being a follower of Webb, while we are followers of Black. (It may be well to state that Webb died in 1882.) On account of making use of the newer knowledge which has been developed during the past twenty years, as well as of the experience gained during these years, a somewhat different interpretation is now given the fundamental principles from those which were given them at the time of Webb. The results of the experiments of the physical properties of the human teeth and filling-materials, the development of our knowledge of stress and its influence on our operations, the development of bacteriology, the setting at rest of the cause of decay of the human teeth, the classification and use of remedial agents, a continual development of our knowledge of the cause of failure of fillings and the conditions of faulty environment, the development of principles of instrumentation, etc., are all factors which have tended to give us a very different interpretation of the essentials from those that we once possessed. But just so long, however, as men are unwilling to make use of the knowledge spoken of, which in altogether too many cases they will not even consider, there will not be harmony among us in so far as this relates to a better understanding of what is necessary. As we make use of the knowledge gained from a constant study of the conditions with which we deal, so are we able to grasp much - better our hold on the fundamental motives for every step of our operations. The profession of dentistry cannot advance until these different things are considered and studied as they should be.

What I wish above all else is that we could persuade Dr. Rhein to spend about a week with the mighty Searl. I have an idea that at the end of this time he would be perfectly satisfied with the knowledge that to be a follower of Black was about the greatest honor man could attain in an ordinary lifetime. The good thereafter which Dr. Rhein would be capable of rendering advanced dentistry would be of incalculable value. But let us to his ideas.

Dr. Rhein has at last recognized the value of having fillings properly seated on a flat gingival wall or seat. From this time forth he will begin to have much satisfaction from noting the stability of the beautiful operations which he is capable of making. The necessity for squaring out the lingual and buccal gingival angles is nicely considered. He recognizes the uselessness of making large and deep undercuts, for these merely weaken the tooth and do not add stability to the filling. The illustrations published in connection with his essay do not, by any means, give us a clear conception of his ideas in regard to an occlusal anchorage. His words, however, cannot be misunderstood when he speaks of the value of right-angle anchorages in the occlusal surface. There is a difference in our methods of cavity preparation, but it is too slight to speak of, with the exception of his treatment of the cavo-surface angle. He trims this angle with a gem stone and then finishes it with sand-paper disks, a method I have observed many men use. Tight margins cannot under any circumstances be made against a smooth margin if gold is the filling-material used. Gold slides over a polished surface, for there is nothing against which it can be restrained in its course. But roughen that margin by planing it with a sharp chisel, and gold will hug that roughened surface, if properly placed, so that water-tight margins can be made. Dr. Rhein, among other things, does not believe in the use of soft or unannealed gold in the gingival third of cavities which we fill in the proximal surfaces of molars and bicuspids. He believes in an all-cohesive gold filling. He anchors his first piece of gold with a small quantity of cement at the junction of the axial wall with the gingival seat,—*i.e.,* gingivo-axial angle. (Dr. Rhein has not been very explicit in the use of terms. I do wish that he had been, so that we could have better understood what he means.) He also believes that after the gingival third of the cavity is filled the filling can be polished; that the matrix can be used; that the gold in the proximal surface should be entirely built up to the step on the occlusal surface; that the electric mallet will pack gold to homogeneous compactness; that those belonging to the Black creed write as though all recurrence of decay is due to non-extension of cavity margins; that we can stop packing our gold into cavities at any point and any number of times, fill the cavity with gutta-percha, and at a subsequent sitting cut down the gold and go on with the operation; that after the cavity is ready for the gold it should be washed with a few drops of ten per cent. solution of formalin, etc. It will not be possible for me to consider these nine subjects in any other than the briefest manner.

Let us, for a moment, look into this matter of using soft or un-annealed gold in the gingival third of cavities in the proximal surface of molars and bicuspids. The most difficult operation a skilled dentist is called upon to perform is the removal of serumal calculus. Following this operation very closely is the ability to make tight margins with cohesive gold, and there are not very many dentists in our profession who can do either perfectly. Any man who has the ability to make a water-tight filling with cohesive gold in one of the proximal surfaces in molars or bicuspids has my unqualified respect and admiration. It is an operation that I would not under any circumstances attempt to make, for I know of the difficulties with which I have to cope. Let me watch an operator place and condense his gold, and I can very quickly tell you whether or not he is making a water-tight filling. On page 526 of the *Dental Cosmos* for 1891 is said all that is necessary about this subject; besides this, I have given you demonstration after demonstration with gold itself. I wish to say that any intelligent person who will watch and make a careful study of the action of cohesive gold under the plugger-point while being packed into a given cavity cannot help becoming impressed with the difficulty of making tight margins with such an intractable material. If we have all this trouble when filling cavities in the mesial surfaces of the upper incisors and cuspids, where conditions are most favorable to success, what can we expect when we deal with cavities in the mesio- or disto-occlusal surfaces of molars and bicuspids? Dr. Rhein has, however, good reasons for his contention. I notice a number of essays in our journals in which the writers advance the idea that a matrix can be placed around a cavity and the whole proximal surface be filled with soft or unannealed gold. Now this is a very common mistake, and it is being made by too many operators. Because a few men advance ideas of this kind is not, in my estimation, a good reason for condemning entirely the use of soft or unannealed gold. Let us take a practical case. There is a cavity to be filled in the lower left first bicuspid. The linguo-bucco-gingival measurement of the cavity is five millimetres. The gingivo-occlusal measurement is 4.5 millimetres. The gingival seat is 1.7 millimetres. The man closes the gnatho-dynamometer to the one-hundred-and-fifty-pound mark. The filling will have an occlusal anchorage. I will take three cylinders made of one-quarter of a sheet of No. 4, untrimmed gold and place them in the gingival third of this cavity and then condense them. On remeasuring the cavity I find that those three cylinders have reduced the gingivo-occlusal size of the cavity 1.5 millimetres. Now, when the cavity is filled the cohesive gold will be 3.5 millimetres thick. This will be amply sufficient for all practical purposes. I cannot conceive what objection there would be to the use of this small amount of soft or unannealed gold. Further, I feel very certain in saying two things: First, that those three cylinders could be placed and condensed before any person could ever mix cement; secondly, that ninety-nine per cent. of operators are more likely to make tighter margins by using soft or unannealed gold in the position named than could ever be made by the use of cohesive gold.

Where patient after patient consults me, in whose teeth I find fillings which have had the gingival third of the cavities in molars and bicuspids filled with soft or unannealed gold, that have done good service for upward of thirty or more years, I am perfectly willing to continue to use it, especially when I am continually seeing failures of fillings which have been made with all-cohesive gold. Several years ago a long line of experiments with cements were published. . Since that time these results have been added to by others who have also made experiments. Now let us consider this matter a little farther, and meet it fairly as men should do. At the present time we have on the market and in constant use cements which are water-logged within two hours after being placed in the cavities in the human teeth; cements which contract and cements which expand. We know definitely that it takes fully five days for cements to obtain their full degree of hardness and settle down into an inert condition. This being the case, I cannot understand how Dr. Rhein can advocate any such method of anchoring his first piece of cohesive gold. Another thing. For a number of years I have removed many gold fillings which have had the first piece or pieces of gold anchored as described by the essayist. In fact, since beginning the writing of this report I have removed three gold fillings which have been anchored according to this method. The cement in these three cases was simply a white powder without structure or form, and this is precisely as I have always found it where this method has been employed. In view of these circumstances, it is deplorable that others are asked to follow a method the ultimate results of which are very far from satisfactory.

Polishing the gold placed in the gingival third of cavites before the entire filling has been made.

Filling part of the cavity with gold and leaving it to be finished; *i.e.*, to continue the placing of gold at another sitting.

Using a few drops of ten per cent. formalin just prior to placing the gold into the cavity.

Anybody who has made experiments with gold fillings knows that the best operations are made where gold is placed against a perfectly clean surface. A clean, freshly roughened surface, such as is made with a sharp chisel, is the only surface gold will hug closely. In fact, it is the only surface against which we can pack gold and make water-tight margins. With this knowledge before us, how is it possible to finish the gold which has been placed in the gingival third, polish it with strips which have been vaselined, and not be compelled thereafter to go over the remaining cavo-surface angle with a sharp chisel. This must be done. Besides this, there will be a bad joint where the filling is continued. Nor is this all. There is a fundamental principle involved which demands some consideration from us, and it is the law governing marginal condensation. If we believe in marginal condensation it is impossible to make a filling of homogeneous compactness in the gingival third only, for the reason that in making the marginal condensation the gold towards the occlusal surface, not being supported, is stretched and driven from its position. How it is anchored in the cavity does not make any difference. It is impossible not to drive the gold in the direction of the least resistance. The gold, not being supported towards the occlusal surface, is spread in that direction to the detriment of the rest of the filling. By following such a method we induce lines of internal weakness in the filling itself. No, I cannot endorse a method of this kind.

After a cavity is once finally prepared, the gold should be placed then and there, or else we should cut a new cavo-surface angle prior to placing our filling-material. And after the cavity is prepared and ready for the gold, no medicine of any nature should ever be placed therein (except, occasionally, when a little varnish may be used on an axial or pulpal wall). When the cavity is finally prepared it is in the best possible condition to make water-tight margins, therefore fill it. I cannot understand the notion possessed by so many operators that all cavities should be washed with alcohol, chloroform, oil of cloves, carbolic acid, or some other agent just prior to placing the filling-material. I view the use of such methods with many misgivings, so far as they relate to the final results.

We have all tried and know what results are obtained where a matrix is used, so far as this relates to making gold fillings. If there is a place in dentistry where they are contra-indicated it is in connection with the use of gold. The matrix and amalgam go hand in hand together, and there let the matter rest. In the fewest possible words, matrices have absolutely no place, nor are they useful adjuncts to employ where we are dealing with gold.

In placing gold in the cavities in the proximal surfaces the best results are obtained if the gold is laminated from the anchorage in the occlusal or incisal surface towards the gingival seat. Surely far stronger fillings can be made by following such methods than by first filling the entire cavity in the proximal surface up to the anchorage in the occlusal or incisal surface. The essayist's remark about keeping gold about even is what has been taught **for** a number of years and his emphasizing this teaching is to be commended.

The essayist says, " In fact, all the members of the Black creed write as though all the recurrences of decay that are found are due to insufficient extension." Now this statement is to be regretted. You gentlemen are intelligent men, and I am very glad that we never hear anything about extending cavity margins. For nearly two years not a man in this Club has said anything to me about applying principles of extension for prevention. This continual harping on this subject is absolutely disgusting. When surgeons meet they do not continually discuss the necessity for sterilizing their instruments, neither are the essays in the medical journals continually dwelling on this one topic. All rational surgeons recognize the necessity for sterilizing their instruments. All rational dentists, who have made a study of their failures, recognize the necessity for the application of principles of extension for prevention. Extension for prevention is simply one of the essentials which it is necessary to consider when we deal with cavities that are in many proximal surfaces. But there are other things besides applying principles of extension for prevention, and these other things call for our most earnest consideration. Cavities at all times must be made accessible, fillings must be properly seated and anchored, gold must be properly placed and condensed, fillings must be trimmed to form and polished, the tooth must be returned to its original mesio-distal diameter, and there must not be a condition of faulty environment left. Each of these subjects is of equal importance, and goes hand in hand with the application of principles of extension for prevention. Ignore one of them, and later on failure will stare you in the face. It was only a short time ago that a patient consulted me regarding the condition of her teeth. The fillings were most beautifully made, trimmed, and polished. The cavities in the proximal surfaces, on account of being refilled so many times, were three-quarters as broad linguo-buccally as the teeth were thick, but there was no contour given the interproximal space, nor could it be done because the teeth were not returned to their original mesio-distal diameter. Within three years these fillings will have to be remade, as there is no possibility on the part of the patient of keeping them clean. No operator, I do not care who he may be, can leave a condition of faulty environment surrounding any dental or surgical operation and expect to obtain

anything else than failure. I hope that so long as I am a member
of this Club we shall never again be called upon to hear anything
about the necessity for the application of the principles of extension for prevention.

There remains, then, but one subject to discuss, and that is
the use of the electric mallet in condensing gold. Like many other
operators, I formerly used the electric mallet. For a number of
months it was in constant use in my office, when it was discon-
tinned. My reasons for this were simply that I could operate more
rapidly by other methods and make much better operations in a
shorter space of time by employing an assistant who used a hand
mallet. Along in 1895 some tests were made with gold fillings
which had been made by using different mallets, different kinds of
gold, etc. In the *Dental Cosmos* for that year, on page 749, can
be found the results of these tests. An expert in the use of the
electric mallet made three fillings for me. The highest specific
gravity reached was 13.2. From an examination of the results
obtained by testing the different fillings, we find that the electric
mallet is not even on a par with the automatic mallet, and until
Dr. Rhein or some other good man will make us some experimental
gold fillings, using the electric mallet for packing his gold, and
give us the benefit of the results of his tests, the results of the
experiments in the 1895 *Cosmos* must be considered standard. I
think that Dr. Rhein may be able to make fillings of 16 or more
specific gravity by using the electric mallet, but it will be necessary for him to give each piece of gold condensed from three to
five minutes malleting. When it is taken into consideration that
twenty seconds of hand malleting on each piece of gold, of a given
and known size, will give a specific gravity of 17 or more, are we
justified in taking a longer time? Are not our operations long
enough, and are they not tedious enough?

I have taken this essay and have made an attempt to discuss it
in a way that was absolutely free from all prejudice. Attention has
been called to a number of things, and they have been discussed as
thoroughly as it has been possible for me to do in such odd moments
as I could obtain from my labors. When it is known that a man
of Dr. Rhein's standing will make changes in his methods to the
extent he has, there is hope that others will do likewise.

I stand for a constant advance in our chosen calling. I have
made a few contentions for that which I considered was of value

in advancing dentistry to the position where I feel it should be. That I have made mistakes nobody knows better than I. Had I not made and recognized them, I could not have discussed this essay in the way I have.

I suppose that you wish me to say something about the gold fillings which we examined this morning. The operations were made by Dr. J. V. Conzett, of Dubuque, Iowa. In the past twenty-five years I have never seen eleven more beautiful operations in the teeth of the same individual which had been made in cavities in the proximal surface of molars and bicuspids. In each operation the cavity margins had been placed in the most convenient position for making as nearly perfect operations as possible. The contour of the interproximal space was as perfect as it was possible to obtain. The contact points were small and correctly placed, with the exception of those made on the fillings in the proximal surfaces of the upper left first molar and second bicuspid. The contact points on these two fillings had been placed a trifle too far towards the disto-bucco and mesio-bucco-occlusal angle, but these two fillings have not been completely finished. At the final finishing it may be possible to alter the position of those two contact points. This is the only comment I have to offer regarding the operations. The knowledge that we have men in this Northwest who have the ability to make such operations and do make them, is an incentive to our ambition. Not only is it a revelation to know that we have men who have ideals and are perfectly willing to carry them out, but examining such operations aids us materially in an educational way, by stimulating us to a higher endeavor. This is the kind of dentistry that I have been trying to interest men in for the last eight years, and I am perfectly satisfied with the results. I cannot speak too highly of the benefits that accrue to a patient who has such operations made in the cavities of his teeth. I have been particularly interested in Dr. Conzett and what he is doing. For the past five years he has given up much time to a study of conditions, in seeking out the cause of his failures, and in having an interchange of opinion with other men in our calling. We are now in a position to judge of his interpretation of the fundamental principles and how he applies his knowledge to the operations which he makes for others. Comparisons are at all times odious, but right in connection with this subject I desire to present for your consideration these two casts. The fillings as outlined in that molar and bicuspid were made some eighteen months ago by a man of national reputation and a teacher of operative dentistry in one of our colleges. As Dr. Searl so nicely says, " The operations made by Dr. Conzett were made to preserve the teeth, and those made by the teacher were made for what mcney he could get. They were not made to preserve the teeth." The patient was thirty years of age, and he was one of the best patients for whom I have ever operated. Whether " skipping corners" in this way, as Dr. Black says, calls for a display of charity is something which you must decide for yourselves. In the operations made by the teacher every fundamental principle was ignored, so far as this relates to those gold fillings. In the operations made by Dr. Conzett we have the application of every known fundamental principle. On this account the operations do not compare very favorably one with the other. Dr. Conzett is an honest dentist. Where to place the teacher, I do not know nor do I wish to know.

All of which is most respectfully submitted.

THE GREAT AMALGAM FALLACY.[1]

BY RODRIGUES OTTOLENGUI, M.D.S., NEW YORK.

At the meeting of the New Jersey State Dental Society, last summer, I presented a paper relative to the filling of children's teeth. In the discussion that ensued I was told by several gentlemen that I was threshing old straw. In reply I pointed out that the chief idea exploited—namely, the filling of children's sixth-year molars with gold, rather than with amalgam—was a theory of practice which I had not seen previously advocated, and I asked those who called my paper " old straw" to indicate where in our literature I could find previously printed papers on the same lines. This was not done then, nor has it been done since, notwithstanding the fact that since that time I have read two more papers on the same subject, one before the new National Association of Canada and one before the Second District Society at Brooklyn. Should similar contention be made in regard to the present paper, it will

---

[1] Read before the Academy of Stomatology, Philadelphia, April 28, 1903.

be incumbent upon the disputants to specify the exact features which are so old as to be beyond further discussion.

In the papers mentioned I decried the use of amalgam in children's teeth, and more especially in cavities which are in the initial stages of decay. One result is that I have obtained something of a reputation as an antagonist of amalgam in general, which impression is erroneous.

In this paper, therefore, undertaking a discussion of amalgam within a realm where the highest attainments in the use of the material should maintain, since the most prominent disciples here abide, I shall hope for a sufficient close attention, so that, in the discussion, what I do say and do mean will receive criticism, rather than that there may be any further mistaken ideas in regard to those theories of practice which I advocate.

A word about the title which I have selected. What is "the great amalgam fallacy"? I take it that the general use of amalgam, as it is employed by three-fourths of the dentists of this country, is fallacious in many vital respects, which I shall endeavor to point out in detail. Of the other fourth of all the dentists, a large percentage use amalgam injudiciously and improperly, in at least some of their operations. Indeed, I venture to believe that not ten per cent. of all the amalgam fillings made are properly inserted—that is to say, placed where they will prove most reliable—and the operations performed in a skilful manner throughout.

The chief fallacy in regard to amalgam, and the one which is the basis of all other errors in connection with its use, is that it is a *cheap* filling. This is a more dangerous fallacy, because it rests upon a modicum of truth. In a large share of cases the amalgam filling will occupy less time than would the insertion of a gold filling in the same situation, and time being the chief measure upon which to base the size of a fee, the fee for amalgam is properly smaller than for gold. But in two important classes of cavities this is not true. In very simple cavities the actual time occupied in placing the gold and finishing the same will be no greater than that required for placing the amalgam, plus the time required at a second sitting for polishing, for on that occasion the dentist must charge to profit and loss all the time from the admission to the discharge of the patient. The exception would be where other work were in progress, but evidently the average dentist begrudges even this minimum expenditure of time, if I may judge by the very small number of amalgam fillings that are polished; and here I mean polished with the same care and completeness as the same dentist would bestow upon the same tooth were it filled with gold.

The second and more important class of cavities are those of large size where the work may be complicated by the difficulties of the environment. I allude particularly to cavities which involve the approximal surfaces and which lie close to or beneath the gum margins. The examination of a hundred teeth with cavities of this character filled with amalgam, removed from the mouth, and compared with a hundred similar teeth filled with gold, will show how inadequate is the usual polishing of such large amalgam fillings. Why? Because the time required in sittings subsequent to that at which the amalgam is placed, for the separation of the teeth and proper polishing, is time lost to the dentist unless his fee is as large as for gold, and he has mistakenly educated his patients up to the idea that amalgam is a cheap substitute.

Let us finish the consideration of this aspect of the case before proceeding farther. There are two methods in vogue for the regulation of dental fees, neither of which alone is adequate. One of these, perhaps the one most used, is the fee system. In this course of business management the practitioner erects a definite, if somewhat elastic, scale of prices. " Small gold fillings, ten cents; medium, fifteen to twenty-five; large, thirty to fifty. Amalgam fillings at half the cost of gold." In many of the smaller towns, even respectable, ethically inclined dentists do not hesitate to print a " scale of prices" on the back of their appointment cards. This system makes of a dentist little more than a shopkeeper, a man with wares to sell, rather than personal services to render for adequate return. The arrangement of fees in accordance with the size of a filling may often deprive the dentist of his merited reward for skilled service, and just in proportion as this becomes true in his practice, will such a man become less skilful. It is exactly in this way that the fee system operates against the best results with amalgam. The low price having been established, the dentist discovers that literally he cannot afford to give his amalgam fillings the same thorough attention as he would devote to gold.

The other system of charges is based upon the time required in performing an operation. The dentist computes the time and charges at a definite rate per hour. Thus he classes himself with the day laborers, the bricklayers, plasterers, and other mechanics. He might well organize a union, and have a fixed scale, with strikes when the community demurs at his charges. This man also finds himself underpaid for his amalgam work, because he does so quickly the actual filling, and because he lacks the courage to include in his bill (or records) a separate item of charge for the time occupied in polishing. Thus by both fallacious methods of charging the amalgam work, being the least remunerative, receives less skill, and I do not hesitate to admit that much of the failure with amalgam is more rightfully chargeable to faulty manipulation rather than to the material *per se.*

How may this be remedied? It appears to me that there is another way of arranging fees; one that is more professional, and which will prove more just to patients and more uniformly satisfactory to the dentist. The charge should be proportionate to the service rendered. The material used, the size of the fillings, and the time occupied may all be taken into consideration in deciding the value of the service, but should never be the sole basis of calculating the size of a bill. For example, let us imagine a difficult cavity in a lower third molar, disto-approximal and morsal surfaces involved. Perhaps, for the sake of the higher fee, a band matrix may be placed in position, napkins adjusted and held with clamps, a saliva injector used, and a gold filling inserted, large hunks of some plastic gold being pushed to place with heavy pluggers, the dentist the while struggling to finish before the tide rises to the point of flood. The same tooth might be filled, with less trouble to the patient as well as operator, with amalgam, and of the two operations the amalgam filling may prove the more durable, because in the environment it was more possible to make a perfect operation with amalgam than with gold. Why, then, should the dentist feel that he is entitled to a larger fee for the gold operation, which in his inner consciousness he knows is not up to even his own standards, merely because the material was of gold, and the operation occupied a longer time? Or, to read the same problem reversely, why should he receive a smaller fee for a perfect operation with amalgam than for an imperfect gold filling?

A joke will sometimes point a moral more swiftly than more elaborate language, and you all have heard of the Irishman who thought his dentist overcharged him for extracting a tooth, because another dentist had taken ten times as long and hurt him a great deal more for the same amount of money on a previous occasion. It is almost as bad to believe that we earn a larger fee by prolonging the time our patients spend in the chair.

I am insistent on this subject, because I truly believe that the tremendous fallacy of basing charges upon the material used in filling teeth has deprived dentistry of the best possible services obtainable with amalgam.

It may seem bad taste to inject the personal aspect into this discussion, but I do so to prove the possibility of my contention. I have for a number of years managed my own business along the lines indicated, charging neither by time, fixed fees, nor for materials used. The result is that I have had all classes of patients, rich and poor, and that from any of them I can obtain a higher price for some amalgam fillings than for many gold fillings. It is a significant fact that the " dental parlor" men, advertising amalgam fillings at fifty cents, can persuade a patient to have a living tooth, with moderate sized cavity, covered with a gold cap, paying five or ten dollars for this abominably bad service. Why, then, cannot the ethical dentist receive as large a fee for properly filling the tooth, rendering a vastly superior service for a fee that will remunerate him for the time and skill expended, even though amalgam be used? Evidently it is a matter of education, and heretofore patients have been improperly educated in this regard, and the dentist has none but himself to thank or blame for his present predicament.

Another serious fallacy in relation to amalgam is that the word amalgam is applied indiscriminately to hundreds of totally different preparations. When we speak of a gold filling, we always allude to a filling made of a metal of a definite fineness. The differences in the various kinds of gold are not very material to the resultant fillings, except, perhaps, as there may be a difference between the old style soft gold and the present day cohesive gold, or between the foils and the plastics. But these differences are well defined and fully taken into consideration in the technique of the operations. This is not true of amalgam. All sorts of alloys are similarly used, and a single alloy may be used in many different ways. What wonder that the results with amalgam have been so diverse. The remedy, as applied to the whole profession, cannot perhaps be found within a brief period. The day when all dentists will use the same alloy, in the same manner, and in the same class of cavities is far off. The remedy for any one practitioner is, however, within his own immediate grasp. Let him select one alloy and use no other, whatever the temptation. In making such a choice, if the dentist be at the outset of his career, I would recommend some alloy that has been continuously on sale for a number of years, rather than any of the newer products. I do not mean that these later-day preparations may not be good, but the older ones would not be still on sale had they not been proved to have some value. Having made a choice, the dentist may soon so familiarize himself with this one alloy as to be able to get the very best possible service from it.

A third fallacy relates to cavity preparation, and is one of the evils following in the rear of the notion that amalgam fillings must be cheap. I take it as sound doctrine that cavity preparation, aside from mere shaping for retention, has no relation to the filling-material which is to be inserted. If it can be shown that the preservation of the tooth from recurrence of decay depends upon a definite extension, such as the removal of infected as well as carious dentine, the trimming away of ragged enamel, the arrangement, shape, and placing of the enamel margins and the polishing of the same, then thorough, honest practice demands the same careful cavity preparation for amalgam as for gold. Indeed, if anything, more care is demanded, since it is generally believed that amalgam suffers an alteration of shape. I know that this will be subject for dispute, and that some will argue that the preparation of the enamel margins alone will be more tedious for gold than for amalgam. But why? Any amount of marginal preparation for gold must be based upon the idea that such shaping will render the tooth safer from recurrence of decay after filling than had this precaution not been taken. It may also be true that identical preparation cannot be made with amalgam. For example, many advocate a bevelling of all margins and overlapping of the same with gold. This cannot be done with amalgam, as, when attempted, the amalgam chips away and invites disaster. But because this is true, it is no good evidence that less careful preparation of the margins should be made for amalgam than for gold, and I am convinced that the best results with amalgam are only attainable where the margins are properly and definitely shaped. Having admitted that one should not bevel edges where amalgam is to be used, it follows logically that all bevelled edges must be avoided and those already bevelled should be altered. I believe that there is no amalgam that has strength to resist the stress of mastication if brought to a feather edge. Consequently all margins should meet the outer surface of the tooth in a strong, but well defined angle, without bevelling. Moreover, the absolute edge should be smooth. Cavity preparations, therefore, may be slightly different for amalgam than for gold, but it is equally requisite that it should be carefully, skilfully and thoroughly done. It rarely is.

A fallacy of some importance, I think, has occurred in the work of our eminent men who have carried on tests for this material. The majority of these tests have been made in matrices of glass or steel, and while much valuable knowledge has been attained in regard to the physical properties of various alloys, and of these alloys when amalgamated, I know of no one who has made tests to give us definite knowledge in relation to the best mode of shaping cavities for the reception of amalgam. I venture to suggest that those who have not considered this matter as one of importance will personally try the experiments which I have made and will now report.

Let me cite, as leading up to the purpose of the experiments, a difficult yet common class of cavities found in every-day practice, and more often filled with amalgam than with gold. Imagine a case where the sixth-year molar has a large disto-approximal cavity, while the adjacent twelfth-year molar has a similarly large mesio-approximal cavity, both involving the morsal surfaces. Preparation of these cavities, so far as removal of carious matter is concerned, discloses the fact that both pulps may be saved alive, but that in both instances the gingival margins must lie at or under the gum. Of course, every gentleman present makes it a practice to properly fill these teeth, even when using amalgam. But let us discuss the work of the men who are not present,—those who get small and stated fees for amalgam.

Different procedures maintain. Some fill both teeth at the same sitting. Of these, a great many polish only the visible and consequently accessible parts of the filling at the second sitting. Still fewer pass a narrow strip of sand-paper along the gingival margins, and polish them in that way, the moisture, blood, and débris, of course, being no hinderance. Another few may next use a steel separator and obtain enough space to polish the contact points, in which case, even though the fillings be polished, they lose their contact.

Following another method, we have those who fill one cavity at the first sitting and polish it at the next, before filling the second. This is better, but the same dilemma maintains when the polishing of the last filling is attempted. Either the contact point remains unpolished, or else it is lost.

Of course, the proper method is familiar to all. The teeth must be wedged apart,—one sitting; one tooth filled,—two sittings; this one polished and the other filled,—three sittings; the second filling polished and the teeth allowed to fall back again,—four sittings. But even with amalgam this kind of work cannot be done for small fees, and that is why it is done so seldom.

I now with some hesitation present a new method of procedure. I do this tentatively only, not giving it a final endorsement, because I have not yet sufficiently tested it. I will say, however, that it seems to promise a satisfactory solution of this difficult problem, and that it allows the filling of the teeth in two instead of four sittings. The cavities are prepared, with the dam in place, of course, the same as for a porcelain inlay, all edges being made sound, smooth, and well defined with small stones. I then make a gold matrix for one cavity, and with the matrix in place fill the tooth with a quick-setting amalgam, building out the approximal contour slightly to an excess. The matrix is then removed with the filling, which is easily done, and of course the matrix suffers no alteration in shape. This is set aside for the time being. The second cavity is similarly treated, and the two are then filled with gutta-percha and the patient dismissed, which ends the first sitting. Each matrix with its contained amalgam filling is then dropped upon a small pile of freshly mixed plaster, which is made to invest the matrices, and then trimmed to satisfactory form for handling. On the following day it will be found that the amalgam can be trimmed to shape and polish, the gold serving as a guide to the true cavity margins. It is best to leave the polishing of the morsal surfaces until after setting the inlays. It is manifest that by this means the gingival margins are easily polished. Some excess is left at the contact points until the patient presents, at which time the dam is again placed and the final polishing and fitting achieved, after which each is separately set as an inlay, and when completed the two amalgam fillings have perfect polish and perfect margins, regardless of the difficulties which would ordinarily be met; moreover, the contact can be made absolute; indeed, the two fillings may be literally wedged between the teeth.

Even if this work is not done in the mouth, it will be most instructive to try a few such fillings out of the mouth. The opportunity to handle the filling, polish it, and replace it in the cavity from time to time for examination will prove more convincing than endless argument that amalgam overlapping a margin has no strength. A thin edge anywhere will be seen to crumble and break under the action of even the finest cuttle-fish disks, and this, more than anything, will satisfy the most sceptical that a definite marginal shape is essential with amalgam. It will also lead him to the thought that the trenches about old fillings which so long have been attributed to *shrinkage,* may in a large percentage of cases more properly be explained by *breakage,* due to overlapping the margins.

One other procedure I will suggest for future trial by the profession. In masticating, or, indeed, in other surfaces where it is desired to retain the filling in the usual way, by retentive shaping, the matrix may still be used, and I think with advantage. In such cases the matrix is first gently pressed into the cavity, getting it as deep as possible without breaking the gold, and then perfectly burnishing to the margins. Next, the gold may be pressed tightly against the floor and walls with spunk, permitting it to break where it will. This restores the retentive shape of the cavity, which is now lined with gold. Into this, without removing the matrix, the amalgam is placed and the excess of gold subsequently torn away. This will give an amalgam filling, but the cavity walls will be lined with gold, which will, I think, permanently prevent discoloration of the dentine by oxidation. Contrary to what might be supposed, the amalgam does not unite with the gold, and the mercury does not penetrate it during setting. I cannot see why it should do so later.

A slight variation of the method will appeal to those who like a cement joint. The matrix being made, but not burnished sufficiently to break it, a thin cement is smeared over all the walls, and the matrix put in the cavity and packed tight with spunk, the excess of cement being carefully forced outward under the matrix and over the margins. After this hardens, the amalgam may be inserted at the same sitting.

There are many other fallacies in regard to amalgam and the methods of its usage, but I believe I have pointed out the more mischievous ones.

THE ADVANTAGES OF CO-OPERATION IN OUR PROFESSION.[1]

BY NED A. STANLEY, D.M.D., NEW BEDFORD, MASS.

MR. PRESIDENT AND GENTLEMEN,—I have called the subject of this short paper " The Advantages of Co-operation in our Profession." Rather, perhaps, let me say, some of the advantages, for they are many and manifold.

We all know that the profession of dentistry in America is an advanced one. We have for many years, if not from the earliest beginnings, when our profession began to engage the whole attention of able men, led the world in new mechanical devices and methods, which go so far towards the success of a large percentage of the operations we are called upon to perform. To what is our position due? In large part to the co-operation of our practitioners. Everybody is familiar with the power of co-operation as it is felt to-day in the business world. With us the value of co-operation in its best sense is seen ; the profession is elevated, made progressive, and every member benefited thereby ; the coming together for mutual aid and benefit ; the talking over of cases and interchange of ideas ; the presentation of some new piece of appliance or method that has simplified difficult operations, and made new ones possible.

In this way the ideas and inventions of individuals have come to be shared by the profession at large. Not only has the operator thus been aided, but his patients have received the direct results of this co-operation.

How much we are indebted to that indefatigable, tireless worker, J. N. Crouse, of Chicago ! How many a head that wears a crown rests easier because of the battles he has fought and won for us,—not for *himself,* but for *us!* And how was this made possible? Only by concerted action on the part of dentists in maintaining the Dental Protective Association. The old fable of the bundle of sticks is here well illustrated : " United we stand, divided we fall." And so the profession has grown to be one of the great professions.

---

[1] Read before the Massachusetts Dental Society, Boston, Mass., June 3 and 4, 1903.

Few occupations call for greater skill, a more delicate touch, or better judgment than our own. Our operations as a whole are much more delicate, and call for greater manipulative skill than do those of the surgeon. It is true we do not share the responsibility of the latter, but we are held responsible for our operations and judged accordingly.

I often think what an unsightly lot of humanity we should be, were it not for the dentist. Nothing can destroy the beauty of the face more than an ugly mouth. To be sure we have those distressing, inexcusable exhibitions, where the abuse of the gold cap has seriously marred the features of the patient and erected a monument to the inartistic, fifteen-years-behind-the-times operator.

We, as dentists, have an important function to perform by teaching that part of the public we see professionally—and indirectly many others—how essential is the proper care of the teeth; and particularly so is this true with children. Here is where a very important work should be carried on, and I feel sure it will not be many generations before the inheritance will be a much stronger dental structure. The present condition of our teeth is one of the penalties of civilization. A return to simpler methods of living and moderation in all things will correct many of the unnatural ills from which we are suffering. Now, how can we best carry out this important work intrusted to us? Our patients are entitled to the best we can give them from our own experience and from the experience of others. If we wish to become representative men, we will not feel satisfied with ourselves until we have become acquainted with and mastered the most approved and most artistic methods at our command.

One of the best ways to grasp these rounds of progress is through society meetings, where something new is always to be seen. And the practitioner who is too indifferent—cannot spare the time—or considers that he is self-sufficient is making a mistake. Much can be derived from reading the reports of meetings, but much more can be obtained by being in attendance at the meetings themselves, for things in this world move rapidly. The present German emperor, when still a boy, took for his motto these words: " If I stand still, I rust."

The man who habitually absents himself doubtless spends very little time over dental literature. I would urge the benefits to be derived from these society meetings. To stand still *is* to rust; it is to go backward.

We must keep pace with the progress of the time, or at least keep within sight of the leaders, with always a receptive mind and a pliant hand, to receive and apply new and better methods.

These are some of the advantages to be derived by us from co-operation: Growth, good-fellowship, new ideas, a day off, and you return to your office refreshed, newly aided, and encouraged.

Reports of Society Meetings.

THE NEW YORK INSTITUTE OF STOMATOLOGY.

A REGULAR meeting of the Institute was held at the " Chelsea," No. 222 West Twenty-third Street, New York, on Tuesday, October 6, 1903, the President, Dr. J. Morgan Howe, in the chair.

The minutes of the last meeting were read and approved.

The President stated that since the last meeting of the Institute one of the fellow-members, Dr. Louis Shaw, had passed away. A committee was appointed to draft suitable resolutions of regret and respect.

COMMUNICATIONS ON THEORY AND PRACTICE.

Dr. Stockton presented a case of irregularity upon which he desired suggestions. Dr. Stockton stated that the question had arisen in his mind whether it would not be better, considering the fact that the boy was in school and objected very much to wearing an appliance, to extract a single tooth and complete the reduction in that manner. He knew that this would raise a storm of objections. However, he would ask the question, " Shall we take out the first bicuspid in this case?"

Dr. Bogue stated that all the light he was able to throw on Dr. Stockton's case would be against any extraction. The teeth being unilaterally dislocated, the easier and more simple method would be to place them in the position intended by nature that they should occupy. Any attempt to thwart nature would be met with indifferent success. Such an extraction would also diminish the nasal cavity, the oral cavity, and the size of the dental arches, diminishing the young man's dignity of countenance.

Dr. Bogue also presented a case of irregularity upon which he invited comment. The left lower bicuspids did not articulate with anything. The right lower second molar was also turned in such a way that it did not articulate, with anything. The upper molars were also both dislocated anteriorly. The teeth all stood apart so that nothing could be gained by extraction, and the upper teeth were so prognathous that the lips could scarcely be closed even with great effort.

Dr. S. E. Davenport wished to say a word to brother dentists who might, during the vacation season, be the means of helping the patients of others out of a difficulty. Dr. Davenport had his acknowledgments to make to a dear friend for services rendered to one of his pet patients during his absence. He wished to couple his acknowledgments with those of the patient for the kind and skilful way in which the service had been rendered. But Dr. Davenport had one fault to find. After the broken tooth had been made comfortable, the patient made her thanks and asked if she might be informed how much she was indebted for the service. The dentist declined to accept a fee, saying that he was glad to be of service to his friend Dr. Davenport. It was upon this point that Dr. Davenport wished to speak. He had always considered that this was a wrong method to pursue in such cases, and it had a tendency to belittle in the patient's mind the value of such service. He believed that a charge should be made as though the services were rendered by the patient's own dentist. So far as he personally was concerned, he should ask his friends so called upon during his absence to make a proper charge in such instances, or, at least, to inform him upon his return of the incident, so that the proper fee might be added to the patient's account.

The President thought the remarks of Dr. Davenport were very proper and timely. Many cases of this kind occur where patients are temporarily relieved by other dentists than their own, without fee, although they expect and desire to pay. He thought this a mistaken idea of conferring a favor upon a fellow-practitioner. No other professional men have such notions, and it seems explicable in the case of dentists only by remembering that as a profession we are young. The value of the service rendered is minimized in the patient's estimation by such practice, and neither practitioner is benefited.

Dr. J. Bond Littig did not think Dr. Davenport had taken just the right view of the matter. If Dr. Davenport's patient came to him for treatment he would say to him that he was not doing this for him, but for Dr. Davenport.

Dr. Wheeler thought it was customary among physicians to do the temporary service and then pass the account over to the physician who rendered the bill. However, he thought Dr. Davenport was right, more especially as by following the opposite course we were putting another man's patient under obligation to us, which we should be averse to do. Personally he would desire any patient of his who received treatment elsewhere to be charged a regular fee.

Dr. Littig said that this was not exactly the point. In rendering this bill the fee might be less than the patient had been in the habit of paying, which might cause dissatisfaction between the patient and his dentist. He thought it better to let the patient's dentist render a bill for the services.

Dr. R. T. Moffatt, of Boston, read a paper entitled "The Art of carving and baking Porcelain Teeth and Crowns."

(For Dr. Moffatt's paper, see page 1.)

DISCUSSION.

Dr. J. Bond Littig did not think he could add anything in the way of suggestions or criticisms, as the essayist had presented the subject in such a concise manner. The paper had carried him back forty years, when the materials for this work used to be ground up by him in a mortar, the quartz, the spar, and the kaolin. At that time very little kaolin was used on account of the opacity it produced. Kaolin was simply disintegrated felspar, having been deprived of its potash and soda, and so was infusible. One great objection to the carved teeth was that they were not as strong as the moulded teeth, because they were not made under such pressure. It used to be a very difficult piece of work to bring out whole one of these carved sections of six teeth after vulcanizing. It was the custom to make a full set of teeth in three sections, the bicuspids and molars in one section and the six front teeth in another. In carving the crown for the space mentioned by Dr. Moffatt, he did not state how much wider it was necessary to make the tooth to allow for contraction after baking.

Dr. C. S. Stockton was astonished to find that what he had considered as almost a lost art was still practised with such success.

However, the question arose, Could we make such a technical knowledge as that possessed by Dr. Moffatt of any value to us, practically, in our every-day practice? He himself had had a thorough training in this work, having carved thousands of sets of teeth, but, from a practical stand-point, to-day the knowledge was useless to him. There were occasions, however, when it was well to know how to carve teeth. He thought it might be made more available now that there had been such an improvement in furnaces, and, inasmuch as the dental course at college had been increased to four years, it would be well to take a little of this time in teaching young men how to carve teeth as the older ones here to-night had been taught years ago.

Dr. Moffatt, in answer to Dr. Littig's suggestion about not using much to make it opaque as to increase the plasticity as an aid in about twenty grains to the ounce of body. It was not put in so much to make it opaque as to increase the plasticity as an aid in carving. Dr. Moffatt thought possibly the carved teeth might not be quite as strong as teeth made under great pressure, but under practical tests in removing the pins from different moulded teeth he had found it more difficult to break carved teeth than "store" teeth. He did not think the question of burning out the color in baking was worth considering, as with a little practice this could always be regulated. Regarding the question of shrinkage in the crown mentioned, the shrinkage in this case took place longitudinally entirely. Dr. Moffatt did not think the age was too fast to appreciate this kind of work. He was sure that thorough work was worth the time given to it.

Dr. Wheeler thought that the proportion of fusible material in a body greatly affected its shrinkage while baking, and that colors were also retained better in the higher fusing bodies, as, for instance, the Parker body as compared with the S. S. White. It seemed to him that this question of carved *versus* moulded teeth was merely the question of work done by an artist compared with work done by an ordinary factory moulder. He thought some of the material furnished us by the supply houses was just about as near artistic perfection as we would expect from a foundry laborer getting two or three dollars a day. The colleges had been playing into the hands of the supply houses in not having such a course in the regular college work. He did not believe that carved teeth were weaker. In his experience they were even stronger. Teeth that were carved contained a larger percentage of body than the moulded teeth, and this would perhaps account for their greater strength, the enamel being much weaker, and in moulded teeth it occupied a much greater proportion. He thought that Boston, with its several practitioners engaged in this work of carving teeth, would compare very favorably with Philadelphia, the Mecca of supply houses, and where, to his knowledge, there was not a single man who could carve a set of teeth.

Dr. Littig thought it required special adaptability to do this work. He did not think, out of an ordinary class of one hundred, over twenty could be taught to do that kind of work. It was hard enough to teach them to make a plaster model. The college takes the trend of general practice throughout the country, and there were very few men now who did this work to any extent whatever.

The President thanked Dr. Moffatt for presenting the subject in such a careful manner and with such illustrations that any one may become well informed in this work.

Dr. Bogue stated that at one time Dr. Moffatt's father was his partner on the other side of the water. He was a man to whom we could all go to school and learn. Dr. Bogue recalled many instances in which Dr. Moffatt, Sr., had tried to teach him to do this beautiful work. He was exceedingly gratified to find that Dr. Moffatt had given the Institute such a paper from which the younger men could gain a knowledge of work that in after years would be their consolation and delight.

Dr. Davenport said he would like to make his thanks to Dr. Moffatt for doing what he had for the Institute. Dr. Moffatt was invited by the Executive Committee to favor the society with a paper, and the result had been most satisfactory. He had brought a great deal of paraphernalia from Boston which perhaps some would have never seen otherwise. Dr. Moffatt had given a clinic during the afternoon attended by at least twenty-five gentlemen, where he had done quite a little of this beautiful work. The members of the society were greatly indebted to Dr. Moffatt for the complete and earnest manner in which he had served them.

Dr. Strang would like advice concerning a very puzzling case he had at present under treatment. About a month ago a lady, thirty years of age, had been sent to him by a physician. The left side of the face was very much swollen and there was considerable discharge exteriorly from a fistula. There had been practically no motion of the inferior maxilla for three months, and she **had** been unable to take solid food. The history was that about one year ago she had had the lower second molar on that side filled, and subsequently the tooth gave so much trouble that it had to be extracted. The swelling began at that time. Dr. Strang had opened into the abscess at one point on the cheek, the pus having come almost to the surface, and had gotten out about a spoonful of what used to be called "laudable" pus. By inserting first a wood and then a rubber wedge he was able to get the mouth open sufficiently in two days to make an examination, and he was convinced that it was arsenical poisoning due to careless manipulation while devitalizing a pulp. There were discharging at the present time three fistulæ opening on the cheek, besides a discharge of pus at the posterior part of the sixth-year molar. He had scraped away a little of the bone that was soft and could be removed without pain to the patient. The temperature had been taken twice a **day,** and remained about normal. The patient is pregnant, **and** expects to be confined early in November.

The question is, Will it be judicious to extract the sixth-year molar?

The President thought the case probably called for the removal of the molar, which may be aggravating the morbid conditions. He supposed from the description that there must be considerable necrosed bone, but that it had not yet shown any demarcation. The removal of the tooth may be a needed preliminary. A sulphuric acid (about 1 in 15 or 20 of water, or the so-called aromatic sulphuric acid) treatment he had found effectual in hastening exfoliation. It was the custom of many surgeons to scrape or bur away the necrosed bone, but he thought it better to let nature's forces cause the separation, which they will do if helped.

Dr. Bogue suggested the cutting process for the removal of a greater portion of the necrosed bone.

Dr. Leo Green said that, inasmuch as three fistulæ were present, marking out a triagular area of which they were the apices, it would seem that the necrotic region had become circumscribed, **and** that the sequestrum was about to be exfoliated. It would be found floating in pus and could be easily removed.

Adjourned.

FRED. L. BOGUE, M.D., D.D.S.,
Editor The New York Institute of Stomatology.

ACADEMY OF STOMATOLOGY.

A REGULAR meeting of the Academy of Stomatology, of Philadelphia, was held at its rooms, 1731 Chestnut Street, on the evening of Tuesday, April 28, 1903, the President, Dr. R. Hamil D.
Swing, in the chair.

A paper was read by Dr. Rodrigues Ottolengui, of New York,
entitled "The Great Amalgam Fallacy."

(For Dr. Ottolengui's paper, see page 34.)

DISCUSSION.

Dr. William H. Trueman.—The essayist, in the opening para-
graphs of his paper, is solicitous that the discussion shall be
strictly confined to the subject presented, and he asks that his
position in regard to it shall not be misconstrued. This is his
right. The paper is now before us; the various suggestions, deductions, and assertions therein contained, and these alone, are our
subjects for discussion. It is important, therefore, that they should
be clearly defined, disentangled, and isolated from the rhetoric
essential to a well-written scientific essay, in order that we may
fully comprehend the ideas expressed and profitably discuss their
merits.

This is the more important from the fact that the essayist has,
in some measure, departed from the well-beaten track, and has
presented his subject in a dress so new that it calls for a discussion
on other lines than those with which we have in the past been so
familiar. We miss the denunciations of the "nasty stuff," the
forceful presentation of its many faults, and the uncomplimentary
expressions in reference to those who use it. If I understand him,
his plea is for better treatment of this long maligned tooth-filling
material. He contends that it is cheap only when cheaply used.
He advises that it is well worth while for every operator to thoroughly study the amalgam question with a view to ascertain the
best composition, the best method of preparing, and when and how
to obtain by its use the very best possible results.

The great amalgam fallacy to which he refers seems to be the
use of amalgam by a large percentage of the profession with but
little regard to these important points.

Acknowledging, as he does, the intrinsic value of amalgam,

his suggestions are directed to giving it a more honorable place in the tooth-saving scheme. As a first step he suggests charging for amalgam fillings a larger fee. Now, it is a question how far a dental society can safely go in discussing this matter of fees. The time was when many dental societies adopted a fee bill, and required their members to observe it as a minimum charge. It did not, however, work well. So many things are to be considered when naming for work like ours a just compensation, that it is difficult, as it is at times injudicious, to attempt to formulate any definite rules. To some dentists, and to some patients, it is merely a matter of education, as the essayist suggests. To many others, however, it is a matter of expediency and ability. Unfortunately, imperative demands upon the earnings of some patients seriously lessen the cash they can command. The question of fees in all its bearings is a problem each operator must settle for himself. No dentist is under obligation to render to a patient a greater service in time and material than the patient is able and willing to pay for, and he is entitled to use his judgment in doing the best he can with the means and opportunity at his command. On the other hand, a dentist is hardly justified in considering his patient a thing to keep appointments promptly, and to promptly meet, without question, any bill that may be rendered. We appreciate and commend the suggestion that if those dentists who can will place upon a well-made and artistically finished amalgam filling the same value that they do upon one equally well done with gold, it will bring this useful material into better repute; it will also bring it more into competition with gold, and will lead to its being much more generally used. It will prove an invitation to both good and evil. Whether it is a wise thing to do is a proper subject for discussion, and as such is presented to you in the paper.

His second point is well taken. It is a fallacy, and a serious one, as he says, to use indiscriminately the many differing compounds included under the word amalgam, without regard to their components, their differing properties, and the special manipulation that these require. I differ with him regarding the remedy. I do not regard the old formula, that of the first alloy placed upon the market and erroneously called " Townsend's," a desirable one to use, notwithstanding that it has been longer and perhaps more generally used than any other. A dentist has a right to know the components of the alloy he uses. He then can ascertain once for all the peculiar properties they confer upon the alloy and upon the resulting amalgam. The market name tells him nothing, the enclosed direction may not be the best for him, and the scientific tests to which it has been subjected before offered for sale were, in all probability, under conditions it will never again meet. I have always made my own. I know what I am using, and am able to trace failings to their cause. There are more things than virtue and merit that keeps these alloys on the market. Properly used in suitable places, the original formula, five parts tin and four parts silver, leaves but little to be desired; nevertheless, it is very far from being a desirable alloy for general use; that it has held its own on the market for half a century or more is due to other causes than intrinsic merit. I would suggest that a dentist, at the outset of his career, make himself familiar with the chemistry and the metallurgy of alloys and amalgams, study closely their properties, learn how to manipulate them and how to make them do him their best service, and insist on knowing the formula of the alloy he adopts in his practice. It is not likely, as the essayist suggests, that the time will soon come when the words "alloy" and "amalgam" will be as definite in their meaning when used by dentists in this connection as is now the word "gold." We have here another thought for discussion.

A third fallacy relates to cavity preparation. Here again the essayist has entered fallow ground. His remarks have, in the main, no relation to the now almost forgottten spheroiding of amalgam. He claims that cavity peparation for amalgam should have at least the same care as that for gold. Aside from mere shaping for retention, he contends that filling-material should not be considered in cavity preparation, that all require the removal of disintegrated and infected tissue, ragged edges, and the same nicety in preparing enamel margins. Owing to the want of edge strength, common to all amalgams, bevelled enamel margins should be avoided. While there are some marked differences in cavity preparation for a material requiring to be welded in position, and one as plastic as amalgam, we can heartily agree with the essayist when he says that it should be carefully, skilfully, and thoroughly done; and he may be right when he adds, "it rarely is."

His further remarks upon shaping and polishing approximal amalgam fillings are worthy of careful attention, and to some extent I can agree with him, indeed, fully in regard to the cases to which he specially refers. It is a high compliment to the tooth-saving qualities of amalgam that it should have attained its present reputation, used and abused as the essayist says it has been. There is room for discussion, whether or not the finish for which he con-tends is really of practical value, or is merely an embellishment. That it is not generally done goes without saying, some, indeed, con-tending that the after-polishing is wholly unnecessary and a waste of time. If this is the case, are we justified in putting the patient to the inconvenience and expense which it entails? Are we profit-ably using our own time and talent? Polishing is necessary when gold is used, because the outer surface of a gold filling is not only rough as left by the plugger, but it consists of imperfectly packed gold which must be removed. Furthermore, in many cases where amalgam proves of much value, the overlaping edges at the cervical border pressing down to the gum tissue, and the large con-tact surface any attempt to polish would remove, are essential to its best service. This is the case where there has been extensive gum recession and where very large interdental spaces exist. The amalgam, filling this space, tends to cleanliness, and its close adap-tation to the surface of the adjoining tooth, where the teeth have become loosened by loss of tooth-supporting tissue, is as important to the patient's comfortable use of the tooth as is its occluding the cavity of decay. The use of amalgam in this way has been criticised as careless and slovenly. When purposely done, with a definite object in view, it is not so; it is then a legitimate and commendable practice. The mere fact that amalgam fillings, thousands of them, have done all the service a filling can do with its contact surface unpolished is very good evidence that it is not a prime essential. There is room here for profitable discussion.

The method of making amalgam inlays does not impress me favorably. It introduces more invitations to failure than it avoids. Lining the cavity with gold-foil is, in some cases, an excellent practice. It does not, however, always prevent discoloration. In some cases the gold remains gold; in others it becomes amalgam, and the tooth discolors more than if it were not there. I find that this is less apt to occur with alloys containing a high percentage of silver than in those in which tin predominates. I find it is not best to be too liberal with the gold. There is danger, if too much is used, that it will not be pressed into close contact with the cavity walls. Why, when gold is thus used in connection with amalgam, the dentine should remain undiscolored, at times for several years, and then, without any apparent cause, discolor, I do not know, but I know it does. Except in the case of frail visible teeth, I see no advantage of a gold lining. It introduces a possible risk of electro-chemical action without any compensating advantage.

Poor amalgam! What a wonderful history it has had!!! The time was, and that not so very long ago, when to confess to its use was professional suicide, and a paper such as has been read to-night would have insured its author a prompt expulsion from his dental society, branded as a quack. We must bear in mind, however, that the amalgam atmosphere of the early forties and that in which Dr. Ottolengui speaks are by no means the same. We now know more about teeth, their surroundings and disorders. Through this has come to pass the great change which has permitted a reputable practitioner to demand that amalgam and gold shall stand side by side, and to merit your applause for so doing.

Dr. Joseph Head.—I have been extremely pleased with the conservatism of the paper. The author's method of preparing the walls of the cavity for the amalgam is that which Dr. Flagg taught us,—that is, that the amalgam should be placed at right angles with the lines of mastication. There was one part of the paper which particularly impressed me, because I felt that I belong to that class of dentists who, according to his definition, work in a slovenly way, not taking proper care in polishing the amalgam fillings. When there is no objection to separation, I prepare the cavities with the floor flat. For the sake of argument we will say that I smooth the edges of the cavities. I then take my amalgam, made plastic in a quantity one-half to twice as much as is required to fill the cavity. When the cavity is dried and sterilized I take a small portion of cement and line the margins, squeezing out all of the cement that I possibly can. I then make the edges free from cement. When that is done I let the cement harden, which takes, with the use of hot air, from three to five minutes. When that is done I squeeze the remaining portion of amalgam dry between my fingers and pack it down into both cavities as though one filling. The consistency is that which Dr. Black requires. That is a matter for the individual dentist to decide upon. Dr. Black carefully explains that too great drying of the amalgam is not an advantage. I now have one large mass of filling-materials between two approximal fillings. I then divide the fillings at the cervices, making a V-shaped space almost reaching the occlusal surfaces, and then with a very fine spatula I divide that amalgam into two fillings, being careful, however, that there shall be a good approximation at the top, so there will be no breakdown from mastication. To prepare two such cavities will not take the average operator more than twenty minutes. Perhaps it is slovenly work, but I cannot see why, with the polishing which can be done later and in ten minutes, these fillings cannot be made perfectly smooth.

The fillings having been prepared and the gingival margins made accurate, the patient is sent away. When he returns, the amalgam, not being as hard as gold, can be readily polished, and by means of little files the gingival margins can be made perfectly true. When we get the gingival margins perfectly accurate and the sides smooth up to the point of contact we can take a sharp spatula and work it backward and forward, spreading the teeth apart just enough to allow them to spring back again after polishing. I polish them not so smooth as glass, but the polish is perfectly good, inasmuch as the contact point is only of metal. When that is done the polishing can be done on the top. From an experience of five or six years I find this satisfactory for all practical purposes. The time required for filling is only about half an hour. The conductivity of oxyphosphate of zinc depends entirely upon the tooth and the person placing the filling. If it is near a nerve, it may not be a poor conductor, though it is certainly a poorer conductor than gold. Its conductivity of heat is in proportion to the ratio of the conductivity of electricity. While there have been many things said against oxyphosphate of zinc, it has been my experience, and I think that of the profession at large, that it is a good preserver of structure, that it will sustain the tooth from shock, and last as long as any known temporary filling.

I think we are not doing justice to our patients in avoiding an easy method of procedure.

Dr. Edwin T. Darby.—When this subject was announced I thought it was going to call forth some pretty spirited discussion, but being privileged to read the paper before it was read to-night, I concluded that Dr. Ottolengui had been so conservative that possibly we should have a tame evening of it, and I am rather inclined to think that he anticipated the same thing, because just before he sat down he threw out a suggestion that I think was intended to warm up the meeting.

I think everything Dr. Ottolengui said in his paper was strictly true. Truth is several-sided, and while everything he said was true, everything that he said might not be expedient. Many things are possible, but they are not expedient. Some of the ideas are perhaps practical, but hardly expedient in all cases. He said that initial cavities in molars were better filled with some other material than amalgam. I think the feeling of the profession at large is that initial cavities in first molars in the mouths of young children are better temporarily filled with amalgam than with gold. I will agree with Dr. Ottolengui when he says that occlusal cavities in first molars are better filled with gold or something else. I believe they are better filled with oxyphosphate of zinc. I feel that by the twelfth or fourteenth year I will have saved these teeth with as little pain as I could have done with anything. I believe, notwithstanding what Dr. Black has said with regard to the hardness of tooth-structure, that clinically the teeth become harder. I know patients become hardened, so that they will bear longer operations at twelve or fourteen than they will at seven or eight.

In regard to the length of time required for filling with amalgam, I think that he is right in the main, and that we could perhaps fill that same tooth with gold and polish it at the same sitting, unless the cavity were too large.

Dr. Ottolengui did not denounce amalgam, as I feared he would. If he would denounce amalgam *per se,* he would meet with a good deal of antagonism from the intelligent body of men before me. It is true that our dental alloys are infinitely better to-day than they were ten years ago. I believe there are better amalgam fillings done to-day than were ever done in amalgam work. I saw fillings to-day which had been done by Bonwill,—four-fifths of them done with alloys. There were four or five beautiful gold fillings. I studied the fillings with respect to the saving qualities of the two materials, and I could not say which was doing the best service. The amalgam work was saving the teeth as perfectly as the gold. I thought then that Dr. Bonwill builded as well as he knew when he used amalgam, and builded as well as any of us know, even though we build with gold. The margins were fine and the contours perfect. That is only one case of many I have seen since he died. His amalgam fillings have been exceedingly well done, and nothing could have saved the teeth better. I am sure that if he were living and here to-night he would emphasize and add very materially to what I have said in respect to amalgam.

With the inlays suggested by Dr. Ottolengui I have never had any experience. I can see that such fillings can be polished out of the mouth, but question the feasibility of removing an amalgam filling that had been thoroughly packed in a matrix of gold. It seems to me it would require great sacrifice of the tooth-structure. It has been said of me that I rush things and have no regard for my patients, but I could not prepare two such cavities in twenty minutes. If I did it well in forty minutes I would think I had worked as rapidly as the good of the patient warranted.

I think Dr. Head's method of separating his alloy after he has packed it is a very good one. That was Dr. Bonwill's method. If we go through the same process with gold, we of course destroy the contour. Dr. Ottolengui has pointed out just the difficulties dependent upon these contour fillings of alloy. It is easier to contour with gold than with plastic material.

I believe that every amalgam filling, no matter where placed should be thoroughly and beautifully polished after it has hardened. Overlapping edges are the cause of many failures in amalgam fillings. They are unscientific, are not beautiful to look at, and they indicate slovenly operators. Amalgam should be trimmed to the margins and finished the same as gold. If this is done I believe it will save the tooth just as long as a good gold filling.

Dr. John C. Curry.—I suppose the doctor would say something in regard to the finishing of approximal fillings. The most satisfactory method I have found is to finish the edges when the fillings are about two-thirds inserted, and then with a piece of thin mica placed between the two fillings polish them. I trim off the mica and leave it between the fillings until they are hard. In that way we get absolute contact, so that the natural spring of the teeth will allow the fillings to come together and it is little trouble to finish them. I find that the thin mica can be readily trimmed and left in place of the matrix, and at the end of two hours removed with a piece of dental floss.

Dr. A. N. Gaylord.—The first part of Dr. Ottolengui's paper would lead us to believe that very few amalgam fillings were ever inserted that were strictly first-class fillings. I think he has overstepped the mark, for I think that, while there are a great many slovenly fillings put in with amalgam, there are also about as many slovenly gold fillings put in. This is not the fault of the filling, but of the man. In my hands it is not a fact that a properly inserted amalgam filling takes as long as a similarly placed filling of gold. I cannot see why it should be. Amalgam is a plastic material and is placed in the cavity with greater rapidity, and after it is put in the polish is certainly more rapidly done, because of the nature of the material itself. Gold is a metal which cuts very hard and heats up very quickly, whereas amalgam is a more brittle metal which cuts quickly under the disk. After an amalgam filling has been placed it can be nearly accurately shaped by rubbing it with a burnisher and brought down to fair shape and contour. The polishing at subsequent sittings is easily accomplished by strips and disks. I admit that the disk is apt to remove the contour, but by using strips I cannot see any reason why the filling cannot be perfectly contoured and left perfectly smooth. I think there is no poorer filling than a poor gold filling, and because of the more easy adaptability of amalgam, an average filling in the back part of the mouth, accurately placed and polished as best we can, will give better satisfaction than the filling of gold which is not properly placed, and many of them are in such position that it is impossible to give them the benefit of the skill and dexterity desired. A chain is no stronger than its weakest link, and the filling is no better than your ability to properly place it. I have put in many fillings which, if I held the tooth in my hand, I would be mortally ashamed of, but, considering the position of the cavity, I have congratulated myself.

I do not think that the young man can at first charge all his patients by the hour. He has patients who are in moderate circumstances, and those patients must know to some extent what their bill is to be. We must have a scale of prices. It is not the fee that makes the dentist less skilful. It is the dentist's conscience. When it comes to the matter of time charge, which I think is the correct one, I do not know but that we are all day-laborers. I know I feel like one to-night. Where is there a successful dentist who is not a mechanic. Dr. Ottolengui suggests another method, which I think is a dangerous one.

The matter of the amalgam inlay does not strike me so favorably that I could try it in my practice. I cannot see how a man could save any time by making an inlay. You must be able to set that inlay downward. It will mean a very extensive cutting of

tooth-structure in order to set such an inlay, and when completed
the weakest link is the cement which holds it. The force of the
mastication on the molar teeth is such that I do not think it
advisable to rely entirely upon cement as anchorage.

I cannot understand how a man with a conscience could subject
the little ones who come to us with the inferior first molars defective
in the fissures, to the long sitting required for the insertion of a
gold filling. The eruption of the tooth in many cases is not sufficient to properly apply the rubber dam without holding it in place
with clamps, which would have to be forced down upon the tissues
and would cause much pain. I think to handle the little ones in
that way is to do them a life-long injury. They grow up with a
natural dread because they remember those first few fillings that
the dentist put in for them, and every subsequent visit to the dentist
is more arduous from a mental stand-point because of the insertion
of those fillings. I do not say that amalgam is the best thing, but
I do believe in doing anything to relieve the young patient of the
tedious sittings required for putting in gold fillings.

Dr. H. E. Roberts.—Gold would be the last thing I would put
in a child's first molar at seven years of age, particularly as we so
frequently first see the child when the cavities have passed beyond
the initial stage.

Dr. E. C. Rice.—Inasmuch as the essayist has treated amalgam
very fairly to-night the remarks I intended to make do not count.
I do not think approximal cavities are ever successfully filled with
amalgam unless a matrix is well and strongly put in. I do not
approve of making fillings after the manner of Dr. Head. I see no
objection to the separation of teeth. I do not think an amalgam
filling can be polished unless a tooth has been separated. It is just
as necessary to make a perfect polish at the point of contact as at
any other. Too many amalgam fillings fail because the operator
depends upon the sensitivity of the molar rather than upon the
conditions of the cavity. A copper matrix can be used which
need not be removed at the same sitting. I think amalgam will
last just as long and give as good service as gold.

Dr. J. A. Bolard.—In the inlay work described by the essayist
I have had no experience. It seems to me there would have to be
cut away a large portion of tooth-structure, which would be unjustifiable. After cutting away so largely I would prefer to put in something that would look better than amalgam. That amalgam will

last without being polished I have evidence in my own mouth. Twelve or fifteen years ago these fillings were put in and never rubbed down. I do believe, however, that they should be polished, and I follow out that idea so far as I can.

I understood from Dr. Ottolengui's paper some time ago at Asbury Park that he never used amalgam. He was criticised at that meeting, and I understood him to say that he never remembered having put in an amalgam filling, and yet in his essay to-night he advocates it when properly employed. If he has been converted I am glad to know it, because I feel there is merit in amalgam. His methods, outside of his inlays, I think are excellent. I am glad if he can get the fees he speaks of; I wish we all could. I do think a man should be remunerated for his services. If we are truly professional men we are not interested in the money alone, but must expect to do for the public a large amount of work for which we get no return. With the paper as a whole I largely agree. If the doctor has had a change of heart it has been in the right direction.

Dr. Ottolengui (closing).—Right next to Asbury Park is the place where conversions take place annually. I would say, however, that I am doing less amalgam work than ever. I think the gentleman misunderstood the Asbury Park paper. I did not say I never put in amalgam fillings, for I have put in many of them. What I said was that I did not remember that I had ever put in an amalgam filling on the occlusal surface of a first molar. The paper reads that way, and has not been changed. In regard to Dr. Rice, when that gentleman's discussion is printed, it ought to be printed in all caps; it is the best thing I have ever heard about amalgam fillings. It is so largely in answer to Dr. Head that I need hardly answer that gentleman. I notice a great versatility of talent, for every time I thought I had to answer a remark, the next man speaking answered it for me. I must, however, say to Dr. Head, that the method he suggests is the one by which I lost a tooth in my own mouth, and the work was done by a good dentist too, a dentist who carried out the method to its limit.

I think a very great percentage of the recurrent decay at the cervical margin occurs around amalgam fillings rather than around gold fillings. I do not think it is because it is impossible to polish amalgam there, but simply that it is not polished there. That the amalgam can be made over when one-half set is one of the greatest errors. In trying to make specimens of inlays I have necessarily done work out of the mouth, and I would like some of you gentlemen to try it for experience, and you will find one error I did not point out. You will find that amalgam is not as plastic as you are apt to think. You could adapt gold to rough edges better than amalgam. You may find that your alloys are in suspension in the mercury, and in forcing them out you force out a lot of mercury and leave some rough margins, and then in putting in the amalgam you never afterwards can get a polish. The little particles chip off and you will have crevices. The gold put in in not too great pieces has a plasticity that the amalgam does not have.

The matter of the inlays I suggested as worthy of trial. Since the discussion I do not think it so worthy. If, however, you do not try it in the mouth, it would be well to try it extra-orally. If Dr. Head would take two teeth with such cavities as he describes, put them in plaster of Paris, file and polish them in the way he has advocated, and split them open, he will find them less well polished than he thinks.

In putting the inlays in you do not have to cut away as much as you imagine. If you desire to have some of the deeper cuts left so that you will not force your matrix in, you could simply fill those places first with cement. Amalgam fillings should always have cement between them and the tooth. I have great faith that fillings of any kind with cement so placed will defy decay longer than any other fillings put in teeth.

I tell my friends in Brooklyn, when they speak in the same way about the cruelty of filling young people's teeth with gold, that I would be glad to take the children off their hands whom they are averse to taking care of, but that I would fill the teeth with gold instead of with amalgam. The only part of my practice in which I place absolute reliance are the grown up people in whose mouths I put gold when they were children. I do not recall having lost a child for whom I filled teeth, except by their having moved from the city or through their marriage. The fact that I have thus retained them is due to the fact that the very time to fill the teeth with the least pain is before they have decayed. The object in putting in gold is that I can prepare the sulci at that time smaller than at any other, and the sulci being prepared smaller, I am safer with the gold filling than with the amalgam, for it is my experience that the cavities can be filled painlessly. You might have a child shrink, and in that case put in gutta-percha and wait. The fact that some teeth are sensitive does not militate against the practice. In those cases I fill with gutta-percha, and in them I ask you to avoid amalgam. The public has been educated to the fact that amalgam is a permanent filling. If you put in gutta-percha, not only does the patient understand that that is temporary, but they are obliged to come back. A good filling can be put in for children of eight years of age and less, and when put in that is the end of it. That tooth never requires to be filled in that place again, and that in itself is a sufficient reason for the practice. It is not because I do it that I advocate the method, because I can name hundreds of men who fill teeth a thousand times better than I do. To get the same effect with amalgam as is secured with gold in these fillings requires greater destruction of tooth-structure, weakening of the walls, enlarging of cavities unprotected by enamel, and in my opinion this invites disaster.

After a vote of thanks to the essayist the meeting adjourned.

OTTO E. INGLIS,
Editor Academy of Stomatology.

MASSACHUSETTS DENTAL SOCIETY.

(Continued from Vol. XXIV., page 893.)

Thursday, June 4, 1903.

THE President introduced Dr. Ned A. Stanley, D.M.D., of New Bedford, who read a paper entitled "The Advantages of Co-operation in our Profession."

(For Dr. Stanley's paper, see page 43.)

DISCUSSION.

Luther D. Shepard, A.M., D.D.S., D.M.D., Boston.—I had the pleasure of reading this paper at my leisure, and I am so well satisfied with it that all I could say would be a word of approbation. It covers the ground, it is concisely expressed, and it states the truth as I have seen it throughout my whole life.

If one would look over the literature of the profession for the past fifty years, he will be convinced that co-operation, the meeting together in societies, has been a great factor for individual growth of the man, extension of his reputation, and the enlargement of the profession by the interchange of valuable ideas.

I could give the names of hundreds who have been active dental society men, and I recall a few instances where men have made their reputation or have impressed themselves upon the world of progress through their activity as society members.

This is such a truism that I wonder at the professional men who keep apart from these meetings. There are among the living a multitude who could be named, but I prefer to speak only of the dead. Our late departed friend, Dr. McKellops, of St. Louis, probably during forty or fifty years gave at least one-twelfth of his time and labor to professional society work. He knew more men and more men knew him throughout the country, and his influence was greater for progress, than any one with whom I have been associated. I could give other examples, but it is not necessary.

The rubbing of man against man, thus reducing their sharp angles, comes from association and co-operation, and this, it seems to me, is a very important factor in the production of substantial growth.

The President introduced Frank R. Mayer, D.D.S., of Worcester, Mass., who read a paper on " Pyorrhœa Alveolaris."

(Dr. Mayer's paper will be published in February.)

The President called upon Dr. Walter E. Decker, D.D.S., of Boston, Mass., who read a paper entitled " A Card System for keeping Dental Records and Accounts."

(For Dr. Decker's paper, see page 19.)

The President then introduced Henry J. Janlusz, D.D.S., of New York City, who read a paper entitled " Suppurative Cleft Palates and Devices for the Same."

(Dr. Janlusz's paper will be published in February.)

There being no discussion on the above papers, the Association then adjouned *sine die.*

WALDO E. BOARDMAN, D.M.D.,
Editor.

Editorial.

WILL GOLD FOIL CEASE TO BE CHIEF OF FILLING-MATERIALS?

THE average dentist cultivated in the art of preparing cavities and filling them with gold-foil will not regard with patience any thought that would indicate an idea that gold, as a filling-material, would ever be relegated to the dust-heaps of memory. The rise of gold as a prophylactic expedient in dentistry has always been held in deep interest by those who regard its past in our work, as not merely of sentimental value, but as the foundation laid by the fathers for the upbuilding of the superstructure which we regard as our profession.

It is appropriate at the opening of a new year, in the first decade of the twentieth century, to review the past and endeavor, through observation of the traces of dental history, to read the future. The man who confines his outlook simply to the present loses that broader horizon so necessary in life's perspective. In the present number our readers will find one of the most earnest advocates of an advanced position in the use of gold-foil as a filling-material condemning the practice of looking backward, and enforces the idea that the outlook must not go beyond the present. This seems to be a narrow conception, leading to an egotistic assumption and imprisonment of mind. It is impossible to understand the present except through comparison with the past, not only in dentistry, but in all the relations of life. Experiences are too closely interwoven to admit of any isolation of periods. The human organism is to-day but the spiritual and physical unfoldment of all that has preceded it, and the dentistry of the hour is the result of the experience of all before this time.

Standing thus, as it were, between two centuries, the nineteenth and the twentieth, we may, with some degree of certainty, not only reason upon the past, but, through it, anticipate the future.

Gold-foil came into our work for the well-understood reason that it presented qualities not possessed by any other metal, and, these being recognized, it became the chief glory of dentistry that it developed processes in its use for the salvation of teeth that

3

actually founded a profession, one improvement leading to an-
er, until what is known as filling teeth with gold has become a
...ex process, requiring not only very decided mechanical skill,
t mental ability of a high order.

For decades prior to 1877 the dentists of the period regarded
...lity to manipulate gold-foil as the standard of excellence. The
...ion prevalent, and insisted upon by the fathers, "that a tooth
...th filling at all was worth filling with gold," was so impressed
...n the dental mind that it required unusual courage to use any
...er material in permanent work. The writer, as well as the
...jority, was thoroughly imbued with this idea, so much so, that
...advocacy of the use of amalgam was regarded as a heresy not
...be tolerated. The amalgam war is now part of a past history,
...ning to some, instructive to others.

It was natural that this consecration of the lines of practice
...and about one material led to an effort to burst these narrow
...ies, and we find a few courageous individuals secretly doing
...which the ethics of the day forbid; but this made no im-
...ion, and these were regarded as unworthy of professional
...cognition.

There came a period, however, in 1877 when a trinity of men
...ed in American dentistry, who took up the gauntlet thrown
...by the fathers and asserted that, "Just in proportion as a
...th needs saving, gold is the worst material that can be used."
...men who thus boldly challenged the faith of the profession
...re not from the ranks, but had been recognized as leaders in
...tal thought. This declaration turned dentistry in America
...no wonder to circumference, and the "New Departure," as it
...called, was denounced upon every side as the creation of a set
...iconoclasts who delighted in tearing down our golden image
...d giving nothing in their place worthy of acceptance. The
...mes of Flagg, Palmer, and Chase were not, therefore, regarded
...an enviable light; indeed, their names and work became a by-
...d and reproach with the unthinking crowd.

It is rare that contemporaneous thought rises to a full con-
...tion of advanced ideas. The mind is narrowed by environ-
...nt, and time alone can raise the mist to a clearer conception
...the possible effect of things new and strange, upon the work

eventually founded a profession, one improvement leading to another, until what is known as filling teeth with gold has become a complex process, requiring not only very decided mechanical skill, but mental ability of a high order.

For decades prior to 1877 the dentists of the period regarded ability to manipulate gold-foil as the standard of excellence. The axiom prevalent, and insisted upon by the fathers, "that a tooth worth filling at all was worth filling with gold," was so impressed upon the dental mind that it required unusual courage to use any other material in permanent work. The writer, as well as the majority, was thoroughly infused with this idea, so much so, that the advocacy of the use of amalgam was regarded as a heresy not to be tolerated. The amalgam war is now part of a past history, amusing to some, instructive to others.

It was natural that this contraction of the lines of practice upon and about one material led to an effort to burst these narrow bonds, and we find a few courageous individuals secretly doing that which the ethics of the day forbid; but this made no impression, and these were regarded as unworthy of professional recognition.

There came a period, however, in 1877 when a trinity of men appeared in American dentistry, who took up the gauntlet thrown down by the fathers and asserted that, "Just in proportion as a tooth needs saving, gold is the worst material that can be used." The men who thus boldly challenged the faith of the profession were not from the ranks, but had been recognized as leaders in dental thought. This declaration jarred dentistry in America from centre to circumference, and the "New Departure," as it was called, was denounced upon every side as the creation of a set of iconoclasts who delighted in tearing down our golden images and giving nothing in their place worthy of acceptance. The names of Flagg, Palmer, and Chase were not, therefore, regarded in an enviable light; indeed, their names and work became a byword and reproach with the unthinking crowd.

It is rare that contemporaneous thought rises to a full conception of advanced ideas. The mind is narrowed by environment, and time alone can raise the mist to a clearer conception of the possible effect of things, new and strange, upon the work of individuals and the world. Thus it was that the ideas of the New Departure advocates fell, apparently, for the time unheeded.

It was only apparent, however, for it was soon evident that the thinking portion of the profession were beginning to ask themselves the question, Have we not been too long worshipping a golden fetish, that has not only been to some extent an injury to our patients, but also to our own loss? It did not take long for the answer to come, and this was demonstrated in an intelligent revision of the entire subject. Amalgam began to be used by the best gold operators where time, money, and strength had been exhansted previously in large gold operations. Plastics of all kinds were adopted where indicated, as the most satisfactory material for the case in charge, and while gold still maintained its preeminence, and the undergraduate was still taught to reverence it as chief of materials in the salvation of teeth, it has measurably fallen from its high estate, and the old axiom is no longer an ethical test to be used by the leaders of dental thought.

If we may judge from the past, taking in view the origin of gold as a filling-material, until the period when it reached its greatest perfection in practice to its decline as an absolute standard of excellence, we may confidently assume that the day will come when its use will be classed as belonging to the barbaric period in dentistry. This may seem an impossible conception, but we have not far to go for a basis upon which to build a prophecy of the future. It is very possible that the present craze for porcelain fillings may eventually reach a lower level than it occupies to-day, but the present indications point directly to the time when it will supplant gold in the large majority of cases coming under dental care, and that plastics, in some form, will subserve dental purposes for the remainder. This, to the gold worshipper, is an inconceivable idea, but if he will only review his dental history he will find, as stated, that there has been a gradual but very sure departure from the old ideas, and dentistry, in this country, could not go back, even if desirable so to do, to the period antedating the new departure creed. Change is in the air and the restless life, ever seeking something new, will drive us on until gold is no longer known as a filling-material for the salvation of teeth.

It seems appropriate that this matter should be discussed at some length, in view of the recent departure of the earnest leader of the three men who made progress in this direction possible.

Dr. J. Foster Flagg was regarded as an extremist, and it is

very true that he was a radical of radicals in his views upon this subject; but while he stood apart among his fellows, it required just such self-abnegation, just that devotion to an idea, which he exemplified, to make an impression. A weak man would· have failed utterly. He, with his colleagues, forced thought, and with thought came action. We may not regard his postulate as being strictly true, but that is unnecessary, for all truth cannot be formulated in a sentence, neither is an oak-tree found entire in the acorn. It is the aggregation of various influences that create revelations. They are not all fully developed at the moment of inspiration.

The writer does not wish to be misunderstood in this connection. He is fully in accord with those who hold to the highest development of gold as a filling-material. It, at present, constitutes that which has stood the test of time, but he recognizes the fact that it is, at its best, but a temporary expedient. What he desires is to enforce the truth, made prominent by the new departure advocates, that age, temperament, quality of tooth-material, and constitutional conditions must all be considered in deciding the question of what is best to use to save teeth. Dr. Flagg answered this when he wrote, in 1888, " For teeth of good structure and with cavities in accessible positions, gold is the king of filling-materials."

If we cannot agree entirely with the iconoclasts of 1877, let us, at least, honor them as earnest men who blazed a path in which the profession must tread reverently. The New Departure has become even now the old departure. The men who originated it have passed to other activities, but the influence they generated will grow and the materials in use in the future will be more in harmony with the structure of which nature has formed the teeth of the human race, and when that time comes the dentist of the period will truly have cause to remember the names of Flagg, Palmer, and Chase as the men who trained the thought from a close adherence to gold-foil to a more reasonable conception of what is needed for the true progress of dentistry and the salvation of all classes of teeth.

Bibliography.

AN EPITOME OF INORGANIC CHEMISTRY AND PHYSICS. By A. McGlannan, M.D., of the College of Physicians and Surgeons, Baltimore. In one 12mo volume of two hundred and sixteen pages, illustrated with twenty engravings. Lea Brothers & Co., Publishers, Philadelphia and New York.

This is another of the Epitome series, and the author says of it, "The purpose is to set forth the accepted and proved facts, forming the basis of the sciences in a manner which, in the author's opinion, will serve best for the clear and easy understanding by the students."

The subjects embraced in this epitome cover physics and inorganic chemistry, hence heat, light, electricity, magnetism, together with those belonging to the latter subject, are very clearly set forth with commendable brevity, yet with a degree of thoroughness that compares favorably with larger works upon these subjects. The author claims no originality, his idea being to bring the essentials in a form adapted for reference and an aid to study.

The diagram of "Metric and Apothecary System Equivalent," giving "comparative scales, showing at a glance the exact equivalent of ordinary weights and measures in those of the metric system and *vice versa*," will prove to the student a ready means of immediate comparison, much more satisfactory than the ordinary table or methods of computation usually given.

Foreign Correspondence.

DR. BRYAN ON PROPHYLAXIS AND CRITICISMS.

BASEL, SWITZERLAND, November 19, 1903.

TO THE EDITOR:

SIR,—In the discussion on my article on "Prophylaxis," in the November, 1903, number of your journal, page 831, reported from The New York Institute of Stomatology, on page 854, I notice with pleasure that there is a growing sentiment in America in favor of these thorough operations which *prevent decay* of the teeth. I also note that there is a misconception of the conditions existing in Europe *versus* those in America. In America, dentistry is sixty years ahead, so far as the public is concerned, in the personal care of the teeth, and with the American patients that I occasionally see there is a decided difference in the way they take care of their teeth and the way representatives of other nations treat theirs. No wonder decay is not on the increase in America. In Basel we have had a long series of American dentists who have trained the people of the upper class in certain things, but still when an American lady comes to me I can tell her teeth from those of any other nation, simply by the way they are treated prophylactically by her (I am not so sure of the masculines). They are *clean,* they are polished like ivory, they have good gold and other fillings, the teeth shine like alabaster. It is a joy and a pleasure to see them, and do the little that is to be done on them, and one has the feeling that the work one does will prove a success for years, and it is a stimulation to *do* good work. One knows that they will brush their teeth as only Americans know how to brush them; that the waxed silk, rinsing, and brushing will remove every particle of food, every night before the patient retires; that they will adopt every suggestion of the dentist, if they do not already know more of the personal care of the teeth than the occasional dentist will tell them between the acts; that they will go to their dentist regularly and never neglect their teeth till they "feel a pain;" in fact, that they will love their dentist and keep his commandments. I do not know whether I should thank the Almighty that I have been sent abroad as a missionary in dentistry or regret the Providence that has removed me from my own people, who are such model patients to prophylaxis or personal care of their teeth.

The above will be sufficient answer to Drs. Gillett and Kimball's criticism of the first paragraph of my paper. I do not have difficulty in doing the "little things" that go to make up the hours of work charged under the heading of "various operations." My people know what they get, and know that these "little things," these "various operations," will prevent more "tedious and expensive operations" in coming years. They already see that the "preventive dentistry" saves them, and especially their children, hours of agony and great expense that they have gone through themselves in former years, when the slightest defect or sensitive superficial decay, that is now stopped with preventive remedies, was bored out with pain and filled with expense. This naturally brings in their friends who have had such a dread that they have never dared to go to a dentist, and their teeth have been left to bacteria and the forceps, under the benign influence of gas, until they need bridge-work or a wabbly plate, which latter should be as much a shame and embarrassment (and usually is) as a wooden leg or a rubber nose.

Dr. F. Milton Smith says "there is nothing new in either the paper of Dr. Bryan or that by Dr. Smith, of Philadelphia." Well, it would be something new if a Dr. Smith of New York would acknowledge that a Dr. Smith of Philadelphia could tell him anything. I have looked pretty carefully for some remedy which was recommended to be applied externally to weak, newly erupted teeth to prevent decay, and have not found it in medical or dental literature for the last fifty years, and I believe this *is* something new, and I believe I have for the Dental Congress in St. Louis some other new things in this line, and will present them there. As for "Dr. Smith of Philadelphia," the profession had better keep an eye on his methods, and also give just a little time to consideration of Dr. Wright's (Cincinnati) suggestion of training feminine assistants to do this prophylactic work, and then you will see not only the Americans who travel abroad, with teeth like pearls, but those who stay at home may gladden the hearts of those dentists who appreciate a clean laboratory,—the human mouth.

Yes, we had polishing with wood points in porte-polishers a generation and more ago, and bathing in the Jordan was recommended long before many Saratogas and Hot Springs were known, and still it's a good thing to recommend the latter nowadays, and it's a new thing under the Western sun.

With greetings to the home brethren, I am yours, fraternally,

L. C. BRYAN.

Biographical Sketch.

J. FOSTER FLAGG, D.D.S.

BY WILLIAM H. TRUEMAN, D.D.S., PHILADELPHIA.

DIED, at his residence, Swarthmore, Pa., on the evening of November 25, 1903, Dr. J. Foster Flagg, after a long and painful illness borne with manly fortitude.

Dr. Josiah Foster Flagg, the only son of Dr. John Foster Brewster Flagg and Miss Mary Waterman Jackson, was born at Providence, R. I., October 15, 1828. He was a grandson of Josiah Flagg, the first native-born American dentist, and the last male descendent of that branch of the Flagg family. The family history dates back to Thomas Flagg, supposed to be a native of Ireland, who arrived at Watertown, Mass., in 1642. It was through his great-grandfather, Lieutenant-Colonel Josiah Flagg, that the family became so closely identified with the rise and progress of dental science in America. Josiah Flagg, then a lad of about eighteen years, was a private in the Elliott regiment, of which his father was an officer, when the American and French troops were encamped in winter quarters near Providence, R. I., 1781-82. The war was practically over, and Joseph Le Maire, a surgeon-dentist from Paris, serving as a surgeon with the French contingent, resumed the practice of his profession. He and Lieutenant-Colonel Flagg became intimate, and the opportunity thus offered for his son to learn this new profession from so skilful a master was promptly embraced. Young Flagg proved an apt student, and achieved a fair measure of success. His eldest son, Josiah Foster Flagg, was educated for the medical profession, but on the death of his father, in 1816, entered upon dental practice.

In 1797 Josiah Flagg married, as his second wife, Miss Eliza Brewster, a direct descendant of the sixth generation from Elder Brewster, who came over in the " Mayflower" as leader of the first contingent of Pilgrim Fathers, thus uniting these two old colonial families. Dr. Flagg's father, J. F. B. Flagg, was the only son of this marriage. His father dying in 1816, when he was only twelve years of age, his education was directed by his elder brother, who exercised over him a fatherly care, and in due time taught him the art and science of dental surgery. On reaching manhood he moved to Providence, R. I., and shortly after married Miss Mary Waterman Jackson, daughter of a prominent citizen of that town. Dr. J. Foster Flagg was their only son. The early education of the latter was received at the schools of that place, and later at a school in Boston conducted by Bronson Alcott. In 1842 his father removed to Philadelphia, and soon became intimate with the more prominent Philadelphia dentists, and was an important factor in inaugurating the movement which resulted in making Philadelphia an important dental educational centre.

On leaving school, Dr. Flagg entered the Jefferson Medical College of Philadelphia, but on account of being under age did not graduate. About 1849 the California gold excitement electrified the country. He had not as yet "settled down," and, with a desire to see the world, he immediately set out for the far distant gold-fields, taking with him an assortment of dental and medical instruments and drugs. The excitement appealed to his active ardent nature, and in due time he arrived at the expected "Eldorado." While there he had varied and exciting experiences. At one time at the gold-diggings, again as a cow-boy on the plains, and later engaged in the first attempt to impound the waters of the mountain-streams for use in mining and irrigation, he and his co-laborers laid the foundation of that which has done so much to develop the industries of that region. It might well be called "a wild life," but J. Foster Flagg knew how to take care of himself; his home training was not forgotten, and his surroundings developed in him a manliness, mentally and physically, that served him well in later years. In camp he was a leader; there was that about him that commanded respect while inviting comradeship; and now and again his well-trained muscles were called upon to administer convincing arguments to those of the unruly element, that he was not to be trifled with.

The dental and medical knowledge acquired before leaving home now came into use, and he soon became a much-sought physician, surgeon, and dentist in treating the disease and accidents of camp life. The much dreaded Asiatic cholera played sad havoc in many camps. On its approach Dr. Flagg instituted strict sanitary precautions, and as a prophylactic adopted the free use of acids, with the result that the disease did not prevail where these precautions were observed. For treatment he advocated giving the sufferers all the water they cared to drink, well dosed with acid, opium only when needed. Pickles were among the camp luxuries, and the surplus vinegar was at times the only obtainable acid. It proved very efficient, and was carefully hoarded, being considered worth " its weight in gold."

The methods of gold-mining then practised required an abundance of water. The supply from the mountain-streams was very irregular, at times deficient, and at other times destructive in its abundance. Dr. Flagg, with a few others, conceived the idea of impounding these streams so as to secure a more reliable supply. While at work solving the engineering problems involved in building a dam to store up water for mining and agricultural purposes, word reached him that his mother was seriously ill, and had a yearning to see once more her only son. His maternal love overcame his ambition, and he promptly decided to at once start for home. This proved a very great financial loss. While he and his partners were well satisfied that their work would prove successful, and in the end profitable, and had embarked their all in the enterprise, it was generally distrusted, and considered a wild scheme. While the desirability of impounding and holding for a time of need the surplus water of the rainy season was fully recognized, its practicability was doubted, and it was prophesied that the first freshet would wipe out all their labor. This made it difficult for him to sell out his interest to advantage; but as he had been there nearly seven years, and was feeling homesick, he decided to leave the Pacific coast for good, and therefore desired to close out all business interests. To do so he was compelled to accept for his share in the enterprise less than he had put into it, and very much less than it was worth, as the sequel proved. His engineering plans proved successful. He had well studied the forces the dam would encounter, and so well planned to resist them that it withstood many freshets, and as a venture was profitable beyond expectation. Enlarged and improved, it continues useful to this day.

His next care was the home voyage. He was informed that a vessel was all ready to sail from San Francisco, but waited to obtain a competent medical officer, and it was suggested to him that his medical experience and reputation in camp might obtain him the position. He applied, and his application was endorsed by some of

his friends. The examination was brief. " Can you treat cholera ?"
" I can," was the prompt and emphatic answer. It was enough.
He was engaged for the voyage and given his passage for his services, with orders to as quickly as possible provide an ample medical
chest at the company's expense. So frequently and so fatally had
the dread disease appeared on former voyages, that no vessel would
sail without a physician; the position was not sought after, and
this vessel had waited days to supply this need when Dr. Flagg
applied. In relating the incident he confessed that the situation
was embarrassing. He had no fear of cholera, unless he himself
should be the victim, and he inwardly prayed that there should be
no other diseases, and but little of that. It was his only chance to
get home quickly. The passenger-list was full, and no other vessel
was expected to sail for a month. Furthermore, the free passage
well suited his finances. He promptly directed and enforced such
proper sanitary precautions as were possible in an overcrowded
passenger-ship, and was the one man in all that ship's company
whose orders were willingly accepted and promptly executed. These
proved efficient. That vessel was one of very few sailing from San
Francisco to Panama at this time which, on arriving at its destina-
tion, was able to report " no serious sickness and no deaths."

Once more at home the question of his life's vocation was
seriously considered. He finally decided to adopt his father's profession, and entering the Philadelphia College of Dental Surgery,
graduated from that institution at its fourth annual commencement, February 29, 1856, in the same class with his distinguished
colleague, the late Professor James E. Garretson.

For a few years he practised in New Jersey, but returned to
Philadelphia in 1860, and located with his father at 1112 Arch
Street. Fortuitous circumstances assisted him to quickly acquire a
satisfactory practice. His genial manners, his professional skill.
and his gentleness in operating gave him a firm hold upon his
patients. Among these was a large number of school children,
whose gratitude he earned by refusing to make appointments with
them on Saturday. He contended it was their holiday, and should
not be broken into even for an hour; the care of their teeth was
fully as important as their education, and should be done in other
time than theirs.

October 31, 1861, he married Miss Mary Craft, who survives
him.

By prudent living and good business management during his active life, Dr. Flagg was able to retire when advancing years made professional duties a burden. At his comfortable, pleasantly situated country home at Swarthmore, with congenial neighbors, his children and grandchildren close at hand, relieved from all care, he enjoyed for a few years a well-earned rest. He was not, however, idle. He continued to manufacture the plastic filling-materials he had done so much to improve, and continued his experiments looking to a still further elimination of their defects, until the inroads of disease compelled him to stop.

He leaves two daughters,—Mary, the wife of Dr. James Price, of Swarthmore, and Lillie, wife of Professor Gummere, of Ursinus College, Collegeville, Pa.

Dr. J. Foster Flagg entered the dental profession determined to succeed; he was energetic, enthusiastic, and a tireless worker. He possessed in full measure the true professional spirit, and held, taught, and practised that every man's interests were best served when each tried to help the other. He promptly became a contributor to periodical dental literature, addressing himself more particularly to those problems usually termed "practical," those which immediately concern a dentist's daily work. His first contribution was upon the construction of artificial teeth (*Dental News Letter,* vol. x., October, 1856, page 209), dealing with the artistic arrangement, and referring to points he had observed to be frequently overlooked. He was a keen observer, quick to appreciate the relation of cause and effect, and resourceful in overcoming the many difficulties constantly taxing the abilities of a dental practitioner. He *knew* what he *did* know, and expressed his convictions with positiveness and confidence, making, however, no pretensions regarding matters of which he was not sure. "I don't know," was with him a frequent expression when conversing upon professional matters; "I think," "It may be so," "I don't understand it," "That is out of my line," etc., were his usual comments upon unsolved problems; but, regarding those which he felt had been solved, his emphatic "I know" admitted of no question and tolerated no doubt. There was in this no egotism, it indicated absolute confidence, nothing more. While holding in profound respect the conclusions of others, especially those which had become crystallized into accepted theories and generally considered safe guides in dental practice, he did not permit them to override or obscure his own observations. He was ever open to new ideas, to consider new theories and new methods upon their intrinsic merits rather than the reputation of their authors. His judgment on these was usually quickly rendered, and generally accurate.

Dr. Flagg began his career as a teacher by accepting the chair of Institutes of Dentistry, in the first faculty of the Philadelphia Dental College at its organization in the spring of 1863, and he outlived them all. The title of this chair was changed at the beginning of the sixth session, 1868-69, to that of Dental Pathology and Therapeutics, a change of name only. He resigned at the close of the seventh session in order to devote his time more fully to private practice, continuing, however, his connection with the college as clinical instructor. With the opening of the seventeenth session, 1879-80, he resumed his old position and continued to lecture until the close of the session of 1895-96, when he finally retired. During this period the Philadelphia Dental College made a decided advance. About 1887 it united with the Medico-Chirurgical College in the erection of a new building for joint occupancy, in order to secure more room and more convenient arrangement to accomodate their constantly increasing classes. Dr. Flagg had much to do with designing the new structure, and skilfully planned the various class- and clinic-rooms to secure the largest capacity without sacrifice of comfort and convenience. During the erection he superintended the details of construction, meeting and solving the many problems that arose as the work progressed. For this he was eminently qualified. He knew what was needed, and his mechanical ingenuity suggested novel expedients which added much to the usefulness of the finished structure, which proved well adapted to its intended use.

As a teacher he displayed marked ability. He had a personal magnetism that attracted and retained the students' attention; he was earnest, enthusiastic, spoke with energy and emphasis, and interspersed in his remarks witty sayings and anecdotes, so appropriate and well told that they served to firmly fix the facts presented in the minds of his hearers. His lectures were not desultory reading of text-books; on the contrary, they were original, well connected, and interesting discourses, and recitals of personal experiences having a direct bearing upon the vocation with which the students were most concerned.

Wherever possible he enforced the spoken word by demonstrating before his class, and constructed for this purpose many ingenious models, among them a rudely formed skeleton of the head, with the teeth and jaws in position. This proved an admirable arrangement for illustrating the position to be assumed in operating, arranging napkin, bandages, etc., and the most convenient way of performing various dental operations. This was duplicated and patented in England as something new more than a score of years after Dr. Flagg had introduced it to his classes.

He had the happy faculty of making himself one with his students without sacrificing the dignity of a teacher. He was approachable, invited their friendship, and made their interests his.

As a writer Dr. Flagg contributed to dental periodical literature all through his professional life. He wrote as he spoke, with emphasis and vigor. His style was quite original, and while it at times lacked scholarly dignity, it conveyed unerringly the writer's thought. He was inclined to be epigrammatic, while wit and sarcasm, pointed, yet so refined as to be thoroughly enjoyed even by those who felt its shafts, flowed freely from his pen. His most notable production is his work on " Plastics," a work that merits a place in all dental libraries.

Dr. Flagg can hardly be considered a professional society man. He could not forget that his father and uncle were compelled to forego membership in the American Association of Dental Surgeons for no other fault than that of declining to sign away their right of using their own judgment in matters of practice. He noted with keen regret that the professional societies held, with all the tenacity of religious bigots, to the accepted tenets of the day. As he once remarked to the writer, he seemed to have been born a professional heretic, and from first to last of his professional career was the subject of adverse criticism, and at times of reproach. He bore it all, however, in good part, and lived to see many of his derided ideas accepted and adopted, and would now and again remark, as he noted in society discussion the once denounced suggestions advanced as good practice, " They are getting up to me; they will be there after a while." Notwithstanding, however, he keenly regretted the spirit of intolerance so frequently displayed in dental societies, and regarded it, as all thoughtful men must do, as a hinderance to real progress. While he frequently attended dental society meetings, thoroughly enjoyed them, and took an active part whenever present, and felt and knew that his remarks were enjoyed and appreciated, he felt more free as a visitor than as a member. That a man remains placid, and replies playfully to adverse criticism, does not imply that he enjoys it. Dr. Flagg did not. He held his membership in dental societies ever ready to slip his moorings to escape expulsion for unwittingly transgressing some part of the *creed* the society itself might shortly expunge.

Early in his career as a dentist Dr. Flagg was impressed with the importance of saving all of the natural teeth that could by any possible means be kept useful and comfortable. He appreciated the difficulties attending the manipulation of gold in teeth badly broken down, and observed that the much decried amalgam seemed to be especially useful in such cases. The expression so frequently used at that time, " Any tooth worth saving should be filled with gold," did not appear to him as a good motto for a dentist who wished to do the best for his patient. To him it seemed more reasonable that any tooth that could be made comfortable and was useful was worth saving, and he realized that this included many teeth that could not be filled with gold by even the most expert operators. The so-called " amalgam war" had just closed; notwithstanding that, however, the leading lights of the dental profession were not converted; they still believed that amalgam was a vile stuff to place in carious human teeth, and had not yet learned that many of the ills credited to it were due to improper or imperfect treatment of the tooth preparatory to inserting the filling. Dr. Flagg's father and uncle, while bitterly denouncing amalgam, quite as bitterly denounced the American Association for provoking the controversy, holding that it had no right to impose restrictions upon its members in their efforts to benefit their patients. Dr. Flagg had been taught to avoid amalgam, many of his professional associates were opposed to it, and he naturally had a prejudice against it. He had not been long in practice, however, when he became convinced that in many cases it was the only available means of prolonging the usefulness of teeth important to the comfort of their owners. He resolved that inasmuch as he alone was responsible for the results of his operations, and that this responsibility could not be shared by those who assumed to dictate what was and what was not in accordance with professional probity, he would be guided in all such matters by his own experience and judgment.

Laying aside as far as possible preconceived notions, he ad-

dressed himself to the problem of tooth-saving. He was thus led
to look upon amalgam as a good thing to use when nothing better
was available. He carefully noted its many defects, and by a long
series of careful observations and experiments sought their elimination. Conducted as this research was, progress was necessarily
slow; it was, however, sure. He first noted the differing behavior
of amalgams made of various alloys, and endeavored to ascertain the
part played by their several components. From his professional
associates he selected a number whom he knew to be skilful, unprejudiced, careful observers, men in whose judgment he had confidence, and whose fields of labor were widely separated, to test the
various alloys he experimentally compounded, asking from them
reports of their behavior as fillings after an interval of several
years. They were requested to carefully prepare a record of the
position, surroundings, and the circumstances attending the insertion of each filling; to place them as far as possible where they
could be frequently seen and their condition noted. Especial attention was asked regarding tooth-saving, integrity, and color. Dr.
Flagg kept a record of the formula of these alloys, and full particulars of the treatment they received before they left his hands.
When reports from these came back to him after an interval of some
years, he was able to collate the experience of many observers, working under varied conditions, and to know far more than could
possibly have been learned by laboratory experiments alone. In
many cases reports were, after a longer interval, revised. An
alloy that was pronounced satisfactory after two years' observation might be condemned a few years later. After years of similar
experimentation he began to learn the varied properties of the
available metals, how these properties were modified by alloying,
and to select and properly proportion them to produce a desired
result. When this point was reached, about 1881, he published the
first edition of his work entitled, "Plastics and Plastic Fillings."
In this work he embodied the results of his labors to date, and
by subsequent editions and corrections he has kept the profession
fully informed of progress made. None but those close to Dr.
Flagg can appreciate the vast labor these researches, continued
more than twoscore years, involved, the care with which they
were conducted, or how cautiously the results were from time to
time announced. Now and again he announced to his friends, "I
have done with it; I have not reached the end, but I have done all

I can; let some one else finish it." He continued, however, his efforts to improve this class of fillings until the very end of his long and useful life. In his last interview with the writer, but a few months before his death, he said that he had just completed some experiments by which he thought he had obtained an amalgam that preserved its color better, and a gutta-percha better able to withstand wear; as soon as he was satisfied with the tests then in progress he intended the profession to have the benefit of it. That was his last effort. He died in harness.

As an unlooked for outcome of these researches the profession was startled about a quarter of a century ago by a boldly announced " New Departure." While making these researches upon amalgam, Dr. Flagg noted that amalgam seemed to have tooth preservative properties apart from those due to its plasticity. Upon examining further in this direction, he observed that in mouths where gold fillings were apt to prove temporary only, decay quickly recurring around the filling or at its cervical margin, amalgam often proved more lasting and more effective in arresting decay. He further noted that with a class of teeth universally termed " soft," teeth that seemed prone to decay, and in which gold fillings required frequent renewal, teeth that dentists in general consider as doomed to be early lost, did far better when filled with amalgam. He still further observed that in cases of recurring decay, if the new decay was removed and the defect repaired with amalgam, the operation was usually more permanent than when the defective filling was removed and replaced with gold, or when the repair was made with gold. These results were unlooked for, and were not inexplicable by any theory then in vogue with the dental profession. It had been before observed that tin was in some cases a better decay arrester than gold, and that gutta-percha was equally effective, if not more so. At first this was explained by the softness of tin and gutta-percha permitting a better adaptation to the cavity walls, but later and more searching observations established that these two tooth-filling materials seemed to be effective in cases where it was known that the cavity adaptation was imperfect, while gold often failed in spite of the best adaptation an expert operator was able to make, and in fillings that seemed perfect.

About this time the late Dr. Stewart B. Palmer, of Syracuse, N. Y., and the late Dr. Henry S. Chase, of St. Louis, Mo. (*Dental Cosmos,* vol. xviii., 1876, pages 244 and 352), both of whom were

4

in correspondence and were working with Dr. Flagg in these investigations, suggested the electro-chemical theory as an explanation. They, indeed, contended that under certain conditions at times present in the oral cavity a filling in a tooth becomes a galvanic battery whose energy depends upon the relation, electrically, between the substance of the tooth and the material of the filling. The farther they are apart, potentially, the more energetic this battery becomes. The result of this electric energy, they contended, was a changed condition of that portion of the oral fluids immediately at the junction of the tooth and the filling, by which they became acid and tooth-destroying. Inasmuch as gold and the substance of the tooth (for convenience in this discussion termed " dentos") are widely separated, on the electro-potential scale, while dentos, tin, amalgam, the cements, and gutta-percha are in the order named closely related, this was presented as an explanation of the mystery. Dr. Flagg made no pretention to knowledge of these intricate matters. The explanation was plausible. He therefore called to his aid scientists well qualified to investigate the matter, and was by them informed that the theory was in accord with recognized principles of electro-chemistry.

These three investigators were now convinced that the failure of gold fillings was not due to defective manipulation, nor yet to an inherent weakness of the teeth themselves, as had heretofore been so strenuously held. Manipulative ability had failed to make gold the tooth-saver the dentist needed in so many cases, and, they felt, it was high time to take a new departure by abandoning this cure-all and using in its place something else for those teeth in which it had so signally failed. The real question was not gold or plastics. They admitted that there was nothing better than gold for all cases where it effectively arrested decay, but contended that its continued use in places where general experience taught it was not effective was not good practice. As was well known, so little are some teeth prone to decay that any kind of a filling will effectively arrest its destruction, while, on the other hand, the best efforts of an expert fails to do more than retard it in others. The first class needs but little help, the second, all the help dental science can give them. Hence the first article of the so-called " New Departure Creed," " In proportion as teeth need saving, gold is the worst material to use," the worst material because by its presence, to a greater degree than does any other tooth-filling material, it brings about a local condition favorable to tooth destruction. That was the theory of the new departure.

Dr. Flagg made a forceful presentation of the subject in an address delivered at a special meeting of the New York Odontological Society, November 20 and 21, 1877. He was well qualified for the task. He felt he was right, and spoke with earnestness and energy. He well knew that the views expressed would encounter a strong opposition, and invite to himself and his colleagues adverse criticism. His purpose was a laudable one. It was to get the profession out of a rut, a slavish following of the old maxim that gold was the only filling-material a respectable dentist should use, and to elevate from the realms of quackery the much abused yet useful plastics. Notwithstanding the tempest his address aroused, it accomplished its purpose, and stimulated a series of improvements in all these plastic fillings that has given them a wider field and increased usefulness. For this the profession owes Dr. Flagg a debt of gratitude.

The value of Dr. Flagg's services in introducing improved formulas for dental alloys and new methods of making and preparing them for use,—and in advocating the use of the non-metallic plastics and acting as their champion on their advent into respectable dental practice in this country, will be more and more appreciated as time goes on. The profession may disregard the theories of the "New Departure," but there is, nevertheless, an unmistakable growing tendency towards the practice he advocated, and a general recognition that it tends to greater success in tooth-saving. Dr. Flagg had reason for now and again facetiously remarking, " They are getting there; they will be up to me after a while."

What an honored place does the three generations of this family occupy in the annals of dentistry in America! The grandfather, the pioneer native-born American dentist; his two sons, distinguished alike as practitioners, teachers, and investigators, who have made the way easier for those who follow; while the grandson's earnest efforts to increase the usefulness of the profession promises to revolutionize the practice of the science. With the death of Josiah Foster Flagg the chapter ends.

Obituary.

MR. WILLIAM ASH.

BORN April 18, 1819; died November 19, 1903.

We regret to announce that Mr. William Ash, the youngest son of Claudius Ash, the founder of the firm of Claudius Ash & Sons, died at his London residence, Tower House, Camden Road, N. W., on Thursday, November 19, in his eighty-fifth year. Born in the parish of St. James's, Westminster, on the 18th of April, 1819, he was educated in London, and in due course joined his father and his brothers George, Claudius, and Edward in business.

For nearly sixty years Mr. William Ash was a familiar figure at Broad Street, and all who remember him will recall his kindly and urbane manner. He ceased to take an active part in the business about ten years ago.

In addition to the business side of his life, Mr. William Ash was deeply interested in the dental profession, and was very closely associated with the Dental Hospital of London from its inception. For a great many years he was an active member of the committee of that institution, and took a prominent part in its removal from Soho Square to Leicester Square, the result of a proposal by Mr. (afterwards Sir) Edwin Saunders. At the annual general meeting of the governors of the hospital in 1873, Mr. Ash proposed an alternative to the Saunders plan. " His idea was to build suitable premises, rather than to convert old ones into the nearest approach to convenience they would allow. At considerable trouble he had procured plans and drawings in connection with sites to be obtained from the Metropolitan Board of Works, on which a hospital could be erected, adapted in all points to the requirements of the managing and medical staff, the students, and also the Odontological Society. . . . His proposal was discussed, but eventually the decision was given in favor of the original plan." [1]

Soon after his twenty-first birthday Mr. William Ash married Sarah, the daughter of Mr. James Matchwick, of Guildford, Surrey, who predeceased him by only sixteen days.

---

[1] Hill's History of the Reform Movement in the Dental Profession in Great Britain, p. 237.

Three years ago a stained glass window was inserted in the church at Heathfield, Sussex, in which parish Mr. Ash had a country residence, as a thank-offering, and in commemoration of his diamond jubilee.

Mr. William Ash leaves three sons and three daughters. Of the sons, William Henry and Claudius James are at present the senior Directors of the firm of Claudius Ash & Sons, Limited.

The funeral took place on Monday, November 23, at Highgate Cemetery and was largely attended by members, relatives, and friends of the family; also by many of the employees at Broad Street and some from the Factory, Kentish Town.

RESOLUTIONS OF RESPECT TO DR. FRANCIS M. ODELL.

THE following resolutions were adopted at a regular meeting of the First District Dental Society of the State of New York, November 10, 1903:

WHEREAS, On October 11, 1903, Francis M. Odell, M.D., D.D.S., an honorary member of this Society and its secretary for some years in its early days, started on that unknown journey;

Resolved, That we, the members of the First District Dental Society, in regular session assembled, testify to the loss we feel in his departure from our midst;

To the loss the community has sustained since he has ceased to be able to give them the benefit of his well-trained mind and his skilful hand;

To his skill, which has preserved thousands of human teeth to remain a comfort to his former patients in their old age, which, in itself, is the highest praise we can bestow.

That we appreciate the work he has done for this Society and the scientific advancement of dentistry during his active career.

That the fortitude and patience he displayed during the last ten years of his life, constantly battling with a dread disease which not only prevented his practising his profession, but entailed untold suffering, makes his character stand out in a manner most creditable and worthy of emulation.

That we condole with his bereaved family; that a copy of these resolutions be sent to his widow, to the dental journals, and also be inscribed on our official minutes.

S. L. GOLDSMITH,
W. E. HOAG,
M. L. RHEIN,
Committee.

Current News.

FORM OF AGREEMENT OF THE STATE BOARD OF NEW JERSEY.

AGREEMENT entered into this ——————— day of ——————, 190 , between the State Board of Registration and Examination in Dentistry of New Jersey, Members of the National Association of Dental Examiners, and the State Board of Examiners of the State of ——————, also members of the same body.

Witnesseth, The party of the first part hereby agrees under the terms of the resolution passed at Asheville, to exchange with the State Board of Examiners representing the State of —————— licenses to practise dentistry, and to issue license to the candidate presenting credentials properly filled out, accompanied with fee such as the laws of each State require.

In witness thereof the president and secretary have signed their respective names and seals in duplicate.

ASHEVILLE RESOLUTION.

"*Resolved,* That an interchange of license to practise dentistry be, and is hereby recommended to be, granted by the various State Boards, on the following specific conditions:

· " Any dentist who has been in legal practice for five years or more, and is a reputable dentist of good moral character, and who is desirous of making a change of residence into another State, may apply to the Examining Board of the State in which he resides for a new certificate, which shall attest to his moral character and professional attainments, and said certificate, if granted, shall be deposited with the Examining Board of the State in which he proposes to reside, and the said Board, in exchange thereof, may grant him a license to practise dentistry."

———————————————
President State Board of ——————— [SEAL]

———————————————
President State Board of ——————— [SEAL]

———————————————
Secretary State Board of ——————— [SEAL]

———————————————
Secretary State Board of ——————— [SEAL]

FLORIDA STATE DENTAL SOCIETY.

THE twenty-first annual meeting of the Florida State Dental Society will be held at Atlantic Beach, May 25, 1904. Following are the officers and standing and special committees for 1903–4:

President, Dr. J. Edward Chace, Ocala, Fla.; First Vice-President, Dr. A. B. Whitman, Orlando, Fla.; Second Vice-President, —Dr. R. L. McMullen, Clear Water, Fla.; Secretary, Dr. D. D. Beekman, Daytona, Fla.; Treasurer, Dr. F. B. Hannah, Jr., Jacksonville, Fla.

Executive Committee.—Dr. Jas. W. Simpson, Kissimmee, Fla.; Dr. Jas. E. Chace, Jacksonville, Fla.; Dr. A. J. Hannah, Umatilla, Fla.; Dr. G. Enloe, Miami, Fla.; Dr. A. B. Stevens, Orlando, Fla.

Operative Dentistry.—Dr. J. D. L. Tench, Gainesville, Chairman; Dr. Edith R. Brush, Daytona, Secretary.

Mechanical Dentistry.—Dr. F. E. Buck, Jacksonville, Chairman; Dr. Jas. W. Simpson, Kissimmee, Secretary.

Physiology and Etiology.—Dr. W. E. Driscoll, Braidentown, Chairman; Dr. Henri Letord, Orlando, Secretary.

Dental Education and Literature.—Dr. W. G. Mason, Tampa, Chairman; Dr. W. S. Taylor, De Land, Secretary.

Essays and Voluntary Papers.—Dr. C. H. Frink, Fernandina, Chairman; Dr. R. L. McMullen, Clear Water, Secretary.

Pathology and Surgery.—Dr. L. C. Elkins, St. Augustine, Chairman; Dr. G. Enloe, Miami, Secretary.

Dental Histology and Microscopy.—Dr. T. J. Welch, Pensacola, Chairman; Dr. R. M. Mason, Sanford; Secretary.

Dental Chemistry and Therapeutics.—Dr. A. B. Whitman, Orlando, Chairman; Dr. E. A. Law, Bartow, Secretary.

Clinics.—Dr. C. C. Collins, Atlanta, Ga., Chairman; Dr. W. McL. Dancy, Jacksonville, Secretary.

Arrangements.—Dr. Jas. Chace, Jacksonville, Chairman; Dr. E. M. Sanderson, Jacksonville, Secretary; Dr. F. E. Buck, Jacksonville.

To investigate Illegal Practice.—Dr. W. G. Mason, Tampa, Chairman; Dr. T. J. Welch, Pensacola, Secretary.

To revise the Constitution and By-Laws.—Dr. C. F. Kemp, Key West, Chairman; Dr. J. E. Chace, Jacksonville, Secretary; Dr. L. C. Elkins, St. Augustine.

The latter committee was appointed to draft a new Constitution and By-Laws more in accord with present needs. Members of the society are urged to make such suggestions to the chairman as may occur to them.

It is urgently requested that all members, whether on a committee or not, will contribute papers or clinics, communicating their willingness to the chairman of the committee to which they wish to be assigned.

Any suggestions which will help to make our next meeting a success will be glady received by the President or Secretary.

J. Edward Chace, D.D.S., *President.*
D. D. Beekman, D.D.S., *Secretary.*

THE INTERSTATE DENTAL FRATERNITY OF THE UNITED STATES AND CANADA.

At the Annual Meeting of the Interstate Dental Fraternity, held at Asheville, N. C., on July 29, 1903, the following officers were elected for the ensuing year:

Vice-Presidents: For Arkansas, C. Richardson, D.D.S., Fayetteville; for California, H. P. Carleton, D.D.S., San Francisco; for Connecticut, James McManus, D.D.S., Hartford; for District of Columbia, Emory C. Bryant, D.D.S., Washington; for Illinois, Hart J. Goslee, D.D.S., Chicago; for Indiana, George E. Hunt, D.D.S., Indianapolis; for Kansas, George A. Esterly, D.D.S., Lawrence; for Louisiana, Edward Kells, D.D.S., New Orleans; for Maryland, B. Holly Smith, D.D.S., Baltimore; for Massachusetts, John F. Dowsley, D.D.S., Boston; for Minnesota, Frank E. Moody, D.D.S., Minneapolis; for Missouri, Burton Lee Thorpe, D.D.S., St. Louis; for New Jersey, Charles S. Stockton, D.D.S., Newark; for New York, F. C. Walker, D.D.S., Brooklyn; for North Carolina, J. A. Gorman, D.D.S., Asheville; for Ohio, Henry Barnes, M.D., Cleveland; for Pennsylvania, I. N. Broomell, D.D.S., Philadelphia; for Rhode Island, Dennis F. Keefe, D.D.S., Providence; for Wisconsin, H. L. Banshaf, D.D.S., Milwaukee.

R. M. Sanger,
Secretary.

THE

International Dental Journal.

| VOL. XXV. | FEBRUARY, 1904. | No. 2. |

Original Communications.[1]

THE VASOMOTOR SYSTEM OF THE PULP.[2]

BY EUGENE S. TALBOT, M.D., D.D.S., CHICAGO.

In 1733 Stephen Hales[3] first published the idea that small arteries changed their caliber. He devised the following ingenious experiment: Tying a brass tube into the aorta of a dog and employing a head pressure equal to the normal aortic tension, he injected water and measured the outflow per minute from the divided vessels of the intestines. He found cold water diminished, while hot water increased the flow. He also showed (by the action of drugs) that one set of agents contracted the vessels and lessened the outflow, while another set widened the vessels and increased the flow.[4]

The chief dominating centre of the non-striped muscles of the arterial system with motor nerves (vasomotor, vasoconstrictor,

---

[1] The editor and publishers are not responsible for the views of authors of papers published in this department, nor for any claim to novelty, or otherwise, that may be made by them. No papers will be received for this department that have appeared in any other journal published in the country.

[2] Read before the American Medical Association, Section on Stomatology, at New Orleans, La., May 5 to 8, 1903.

[3] Statical Essays, 1733, vol. xi.

[4] A history of some of the experiments from this period to the present time may be found in Text-Book of Physiology, by E. A. Schäfer.

vasohypertonic) lies in the medulla oblongata. The nerves which pass to the blood-vessels are known as the vasomotor nerves. Without mentioning the experiments which have been made, I might say, in a general way, stimulation of this nerve-centre causes contraction of all the arteries, resulting in great increase of the arterial blood-pressure and swelling of the veins of the heart. Paralysis of this centre causes relaxation and dilatation of all the arteries, resulting in an enormous fall of the blood pressure.[1]

The sympathetic nerves consist of two chains of ganglia, one on each side of the spinal cord. Their function is to stimulate the viscera, glands, heart, blood-vessels, and unstriped muscles of the body generally.

There are four small ganglia [2] connected with the fifth nerve. The ophthalmic, spheno-palatine, otic, and submaxillary. Each has three roots derived from motor, sensory, and sympathetic nerves respectively, and varying members of branches of distribution. These cells are multipolar, thus resembling the cells of sympathetic ganglia and differing from those of the ganglia of the posterior spinal nerve-roots and Gasserian ganglion.

Each ganglion is a reddish-gray color, soft in consistence but enclosed in a strong fibrous sheath. It is connected above and below by an ascending and a descending trunk, and with at least one spinal nerve by one or two communicating branches. Each ganglion distributes different branches, which either directly or through the intervention of a secondary plexus supply blood-vessels.

The second or superior maxillary division of the fifth pair of nerves gives off the posterior superior, middle superior, and anterior superior dental nerves. These three nerves form a plexus and loops of filament which pass to the tips of the roots to form the dental pulp. The third division of the fifth, the inferior maxillary, a mixed sensory and motor nerve, enters the inferior dental canal, passing forward towards the symphysis menti, supplying branches to the teeth and gums.

The Gasserian ganglion received filaments from the carotid plexus of the sympathetic. Connected with the fifth are the four small ganglia already mentioned, which form the whole of the cephalic portion of the sympathetic. With the first division is

---

[1] Landois and Stirling, Human Physiology.
[2] Gerrish Anatomy.

connected the ophthalmic ganglion, with the second, the sub-maxillary ganglion. All the four receive sensitive filaments from the fifth, motor and sympathetic filaments from various sources. The ganglia are also connected with each other and the cervical portion of the sympathetic.

According to the "American Text-Book of Physiology," the vasomotor apparatus consists of three classes of nerve-cells.[1] The cell bodies of the first class lie in sympathetic ganglia, their neuraxons passing directly to the smooth muscles in the wall of the vessels; the second are situated at different levels in the cerebro-spinal axis, their neuraxons passing thence to the sympathetic ganglia by way of the spinal and cranial nerves; the third are placed in the bulb and control the second through interspinal and intercranial paths. The nerve-cells of the first class lie wholly without the cerebrospinal axis, the third wholly within, while the second is partly within, partly without, and binds the remaining two together.

The vasomotor fibres for the face and mouth have been found in the cervical sympathetic by Dastre and Morat, leaving the cord [2] in the second and fifth dental nerves and uniting (at least for the most part) with the trigeminus by passing, according to Morat,[3] from the superior cervical sympathetic ganglion to the ganglion of Gasser, and thence to the fifth nerve. The nerves of the cerebrospinal system, with the exception of the olfactory, are medullated nerves.

The vasomotor nerves are axis cylinder processes of the sympathetic ganglion cells. They follow for a time the course of the corresponding spinal nerves. Intermingled with the medullated fibres are always found gray or non-medullated fibres. According to Shäfer,[4] these fibres frequently branch; the medullated fibres rarely do, except near their termination. The sympathetic nerves are largely made up of these fibres as they approach their peripheral distribution, and possess a thin medullary sheath.

From what has been said it will be seen that the intimate rela-

---

[1] By "nerve-cells" is meant the cell body with all its processes,—namely the neuraxons, or axis cylinder processes, and dentrites, or protoplasma processes.

[2] Dastre and Morat, 1884, pp. 116, 120.

[3] Morat, 1889, p. 201.

[4] Essentials of Histology, p. 118.

tion of the fifth nerve is a motor nerve in mastication and a sensory nerve to the great surface, both external and internal, which belongs to the face and the anterior part of the cranium. From the great size and the large portion of the medulla with which it is connected, there can be no question but that its sympathetic and vasomotor connection is established.

The nerve-trunks as they pass through the lower jaw are made up of nerve-fibres gathered together into bundles or funiculi, held together by connective tissue and called the perineurium. The connective tissue which unites a number of the bundles of funiculi is called epineurium. The cut ends under the microscope resemble very much the end of an ocean cable, the wires representing the nerve-fibre, and the rubber covering the connective tissue sheath.

From this nerve-trunk, smaller medullated nerve-fibres are given off at the nodes of Ranvier, which pass up and into the apical foramina of the roots of the teeth. Sometimes there are two and again three or ten to twenty-five nerve-fibres entering the foramina. The number depends upon the size of the opening. In my paper last year on " The Evolution of the Pulp," I demonstrated that in animals whose teeth were in continuous eruption during life, the pulp was larger at the opening than in the pulp-chamber. In ascending to man, the second teeth have small openings, especially later in life. In the very nature of things, as the root calcifies, especially in exostosis, the openings grow smaller. The number of nerves entering the foramina, then, will depend upon the size of the apical opening.

In a general way the motor, sensory, and the sympathetic nerves have been traced from their source to the roots of the upper and lower teeth. Text-books demonstrate the peripheral end organs to other structures of the body. In no case (to my knowledge) has the character of the nerves of the pulp been demonstrated.

At the meeting of this Section last year, Dr. Vida A. Latham, in a paper entitled " Résumé of the Histology of the Dental Pulp," showed the nerve supply to the pulp in different forms and also one illustration of the vasomotor system of the pulp. Part of our special work in the laboratory this year has been to demonstrate the character of the nerves of the pulp.

Pulp study has been conducted by Dr. Latham and myself in different laboratories for the past four years. For this work, teeth

FIG. 1.

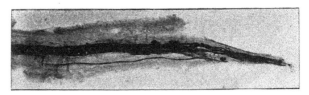

Nerve-fibres torn from main nerve-trunk and entering the canal through the apical foramen. × 50.

FIG. 2.

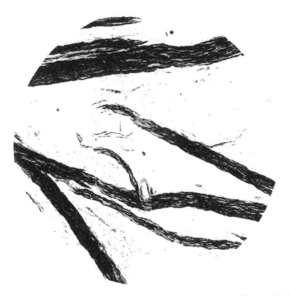

Bundles of nerves in the pulp showing vasomotor system. Nerve-fibres encircling an artery, showing terminals. 50.

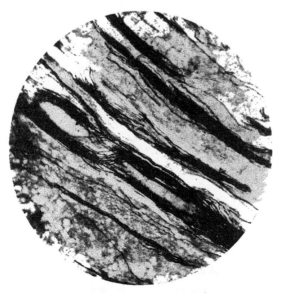

Bundles of nerves in the pulp showing the vasomotor system. Crossing of nerve-fibres m one bundle to another. These extend along and around blood-vessels. Degeneration sue at lower border.   ⸝ 50.

FIG. 4.

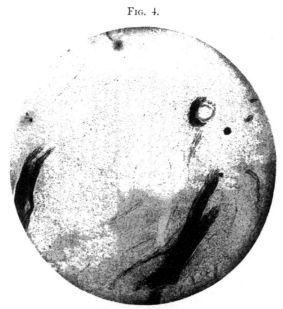

undles of nerves in pulp showing vasomotor system. Nerves around a cross-cut artery.
V-shaped artery in centre showing terminals   ⸝⸝ 50

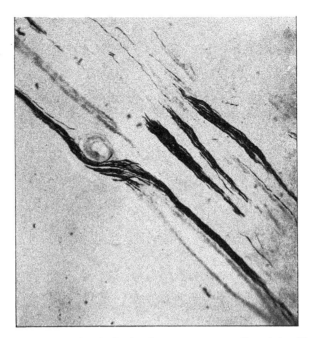

Bundles of nerves in the pulp showing the vasomotor system. Five arteries with nerve-res running lengthwise, also cross and long section of artery with nerve-fibre around it. hic ening of arterial walls, showing terminal nerve-fibres. 50.

Fig. 6.

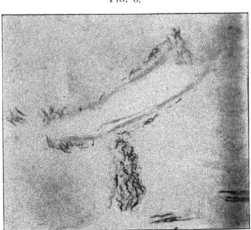

Bundles of nerves in pulp showing vasomotor system. Nerves extending along the arterial wall. At right angles may be seen the muscular coat of an artery filled with terminal nerve fibres. × 60.

FIG. 7.

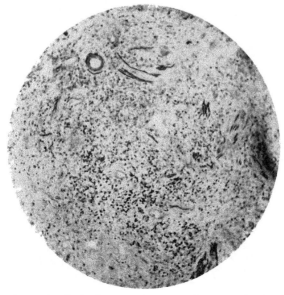

Bundles of nerves in pulp showing vasomotor system. Cross-cut section showing ends of nerve-fibres, also nerve encircling cross-cut artery. × 25.

FIG. 8.

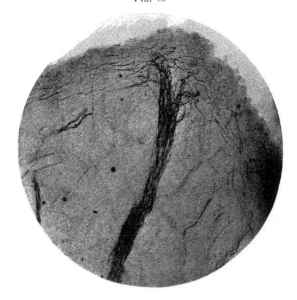

have been collected to the number of over four thousand. These have been cracked open and over two thousand specimens of pulps have been placed in different fluids ready for cutting, staining, and mounting for the microscope. All the different methods of preparation of nerve-tissue have been used as reported by Dr. Anderson in a paper entitled " Notes on Pulp Technique."

The nerve-fibres, after leaving the main trunk in the jaw, evidently enter the apical foramina in single nerve bundles. In many cases these nerve bundles continue the entire length of the pulp without branching. On the other hand, the branching in many cases begins after the trunk nerves have passed through the apical foramina. In Fig. 1, when the tooth was extracted the pulp protruded from the end of the root, the opening being quite large. In this illustration the nerve-fibres are shown from the inferior dental nerve extending through the apical foramina in the root-canal of the tooth. These seem to run in a bundle or funiculi, with the exception of one fibre, which is isolated at the root. Fig. 2 shows bundles of nerve-fibres loosely arranged running in different directions. Between these bundles may be seen many single nerve-fibres running in all directions. In the centre of the field is an artery cut crosswise with terminal fibres encircling it two-thirds around. Fig. 3 beautifully illustrates the vasomotor nerves in their relation to the blood-vessels. The blood-vessels and nerves run in the same direction. In the centre of the field may be seen four arteries. Nerve-fibres are notably running the entire length between, but they cross and recross at different localities. Nerve-fibres in bundles and singly cover the entire field. Fig. 4 shows bundles of fibres, with many single fibres throughout the field. In the centre may be seen an artery cut lengthwise branching in two directions. The most interesting of all, however, is an artery cut crosswise with vasomotor terminal nerves encircling it. Fig. 5 demonstrates the vasomotor system more thoroughly. In the centre of the field may be seen nine arteries cut lengthwise and one cut crosswise. Bundles of nerve-fibres run between the arteries and along the arterial walls. Nerve-fibres are seen crossing and recrossing the arterial walls, sometimes in bundles and again in single terminal fibres. In the cross-cut artery a nerve-fibre may be seen almost encircling it. Fig. 6 shows an enlarged artery cut lengthwise, while just below it may be seen an artery running towards it at right angles. In this artery only the outer surface

is seen. In both arterial coats terminal nerve-fibres are well
shown. Fig. 7 shows the ends of the nerve cut crosswise. An
artery may also be seen with a nerve encircling it. Fig. 8 illustrates the crown end of the pulp with a bundle of nerve-fibres
which have extended intact the entire length of the pulp and is
distributing its fibres throughout the odontoblastic layer.

In consideration that the blood-vessels and nerves pass through
the pulp in a wavy direction and not in straight lines, to have
been able to obtain so many beautiful specimens showing so clearly
and distinctly the vasomotor system is fortunate.

I am obliged to Dr. Ludwig Hektoen for verifying these illustrations, and to Dr. Martha Anderson for valuable services.

THE RELATION OF THE CHEMISTRY OF THE SALIVA (SIALO-SEMEIOLOGY) AND NASAL SECRETIONS TO DISEASES OF THE MUCOUS MEMBRANE OF THE MOUTH AND UPPER RESPIRATORY TRACT.[1]

BY D. BRADEN KYLE, M.D., PHILADELPHIA.

MR. PRESIDENT AND GENTLEMEN OF THE INSTITUTE OF STOMA-
TOLOGY,—I know of no subject in which the dental and medical
profession should be more intimately interested than the one of
sialo-semeiology. That the various chemic compounds introduced
into or secreted within the mouth have a direct action on the teeth
and adjacent structures cannot be doubted. If, then, a secretion
has been perverted from the normal, and in this perversion there
is eliminated or precipitated some irritating material, such material will not only have a deleterious effect on the teeth, but when
taken back into the system will in turn produce some pathologic
alteration in other structures.

In the chemic study of the nasal and salivary secretions we may
conveniently classify them under three varieties: First, secretions
—non-irritating *per se*—which on exposure (when coming to the
surface) undergo some chemic change producing an irritant; this
may be noted in either an acid or alkaline secretion. As I will

---

[1] Read before The New York Institute of Stomatology, November 6, 1903.

show later, an exceedingly alkaline secretion is decidedly more irritating and productive of a more destructive pathologic process than even a strongly acid secretion. Second, secretions which are irritating *per se* when poured out on the surface. Third, secretions which come to the surface in a non-irritating form, but on coming in contact with extraneous material are rendered irritant. While my observations have been more from a medical stand-point, yet many of the principles involved are applicable in many pathologic lesions as observed by the dental profession.

Two great principles which have been satisfactorily demonstrated are these: In highly alkaline conditions there is an exaggerated oxidation process and the chemic change takes place in the secretion after it is poured out. This is of the greatest importance in nasal, laryngeal, and pharyngeal lesions, and is also of immense significance in pathologic changes in the gums and about the teeth, as highly alkaline secretions will cause necrosis more quickly than an acid secretion. In highly acid conditions the oxidation process is incomplete, hence there is a greater tendency to a precipitation of material within the tissue, with the necessary pathologic alteration—an infiltration process. This as applied to the teeth would produce a class of diseases in which the structure of the tooth is altered through faulty nutrition with a tendency to infiltration, or, in other words, the alkaline condition would produce external alterations going from without in, while the acid condition would produce lesions within with a tendency to come to the surface.

Any one familiar with laboratory investigations involving organic chemistry will appreciate the many hours spent over chemic formulæ and analyses in which the results are negative, through faulty lines of investigation, due to the fact that we are dealing with organic chemistry and searching for unknown quantities. I have purposely omitted from this paper the tedious laboratory details and chemic formulæ, dealing entirely with the practical side of the subject, and I hope at some future date to publish the laboratory formulæ to be used in obtaining reactions of certain pathologic materials which I have found present.

Being so impressed with the import of the study of not only the excretions from the intestines and kidneys, but also of the saliva and various secreting glands, I devoted a number of lectures to this subject during my course on pathology in the Jefferson Medical

College, 1895–96, since carrying on, as time would permit, investigations in this line in my own private laboratory.

Michaels, of Paris, in his admirable paper read before the International Dental Congress, August 9, 1900, was the first, I believe, to call attention to this subject, not in medicine, but in its relation to dentistry; also, Kirk, of Philadelphia, has taken up the investigation.

Naturally, it was necessary to investigate the histo-chemistry of normal saliva, concerning which subject the literature is very meagre. The saliva is the mixed secretion of the parotid, submaxillary, and sublingual glands and the small mucous glands of the mouth. Physiologically, three kinds of secretion may be distinguished,—a serous from the parotid, a mucous from the mucous glands, and a mixed secretion from the submaxillary and sublingual glands. Mixed saliva is opalescent, tasteless, generally alkaline, and has a specific gravity of 1004 to 1009. Saliva contains serum albumin, globulin, mucin, urea, an amylolytic ferment called ptyalin, and a proteolytic and lipolytic ferment; also salts, the most important of which is the ammonium and potassium and the sulphocyanide combinations derived especially from the parotid gland. The proteolytic and lipolytic ferments are not important. It is possible that any other fermentation save the amylolytic is due to bacteria. The amylolytic ferment is most important. The irritating materials produced by this ferment are most significant in causing dental lesions.

The ammonium salts and sulphocyanide in healthy saliva are in equal proportion and in very small quantities; in the hypoacid condition the ammonium salt exists in greater quantities than the sulphocyanide, and tends to rapid decomposition. In the hyperacid condition the sulphocyanide is in excess, and the tendency to decomposition is not so great as in the hypoacid condition until exposed to moisture or air; in other words, after secretion has taken place and chemic action has caused alteration of the compound.

In hyperacid conditions the sulphocyanides are in greater proportion than the ammonium salts, and the secretion is less irritating; while in the hypoacid state the ammonium salts are in excess of the sulphocyanides and the secretion is decidedly irritating, and in many cases in which I have been able to examine the secretions, especially of hay-fever patients, this hypoacid condition has existed.

My studies of the saliva have been very much in the same chemic line as Michaels's. First, the study of the normal healthy saliva; second, the saliva from hypoacid individuals; third, the hyperacid condition. To this I have added the neutral or irregular cases, which are neither normal, hyperacid, or hypoacid.

From my investigations I found that the reaction of the salivary secretions as given by the ordinary litmus test was often faulty and misleading, that owing to chemic changes which had taken place after the secretion is poured out on the surface of the membrane the reaction of the secretion changed. This was of the greatest import from the stand-point of treatment, as the reaction might show precisely the opposite as existed in the secretion as it came from the gland proper.

The condition of normal, hypoacid, and hyperacid conditions can best be illustrated by cases.

(1) Strongly alkaline conditions. The following case illustrates this condition. Dr. B., who had been suffering from an irritating rasping cough since September, 1902, was referred to me in January for an examination of his throat. The symptoms presented were principally the cough, with hyperæmic and irritated mucous membranes, though the congestion and swelling were not in proportion to the severity of the cough. The cough was persistently spasmodic, resembling almost paroxysms of whooping-cough, except more often repeated. There was decided hoarseness and congestion of the vocal cords. The chest examination was negative, with the exception of slight bronchial râles. Here and there on the mucous membrane were small hemorrhagic spots, which I believe had been produced by the violent irritation caused by the spasmodic cough.

In so many cases in which the objective symptoms were in excess of that which the local lesion would justify, I have found that the irritation was brought about by some altered chemistry of the secretion, and that the local lesion was merely a manifestation and result of this alteration. Thus, on examination of his saliva it was found to be hypoacid, the ammonium salts being in excess, and when the secretion came to the surface there was liberated free ammonia gas, which was in sufficient quantity to produce the irritation. On this basis the treatment was administered, all the organs of elimination were stimulated, and the chemistry of the secretion was changed to acid or neutral reaction, following which change the cough disappeared within a few days and the irritation rapidly subsided, and in ten days all inflammation had disappeared with the exception of some slight localized areas, which probably had been brought about by the persistent coughing, and these areas rapidly yielded to local treatment.

To review the chemistry, ammonium is a hypothetical alkaline base, having the composition of NH_4; it does occur in a free state, however, in the form of ammonia gas, NH_3, the inhalation of which is very irritating to the mucous membrane and causes suffocation and œdema of the glottis. As the ammonium salts usually exist in combination with other materials, is it not likely, in certain conditions in which the secretions are hypoacid, that when the secretion comes to the surface of the mucous membrane, owing to its chemic combination with oxygen, there is liberated NH_3, the irritating ammonia gas; surely the symptoms in many cases justify this conclusion, and the chemic study of the secretions supports this view.

Some cases of hay-fever further illustrate this point. The numerous theories as to the etiologic factor in this disease proves conclusively that as yet there has not been established a definite cause. It may be that different conditions act as etiologic factors; in fact, it is my belief that not all cases which we call hay-fever, or hyperæsthetic rhinitis, are due to any one cause; or, if to any one factor, that factor must be in the altered chemistry of the secretions of the individual. In fact, I am persuaded, after making a series of examinations of the saliva in certain individuals afflicted with hay-fever and those not so afflicted, that in some cases the causes, direct or indirect, of local irritation in the nasal mucous membrane are brought about by some chemic change in the constituents of the secretions of the mucus-secreting glands, and that in such cases the reaction of the secretion is strongly alkaline. Treatment based on this view was certainly most effective. Sensitive areas within the nasal cavities, or irregularities in formation of the cavities themselves, are factors in some cases, yet such areas or irregularities, instead of being etiologic, are merely auxiliary factors, which render the individual more susceptible to the irritant from within.

(2) The cases in which the secretions are hyperacid. The following case is an illustration: Mr. C., aged forty-two, consulted me in regard to what he supposed to be a catarrhal condition asso-

ciated with ozena. His breath was surely most offensive, but, although pronouncedly so, it was not the penetrating, clinging odor observed in atrophic rhinitis with ozena. He had observed the condition rather suddenly, and it had existed continuously for some four or five years. His history was absolutely negative as to any catarrhal condition other than an occasional cold. He had consulted specialists both in this country and abroad, not only as to the possibility of the odor coming from the nose or some of the accessory cavities, but had also consulted specialists on diseases of the stomach, as well as having had a thorough inspection of all his teeth. He had been told that he had practically no catarrh, and as his digestion was good and nothing found wrong by analysis of the contents of the stomach, it was quite puzzling as to the source of this odor. After a thorough examination, and knowing that the men under whose care he had been were most thorough and competent in their line, I reasoned that there must be some source of the disagreeable odor outside of the parts already mentioned. As this was in the winter of 1895, and as my attention had been called to the import of the secretions by other conditions, as well as a statement made to me by the patient, I decided to investigate the saliva. The statement which he made to me, which was most significant, was this: That while his appetite was very good, and when his olfactory nerve was stimulated by the odor of a delicious meal, causing his mouth to water, the disagreeable odor and taste became so pronounced as to almost nauseate him. I collected then some of the saliva. The method I used for its collection I learned from my experience in a dentist's chair: that while sitting with your mouth wide open for a few minutes you have a most profuse flow of saliva. This method, practised just before meal-time, enabled the collection of quite a large amount of the secretion. The offensiveness of the secretion was at once detected.

In order to explain the chemic source of the offensive odor it is necessary to take up the chemistry of the sulphocyanides. As to the sulphocyanides which are present in the saliva, it is a chemic fact that most of the cyanides are actively poisonous and that a cyanide is formed or is a compound of cyanogen with a metal or radical. A sulphocyanide is a salt in which the sulphur takes the place of oxygen in the acid radical. Cyanogen is a radical molecule having the structure CN, an acid compound of carbon and nitrogen. A radical is a group of atoms having unsatisfied valency, an unsatisfied molecule which goes into or out of combination without change to itself and which determines the character of compounds. A sulphocyanide is a combination, then, denoting the chemic combination of sulphur with a radical. When a sulphocyanide is eliminated the secretion in which the ammonium salts are in excess is alkaline, but when it comes in contact with the air, owing to the chemic change which takes place, it becomes an acid radical.. Hence in many instances in which from our test we believe the secretion to be acid, it is really hypoacid (alkaline). This is most important, and in many instances in which from the test reaction we are led to conclude the reaction to be acid, it is in reality in the system an alkaline reaction, and only becomes acid when, owing to chemic action due to exposure to air, certain materials are eliminated and the reaction changed. In some of the sulphocyanide combinations in which we get the bad odor, as illustrated in the above case, the chemic change causing such odor is as follows: Sulphur itself is an acid element, which unites with oxygen to form an acid radical, but in a sulpho-salt the sulphur takes the place of the oxygen in the acid radical. The sulphocyanide itself would be a sulpho-salt in which, in combination, the sulphur would take the place of the oxygen and give off sulphuretted hydrogen. In a sulpho-salt the sulphur takes the place of the oxygen in combination to form an acid. A sulphocyanide is a sulpho-salt, and when the sulphocyanide is in excess, when liberated and coming in contact with the secretion which contains moisture (H_2O), the sulphur would unite with the hydrogen, giving off free oxygen, and form hydrogen sulphide. A radical is a group of atoms having an unsatisfied valency, and is really unsatisfied molecules which go into or out of combination. It is possible, then, to have in a hyperacid condition many chemic combinations take place. This chemic result surely verified the olfactory diagnosis in this case.

(3) The cases neither hypoacid nor hyperacid. That cell nutrition depends upon the chemistry of its supply is illustrated in disease processes associated with any form of infection or rise of temperature. This opens up an enormous field for speculation and investigation. The amount of infection, the peculiar chemic change produced by temperature, the materials absorbed into the body from infective processes, or the autoinfection from the intestinal tract, would in each condition produce its own peculiar chemic compound. Yet I believe a general basis or standard can be reached,

at least sufficiently accurate, from which to draw chemic and clinical deductions. For example, of peculiar effect on various structures in the body, brought about by an altered chemistry, in which the secretions may be neutral or irregular, I will quote from an article which was published in *American Medicine,* February 8, 1902, in which I reported a number of cases of enlargement of the thyroid gland in which the cellular elements of the thyroid structure were increased, the enlargement not being due to distended vessels, cystic condition of the gland, or new growth. I reasoned the matter out as follows: It is a well-known physiologic and therapeutic fact that certain drugs have a selective action on certain tissues or organs of the body; *e.g.,* belladonna, with its selective action on the pharyngeal surface; sodium phosphate, with its selective action on the liver, etc. It is also a physiologic fact that the normal chemistry of the body controls the normal secretions from the various secretory·organs, that any perversion from the normal necessarily alters the character and chemistry of the secretion, and that the products of such alteration act as irritants to certain parts of the body; the difference between this and drugs administered is that one is introduced into the body and one is manufactured within the body. I therefore reasoned that under certain conditions there is precipitated—due to perverted chemic reaction—a certain material which, circulating through the blood, had a selective action on certain tissues; in the cases observed such selective action occurred in the thyroid gland, acting as an irritant to that gland. While the treatment of these cases reported was somewhat theoretical, I believe, however, that the drug introduced into the body, by its chemic action, altered the chemistry of the material which was acting as an irritant, either rendering that irritating material inert or forming a compound which was non-irritating.

In regard to the pathologic chemic process producing such reactions of the secretion, it is a well-known clinical and laboratory fact that a study of the products of the secreting organs, which in their excretory functions throw off waste material, gives us by deduction a fair idea of what process is going on within the body. Yet this excretory secretion or material is altered in its chemic composition and controlled by the chemic constituents within the body proper.

There is no question that under certain conditions,—for example, when the secretions are acid or alkaline,—the chemic process taking place within the various secretory glands must vary, and the product of such variation in these unknown quantities must be somewhat the same as the variations we would obtain in dealing in the laboratory with known compounds. In other words, that the body is largely a chemic laboratory, having on hand a certain amount of material and having added to it daily ingredients through the respiratory and alimentary tract. Now, any perverted condition from what is known as the normal chemistry may bring about a series of changes and produce chemic products which may be harmless or productive of disease processes. On no other basis can we explain the various diatheses and the precipitation of certain materials in the tissues of the body.

The altered chemistry of the saliva presents many possibilities from an etiologic stand-point. Many forms of lesions of the mucous membrane of the nose, nasopharynx, larynx, mouth, and gums, as well as diseases of the stomach and intestines, may be brought about by the altered chemistry of the saliva. A great many morbid processes are traced to uric acid in some of its many forms, but I believe that many other substances, especially in hyperacid conditions, equally important are deposited and eliminated, which substances act as irritants, producing apparent local lesions. It is a well-known clinical fact that saliva from certain individuals is exceedingly poisonous, as is indicated by the infectious wounds produced by the bite of such individuals, showing that the saliva may be the site of poisonous pathologic, as well as physiologic, compounds.

Unquestionably the chemic reaction of the secretions of the body is an important factor in the susceptibility of individuals to disease. I think there is no doubt that the fact that at one time the individual resists disease and at another time succumbs can be largely explained on this basis. To be sure, it is a question of resistance on the part of the individual, but that resistance is largely controlled by the chemistry of the cell or secretion. It also demonstrates the fact of the accumulative phenomena of certain of the diseases, as is illustrated in uric acid diathesis, which Haig has described as uric acid storm. There is no reason why these same phenomena could not occur as the result of the accumulation of other materials brought about by chemic changes which lessen oxidation and tend to precipitation and accumulation of various morbid products.

The administration of drugs for the relief of, for example, an infective process probably affects such a process beneficially, owing to the fact that in its action it changes the chemistry of the secretions and blood constituents, thereby producing a chemic compound which either prevents the formation of infectious material or alters the nidus of infection to such an extent that it is not suitable for the growth of bacteria.

While my investigations are incomplete and fragmentary, I am convinced that from the study of the saliva we can determine to a great extent any variation in the chemistry of the body. As these various secreting glands receive from the blood the supply from which they elaborate certain chemic compounds, if an analysis were made of the composition of such secretion it would give a good index to the general condition of the individual, and while in many cases the deductions have to be based on, or rather associated with, clinical observation, I soon found them to be of immense value from a stand-point of diagnosis.

The fact that the reaction of the secretion may be apparently acid when there really is present an alkaline condition explains to us many of the cases in which from an acid basis our treatment has failed. That such a condition may exist has been shown by Douin and Gautrelet in their studies of the blood; that the reaction of the plasma is really acid, and if waste products are not eliminated this acidity is increased. The secretions and excretions then also become of an acid reaction.

The irritating gases which form in the stomach and intestines and produce laryngeal and pharyngeal irritation are the result of chemic changes in the intestinal secretion, and such chemic change in the secretion can be demonstrated by a study of the saliva. That autoinfections and chemic changes in intestinal secretions have a marked general effect on the individual is well known. Such material absorbed into the system will unquestionably alter the chemistry of all the secreting glands, and the compounds formed by such alteration which affect the individual can only be determined by the study of organic chemistry. The asthmatic conditions which are not associated with any organic lesion I believe can all be explained on this basis, and when treated accordingly can in many instances be relieved.

In examining the secretion and excretion of the body, we can obtain as good an index of the systemic condition of the individual

by a study of the saliva as by a study of the urine; in the urine
we have only an index of the waste material, while in the saliva
we have products of elimination which return into the body to
perform a physiologic process. Another important factor to be
worked out is the different chemic changes which take place in
individuals suffering with the so-called functional diseases and those
suffering from organic or structural changes. In the functional
we have a perverted chemistry, which may be brought about by
many causes, such as faulty elimination from the kidneys or liver,
and perversion of secretion from the intestinal tract, autoinfection
from the intestinal tract; also chemic changes of the secretion
illustrated in mental tension, from fright, worry, and anger; while
in the organic lesions we have to deal with a structural change in
tissues with retrograde metabolic changes, in which there is also
associated inflammatory processes with their accompanying phenomena and physiologic and pathologic effect on the individual.

What deductions can be made from the stand-point of the dentist? What effect does the hypoacid condition have on the teeth
and alveolar processes? How does it differ from the hyperacid
secretions? My own observations have shown that in many cases
with highly alkaline secretion there has been irritation of the gums,
in some cases amounting to a spongy condition, and in not a few
cases pyorrhœa alveolaris, with a tendency to decomposition around
the teeth; while in the acid condition the alterations occurred
more as a direct lesion of the tooth or nerve, the process beginning
from within. This confirms the observations as to the oxidation
process. Are these changes due to the altered chemical conditions
or to some other cause? I leave it to you, gentlemen, to make the
deduction, and, if you find any suggestion worthy of consideration,
to apply the same to the pathologic processes occurring within the
field of dentistry.

A SUSPENSION PARTIAL DENTURE.[1]

BY DR. P. B. M'CULLOUGH, PHILADELPHIA.

THE artificial substitution of the two upper bicuspids of either side in a fixed denture, supported by a crown or other device upon a first molar, with the artificial teeth resting upon and forming a water-tight joint with the gum.

The striking natural adaptability of the soft tissues to artificial dental appliances, together with the astonishing tolerance of even abusive measures in the mouth, offers pregnant suggestion of the possibilities in taking righteous advantage.

The natural toughness of the gums, the severe use which they will stand after the loss of the teeth and, as Gray says, of the mucous membrane covering—" remarkable for its limited sensibility"—are physical reasons that make the wearing of artificial dentures possible.

If inflammation without the presence of pathological bacteria is impossible, then it is a reasonable inference that the application of a foreign body to a studied limited surface of gum tissue, with the related surfaces sterile at the time contact is made, with the adaptation so perfect as to form a water-tight joint, that the joint so effected will be a mechanical dam against infection, and that the surfaces so united will remain surgically clean as long as the dam remains complete.

In contemplating the practical application of a method the success of which depends so much upon cleanliness, only such means as will insure absolute accuracy in every detail of the mechanical work is to be entertained.

To this end therefore, to parallel the walls of the first molar, to envelop it with a gold crown, and form an accurate joint below the free margin of the gum is, with the devices at present known, a practical impossibility.

When the case presenting is one where the first molar is without decay, with a stone a cavity is made in the mesial surface with parallel walls and involving the occlusal surface, it is extended on the latter surface with a narrow stone cutting in a straight line

---

[1] Read before the Academy of Stomatology, Philadelphia, October 27, 1903.

distally and terminating in the ridge which connects the disto-buccal and the mesio-palatal cusps, into which it is dovetailed lat-erally. The cavity must be of sufficient depth and the walls diverge slightly from the floor. In the cavity thus formed is adapted platina-foil, forming a matrix after the methods in vogue for por-celain work.

After the matrix has been formed, a thin coating of 22-karat gold is melted in and again adapted to the cavity, and repeated after each melting until it no longer yields to burnishing, the walls being first built up, then the middle.

If borax should accumulate to such an extent as to interfere with the work, it should be dissolved by boiling in dilute hydro-chloric acid in a test-tube. If, by chance, the gold should flow to the under surface of the matrix, the gold within should be covered with wax and the plug immersed in nitrohydrochloric acid until clean.

With the finished plug in place, a plaster impression is taken that will include the molar and at least the cuspid tooth, when it is not necessary to take the occlusion or bite. The method of attaching the porcelain teeth is the same as hereafter provided for the gold crown.

When the first molar is in such a condition as to suggest any doubt as to the pulp remaining vital any considerable time, it should be devitalized and the entire crown removed, and if pulp-less, the crown should be likewise ground off below the free margin of the gum.

The only crown deemed fit for this character of work is the one published in the transactions of the Academy under the name of the " Burnished-Cap-Crown." [1] The only change made since then is in the use of formaldehyde as a separating medium for the cement instead of the mixture then recommended. The impres-sion is immersed for five minutes in the solution.

By virtue of the typical platina cap in this crown, when fin-ished, it is possible to line the inner edge of the cap with temporary stopping and by pressing it to place while soft the impression of the root in the stopping will show the operator the direction in which the crown must be pressed to insure its fitting the root exactly as designed. It is particularly necessary to observe this precaution

---

[1] INTERNATIONAL DENTAL JOURNAL, August, 1902.

when the crown presses against the second molar, which it should when the relation is normal.

Preparatory to taking the impression, the crown is filled to the inner edge of the cap with plaster, and the pulp-cavity with temporary stopping, when the crown is set with a quick-setting brittle cement and held under pressure until the cement crystallizes.

As it is the purpose in this operation to reproduce the natural lines of the bicuspids, and as the artificial teeth should not be ground before soldering, except as hereafter provided, it is often sufficient to have only as a guide in fixing the length and angle of the teeth a model that will include the crown and cuspid tooth. It is well, however, that it include also the lateral and second molar. When it is deemed advisable to have a model of the occluding teeth, it is necessary to take full impression of the teeth of both jaws, as partial models cannot be accurately articulated. Before the plaster impression is filled any cement adhering to the crown should be cleaned off.

Of the teeth at present manufactured, only the Ash tube-teeth can be used for this denture. They are ground to fit the model with their buccal surfaces parallel with the crown and the plaster cuspid, and one-sixteenth of an inch longer than what it is designed their fixed length shall be. In this position, with a narrow knife-blade, a line is marked on the plaster around each tooth, then the teeth are removed, and with a suitable instrument the plaster is cut away inside of these guide-lines to the depth of one-sixteenth of an inch, forming depressions in which the teeth should fit.

The teeth are then placed in position, having care that there be space between their approximal surfaces equal to double the thickness of a postal-card, and that the same space be between the second bicuspid and the crown. The spacing is to provide for the contraction of solder. With the teeth so held they are waxed together by coating their palatal and buccal surfaces freely with hard wax, having care to avoid the plaster model.

When the wax has become hard the teeth are taken from the model and, with a square-edge corundum stone in the engine a little thicker than the diameter of the tubes, a groove is cut between the cusps from the mesial surface of the first bicuspid to the distal surface of the second, and involving these two surfaces, with the sides and bottom of the groove forming straight lines. This groove should be of a depth not less than the sixteenth of an inch at its shallowest points. (Fig. 1.)

The teeth are then returned to the model, the sides of the groove marked on the occlusal surface of the gold crown, the teeth removed, and a groove cut in the crown extending distally over its occlusal surface at least one-eighth of an inch, replacing the teeth as required to insure the edge of the groove being continuous with the groove in the teeth.

A piece of half-round clasp gold wire heavy enough to fit the groove loosely is cut long enough to extend its entire length and into the gold crown, then, with the teeth free from the model the bar is held in the groove and the position of the tubes marked on the bar by passing through the tubes a steel pin with a flat sharp edge. Holes are then drilled in the bar at the points marked.

Two pieces of round clasp gold wire, long enough to extend beyond each end of the tubes and of a diameter that will fill them loosely, are placed in the tubes and through the holes in the bar; in this position they are hard waxed to the latter, removed, invested, and soldered with 18-karat solder. (Fig. 2.)

With the teeth on the model the bar is pressed to place to mark in the plaster the points where the posts extend beyond the tubes, then the teeth are removed and holes drilled at the points marked. Extending the posts beyond the tubes is designed to draw the solder.

The teeth are then cleaned with boiling water, and, with the bar and posts in place, returned to the model and firmly tacked to the latter by applying hard wax only to the palatal and lingual surfaces of the teeth.

When the wax has become hard the bar is removed and crown metal, two one-thousandths of an inch, with the gold surface next the porcelain, is thoroughly adapted to the groove with wet spunk and orange-wood sticks, frequently annealing.

The metal must be large enough to extend beyond the mesial surface of the first bicuspid one-eighth of an inch, where the plaster cuspid is cut away, and above the occlusal surface one-fourth of an inch, and into the groove in the crown one-sixteenth of an inch. After the metal has been perfectly adapted, with the pencil-point of an orange-wood stick it is burnished over each tube until punctured, then with pressure and a turn of the stick the extended edges of the punctured holes are burnished to the inner surfaces of the tubes. Thus the porcelain is protected. Before the metal is fixed

FIG. 1.

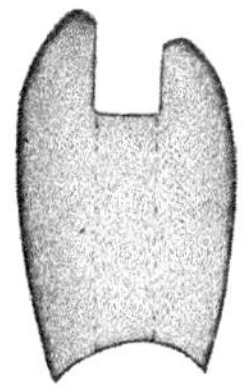

FIG. 2 (upper).

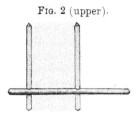

FIG. 3 (upper).

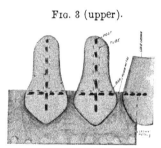

FIG. 4.

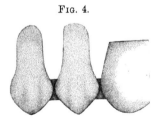

FIG. 5.

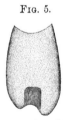

Showing mesial surface of first bicuspid.

in place holes are punched along the two edges extending above the teeth, which, when filled with the investing material, will keep the metal from warping.

The bar with posts is then dropped in place to see that the position of the teeth has not changed during the burnishing, then removed, and a small quantity of hard wax placed in the metal groove, the bar heated and dropped in place to carry the wax through the tubes, then hard wax is added until the metal matrix is nearly filled and the bar thoroughly waxed to the crown. (Fig. 3.)

After the wax has become hard the wax holding the teeth to the model is carefully cut away, the crown pried off, with the teeth attached, and invested.

When the investment is set the wax is cleaned off by " pouring" boiling water, then a drop or two of borax finely ground in water is carried with a stick to the tubes and around the bar at the joint with the crown, then, piece at a time, the 16-karat solder is taken from the plate, each particle wet with borax, and applied until all the solder that will be required has been placed.

The case is then placed upon a charcoal bed so that the blow-pipe can be held to one side, directing the flame under the investment. The flame at no time should be directed on the metal before the solder melts. The heat, of course, must be increased gradually; it, however, should not take longer than from ten to fifteen minutes to solder. The practice of long drying out and heating up is not only unnecessary, but probably harmful.

The metal surface should be immediately covered with a piece of glowing charcoal and the case left undisturbed for from twenty to thirty minutes to cool, when, after removing investment, the case is placed in dilute hydrochloric acid in a test-tube and boiled; thus the borax is quickly removed, and, what is more important, the teeth are annealed.

The only care necessary to observe in finishing is that the metal be not cut too thin where it bridges the spaces between the teeth, and particularly at the crown, where the strain will be greatest. (Fig. 4.)

The ends of the posts extending beyond the tubes at the surface fitting the gum are ground down flush with the porcelain surface and the latter polished, finishing the edges with emery and cuttle-fish disks. (Fig. 5.)

While a pulp-cavity of retentive shape will be sufficient anchorage for any molar crown of the referred-to system, it is not enough when other teeth are supported; therefore dowels or pins must be placed in the three canals long enough to extend into the crown, and they should be made as described for the dowel crowns of this system.

They should be set with the same mix of cement that holds the crown, as, by this means, with the pressure the cement will be better packed around the pins.

Great pressure should be used to force the crown to place and maintained until the cement hardens, which, with some cements, requires from ten to twenty minutes.

Should the porcelain teeth press so hard upon the gums as to make it impossible to force the crown to place, then they should be ground off; care, however, must be observed that the surface is evenly ground and that the arc of the concavity fitting the gum is not changed.

It is well to oil the surfaces of the teeth fitting the gum, then any cement between the teeth and the gum can be removed by passing the end of a piece of binding wire through one interdental space and out the next, thus forming a loop which can be drawn over the top of the tooth.

In the same way a loop is made with linen or silk thread, then saturated from a cotton with formaldehyde, and pulled through between each tooth and the gum. Should the lower teeth " strike," the points of contact should be marked with articulating paper and the spots ground off the lower teeth; the cusps of the artificial teeth may be ground, but care should be observed that if the gold is cut it should not be at points that would weaken the denture.

It is designed that the extent of gum surface covered shall be equal to that displaced by the natural teeth; thus the area involved will be less in proportion to the degree of shrinkage.

OSTEOMYELITIS: A CASE IN PRACTICE.[1]

BY DR. H. B. HICKMAN, PHILADELPHIA.

THE case I wish to bring before you is that of a man, aged forty-three years, weighing one hundred and sixty pounds, five feet six inches tall, with no apparent evidence of any specific disease, although his mother died of some form of tuberculosis.

Up to within six months of the time when this second bicuspid started to give trouble, he was in fairly good health, being manager of a large business and with a superabundance of energy, although he had not taken a vacation for eighteen years.

His wife had been in bed with an incurable disease for over a year; he was needed abroad to attend to very important business, but his wife would not consent to his going away even for a short stay; and since his wife had been sick he had been forced to give up his only recreation, music. The strain at home and office, with no rest, began to manifest itself by his being very nervous, having lost appetite, being easily fatigued and anæmic.

I was able to watch the change in the condition of this man because he was a very intimate friend, and also because his teeth gave him a great deal of annoyance during this period; but he would not listen to advice as to rest, tonics, etc.

This brings us to the time he called at the office with the right lower second bicuspid very sore, aching, and slightly loose. I diagnosed pericementitis caused by a putrescent pulp. After chilling the tooth with chloride of ethyl spray, which relieved the pain, I opened through a small amalgam filling and found the pulp-chamber and canal filled with gutta-percha; then the patient remembered that it had been treated and filled ten or fifteen years before. After removing the root-canal filling I was able to pass a broach through the apical foramen, which opening gave only momentary relief.

I prescribed a laxative and anodyne, with the usual treatment for pericementitis, feeling sure he would be better the next morning.

On the day following he returned to the office. The tooth had ached continuously and he wished it extracted, which was very

---

[1] Read before the Academy of Stomatology, Philadelphia, October 27, 1903.

nicely done, under nitrous oxide gas, by a specialist, who cleansed the mouth with an antiseptic solution both before and after extracting. I examined the root and found it slightly exostosed. The socket was packed with phenol sodique and cotton.

The pain returned before he reached home, and his physician, who had been summoned, could not relieve him. His physician wished him to go to bed there and then, but he suffered so much more when lying down that he slept in a reclining-chair.

I saw him at his home the following day at noon, and found that a saturated solution of carbolic acid on cotton gave him relief for eight hours, when the pain returned with renewed force.

This condition continued for ten days, the socket being packed every eight hours with carbolic acid, at the same time using fifty per cent. phenol sodique as a mouth-wash.

Sulphate of zinc was tried in the socket with only partial relief.

By this time the patient was in bed with a temperature varying from 102° to 104°. The legs and body were covered with pustules resembling chicken-pox, which disease the physician led the family to believe he had.

At this time there was some swelling or puffiness of the gum tissue around the socket, which had not filled up very much. The temperature was about 103° to 104°. There were rigors alternating with flashes of heat, followed by copious sweats, which had rather a disagreeable odor. He had an exceedingly irritating cough, especially when he talked or became the least excited.

At the end of six weeks, a mere shadow of his former self, he died, having been delirious the greater part of the last five weeks.

According to one physician it was called general nervous collapse, but others thought it was septic meningitis that caused his death, superinduced by the osteomyelitis and the very low state of his health.

SUPPURATIVE CLEFT PALATES AND DEVICES FOR THE SAME.[1]

BY HENRY J. JANLUSZ, D.D.S., NEW YORK CITY.

MR. CHAIRMAN AND GENTLEMEN.—It gives me great pleasure to appear before you on this occasion, and I assure you that I most thoroughly appreciate the courtesy and honor conferred upon me by being invited to deliver an address before you. My anticipations were very great when I knew I was to attend this meeting, but the fruition far exceeds anything I could have imagined. It is always most pleasant to come in contact with those who are interested in my work, or those whom I may interest.

The subject I wish to discuss to-day is one that admits of a most comprehensive description, readily and easily understood, and while it is in the nature of an innovation, I am quite confident I can bring clearly before you my method of treating certain forms of cleft palate. My work in this direction, and I say it without any flattery to myself, fills what I consider a long-felt want. It is a decided digression from the regular line of dentistry, but one of which I have made a deep study and a specialty. In my work I have sought neither praise, honor, notoriety, nor distinction. I am free to confess I have been inoculated with a certain amount of self-conceit, and while I do not look upon myself in the light of a beatified good Samaritan, I do consider that I have brought joy and happiness into many a discouraged brother's life, and, my friends, you can do the same. I am sure there is not one present who would not be willing to put aside all sensitive feelings if he could be assured that by so doing he would better the condition of suffering humanity.

But will you pardon this digression? I can only plead in extenuation of the fault that I feel so enthused with my work I am always most anxious to interest others, and for this reason it is often difficult to me to refrain from being too verbose.

I have made a specialty for some considerable time of treating cases of cleft palate where they were the result of either hereditary or acquired syphilis, a phase of the work about which little has been

---

[1] Read before the Massachusetts Dental Society, June 3 and 4, 1903.

written and almost as little done for the people upon whom this dread disease has been inflicted. I am free to confess that cases of this nature are far from inviting to handle; in fact, unless the greatest care is exercised the gravest results will occur. But there are other as dangerous patients with whom we come in almost daily contact in our profession, and only cautious care and watchfulness is necessary to ward off any evil results. You will readily understand that tools used for clients of this class can not properly be used for others, even though there be no danger, but the idea would be most obnoxious. Implements must be more than carefully cleaned and left for a long time in glyco-thymoline. Never fail to have the hands most carefully protected with rubber gloves, and under no circumstance ever bring them in contact with the lips or eyes. Glyco-thymoline will minimize the possibility of infection, and very often in the course of my work I immerse my glove-covered hands in this preparation.

I have always found it best to become, to a certain extent, well acquainted with my patients, for such I consider them, for the simple reason they will understand your interest in them, will have every confidence in you, and more readily and earnestly follow your every direction to the most minute detail. As a general thing I have found people afflicted with this disease decidedly diffident about speaking of their affliction, but once their confidence is gained they have no hesitancy about going into every detail that may be required to insure perfect success in your work.

Having everything carefully prepared for taking your impression, the cavity should be carefully cleansed with glyco-thymoline and then smeared thoroughly with sweet oil. Into the cavity is then placed some wax which has been softened, in this way securing an exact impression. Carefully remove this and cool it. Replace it, and with a napkin wrung out of hot water smooth the under surface of the wax until it is flush or even with the natural palate. Insert some little wire hooks into the wax so that the loops hang down to be readily embraced by the impression material, which is now used to take an impression of the mouth in the usual manner. It is absolutely necessary that the cast become perfectly hard before removal, so that when taken from the mouth the wax plug comes with it. It is now plain to the meanest comprehension that you have an accurate impression of the mouth and cleft, and no difficulty should, of course, be experienced in making a model.

No other material but gold should be used for the plate, and before moulding the model the cleft should be filled with wax, so that the plate is swaged across it. I know that in some instances rubber has been substituted, but I would not recommend this for an instant, as in cases of this kind absolute cleanliness should be the key-note, and this cannot be gained if rubber is used, no matter what care and precaution may be exercised.

As is well known, there is a great deal of discharge of an exceedingly disagreeable nature from the cleft palate of a syphilitic patient, and in order to arrange for this, and to obviate the necessity of this mucus passing again into the system, I have arranged for an appliance in the nature of a small cup or receptacle for the retention of a tiny sponge or bit of gauze of the finest texture. It is necessary, for obvious reasons, that this appliance of which I speak be removable, and this is accomplished by having it fitted to the plate by means of a slide or screw.

In order to secure the appliance referred to you have simply to fill in the abnormal cavity of the cleft, which appears in the model, with wax, and then proceed to make a Babbitt's metal cast as you would an ordinary gold denture.

It is not my desire to be prolix or to weary my listeners, but I wish to call your attention to a few special cases which I have treated during the past two years, and which I trust may be of some interest to you.

CASE I.—Mr. P. S., aged sixty-four, was inoculated many years ago. I met the gentleman for the first time about seven years ago. I show you the condition of the maxilla as it was then. Mr. P. S. engaged an advertising dentist to make him an obturator, which was nothing but a vulcanized rubber plate, with a considerable amount of soft rubber to fill out the cavity. You can imagine the suffering of this unfortunate man, the soft rubber destroying the maxilla in a most terrible manner.

I now show you the present condition of the maxilla. The plate I show you here is but a copy of the original, consequently it is not as fine as the plate which he is wearing. You will notice a hollow box soldered upon the plate proper, which holds the contrivance with a screw. The patient removes the sponge daily, changing it for a fresh one soaked in glyco-thymoline, which keeps the cavity clean and wholesome. Prior to my making this palate for the patient, he swallowed the mucus flowing from the cavity, a rather disagreeable state of affairs. But since wearing this appliance he tells me he feels like a new man.

CASE II.—S. G., aged forty, American birth; father, American, perfectly healthy; mother, American, syphilitic. I could not receive any further information.

The cleft made its appearance for the first time about three years ago. Teeth intact, free from caries, perfectly sound. Originally I made a gold plate with my usual appliances. About eight months afterwards an ulcer made its appearance on the uvula. You all know the difficulty of retaining a dressing upon it. As you perceive, an extension soldered to the plate proper upon which a movable slide was soldered permits the patient to change the dressing according to the direction of the surgeon. After several weeks the ulcer healed, the slide was removed, and the plate is worn at present without it, giving the patient entire satisfaction and enabling him to speak plainly.

CASE III.—L. W., aged fifty-one, sailor by profession, an illiterate man, from whom I could not elicit sufficient information regarding family history.

When twenty-one years of age he married a Malay woman whom he brought to this country. He claims that the parents of the woman were inoculated with the disease. In all my experience with difficult cases this was no doubt the most severe. The duplicate of the plate which I show you has two distinct appliances. One serves as a holder for the sponge, which the patient removes before retiring, the other is used during the night, medicated cotton being applied.

It is hardly possible to exaggerate my success in this particular case; but if there is one person in this world who appreciates my work and is thankful he made my acquaintance, it is this man.

CASE IV.—A well-known dentist of New York City, some two years ago, sent me a man, English by birth, who had an acquired syphilitic cleft palate. As this man had but six hours time before his departure, I could not make him a plate according to my original idea. He wore a gold plate made in England, to which the old-fashioned Ash & Sons' tubular teeth were fastened. The little appliance which you perceive here is nothing but an ordinary neck-tie holder, as I had no time to make him a proper appliance, and accidentally had the neck-tie holder in my possession.

I wish to state that there was a constant flow of mucus. Imagine, gentlemen, a man swallowing this discharge constantly. My idea was not to permit the mucus to run down his throat. I simply took an ordinary vulcanized hollow rubber finger, which he placed into the catch, allowing the mucus to run into this rubber finger, which was replaced by a new one whenever necessary. You can imagine how happy the man was after having found relief. Several months later he visited me, accompanied by his daughter, a very pretty young woman, aged twenty-two, but who has never been in the possession of a set of teeth. I show you the copy of the plate I made her. The discharge in her case was not as severe as her father's.

CASE V.—This is a case of unusual interest. N. M., male, aged forty-four. The case is similar to any other syphilitic cleft, with the difference that both sides of the maxilla were destroyed. The six teeth, two bicuspids and two molars on each side, were worn down to such an extent that it was necessary to crown them to lengthen the bite. This plate is like all others, simply a copy; the slides are removable, serving as the holders for the dressing or sponge. This patient wears the plate with absolute comfort and perfect satisfaction.

CASE VI.—J. L., West Indies British, informs me that syphilis has been prevailing in his family for years past. This was an absolutely dry case, only at times a very small quantity of mucus making its appearance.

CASE VII.—This is also a very interesting case, that of a lady, E. S., whose husband acquired syphilis while a young man. He committed suicide about four years ago, having lived a very miserable life. The poor victim, his wife, who, as she claims, was absolutely healthy, of American parentage, suffers for the vices of her late husband. I have made the woman as comfortable as possible, but I have little doubt that eventually she will die a miserable death. I have also made for this patient an artificial nose, but as she feels delicate about the matter, I am unable to give you a *fac-simile,* or rather a *prima facie* evidence, but I can assure you that the woman is as comfortable as possible under the circumstances.

CASE VIII.—B. F., who has been a sufferer from syphilis for the past sixteen years. Though caries has troubled him, I could not prevail upon him to have the six anterior teeth removed, although they are not of much use to him. You will notice that I could place but four teeth on each side. On the plate proper I have a box made of pink rubber, in which an antiseptic is placed. This receptacle catches the discharge constantly. Whenever it is filled the patient uses a syringe, cleansing the receptacle by putting in another piece of cotton saturated with glyco-thymoline or a weak solution of carbolic acid. Naturally it is not a pleasant thing for a patient to wear a plate of this nature, and I have made an improvement on the second plate. Instead of making a rubber box, I simply cut an ordinary rubber ball in two portions, and fasten it to the plate proper, permitting the mucus to be drained into it. The rubber ball is replaced every second or third day. It makes the plate lighter and more pleasant to wear, but I dare say that at best it is but a palliative measure.

CASE IX.—This represents a simple case of syphilitic cleft palate. I wish to say, gentlemen, that my purpose is not to show beautiful workmanship; I simply wish to convey my idea, because I have made it a practice to always make a duplicate of each case. The original of this copy is far lighter and much prettier in form, etc. The manner in which this was made is as follows: when you are packing a case of this nature, though I very seldom use rubber for cleft palate work, after you have the surface packed, put a piece of ordinary rolled cotton into the cavity, covering it with rubber, then proceed by pressing the same as you would in an ordinary denture. Examine the work, if you should suspect that it may vulcanize porous. I usually make the so-called plumpers when I work to fill out the cheeks. In this case you will perceive the slide on the back part of the plate proper, which holds the sponge or any dressing which you may care to use.

Fellow-workers, I thank you for your attention and the interest you have manifested. A stranger,—a foreigner,—I have much with which to contend in an endeavor to make myself thoroughly understood, for I have not only to overcome the difficulties of proper enunciation, but also the rules of prosody and syntax. If there is any one point on which any member wishes more explicit detail it will be my pleasure to give the same either in public or private. Again expressing appreciation of the courtesy accorded me, I will only add that I will feel more than repaid for my trite efforts if I have placed my subject in such a light that some fellow-practitioner may bring relief to at least one afflicted sufferer.

Reviews of Dental Literature.

SOME OBSERVATIONS UPON SUPPURATION OF THE MAXILLARY ANTRUM; WITH SPECIAL REFERENCE TO DIAGNOSIS AND TREATMENT.[1] By Herbert Tilley, M.D., B.S. (Lond.), F.R.C.S. (Eng.).[2]

The natural opening of the antrum into the nose is situated in the membranous upper portion of the inner antral wall. Seen from within the nasal cavity, it will be noticed that it opens into the channel of the infundibulum in the middle meatus of the nose. The high situation of the opening renders it very unsatisfactory for purposes of drainage. (Diagrams were shown illustrating these points.)

I would ask you to particularly bear in mind two anatomical features which have an important bearing upon the pathology and treatment of nasal accessory sinus suppuration. The first is the relation of the maxillary antrum to the frontal sinus. It will be noticed that the infundibulum terminates at or in the antral opening, and that a fold of mucous membrane extends upward from the foramen, forming a pocket, at the bottom of which is the antral foramen, the fold referred to being on the inner side.

It results from this that a discharge issuing from the frontal sinus would tend to fill the antrum before the latter began to overflow into the nose, and hence the lower sinus may act as a reservoir for discharges from the ethmoidal cells or frontal sinus, without being itself primarily diseased.

Again, Tillaux has shown that if water be injected into the frontal sinus a considerable quantity of it flows into the cavity of the antrum. Hence, the fact that an antrum contains pus does not necessarily mean that it is produced there, for it may be merely acting as a reservoir rather than as a generator of the discharge. The following case will illustrate my meaning:

---

[1] Abstract of a paper read before the Odontological Society of Great Britain, November 23, 1903.

[2] Surgeon to the Hospital for Diseases of the Throat, Nose, and Ear, Golden Square.

Mr. F., aged fifty-four, had for five years suffered from a purulent nasal discharge, associated with nasal obstruction due to large polypi within the nasal cavities. On several occasions the polypi were removed, but the discharge continued as freely as before, and it was ascertained that it proceeded from the frontal, ethmoidal, sphenoidal, and antral sinuses. Both maxillary antra were drained by the alveolar method, and for two years were irrigated twice daily with antiseptic lotions. The purulent discharge, although lessened in amount and robbed of its fetor, continued to flow, and the patient used on an average fifty handkerchiefs a week. He finally decided to submit to radical operations upon the different sinuses, with a view to the discharge being entirely cured.

Last June I operated upon both frontal sinuses, and to my astonishment found that it was not necessary to further treat the antra, for from the day on which the operation on the higher sinuses was performed not a single drop of pus could be washed from the antra. Surely it is a remarkable thing that these sinuses (antra) could have merely acted as reservoirs of pus for so long a time without themselves becoming actual generators of the same.

The last anatomical feature to which I would like to draw your attention is that sometimes, as is shown in the diagram, some of the lower anterior ethmoidal cells spread outward in the bony floor of the orbit, and infection may spread from these into the antrum. It is of the utmost importance in the radical operation for the cure of chronic suppuration to see that these cells (if they exist) are not overlooked; for if left behind in a septic condition they would reinfect the antral cavity.

Causes of Antral Suppuration.—As many of you are aware, it used to be thought that all cases of antral suppuration were caused by diseased teeth, but during recent years it has become an equally well-established fact that many cases arise by infection from the nose, and this is especially likely to occur during the course of one of the acute specific fevers. Influenza has proved a prolific parent of suppuration within the nasal accessory sinuses, while in a smaller number of cases erysipelas, scarlet fever, measles, diphtheria, typhoid, and pneumonia have been definitely proved to be the cause of the infection. A certain amount of catarrh of the nasal mucosa is frequently present during the course of these diseases, and since the nasal mucous membrane is continuous with that lining the accessory cavities, the latter are very prone to become affected by simple·extension of the catarrhal process. Hence we can easily understand that an acute nasal catarrh may be followed by a similar condition, with retention of the secretions in the accessory sinuses, a condition possibly accounting for some of the frontal discomfort experienced during an acute " cold in the head." If owing to inefficient drainage such secretions be retained under tension, an increase of inflammation may result, and should certain micro-organisms gain access to the suitable medium thus provided, suppuration may occur—it may be in the antrum, in a single ethmoidal cell, in a frontal sinus, or in any combination of these cavities.

If we suppose an ethmoidal cell to be affected, and to have become the focus of suppuration, it is at least possible that the contained pus may find its way into the maxillary antrum, or even into a frontal sinus, and *vice versa.* So that—given an acute or chronic catarrhal condition of the mucous membrane acting as a predisposing cause—the exciting cause of empyema may be organisms associated with influenza, syphilitic nasal lesions, insanitary surroundings, or convalescence from long illnesses, especially acute infectious diseases; while, as will hereafter be stated, most cases of antral suppuration are due to septic infection starting from the root of a diseased tooth, especially the second bicuspid or one of the molar teeth.

Traumatisms will account for a certain number of cases,—possibly more than we are inclined to admit,—and I fear that the dental as well as the nasal surgeon is not always free from blame. For example, I have a vivid recollection of three or four cases where symptoms of empyema have immediately followed the attempt at extraction of a tooth, in which the history would seem to suggest that a portion of a dental root was broken into the antrum. Or again, the symptoms appeared shortly after a tooth had been " filled," and were preceded by intense toothache, followed by a sudden relief which was associated with a foul smell within and a purulent discharge from the nose. Under such circumstances it is probable that the cavity within the tooth had not been rendered perfectly aseptic before the " filling" had been inserted, and the resulting suppuration had followed the path of least resistance and found its way into the overlying sinus.

On the other hand, I have known antral suppuration to follow upon the careless use of the galvano-cautery in the middle meatal region of the nose; and in two other instances it complicated the

5

convalescence of an operation undertaken for the removal of an outgrowth from the nasal septum. Under the latter circumstances, when the nasal mucosa are in an irritable condition, and septic accumulations lie within the nasal cavities, it is particularly easy for a patient in blowing the nose to force such material into the neighboring sinuses and thus to start a chronic suppurative condition.

The question, however, which I feel sure many of you will ask me will be, What proportion of cases of chronic antral suppuration do you consider arises from dental causes?

I am afraid it is impossible for me to give you anything like a direct answer, but this statement may interest you,—namely, that with one exception, in each of the sixty-four cases upon which this paper is based, diseased bicuspid or molar teeth were present (or by their absence implied previous removal for disease) upon the side corresponding to the antral suppuration. I would even go farther, and say that during the past ten years, during which I must have seen at least three hundred cases of " antral abscess," I have only met with one patient (a girl, aged twelve) in whom the teeth were quite healthy.

These are somewhat startling facts, but I am able to substantiate them, even though there rings in my ear the statement of Grünwald, of Münich, that, out of ninety-eight cases of antral suppuration, in fourteen only could he trace with certainty their origin from diseased teeth. How does this curious difference in large experiences arise? Possibly in this way. You will notice that in my statement it is asserted that " diseased" teeth were present in all cases, and by " disease" is meant any departure from the normal, ranging from a tiny carious cavity in the crown of a tooth to a septic condition involving the crown, roots, and surrounding alveolar sockets. In a few of my cases it was difficult to believe that the antral suppuration had been influenced in any way by a small carious cavity in the crown of what (with this exception) was a sound tooth, and it is probably all such mild cases of dental disease which Grünwald excluded from his statistics. Nevertheless, the constancy of the association between the diseased teeth and the sinus suppuration would seem to me to be more than mere coincidence.

Or can we explain the facts in this way? That in this country there are very few people beyond the age of puberty whose teeth are absolutely sound, and therefore the chances of any one individual who is suffering from chronic antral suppuration (relatively a much rarer condition) having unhealthy teeth on the same side are very great. .

Or again, may we not reasonably suppose that a small amount of disease, limited even to the crown of a tooth, will probably set up a certain degree of irritability of the mucous membrane of the antrum in the neighborhood of the root of that tooth—shall we say an increased vulnerability, which renders it more liable to infection from the nose? Unless it be assumed that my figures are the result of mere coincidence, I fear we must adopt some such explanation as this, and in this connection would quote what Grünwald says, in spite of his opposition to the frequency of dental disease as a cause of antral suppuration. He says, " I would especially emphasize the fact that a tooth must not be considered harmless because the socket is not diseased. Infection creeps along the lymphatics of healthy bone, and a focus of infection in the crown of a tooth is by no means to be despised, for even if an empyema of the antrum be due to another cause, yet disease of the crown of a tooth is calculated to maintain such a state of irritation in the mucous membrane as may frustrate all attempts at cure."

Symptoms.—The symptoms of acute antral suppuration are so well known to you that I need scarcely do more than mention the acute throbbing pain in the cheek and supraorbital region, tenderness of one or more teeth and their immediate neighborhood, especially that of the canine fossa. Sometimes the soft tissues of the face and cheek are also swollen and tender, while fever and the constitutional symptoms associated with it add to the sufferings of the patient. Relief comes when the abscess bursts into the nose, or is relieved by extraction of the inflamed tooth and (if necessary) perforation through the alveolar socket.

A patient suffering from chronic antral suppuration will, I take it, consult the dental surgeon only when dental symptoms are prominent, but the medical attendant is often appealed to for the relief of symptoms which do not at first sight suggest the antrum ; *e.g.,* " an offensive discharge from the nose," a frequently recurring " disagreeable taste," " increasing difficulty in breathing through the nose," due to the formation of polypi, " chronic nasal catarrh," " headache," " brow ague," feelings of " weight over the forehead," or " round the eyes." In other cases the digestion is impaired owing to more or less severe forms of gastritis, brought about by the swallowing of pus into the stomach; while absorption of the purulent material into the general circulation has a very subtle effect on the nervous system, inducing a lack of energy and general condition of depression, which may perhaps be best exemplified by the following passage taken from a patient's letter two months after the antra had been drained. She says, " Before the operation I was always depressed, and often cried several times a day; if I walked a mile I was tired out, but now I can walk eight miles without any fatigue whatever."

If the dental symptoms be associated with a " discharge of offensive matter from the nose," coupled with a " sickly taste" in the mouth, and at the same time there are frequent attacks of supra-orbital headache,—possibly of greater severity during the earlier hours of the day,—especially if these symptoms should be associated with any of those I have already mentioned, under such circumstances you may reasonably entertain a strong suspicion that the antrum is diseased, either alone or in combination with the other accessory sinuses.

Diagnosis.—Here, again, we must not dwell upon fine details, because, in order to recognize the chief diagnostic features of chronic antral suppuration as seen within the nose, I should have to presume that you had an intimate acquaintance with the appearances of the nasal cavities both in health and disease. Still less is it necessary for me to discuss the diagnosis of those difficult cases in which more than one of the accessory cavities are simultaneously affected. Two tests, however, which you may often apply with advantage are the following:

(1) Ask the patient to blow his nose thoroughly upon the affected side until no pus is expelled. Then let him rest for from three to five minutes with the suspected antrum uppermost, during which time the pus will probably flow into the nose. On again blowing the nostril, the yellow and often offensive discharge may once more be seen upon the handkerchief.

(2) Let the patient place the feet close together and endeavor to touch his toes without bending the knees. If this position be maintained for from one to two minutes, considerable congestion of the head will be caused, and aching of the inflamed tooth or diseased antrum, or corresponding frontal region, may be induced.

As I stated just now, the appearance of pus in the middle

meatus of the nose, the presence of polypoid granulations or hypertrophies in this position, or the well-known swelling of the mucosa covering the uncinate process of the ethmoid ("Kaufmann's cushion"), cannot be discussed with any advantage upon this occasion.

Presuming we are dealing with an uncomplicated case of unilateral suppuration, there is one test which, whilst not by any means infallible, may give you strong confirmation of your suspicions of antral mischief, while it is painless and usually of considerable interest to the patient. I refer to transillumination by means of a small six- to ten-volt electric lamp placed within the patient's mouth, while the room is darkened or the head covered with a dark cloth, in order to obtain the fullest contrast between the lights and shades provided by the test.

If there be pus within the antrum, it will be noticed that there is no infraorbital "light crescent" upon the diseased side, or a much less definite one than on the healthy side. This infraorbital opacity is due, in my opinion, to a chronic inflammatory process in the bony walls of the antrum, because not only is it present immediately after the pus has been washed out, but may sometimes be seen forty-eight hours after the radical operation has been performed, and when the sinus cavity is without any membranous lining at all. Unfortunately the test is not always reliable because a similar opacity may be noted in healthy but thick-walled antra, and of course its value is diminished when both sinuses are diseased. Other conditions may also modify its reliability, but in the great majority of cases it may very materially assist you in *confirming suspicions* founded upon other symptoms presented by the case.

(A practical illustration of transillumination in a patient suffering from chronic antral suppuration was given.)

There is only one absolutely certain means by which you can demonstrate the presence or absence of pus in the antrum, and that is by exploration of the cavity. Formerly it was (and I fear, in many quarters still is) the custom to perforate the alveolus under nitrous oxide anæsthesia and, if necessary, to remove a tooth for the purpose. Should the exploration demonstrate the absence of pus, the patient will possibly have lost a useful tooth, to say nothing of the inconvenience of the anæsthetic, and of—not improbably—a considerable amount of after-pain and discomfort in the jaw.

All these disadvantages can be obviated by making a puncture within the nose. This little operation is practically painless. It needs no general anæsthetic, it may be done in the consulting-room, and its evidence is absolutely reliable.

A small dossil of wool is moistened with a ten per cent. solution of cocaine and applied by means of a probe to the inner wall of the antrum underneath the anterior end of the inferior turbinal bone. In a few moments a (Lichtwitz's) fine trochar and canula are passed outward, backward, and slightly upward, through the inner antral wall. The trochar is withdrawn, leaving the canula in position, and to its proximal end is fitted a rubber tube through which some warm boracic or normal saline solution can be injected. If there be any pus in the sinus it is at once demonstrated by this simple, bloodless, and absolutely reliable method. Curiously enough, in a number of cases in which I have used it, immediately the antrum had been perforated the patient at once complained of aching in one of the diseased teeth upon the same side. This was very valuable information, for it at once suggested which one, of perhaps several unsound teeth, was the real cause of the trouble.

Treatment.—The treatment of acute antral suppuration need not detain us long. The painful symptoms rapidly subside if free drainage be provided, either through a tooth socket in the alveolus, or through a large opening in the inferior meatus of the nose. If the antrum be irrigated daily with some mild antiseptic for ten days to a fortnight, the suppuration will cease and the opening in the alveolus may be allowed to close. Very occasionally one irrigation will suffice and the insertion of a drainage-tube will be unnecessary. It is a moot question whether any tube is necessary in acute cases or whether they will not do better if only a moderate-sized alveolar perforation be made. Personally, I prefer a tube, because we can be sure of efficient drainage until it is certain that suppuration has ceased, whereas, should the opening close before the discharge has quite disappeared, it might be necessary to open up the alveolar perforation for a second time.

With regard to chronic suppuration, you will gather from what has already been stated that in the treatment of every case the first desideratum is that the teeth be attended to, and this even when the history may seem to indicate that the primary infection entered by way of the nose. However clear such a sequence may be, a diseased tooth may add such irritative factors as to rob any other methods of treatment of complete success, and hence the reason why your services should be requisitioned.

Next will come the question, What form of local treatment shall be adopted for checking the suppuration within the antrum? Will you pardon me if I presume to remind you that we are dealing with a bony-walled cavity which is lined by a pyogenic membrane, and that our first endeavor should be to restore the latter to its natural condition, or, failing this, we must adopt other means to cure the patient's symptoms. In any case we must be guided by those well-known principles of surgery which are adopted in other regions of the body in the treatment of abscess cavities. I would not emphasize this point had my experience not amply proved to me that such principles are often more honored in the breach than in the observance. Now there are three principles which should influence us in the treatment of all our cases:

(1) *Efficient drainage,* the ultimate success of which will be accelerated by frequent irrigations of the unhealthy mucous membrane with mild antiseptic washes.

(2) *More or less obliteration of the diseased cavity.* This last method will be the final one if failure attends a fair or lengthy trial of simpler measures.

(3) *Attention to the general health of the patient.* We must never forget that defective hygienic surroundings and excesses in eating, drinking, and smoking have a very great influence for evil upon the general progress of the case. Immoderate use of alcohol or tobacco have a great tendency to induce congestion and chronic catarrhal conditions of the mucosa of the upper air-passages, conditions which are very adverse to rapid recovery after operative interference in these regions. Occasionally two or three grains of calomel over night, followed in the morning by a saline draught, will produce more improvement than all those new antiseptics of " high destructive power," the advertisements of which form an increasing constituent of our waste-paper baskets.

Drainage (alveolar method).—Since efficient drainage can only take place when our opening is situated at the lowest level of the abscess cavity, it need scarcely be said that an alveolar perforation is better than drainage through the canine fossa, or through the inferior meatus of the nose. Drainage through the canine fossa is inefficient, and the tube or plug often causes great irritation of the mucous membrane of the cheek or gums, while any but a large opening in the inferior nasal meatus has a very great tendency to close, in addition to which the patient nearly always finds a difficulty in carrying out the necessary irrigations.

You all know the many and ingenious alveolar drainage-tubes which from time to time have been invented. Those seem to answer best in which a plate fixed to adjacent teeth supports a metal tube, the lumen of which is about the size of a crow-quill, and which is occupied by a split plug which can be inserted during meal-times in order to prevent access of food to the antrum. I have also seen cases do equally well in which a solid plug takes the place of the tube. Whichever form of tube you adopt, be careful that its upper end, when it is in position, does not stand high above the level of the antral floor, under which circumstances its very function as a drain will be destroyed.

As to the irrigating lotion which the patient shall use, I can only say that I am wedded to no one in particular, and am certain that the best results will be attained by constantly changing the nature of the antiseptic. A saturated solution of boracic acid, chlorate of potash (twenty grains to the ounce), carbolic lotion (1 in 60, for the early treatment of offensive cases), lysoform, the active principle of which is formalin, in strength five minims to a tumblerful of water, peroxide of hydrogen, ten per cent. solution, sulphate of zinc (two grains to one ounce), and finally normal saline solution,—all these may be found useful. In the later stages, after washing out the antrum, it may be well to inject and leave within the cavity one-half drachm of an alcoholic solution of boracic acid (pulv. ac. boracic, ten grains; spir. vini rect., aq. destill., of each, two drachms).

At the outset the patient should wash out the antrum twice daily; as the discharge lessens, once daily; with further improvement, every second or third day; and finally, if after an interval of ten days no pus returns upon irrigating, then the case may be considered cured and the tube removed.

Remember: (*a*) Always use the solution warm; (*b*) never use warm water alone, even when sterilized. Its density is different from that of blood serum, and will often induce a free discharge of mucus, and sometimes cause pain.

Three questions now suggest themselves:

(1) What is the result of such treatment?

(2) How long should it be continued?

(3) To what class of case should it be applied?

(1) With regard to the result, my experience is that in nearly all cases—even those of long duration—alveolar irrigation rapidly diminishes the amount and fetor of the pus, together with those more general symptoms which have been described; but that in cases of more than a few months' duration it is extremely difficult to get rid of the last trace of discharge, so that you can feel justified in removing the tube altogether. I have recently ascertained that out of twenty-seven of my patients in whom the alveolar treatment was adopted and irrigation patiently persevered in, only five have been able to give up their tubes. The rest still find a small amount of purulent secretion comes away on irrigation, and if they fail to carry on the treatment an increase in the amount of discharge is rapidly noticed.

(2) How long should the treatment be continued? Until the discharge entirely ceases, or until the failure of simple measures renders it obvious that, if the patient desires an absolute cure, some further and more radical treatment will be necessary. Out of my twenty-seven alveolar cases seen during the past two years, fifteen of them have worn the tube and carefully irrigated for at least six months. One patient had been doing so for ten years, another for three and a half, and a third for two years. Many of them found the tube caused no inconvenience, and preferred to go on with the irrigation. Five, however, elected to have the radical operation, and I am glad to say that they have without exception been cured, and by the term "cure" I mean that not a trace of pus can be found within the nose.

(3) To what class of cases should the alveolar treatment be applied? Certainly to all those the duration of which has been a matter of months rather than of years, and possibly as a first measure in most of the chronic cases, because now and again, even in these, alveolar drainage and irrigation have resulted in a rapid cure.

The advantages of the method are its simplicity, and in this respect it is scarcely a more serious operation than the removal of a tooth. The after-treatment can soon be carried out for long periods by the patient himself, and the general improvement which is effected is very great, even if the measure be not an entirely curative one. To the very old, the broken in health, the nervous, the busy man with the cares of a family and an exacting occupation, and to whom a week or ten days' lying up is a very serious matter, the alveolar method has many advantages. On the other hand, we meet with cases of long-standing suppuration, in which— no matter how persistently or with what variety the irrigating lotions are used—the discharge of pus from the nose into the mouth is still profuse, the patient becomes tired of irrigating, and wants to know " if something cannot be done to cure him once and for all ?" Or, perhaps, he or she will be one of those impatient indi- viduals who " do not want to be bothered with tubes," but fret day by day because they " can blow matter from the nose, and always have a nasty taste in the mouth." For this class of patients we may adopt other and more radical measures.

   The Radical Operation.—An aseptic sponge having been passed into the nasopharynx and a second one placed between the cheek and teeth on the affected side, in order to prevent any flow of blood into the larynx, the anterior end of the inferior turbinal bone upon the diseased side is removed by a pair of angular scissors and a wire snare. An incision is then made in the gingivo-labial groove and over the canine fossa parallel to the alveolar process of the jaw, and extending from the malar process of the superior maxilla to the canine ridge. The soft parts and periosteum are turned up and the anterior wall of the antrum, as represented by the canine fossa, is removed by gouge and mallet. An opening is made in the canine fossa, between the size of a sixpence and a shilling, the larger within reason the better, but care should be taken not to wound the infraorbital nerve. The diseased mucous membrane is then care- fully and thoroughly curetted away, the free hemorrhage which interrupts the procedure being checked by means of a good supply of sterilized strips of gauze. The same end may be more rapidly attained if, after having curetted away most of the diseased mem- brane, one or two strips of gauze be moistened in adrenalin chloride, or hydrogen peroxide solution, and tightly packed into the sinus and allowed to remain for from three to five minutes. The time thus lost will be more than regained by the greater ease with which subsequent proceedings can be carried out.

   At this stage we have to decide how much of the inner antral wall shall be taken away in order to provide free drainage from the sinus into the nose. The following considerations should guide you. If the diseased mucous membrane be mainly confined to the lower half of the antrum and the middle meatal region of the nose be healthy, it will suffice if a counter-opening be made in the lower anterior region of the naso-antral wall; this opening should at least be as large as a sixpence because of the great tendency to cicatrization which characterizes wounds in this neighborhood.

If, on the other hand, the whole of the lining membrane be diseased, and especially if polypi or mucous membrane hypertrophies be seen in the middle meatus of the nose, the whole of the inner antral wall should be removed, and it is this modification of the simpler operation which has yielded me my best results. The reasons for this extensive ablation are twofold,—the lower half being removed for drainage purposes, the upper half in order to destroy that membranous portion of the inner wall which is often in a polypoid condition, and also to gain access to any lower ethmoidal or maxillo-ethmoidal cells which are so frequently diseased, and which, if left untouched, will reinfect the antrum. The sinus cavity is finally mopped out with strips of gauze soaked in carbolic lotion (1 in 20), and the operation is completed. It is unnecessary to insert any packing unless the hemorrhage be unusually free; in any case only a loose strip of gauze will be necessary, which should be removed forty-eight hours after the operation and not replaced. In a straightforward case the operation may be completed in from thirty to thirty-five minutes.

The after-treatment consists in douching out the nose, and by this means also the antrum, twice daily for two or three weeks with some mild antiseptic wash. The patient can sit up on the third day after the operation, and may usually go out within ten days. The bucco-antral wound heals very quickly (seven to ten days), and no deformity or falling in of the cheek occurs. I would particularly emphasize the latter point, because one of the objections which have been raised against the radical operation is the deformity which may result. During the past two years I have performed this operation thirty-seven times, and have kept myself intimately acquainted with the progress of each patient, and it is with no small feeling of satisfacton I can record thirty-four successful cases as against three imperfect results (*vide* " Synopsis of Cases"). The three patients to whom I refer were not operated upon by quite the same method as I have just detailed, and therefore cannot be said to detract from the value of the operation which I am advocating. The failure to produce complete cure in the patients referred to was due, I think, to the fact that no counter-opening was made into the nose.

Excepting for a troublesome neuralgia, which occurred in four cases and lasted for from four to ten days, I have met with no complication.

To the question, " What circumstances would guide you in advising a radical operation without preliminary trial of simpler measures?" we may answer, " The appearances presented by the middle meatus of the nose." If in a long-standing case this region be filled with polypoid granulations or swollen and œdematous mucous membrane, then it is fairly certain that the antral mucous membrane is also in an advanced state of chronic degeneration, and nothing short of radical treatment will effect a permanent cure.

You may quite naturally ask, " What is the condition of the antrum in a successful case, six months after operation?"

There can be no doubt that it is partially obliterated by the granulations which spring up over the bony walls uniting with those which grow inward from the soft tissues of the cheek through the large opening in the canine fossa. This mass of granulation tissue becomes covered with epithelium which spreads inward from the circumference of the naso-antral opening, because without this natural method of healing suppuration would inevitably continue.

It is only necessary to examine a patient four or five months after operation with a small mirror passed within the nose, or by means of a curved probe, to satisfy one's self that the original antral sinus is partially obliterated and is only represented by a concavity upon the outer side of the nasal fossa, which is very much smaller than the original antrum.

Reports of Society Meetings.

THE NEW YORK INSTITUTE OF STOMATOLOGY.

A MEETING of the Institute was held at the " Chelsea," No. 222 West Twenty-third Street, New York, on Friday, November 6, 1903, the President, Dr. J. Morgan Howe, in the chair.

The minutes of the last meeting were read and approved.

Dr. Wooley, as chairman of the committee, presented a memorial to the late member of the Institute, Dr. Louis Shaw. The memorial was adopted and ordered recorded in the proceedings of the society. The secretary was instructed to send a copy of the same to the family of the deceased.

Owing to the importance of the paper of the evening, the communications on theory and practice were omitted.

Dr. D. B. Kyle, of Philadelphia, read a paper entitled " The Relation of the Chemistry of the Saliva (Sialo-Semeiology) and Nasal Secretions to Diseases of the Mucous Membrane of the Mouth and Upper Respiratory Tract."

(For Dr. Kyle's paper, see page 94.)

Dr. Kirk wished first to express his thanks to the Institute for the privilege of being present and listening to such an instructive and interesting paper. His own interest in the subject had extended back about three years, and his researches and study had been confined principally to one aspect of the subject only,—the hyperacid diathesis. He had learned a great deal to-night about the chemical side of the hypoacid diathesis. Dr. Kirk was pleased to confirm, from his own observation, the chemical aspect of the problem, so far as the essayist had stated it.

Speaking of the susceptibility to necrotic conditions in hypoacid cases, Dr. Kirk asked if the essayist meant to imply that the necrosis was chemical and not bacterial. He thought it generally conceded that the hypoacid case was the one most susceptible to bacterial infection. He did not think the essayist intended to convey the idea that necrotic conditions were produced by the hypoacid condition, but that diathetic hypoacidity was a condition that made these cases susceptible to bacterial infection, which infection caused the necrosis. Dr. Kirk thought there was a direct relationship between the food habit and the diathetic state. It had been recently shown that in Oriental countries, where the diet was chiefly vegetable, while caries of the teeth was not prominent, pyorrhœa alveolaris existed to a tremendous degree. A starchy diet evidently tended in certain cases to the production of a hypoacid condition.

Regarding the exact interpretation of the microscopic appearances of crystallized saliva deposits, Dr. Kirk had for some time been endeavoring to determine, one at a time, the chemical nature of some of the substances that we see. The essayist had developed the thought that a high ammonium content in saliva indicated a hypoacid diathesis. From his own point of view he had settled upon large quantities of the so-called neutral sodium phosphate rather than the ammonium as indicative of the hypoacid diathesis. Sodium phosphate is an extremely interesting compound. The early writers on the chemistry of the saliva and the urine had gone astray in their interpretation of its appearance under the microscope. Chemical investigation in this field by the ordinary methods of the laboratory is extremely difficult. In many respects it is beyond the reach of such methods. When Michaels suggested the use of the polariscope he gave us a means in advance of anything that had been accomplished. The neutral sodium phosphate occurring so abundantly in the hypoacid conditions had been put down in earlier works as ammonium chloride. The appearance of the two compounds is very similar until a special study has been made of them. However, the so-called neutral sodium phosphate is really alkaline, and the alkalinity of the normal saliva may be measured in terms of sodium phosphate, with sodium carbonate and bicarbonate. Both are found in normal and in hypoacid saliva, but in different amounts.

When we came to the hyperacid individual we had an entirely different aspect. Here we had an individual producing large quantities of CO_2, and more rapidly than it can be eliminated, the excess being dammed up in the plasma of the blood, existing as H_2CO_3. The normal reaction by which this over-acidity is taken care of by the renal epithelium is $H_2CO_3 + HNa_2PO_4 = H_2NaPO_4 + HNaCO_3$, but when the conditions are such as to produce larger quantities of carbonic acid than the kidneys can eliminate as sodium acid phosphate, other epiblastic structures take on the same action and there is a higher acidity of the saliva as well as the urine. A curious chemical feature of this matter was that the acid sodium phosphate and the neutral sodium phosphate might exist in the same solution without neutralizing each other, giving a solution that would turn blue litmus-paper red and red litmus-paper blue, the so-called amphoteric reaction. Thus we sometimes find saliva that would give both an acid and an alkaline reaction.

Certain conditions of the teeth exist in these hyperacid conditions, in the shape of erosions of the teeth. The teeth themselves were also of a peculiar character, becoming over-calcified and hard, translucent and vitreous in texture.

The appearance of the lactophosphate of calcium in the saliva and urine indicates certain diseases of the liver. Dr. Kirk had been led to this conclusion from reading the researches of Minkowski, who had found, in a series of experiments upon geese, where he had removed the liver, that they then excreted, instead of uric acid and the urates, the ammonium lactate, and he deduced from these experiments that one of the functions of the liver was to convert ammonium lactate into urates; so the appearance of lactates in excessive amounts in the excretions, especially in the urine, is indicative of a disordered liver function.

Dr. Kirk also called attention to the coincidence of neurasthenic states with the appearance of oxalic acid in combination with sodium, both in the saliva and in the urine. He had determined to his own satisfaction that the presence of these oxalates of the alkali bases in the secretions was metabolic in origin, and that the oxalic acid was not derived from the ingested food, for he found them to persist in patients from whom all oxalate-carrying food-substances were excluded. The oxaluria of sodium oxalate was only possible of determination by the polariscope and a stage of the disorder considerably antedating the period when calcium oxalate makes its appearance in the urine and saliva. The nervous phenomena coincident with the sodium oxalate oxaluria are constant and pronounced.

In conclusion Dr. Kirk stated that he was doing all he could in this direction, and that he was glad to learn that Dr. Kyle was also interested and had taken up the work along the same line.

The President asked whether there was any test, readily applied, by which the hyperacid, the hypoacid, or the normal condition of the saliva could be ascertained.

Dr. Bogue thought that if Dr. Kirk would consent to tell us the methods by which the various oxalic acid compounds could be detached by means of the polariscope, a partial answer would be given to the President's question.

Dr. Kirk stated that in the saliva of the hypoacid cases and in the saliva of the normal individual he had never found the oxalates, acid phosphates, and urates. In the hypoacid individual there was a preponderance of the neutral sodium phosphate, with ammonium salts and chlorides, and the individual himself was of a different type from the hyperacid, in whom there was an absence of caries and a tendency to erosion.

He could not very well describe the polariscope. It so happened that many of the waste products of the urine and saliva had the property of rotating the plane of polarized light. Hence these waste products of abnormal nutrition were readily recognized by the polariscope. The abnormal ones were the most readily polarizable. Under the microscope without the polariscope there was very little to distinguish them.

Dr. Kyle, in closing the discussion, stated, in regard to the relation of the hypoacid state to necrosis, that the strongly alkaline condition of the saliva was more irritating to the mucous membrane than the hyperacid condition. This irritation would make the tissue more susceptible to bacterial infection and beginning necrosis. Of course, necrosis does occur without bacterial infection. What he meant, however, was that this alkaline condition was a strong predisposing factor.

He was pleased to hear from Dr. Milliken's report a confirmation of his theories. He was glad also to see from Dr. Kirk's statements that, although not working together, their results were practically the same.

He was extremely interested in the statements of Dr. Kirk relative to the determining of lesions of certain organs by the chemic constituents of the saliva. He believed this would be a very valuable means, in time, of determining the position and character of organic lesions.

Dr. Kyle closed by thanking the Institute for his kindly reception.

Dr. F. Milton Smith did not feel competent to discuss the paper, but he wished to express his sincere gratitude to the gentlemen who had taken part. He thought he could appreciate the embarrassment under which such men worked, and the fact that so many times they worked long and diligently with little apparent reward other than the feeling in their own hearts that they were doing the right thing and were bringing things to pass, although they might not seem to be appreciated. For this reason he wanted to express his great appreciation for the papers that had been read and the words that had been spoken. He would also relate a little experience that might give one of the gentlemen present a feeling of satisfaction.

Some ten years ago he had had the pleasure of hearing Dr. Kirk read a paper upon a subject which at that time seemed somewhat foreign to dental matters. The subject was " Infantile

Scorbutus." At the time he did not expect to meet with any such case in his practice, but within six months a lady came to him with a little one thirteen months old with a condition that he was able, from Dr. Kirk's description, to diagnose as infantile scorbutus. The child had been treated by various physicians for dental paralysis and rheumatism, but none had been able to recognize the true cause of the trouble. Following the suggestions of Dr. Kirk's paper, Dr. Smith suggested a course of treatment, and in six weeks' time the child was practically well. She had shortly been in his chair, and while there her mother had asked if she remembered Dr. Smith. The child had said that she did not. The mother said, " Dr. Smith saved your life." Dr. Smith stated that if any one saved the life of that child it was Dr. Kirk, for she certainly would have died had she not received proper treatment, and that speedily. He also said that we really did appreciate their work even if we did not discuss it as we would like to do.

Dr. C. F. Allan stated that it had been a great favor to the society to have this paper presented. It had been a great favor for Dr. Milliken to come so far in order to present his valuable clinical evidence, and it had also been a great favor to the society for Dr. Kirk to come here to-night and give us this information about the investigations he was making. Dr. Allan moved that the thanks of the Institute be extended to these gentlemen.

Motion carried unanimously.

Adjourned.

FRED. L. BOGUE, M.D., D.D.S.,
Editor The New York Institute of Stomatology.

ACADEMY OF STOMATOLOGY.

A REGULAR meeting of the Academy of Stomatology, of Philadelphia, was held at the rooms of the Academy, 1731 Chestnut Street, on the evening of Tuesday, October 27, 1903, the President, Dr. L. Foster Jack, in the chair. A paper was read by Dr. P. B. McCullough, entitled " A Suspension Partial Denture;" also one by Dr. H. B. Hickman, entitled " Osteomyelitis: A Case in Practice."

(For Dr. McCullough's paper, see page 105; for Dr. Hickman's paper, see page 111.)

Dr. J. H. Gaskell.—I have been very much interested in Dr. McCullough's paper, but I cannot but feel that it is a mistake to saddle or have a broad surface of the mucous membrane covered by a permanent fixture in the mouth. No matter how accurately it may be attached, the gum is a tissue which is more or less yielding, and the pressure is bound to force food between that fixture and the mucous membrane. If it is placed permanently the pressure will cause absorption, so that in time the gum will not be as firm as when the fixture is put into place. I have seen results from bridges made very similar to the one described by Dr. McCullough. I have had occasion to take one out which had been in for two years. The tissue had become infected, and was inflamed and swollen, and when I took off the bridge the periosteum was entirely exposed.

Dr. William H. Trueman.—The conditions we have to meet in crown- and bridge-work are so different that we need all the light we can obtain. There is no doubt that in many cases the method described by Dr. McCullough will answer a good purpose. It also has in my judgment some weak points. When put on a molar or bicuspid, my experience has always been that the apparatus gave way. In one case I had made a joint that I thought could not possibly open; nevertheless it did it very promptly. When the pressure is all exerted towards the gum such an attachment may answer for a long time, but it does not answer when side pressure is exerted. I always prefer to have some kind of a band around the tooth to hold it firmly. The point which the doctor makes about pressing the gum is a good one. A nice adaptation is made and the area of pressure is limited, and absorption does not take place to any great extent. I hardly think the attachment is safe made between the two bicuspid teeth, where we are told the strain exercised is several hundred pounds. It is always well to remember that in these cases it is the impossible that generally happens. Unless all the force of mastication is brought against the gold there is lack of durability, and in this respect the method shows a weak point. With the second bicuspid and molars it is wiser to dispense with the porcelain and make an open bridge. I am in the habit of doing this, and the method is satisfactory.

There are points in the doctor's paper that can only be taken in as we read and think over it. There are many cases in which

.the method has a practical application. We cannot tie ourselves to any one system, but must do the very best we know how for the patient.

Dr. E. C. Kirk.—I do not want to betray confidence, but would say that some years ago Dr. Henry C. Register showed me a bridge appliance which had one feature in common with those described by the essayist: the crowns fitted the mucous membrane very closely, and Dr. Register has evidently had experience as to the tolerance of this mucous tissue of the contact of foreign bodies. The method employed by the essayist seems to be, in a measure, a theoretical one after all. The tolerance of the gum tissue, which has been by one speaker condemned, has been by another approved.

Dr. H. C. Register.—I hesitate to talk upon the subject, but feel that I must express myself entirely in favor of small open bridge-work.

I commenced the bridging of teeth certainly eighteen or twenty years ago. I took off two saddle bridges this last winter that had been doing service for eighteen years. It is a decided mistake, in speaking of the saddle, not to define it very carefully. The saddle represented in Dr. McCullough's first figure is about the proper thing; it is absolutely clean. Many persons, in speaking of a saddle, mean a continuous saddle. I have used in certain cases a very narrow saddle, and have not confined it to the tooth, but made it a continuous one. Even in those cases I have never had any serious trouble.

I think Dr. McCullough's plan very desirable in its application to the bicuspids in these cases, as we find it very difficult without destroying two teeth to get sufficient anchorage. Teeth of this character placed in the mouth are much more comfortable to the patient than those made on the ordinary lines of bridge-work. In the case of the two bridges I spoke of I replaced with the more approved style of bridge-work, having the tip of the tooth touch the gum and without the lingual contour of the natural tooth. Both cases went to Europe, and I have received three or four letters from each saying how much more comfortable the old appliance was than the new.

Dr. A. N. Gaylord.—In my experience the so-called clearing space in bridge-work is in reality a place for the collection of food. Dr. McCullough's idea of fitting the tooth against the gum seems preferable. I have yet to see a bridge, where the surface bevelled from the inner cusp'to the outer gum margin, which was not covered with more or less deposit. It is difficult, and in many cases impossible, to keep such a place clean, besides being annoying to the tongue. I have not received a sufficiently clear idea of the method of the essayist to endorse or speak against it. I would like to see a case that I might study it more fully. However, I am much in favor of removable bridges. I would ask Dr. McCullough the comparative time required in making this appliance and an ordinary bridge. I should imagine it much greater. If so, I should prefer to spend the extra time making a removable appliance, which could be cleansed in the hand and replaced. Such appliances are cleanly and satisfactory in every way.

Dr. McCullough.—Should a fair test of the principle here elucidated, of covering a limited area of gum tissue with a fixed denture, for pathological or mechanical reasons, prove impracticable, then the only change necessary to be made in the method of construction to insure success will be to make the surfaces of the teeth next the gum, mesio-distally, convex, and support the bridge anteriorily by a lug forming a movable joint with a filling in the cuspid.

This is the most conservative method, involving the cuspid, that can be used. By it the pulp is not involved, the natural independent mobility of the natural teeth is not impaired, and the bridge is more artistic, cleaner, and more acceptable to the patient than the modern bridge for the same space.

Presupposing the cuspid tooth sound, to substitute the two bicuspids without involving the cuspid leaves as the only alternative the resting of these teeth upon the gum.

When it is proved that the principle of covering the gum, as here interpreted, is unscientific, then I am unwilling to believe that any form of fixed saddle-bridge can have dental merit.

Justification for the belief in its possible practicability may be found in the following three cases of a number observed in practice.

One, showing the importance of imitating the forms of the natural teeth as a purely moral factor, is that of a woman for whom I made an upper vulcanite plate with five or six teeth. On the right side the only artificial tooth attached to the plate was the first molar. When this plate was placed in the mouth it seemed to have every point of merit that could be desired.

In a few days the patient returned and in a very positive manner stated that the plate did not fit.

After some fruitless questioning, I asked the patient, " On which side, in your opinion, is it that the plate does not fit? She indicated the right side. Here I observed that the buccal face of the artificial tooth extended out of line of the buccal faces of the two adjacent natural teeth. After grinding the artificial molar to alignment with the natural teeth and changing the plate, and in no other way, the patient left satisfied.

The next case is that of a physician, showing natural tolerance, for whom I made a bridge of a lateral and a cuspid supported by a crown on a loose first bicuspid, the near central being too loose to support one end.

The bridge was made with a gold plate three-eighths by three-fourths of an inch extending from the palatal surface of the lateral over and engaging the ridge. Clearly this is not clean, the bridge and plate moving with the loose bicuspid supporting it; nevertheless there is no sign of an inflamed area around this plate, and after three years it is still worn comfortably.

A case showing natural adaptability is a bridge for a young man consisting of the upper four incisors supported by the cuspids. In this case the absorption and consequent gum shrinkage was extreme, requiring the use of gum teeth, which could not be made to touch the gum and bear the normal relation to the lower teeth.

When this bridge was set temporarily, the space between the gum and the gold backing was at least three-sixteenths of an inch.

After it had been worn for two days the frænum was considerably lacerated by the porcelain gum being too high. This was remedied by grinding. Later the patient was annoyed by liquids and small particles of food passing between the gum and bridge, over the latter and under the lip. Three days later the patient reported no further annoyance from the space. Upon examination I found that the gum, without sign of inflammatory process, had extended out to the bridge until the space was entirely closed.

In conclusion, I beg to state that it has long been observed that the absorption of process is less when artificial teeth are substituted than when they are not.

This fact would tend to suggest the possibility of the process, under these bicuspids, increasing in density under the stimulus rather than its being absorbed. In my opinion this is not a space for a removable bridge. The application of this denture presupposes the two bicuspids the only missing teeth.

If the masticating area of six molars and two bicuspids is taken in the aggregate and compared to the masticating surface of these two bicuspids, the strain upon the latter in comparison will be found to be small. There is present this evening a young man wearing a denture like the one described, which I will be glad to have the members examine.

Adjourned.

OTTO E. INGLIS,

Editor Academy of Stomatology.

"F. D. I." INTERNATIONAL DENTAL FEDERATION.

INTERNATIONAL GROUPING OF DENTAL INTERESTS.

(Circular to the Presidents of National Dental Societies.)

OFFICE OF THE SECRETARY-GENERAL,

45 RUE DE LA TOUR D'AUVERGNE,

PARIS, September 18, 1903.

· DEAR SIR AND HONORED CONFRERE,—The International Dental Federation at its meeting held in Stockholm in August, 1902, in accordance with the powers that had been conferred upon it, decided that the Fourth International Dental Congress be held at St. Louis, Mo., in August 1904, at the time of the holding of the St. Louis Universal Exposition. The decision thus reached followed the receipt of invitations regularly addressed to the F. D. I. by the National Dental Association, the Odontological Society of St. Joseph, the National Association of Dental Examiners, the Odontographic Society of Missouri and Western Kansas, the Society of Dental Science of St. Louis, the Committee appointed by the Missouri State Dental Association, the Dental Society of St. Louis, the city of St. Louis, the government of the State of Missouri, and the authorities of the Louisiana Purchase Exposition. This decision was confirmed at the session of the F. D. I. held in Madrid in April, 1903.

The officers of the executive Council of the F. D. I., in accord with the authorities of the Exposition and the Committee of Organization of the Congress, have determined the conditions under which the Federation will take part in the organization of said Congress, and we are now officially advised that the Fourth International Dental Congress will be held in the city of St. Louis in 1904, from August 29 to September 3, inclusive.

The purpose of this circular is to inform you that the International Dental Federation has decided to lend its entire support to the organizers of the Fourth International Dental Congress, and, in view of assuring the perfect success of the Congress, we therefore request you to appeal to the several dental societies in your country to take part in the said Fourth International Dental Congress.

It seems unnecessary to call your attention to the importance of all dental societies the world over being appropriately represented at this gathering, both scientifically and professionally. We think it, however, desirable to call attention to matters which the delegates of the different federations and national societies will be called upon to discuss with reference to the organization of the second term of the International Dental Federation,—that which will be comprised, namely, in the period between the fourth and fifth international dental congresses.

During the first working period of the F. D. I., comprised between the Third International Dental Congress held in Paris in 1900 and that of St. Louis to be held in 1904, the members of the Executive Council of the F. D. I. who were appointed in Paris by your representatives have fulfilled to the best of their abilities the mission with which they had been intrusted by the members of the Third International Dental Congress, of which you may have been able to judge from perusal of the printed transactions of its different meetings.

They have assured the holding of a Fourth International Dental Congress (resolution No. 13).

They have created an International Commission of Education, which presented a programme of international dental education at the sessions held in London, Cambridge, Stockholm, and Madrid (resolution No. 16).

The International Commission of Dental Hygiene, organized at the Cambridge session, will at the St. Louis meeting complete the programme of international dental hygiene to be recommended to the public authorities.

Other projects of interest to the evolution of dentistry—such.

for instance, as the publication of an international dental review—
are being carefully studied in view of future realization.   Reports
have been prepared and presented on the federation of schools; and
other propositions are now under consideration, such as the creation
of a universal nomenclature, and also of a code of ethics to be
universally accepted.   The execution of these projects will fall on
our successors in the subsequent terms of the F. D. I.

It will be the duty of the delegates to the St. Louis Congress to
ratify the constitution of the F. D. I., to introduce such amend-
ments as may be necessary, to appoint the members that will represent the different countries in the Executive Council, and to
decide on the programme of the second period of the F. D. I.

Appreciating the importance of the great international gathering to be held in St. Louis in August, 1904, we are convinced that
you will be able to induce the National Dental Association and the
other dental societies of your country to take part in the Congress
by sending delegates and by contributing scientific papers.

We request that this circular be published in all the dental
journals of your country.

Please accept, dear sir and *confrère,* the assurances of our fraternal sentiments.

Dr. Ch. Godon, *President.*
Dr. E. Sauvez, *Secretary-General.*

Editorial.

WILL THE DENTAL COLLEGES REVERSE THEIR DECISION?

Twenty years in the past the organization known as the National Association of Dental Faculties was born, or, to be exact,
August 4, 1884.   From that time to the present year there has
been a constant struggle to legislate for a higher standard of dental
education in this country.   Through a fifth of a century, step by
step, the culmination of all these years of anxious labor was reached
when the vote was finally announced in the Faculties Association
that the resolution requiring that four years of seven months in

each course had been adopted, and that all the colleges in membership with the organization were expected to faithfully comply with its demands. The unanimity of this vote was not the least pleasing feature of this advanced stand taken in dental education. It seemed to imply something more than a passing resolve that might possibly lead to a change from varied motives, but indicated that dentistry had made, practically, its final stand in the United States for thorough training, and from this decision there could be no retrograde movement tolerated.

The meeting preceding the enforcement of this resolution was that held at Asheville, N. C., in August last. Rumors were rife that this session would witness a change of opinion and possibly an effort might be made to rescind the former action. The vote, however, on the Harvard application, refusing permission for that school to remain at three years, seemed to settle all fears in that direction, in the minds of those present, as to the stability of the four years' course.

Three months subsequent to this meeting rumors were again heard that an effort was being made in certain quarters to call a meeting of the Association of Faculties at Buffalo during the session of the Institute of Pedagogics, to consider the necessity of returning to a three years' course. Even then it was not supposed that the active workers in this move would carry this out in violation of all precedent traditions, and in actual repudiation of established rules of the organization. Those who thus regarded the matter were doomed to disappointment, and were startled to receive a notice, in due form, from the chairman of the Executive Committee, that upon the demand of five members (colleges) belonging to the Association a meeting of the National Association of Faculties would be held in Buffalo at the time named. This meeting has since been held, and hence, whether for good or ill, its work has passed into history.

The fact that this was done cannot be lightly passed over. Dental education is the most important topic to claim the consideration of broad-minded men in dentistry, and to permit this attempt to lower its standard without journalistic comment would be to render valueless all periodical literature, for herein lies its especial duty.

This meeting must have been a disappointment to those who anticipated much from its decisions, for in this respect it was inconclusive, and this should have been anticipated before a single notice had been sent forth. If this were understood in advance of action, then those who engineered the meeting must have been fully cognizant that it would resolve itself into a conference—politically, a caucus—and thus crystallize sentiment to enable them to carry the backward movement with a hurrah at the annual meeting to be held the present year. With this motive, if held, the writer has nothing to do, for the importance of the main issue transcends all seeming sinister motives, for it strikes at the very root of dental education in this country, and, if successful, will place this where it stood twenty years ago. One retrograde step is simply the forerunner of another. This is the lesson of history, and must not be forgotten or be overlooked.

The immediate injury, however, while destructive to dental education in general, will be equally injurious to the association that represents it, and here the writer desires to dwell for the time being.

When persons join an organization, of whatever character, they become by both word and deed bound to obey the rules of said body, and under no circumstances, however tempting, should they even offer to violate these. For what, then, have these members become responsible in calling this meeting?

First, the Executive Committee has never been given power to call a special meeting of the Association of Faculties. No provision has ever been made in its rules for any such meeting, for its whole spirit since its origin has been adverse to the possibility of a snap judgment upon vital questions. No such meeting in its entire history was ever contemplated or desired. The article in the constitution giving that committee power to call the regular meeting at "such time and place" as might be deemed necessary was a wise provision to give liberty to change in case the Executive Committee of the National Dental Association selected a different time and place of meeting for that body, a change frequently found desirable. The intention was that the Faculties should always meet at the same time and place with this body. This was done largely as a matter of convenience for those members who belonged to both organizations, to avoid unnecessary travel and expense. The only time in the history of the Faculties that it met independently was at Chicago in 1885, when the then national body, the American Dental Association, met at Minneapolis. This proved the least valuable meeting of the entire series, and this was altogether due to the fact that the work was hurriedly passed upon by the members, so that they could proceed to the aforesaid national gathering. Some of those-present at these Chicago sessions have been in opposition to any meeting separate from the national body since that day.

The present meeting was called at the request of five colleges. As before stated, there is no authority for this. It is presumed some had been reading the report of the Committee on Codification of the Rules, presented at the Asheville meeting, and in which the said committee interpolated a provision for the calling of special meetings, but, as this report was laid over for action at the regular meeting in 1904, it has no force until its adoption, and therefore the Executive Committee exceeded its powers in consenting to the request of the five members (colleges). In the call for special meetings in all organized bodies, when these have rules providing for them, it is necessary to state in the call the subjects to be acted upon, and this was not neglected upon this occasion, and it was, perhaps, the only regular part of the proceedings. The members were fully notified that the " Four-Year Rule," together with the " Count" question, would be considered. It must have been well known that the first had no legal status in such a meeting, for all subjects affecting the interests of dental colleges connected with the Association must lie over for one year before action, and due notice must be given to this effect in the official report. This applies with equal force to the second proposition. This being understood, it is not surprising that the special meeting resolved itself into a discussional gathering and resulted in a fiasco, as far as dealing finally with the problems named. From what has been gathered from reports, not much comfort was derived for those who advocated a course of three years with nine months in each session, for the general spirit was antagonistic to even this compromise. There seemed to be an entire want of harmony of purpose with those who desired retrograde action.

The writer feels that a wrong has been done the Association of Faculties, first, by calling this meeting without authority, and, second, in the attempt to lower the standard of dental education it had so carefully secured through years of constant struggle; and, further, in thus attempting a retrograde they have tried, whether intentional or not, to make dental education in this country a subject for reproach throughout the professional world.

Will this effort to effect a return to three years be successful? The answer to this question can best be given after the close of the next regular meeting of the Faculties. That the effort will be made by the colleges interested in this retrograde movement is self-evident, but it is not possible that it can be successfully carried through. The writer has not lost faith in that professional spirit that looks to higher results than the sordid accumulation of money. It is believed that there are a sufficient number who will stand solidly for the advanced standard already established. If, however, this trustful feeling should not be realized, and the next meeting should show that the National Association of Dental Faculties had reversed its position on the question of dental education, then may the dental profession in the United States mark the beginning of decadence of the professional character so earnestly striven for during the past half-century, and, in addition, it will present a spectacle for a jeering professional world. May our colleagues seriously consider the situation, and come prepared at the annual meeting to uphold, at all hazards, the honor of American dentistry.

It was suggested at the Buffalo, so-called, special meeting that the Faculties be called together in June instead of August, possibly at Louisville, Ky. In view of what has been already stated, this is simply a usurpation of power on the part of the Executive Committee, for the meeting, as organized, had not the slightest authority to change the original intention of meeting at St. Louis. It is to be hoped that the Executive Committee will not fall twice into error in one year. It must be remembered that probably all the members will desire to visit St. Louis during the Exposition and the World's Dental Congress. This membership extends from New England to California, and it is unreasonable to ask these widely separated members to travel long distances in summer, in some cases across the continent, to attend two meetings. The experiment of holding a separate meeting has already been considered, and the injurious effect demonstrated then will be intensified during this year if this be attempted. The men who will actively manage the World's Dental Congress are those mainly interested in dental education, and their interests should be considered. Those who will attend the Congress at St. Louis will naturally arrange to spend several weeks there. This was the experience of those in attendance at the Columbian Exposition at Chicago, and no difficulty was found then in holding the meetings in advance of the great world's dental convocation. It is very true that the success of this must be assured regardless of what may be termed local interests, but if it is desired to injure the Congress, there seems no better way than to decentralize the various meetings of the year. A much better plan would be to postpone all the national meetings until 1905, for nothing would suffer by this action, while it would concentrate effort on the one meeting that should and doubtless will represent the dentistry of the world as it exists in 1904.

NOVEL METHOD IN CONFERRING DEGREES.

THE traffic in diplomas has evidently started in a new section of country, if the following quotations indicate that which is implied by the text. It has been rumored for some time that a college in Toronto, Dominion of Canada, would accept legally registered practitioners from any part of the British Colonial possessions and upon an examination confer the degree of Doctor of Dental Surgery (D.D.S.). This, taken at its face value, would seem a harmless proceeding, but when analyzed it assumes special importance and worthy the attention of all interested in keeping the degree in dentistry fully up to the standard established by the National Association of Dental Faculties.

The following is taken from the published announcement of the " Royal College of Dental Surgeons of Ontario :"

" Students of Dentistry *not desiring to qualify for practice in the province of Ontario,* by obtaining the L.D.S. of the R.C.D.S. of Ontario, *may avail themselves of all the privileges of the school of dentistry of the R.C.D.S.* and proceed to the degree of Doctor of Dental Surgery, either in the University of Toronto, or in Trinity University, on compliance with the requirements of their curriculum in dentistry."

The requirement in the announcement of Trinity University, Toronto, is as follows : " All legally qualified practitioners of Dental Surgery of Great Britain, or of any portion of the British empire, will be admitted to the final examination without passing further matriculation and without *further attendance on lectures.* Fee for registration, $5. Fee for final examination, $10. Fee for degree of D.D.S., $15." (Italics ours.)

In a private letter from a prominent official, in another school, to an applicant, the writer warmly endorses this university and its methods.

One of the singular conditions demanded in conferring this degree is to be found in the fact that the recipient is not to make use of it in the Dominion of Canada, but it is available only in other portions of the colonial possessions of Great Britain; in other words, it is not quite good enough for Canada, but will answer very well for outlying districts. This appears to be a remarkable assumption of authority, especially as there is no indication that the people in said sections of the empire have been consulted in the matter. This, however, can be settled by the colonial residents without interference from this side of the boundary line.

It is not supposed that the active originators of this novel method of conferring a degree thought for a moment that they might be imitating the dealers in fraudulent diplomas, but their action comes perilously near to the standard set up by these individuals.

The diplomas sent out from Chicago were not dealt out to persons in the United States, but were considered most suited to the residents of foreign climes. In justice to the schools in Toronto it must be stated that they do require a certain amount of attendance sufficiently long to make an examination. This was not regarded as important by the Chicago diploma manufacturers.

In some of the colonial possessions of Great Britain dentists are trained solely in private practice, and after a certain time are permitted to come up for examination, attendance at a dental college not being required. This is true of New Zealand, where a three years' private preceptorship is demanded, and nothing further except the government examination.

With these facts known to all dental educators, how is it possible for men having a supposed interest in higher dental education to continue such objectionable methods? Whether this plan will tend to attract many from Australia, New Zealand, or South Africa is not important to those dwelling this side of the Dominion, but it is important to these that the degree which originated here be kept unsullied and free from the taint of commercialism. From its adoption as a test of ability, the effort has been to raise its value, and the degree of Doctor of Dental Surgery (D.D.S.) received its highest valuation when a four years' course was demanded of the undergraduates. That the schools in the Dominion of Canada should offer an easy path to its acquirement is not only discreditable, but is in direct violation of the ruling of the National Association of Dental Faculties. To preserve this degree in its purity has been the aim of this organization from its origin, and it cannot view with complacency this open attempt to lessen its value through methods that must be condemned by all dental educators throughout the world.

CORRECTION OF A SERIOUS ERROR.

FROM a number of letters received at this office, it is inferred that a very erroneous opinion exists in the minds of many of the good friends of the INTERNATIONAL that this journal has been sold to the J. B. Lippincott Company, and, to that extent, has ceased to be a professional journal. We beg to assure those interested in the JOURNAL's welfare that it remains exactly as it has during the years of its existence, in the ownership of the stockholders who originally established it under its present title. Some business arrangements were entered into, to render it, it is hoped, of greater value to the dental profession, but beyond that it will remain, as it always has, free from trade complications, an outspoken vehicle of independent thought and an earnest advocate for that which tends to elevate dentistry wherever it is practised as a profession.

Bibliography.

Hale's Epitome of Anatomy. A Manual for Students and Physicians. By Henry E. Hale, A.M.., M.D., Assistant Demonstrator of Anatomy College of Physicians and Surgeons (Columbia University) New York. In one 12mo volume of three hundred and eighty-four pages, with seventy-one illustrations. Lea Brothers & Co., Publishers, Philadelphia and New York, 1903.

This volume covers three hundred and eighty-four pages and seventy-one engravings, yet the matter is so carefully condensed that, like the others of the Lea series, it can be carried in the pocket for ready reference.

Every medical and dental student regards his Gray with peculiar reverence, but this large volume, wonderful in its simplicity and teaching force, cannot readily be handled at all times, and the student needs just such an epitome for his daily work. The foundation study of anatomy must necessarily be the same, whether it be derived from larger or smaller work, but there are manuals and manuals, each one aiming to give the subject in condensed form, but this one, like the others of the series, shows a marked ability in condensing without loss by abbreviation. The subjects follow each other in orderly sequence, and subjoined to these are a series of questions. These may, possibly, be of more value here than in the other books of the series, in that they enable the student to give a self-examination at the critical periods of college and State examinations. The condensed thoroughness of this book makes it, as well as the others, of very great value.

Domestic Correspondence.

AN APOLOGY TO DR. L. C. BRYAN, OF BASEL, SWITZERLAND.

To THE EDITOR:

SIR,—Will you kindly permit me, through the JOURNAL, to make my humble apology to Dr. L. C. Bryan for what appears to me, as I read it in cold type, a little discourteous.

Dr. Bryan in his reply (see January INTERNATIONAL DENTAL JOURNAL, page 69) to the discussion at the meeting of the Institute of Stomatology, held May 5, 1903, upon his paper, which was read and discussed that evening, says, " Dr. F. Milton Smith says ' there is nothing new in either the paper of Dr. Bryan or that by Dr. Smith, of Philadelphia.' "

By reference to the discussion I read (INTERNATIONAL DENTAL JOURNAL, November, 1903, page 857), " Dr. F. Milton Smith stated that it seemed to him that the whole thing was a matter of thoroughness. He could not see that there were any very new things suggested either by the paper of the evening or by Dr. Smith, of Philadelphia. It seemed to him that if Dr. Smith had announced that we were at times a little careless and that we ought to be more thorough, he would have hit the nail on the head. To this charge he [Dr. F. Milton Smith] would plead guilty."

My apology to Dr. Bryan is not for these remarks. I think any fair-minded man will see in them at least a little more courtesy than Dr. Bryan's *quotation* would seem to indicate.

Dr. Bryan also in his reply states that " it would be something new if a Dr. Smith of New York would acknowledge that a Dr. Smith of Philadelphia could tell him anything."

As to this, may I at this time say publicly that which I have spoken many, many times in private,—that through the courtesy of Dr. D. D. Smith, of Philadelphia, I was permitted to inspect, in his office, the mouths of probably ten or twelve people who had been under his treatment for some years. These patients represented almost every class of dental service. As an exhibition of magnificent *thoroughness* in cleansing and polishing, in gold fillings

6

and bridge-work, and in amalgam (I think), in fact, in almost every class of work, I have never seen its equal; and I further say that I very much doubt if five men in the whole world can show such a beautiful result of thoroughness in all-around dental service, including oral prophylaxis.

This, of course, is only my opinion. In the sense that I had never seen such a beautiful dental exhibit before, I am compelled to say that Dr. Smith did show me something new.

To admit, however, that Dr. D. D. Smith has discovered an entirely new process, a sort of " Aladdin's lamp," so to speak, that by its magical power changes poor broken-down teeth into perfect glistening pearls, I am not willing to admit. I will admit that Dr. Smith has certainly provoked me to be more thorough and careful, and for this I am profoundly grateful to him.

But the remark for which I desire to apologize to Dr. Bryan is found on page 858 (INTERNATIONAL DENTAL JOURNAL), sixth and seventh lines: "He [Dr. F. Milton Smith] believed there were thorough men outside of Philadelphia and this side of Switzerland." This was certainly superfluous and, as it appears to me, not quite in tune with that high standard which every true gentleman should seek to attain unto.

I make my humble apology to Dr. Bryan, and promise him in the future I will try to be a more *thorough* gentleman.

F. MILTON SMITH.

NEW YORK CITY, January 9, 1904.

Obituary.

DR. T. B. WELCH.

DIED, at Overbrook, near Philadelphia, Pa., December 29, 1903, Thomas Bromwell Welch, M.D., aged seventy-eight years.

Dr. Welch was born in Glastonbury, Somersetshire, England, December 31, 1825, and came to this country when quite young. His education was obtained at the public schools of Watertown, N. Y. After a course of study at the Gouverneur Wesleyan Seminary, he entered the Wesleyan Methodist ministry, and served several charges in New York State. Later he entered a medical college and graduated with the medical degree when in his twenty-sixth year. After a few years' medical practice he decided to practise dentistry, settling in Winona, Minn., about 1856. In 1865 he removed to Vineland, N. J., where he continued dental practice. About 1869 he originated a method of preserving grape-juice absolutely free from alcohol, especially designed for church communion and medical uses. This grape-juice became more and more popular as the years went by, and is now well known all over the world.

Dr. Welch was first brought prominently to the notice of the dental profession as the manufacturer of an improved alloy for amalgam. Shortly after the late Dr. Flagg and his colaborers had announced their "New Departure" theories, there was a demand in the profession for something better than the alloys then on sale at the dental depots. Dr. Welch had prepared an alloy for his own use, samples of which he distributed to some of his professional friends, who were much pleased with it. This was brought to the notice of the New Jersey State Dental Society, of which Dr. Welch was then a member, at the meeting held July, 1878, and resulted in a resolution requesting Dr. Welch, or any other of its members, to place on the market an alloy, reliable, and yet at a reasonable price. In response to this, Dr. Welch began the manufacture of his Gold-and-platina alloy; and that it was "reliable" is attested by its quickly becoming, and still remaining, notwithstanding its many competitors, the stand-by of many excellent operators.

At the same time he began the publication of a bi-monthly dental journal, mainly as an advertising medium, entitled *Items of Interest*. This first appeared as a four-page folio, June, 1879. As its name indicated, it was made up of "items of interest" to dentists, and as Dr. Welch possessed the rare, yet happy faculty of quickly discerning, condensing, and properly presenting items of interest appearing in dental and other journals, his unpretentious little journal soon made for itself a place in dental literature. The second volume terminated with the December number (No. 4), 1880, in order to begin Vol. III. with January, 1881; and with the third number, May, 1881, it became, and has since continued, a monthly. Beginning with Vol. IV. the number of pages was increased to sixteen, and their size reduced from folio to quarto. The first number of Vol. V. was issued in quarto form, but with the

February number it was changed to an octavo of forty-eight pages, and later the January number was reissued to correspond. The yearly subscription of Vols. I. and II. was fifteen cents, Vols. III. and IV., fifty cents, and with Vol. V. it was raised to one dollar. While still at Vineland, Dr. Welch enlarged his business to include dental supplies, and early in 1881 removed to 1405 Filbert Street, Philadelphia, where, under the firm name of Drs. T. B. Welch & Son, he opened a dental depot. In a few months he moved to 1413 Filbert Street; in June, 1885, the firm-name became "Welch Dental Company," and this, in March, 1889, gave way to the "Wilmington Dental Manufacturing Company." In July, 1896, this corporation became financially embarrassed and terminated, and the journal Dr. Welch had so long edited passed into other hands. Dr. Welch then began the publication of a dental journal in much the same style entitled *Welch's Dental Journal,* which later, in other hands, became the *Dental Brief.* Dr. Welch was a ready writer. He earnestly urged the importance of terseness and clearness upon contributors to his journal, and set a good example in these respects by his own contributions.

Dr. Welch was a strong advocate of total abstinence, and took an active part in the work of seeking out and prosecuting illegal liquor selling. He was also interested in the so-called spelling reform, substituting phonetic, or sound spelling, for the arbitrary method in general use.

Dr. Welch possessed a kindly disposition, and delighted in doing good. He was a devoted and prominent member of the Methodist church in Vineland, where he so long resided, and where he was buried.

After the death of his wife he married, in 1895, Miss Sherburne, of Vineland, who survives him. His surviving children are Drs. George and Charles E. Welch; Mrs. Dr. Emma Slade, Mrs. Dr. Thomas, Mrs. Professor Murray, and Mrs. Milo Gould.

W. H. T.

Miscellany.

RETAINING PORCELAIN INLAYS.—Erich Schmidt, of Berlin ("The Filling of Teeth with Porcelain," by Walter Wolfgang Bruck, page 49), suggests a novel method of forming the retaining grooves in porcelain inlays. Before filling the matrix with the porcelain paste he places upon the floor of the matrix small pieces of copper wire, and after the inlay is fused he places it into nitric acid, by which the copper is quickly dissolved, leaving grooves well adapted for retention. For inlays fused at a lower temperature than that at which copper melts this will prove an excellent idea, as it enables the operator to form the retaining grooves in positions where they could not be cut with a disk, and of a form more retentive than can be made with a revolving tool. The presence of the copper does not seem to impair the color of the inlay.

ASBESTOS AND ALCOHOL AS AN INVESTMENT.—In some cases alcohol is much to be preferred to water in forming ground asbestos into a paste when it is used as an investment. As soon as the investment is complete, by setting the alcohol on fire, it is dried out quickly, and can be immediately subjected to heat without risk of displacement. When water is used the heat must be applied cautiously, especially in delicate work, to avoid displacement by the water boiling.

A DANGEROUS FEATURE OF ARSENICAL PASTE.—An editorial in the October number of the *Dental Cosmos* (1903) invites attention to several cases in which serious trouble has followed the use of this agent in devitalizing a dental pulp and afterwards filling the tooth temporarily or permanently, without removing the devitalized tissue. In all these cases a mummifying paste had been used. In each case, shortly after the operation the patient had returned to the operator complaining of a continued dull throbbing pain and swelling and tumefaction of the tissues about the socket of the treated tooth, the pain extending deeply into the jaw. This was followed by severe inflammation, exfoliation of the tooth, and much distress during a long period of repair. The writer suggests that this may be due to the arsenic absorbed by the proteid elements of the pulp-tissue and by the hæmoglobin of the vascular supply to the organ being liberated by a breaking down of these tissues and diffused throughout the structure of the root until it sets up an arsenical necrosis in the pericementum. He advises, and urges, great care in the use of this agent, the prompt removal of the devitalized tissue, and a more general use of strictly surgical methods of pulp extirpation under cocaine anæsthesia.

He also suggests that it is highly probable that ingredients of the mummifying paste, when applied to arsenic-saturated pulp-tissue, by virtue of their affinity for proteid matter, upon which their tanning property or their power to bring about the fixation of animal tissue depends, contributes to the result by liberating the arsenic from its original proteid combination in the pulp, thus setting it free to work out its destructive results upon the retentive tissues.

W. H. T.

LEAD-PENCIL ERASING POINTS AS DENTAL TOOLS.—Dr. C. H. Land (*Dental Cosmos,* vol xlv., August, 1903, page 617) recommends the rubber erasing points of Dixon's Secretary lead-pencils, No. 2, and his Cabinet, No. 2—724, as useful tools in forming the matrix for inlays. He suggests that the operator be provided with a half-dozen of each, trimmed into suitable sizes and shapes by means of a coarse emory disk in the dental engine. The rubber of which they are made is a soft variety, and especially desirable for this purpose; they are, moreover, purchasable at any book or stationery store, and are inexpensive.

A USEFUL PAIN OBTUNDENT.—Chloretone dissolved in chloroform is a convenient pain obtundent in preparing cavities of decay for filling, preparing roots for crowning, and for extracting. Chloretone dissolves sparingly in water, but quite freely in chloroform. A few of the crystals dissolved in a few drops of chloroform forms an effective solution quickly made when needed. A pellet of cotton saturated with this and placed in the cavity for about a minute, makes a very perceptible difference in the pain of excavating. Applied in like manner about a root makes its preparation for crowning far less painful, and assists in extraction. It is also a germicide. It cannot be safely used hypodermically.

EXCESS OF SOLDER TO BE AVOIDED IN PORCELAIN WORK.—In an article upon "Porcelain Dental Art" (*Dental Cosmos,* vol. xlv., August, 1903, page 617) Dr. C. H. Land emphasizes the importance of care in avoiding an excess of pure gold used as a solder in constructing platinum jackets and other devices used as a base for porcelain restorations, and, indeed, all work over which porcelain is to be fused. In the first place, an excess is apt to cause discoloration of the porcelain. Secondly, if the platinum is very thin there is danger of the pure gold alloying with it and melting a hole when the work is subjected to the intense heat of the porcelain furnace, just as the base metals will do at a very much lower heat. Thirdly, it is apt to cause warping. Hence it is important to make all joints fit closely and neatly, so as to reduce the amount of pure gold needed as solder to a minimum.

Current News.

THE NEW YORK INSTITUTE OF STOMATOLOGY.

THE following officers of The New York Institute of Stomatology have been elected for 1904:

President, A. H. Brockway; Vice-President, C. O. Kimball; Treasurer, J. Adams Bishop; Recording Secretary, H. L. Wheeler; Corresponding Secretary, J. B. Locherty; Curator, S. H. McNaughton; Editor, F. L. Bogue; Past President, J. Morgan Howe.

Executive Committee.—S. E. Davenport, Chairman; Charles F. Allan, F. Milton Smith.

SOUTHERN BRANCH, NATIONAL DENTAL ASSOCIATION.

THE next meeting of the Southern Branch of the National Dental Association will be held in Washington, D. C., February 23 to 26, inclusive. The Association will meet conjointly with the District of Columbia and Maryland State Dental Associations, in response to an invitation from those local organizations.

The opening meeting will be held in Columbian University Hall, Fifteenth, corner H Street, N. W. The clinics and other meetings of the Association will be held in the Medical and Dental Department building of Columbian University on H Street, between Thirteenth and Fourteenth Streets. There will be a banquet at the New Willard Hotel on Thursday evening, February 25, given by the Maryland State Dental Association and the District of Columbia Dental Society, complimentary to the Southern Branch of the National Dental Association as their guests.

The Southeastern Passenger Association grants a rate of one and one-third fare, plus twenty-five cents, from all points in territory south of the Ohio and Potomac and east of the Mississippi. The hotels of Washington have granted reduced rates, as follows:

The New Willard (head-quarters), $2.50 and up, European plan; the Raleigh, $2 and up, European plan; the Ebbitt, $3 and up, American plan; the Riggs, $3 and up, American plan; the Oxford, $2 and up, American plan; the Hamilton, $2 and up, American plan.

Ample provision will be made at the University for clinics and exhibits. All practitioners who conduct themselves according to the code of ethics are cordially invited to attend.

L. G. NOEL,

Chairman Programme Committee.

[The foregoing notice of the Southern Branch of the National Dental Association was received as we were about to go to press, and too late for the insertion of the list of papers and clinics. This is an unusually full one, indicating the promise of an exceedingly interesting meeting at Washington, D. C.—ED.]

THE

International Dental Journal.

| VOL. XXV. | MARCH, 1904. | No. 3. |

Original Communications.[1]

SOME HISTOLOGICAL FACTS THAT CONTRADICT THE GENERALLY ACCEPTED ODONTOBLAST THEORY.[2]

BY MICHAEL MORGENSTERN, STRASSBURG, GERMANY.

MR. CHAIRMAN AND MEMBERS OF THE SECTION,—The committee of the Section on Stomatology of the American Medical Association has been kind enough to invite me to address you on the subject of my investigations on the pulp. While I feel very much honored by your kind invitation, I nevertheless approach my task with some trepidation, because my histological examinations lead me to conclusions that are considerably at variance with those that others who have worked along similar lines have arrived at in the course of the past years. It is this fact that makes it somewhat embarrassing for me to address you. In Germany I have for the present only a small number of followers, and I fear that the majority of you who are assembled here to-day are also fanatic

---

[1] The editor and publishers are not responsible for the views of authors of papers published in this department, nor for any claim to novelty, or otherwise, that may be made by them. No papers will be received for this department that have appeared in any other journal published in the country.

[2] Lecture with lantern-slide demonstration, read before the American Medical Association, Section on Stomatology, at New Orleans, May 5 to 8, 1903.

adherents of the old odontoblast theory; consequently I assure you that I expect only a moderate amount of applause and of approbation at your hands.

But it is in your country precisely that the first voices were raised years ago against the prevailing views in regard to the rôle of the odontoblasts, and while I do not fully share the views of Heitzmann, Bödecker, Abbott, and Andrews, I nevertheless recognize in these men brave pioneers, and their example inspires me with the courage to appear with my results before an audience that is composed of the greatest investigators in our particular field of research.

Fig. 1.

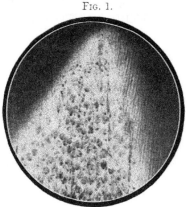

Multiple layer of odontoblasts at the tip of the dentine germ from the cuspid tooth of a new-born infant. Longitudinal section.

According to the views that are prevalent in regard to the rôle of the odontoblasts, the surface of the pulp is covered with a single layer of cells that are in intimate contact with each other like epithelium; these are the dentine cells, or odontoblasts, each one of which sends a protoplasmic process (dentine fibre) into the dentine. It is claimed that these odontoblasts are perennial,—*i.e.,* that they persist during the formation of the dentine, and are neither reduced in number during this process nor replaced by other cells. It is further claimed that the nutrition and the sensation of the dentine is exclusively bound to these dentine cells and their protoplasmic processes. All subsequent formative changes in the dentine, as, for instance, the genesis of the transparent zone in caries and the broadening of Neumann's sheath in senile teeth, are also believed to be exclusively due to metaplastic activity going on in the protoplasmic processes of the odontoblasts.

The great advantage of this theory is its simplicity, for the most complicated physiological processes can be explained on a very simple, one might almost say, unitarian histologic basis. The very fact, however, that everything seems so simple should lead us to be sceptical. Recent investigations into the structure and the composition of the albumins teach us that things that appear exceedingly simple are nevertheless most complicated, and it seems hardly prob-

FIG. 2.

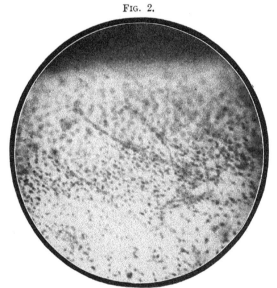

Multiple odontoblast layer in process of degeneration, from the pulp of an incisor tooth of a new-born calf. Longitudinal section.

able that different physiological processes can be explained on the basis of one histologic unit. True, the adherents of the odontoblast theory point out that in the lower orders of animal creation a single cell or group of cells may occasionally assume all the functions of the organism and that similar conditions might obtain in the case of the odontoblasts; against this argument we can formulate the objection that the odontoblasts are simply parts of a more complicated organism, and that in higher orders of animal creation the anatomic differentiation proceeds *pari passu* with the physiologic division of labor that becomes operative in complicated organisms; one might further object that in no vertebrate is any other cell variety known to exist whose protoplasm can at the same time perform the functions of nutrition, of sensation, and of metaplastic transformation.

These theoretic objections alone do not, however, lead me to doubt the correctness and the validity of the odontoblast theory as it is accepted to-day; I have, moreover, been able to discover a number of histological facts that cannot be reconciled with this

Fig. 3.

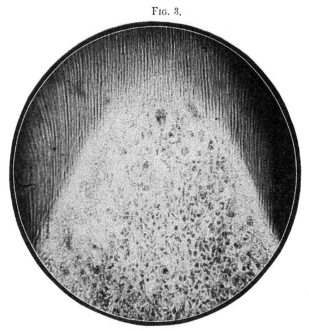

Total degeneration of the multiple odontoblast layer at the tip of the dentine germ of a temporary molar tooth of a new-born infant. Longitudinal section.

theory. It is the main object of this address to demonstrate these histological facts to you with the aid of lantern-slides that I have made from my microscopic preparations.

1. I have frequently seen, in the so-called pulp-horns of the dentine germ in the fœtus and the new-born, the dentine cells arranged in a multiple layer. Fig. 1 is one of a series of sagittal sections through the anterior dental germs of a new-born child. You will notice that each dentine cell is pear-shaped; you will also

notice the direction of each dentine fibre and of the capillaries, for all these features show that we are actually dealing with a longitudinal section and not with a diagonal section in which the multiple arangement of the cells might be simulated. The layer I am discussing consists of ten to twenty rows of cells. The individual cells show no trace of lateral flattening from mutual pressure; on the contrary, capillaries and fibrillæ will be seen running between the different cells in a direction that is parallel to the longitudinal

Fig. 4.

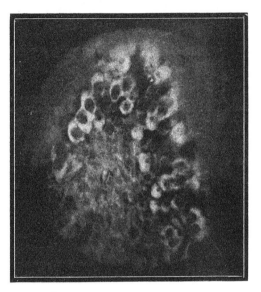

Changes in the odontoblasts before the beginning of dentiuogeuous disintegration. From the tip of the dentine germ of an incisor tooth of a sheep's fœtus.

axis of the dentine germ. It is clear, therefore, that the cells are not arranged in several layers on account of crowding or lack of room and mutual pressure.

The structural changes in the dentine cells also call for discussion. It will be seen that the cells become paler from the bottom towards the surface of the layer, that the nuclei disappear, and that the cell boundaries become indistinct, until finally near the margin of the dentine hardly any cell remnants can be seen; for in this zone the changes in the substance and the structure of the cells are so far advanced that the dentine cells have become fully disintegrated and have disappeared from view.

FIG. 5.

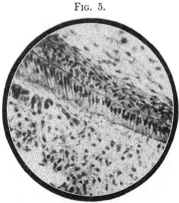

From the longitudinal section of a portion of the pulp from a normal premolar tooth of a girl of twelve years. Multiple layer of odontoblasts and demonstration of all the vessels and nerves of the pulp. particularly of the spindle-shaped cells of Ranvier.

If we compare Fig. 2, made from a frontal section through the pulp-ridge of a young tooth, with Fig. 1, we will find the same

FIG. 6.

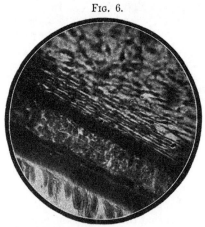

Last stage of conjugation of dentine cells, from the tip of a molar tooth of a young rabbit, the tip having undergone partial calcification.

conditions. Here again we see a broad layer of oval and round cells, that are already beginning to become pale, extending up to the edge of the dentine; the layer here consists of some twelve rows of cells. These cells are odontoblasts in a state of dentino-genous metamorphosis, and show evidence of beginning disinte-gration. Between the cells we see capillaries running in the same direction as the dentine canaliculi. Below this zone we see the pulp-cells in close aggregation, arranged in rows and extending their processes into the layer of disintegrating odontoblasts; these cells are in a state of conjugation or of disintegration. These processes lead to the formation of odontoblasts.

FIG. 7.

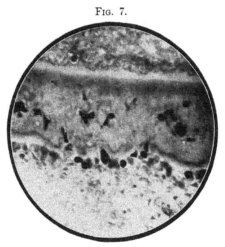

First stage of conjugation of the mesodermic cells of the dentine germ for the forma-tion of odontoblasts; also some preformed dentine fibres in places where no odontoblasts as yet exist. From the dentine germ of a human fœtus.

In preparing a tooth-germ according to the method of Koch-Weil, and in making a section without decalcification, spherical solid structures are seen in place of the pale disintegrated odonto-blasts; these spheres were formerly considered to be dentine spheres or globular masses, and were described by these names. In another stage of the formation of dentine a transparent homogeneous layer composed of single trabeculæ is occasionally seen in place of the disintegrating odontoblasts.

If a tooth is still in a developmental stage, and is only incom-pletely decalcified, spherical structures are also seen in the place of disintegrating odontoblasts; many of these little globules, how-ever, contain remnants of cells and nuclei; in injected specimens

I was even able to detect capillaries between the spheres. These capillaries could be sharply differentiated from the colorless spheres of dentinogen by their intense color.

After this discursion you will be able to understand Fig. 3, prepared from a frontal longitudinal section through the germ of a molar tooth in a new-born infant. The preparation was decalcified until all the calcium salts were removed. In the natural state dentinogenous masses of spheres were found throughout the whole visible portion of the pulp; after careful and thorough decalcification a wide layer of disintegrating cells was seen instead, in which

FIG. 8.

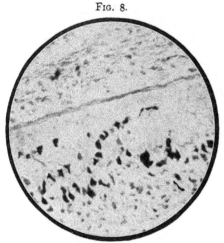

First formation of dentine and trabeculæ of odontoblasts without nuclei. From a longitudinal section of the dentine germ of a cow's tooth.

odontoblasts could no longer be found. Towards the centre, pulp-cells are seen that are odontoblasts and that send processes or fibrillæ into certain portions of the area of disintegrating cells and through this zone into the dentine.

In a later stage of formation dentine appears in the place of the mass of globules and the pulp-cells are seen to have undergone metamorphosis into trabeculæ of odontoblasts; some of them become distended and appear as cartilage cells that are surrounded by a light areola. This is the stage that preceded the disintegration or the dentinogenous formation of globules and that is illustrated in Fig. 4. This specimen is prepared from a longitudinal section through the dentine germ of a sheep's fœtus.

As long as the formation of dentine continues, the arrangement of dentine cells in multiple layers can be demonstrated. In Fig. 5, made from the longitudinal section through a normal bicuspid in a girl of twelve years, the layer of odontoblasts still consists of seven to eight rows of cells. I have been able to show that innumerable rows underneath each other are merely different layers of a single row that have become displaced so as to lie below one another, but really consist of several rows of cells. In Fig. 6, representing the partially calcified pulp-horn from the back tooth

Fig. 9.

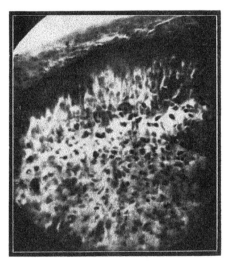

Narrow layer of dentine, with inclosed odontoblasts, from the root of a young cow's tooth. Transverse sections. Total metaplastic transformation of some of the odontoblasts of the odontoblast layer.

of a rabbit, you can see, particularly in the centre of the slide, how the arrangement in rows develops and how a single fibrillar process starts from several odontoblasts. The light spots between the cells are young dentine, so-called secondary dentine.

I have been able to demonstrate this conjunction of pulp-cells for the purpose of odontoblast formation in the earliest developmental stages. In Fig. 7, made from the tooth-germ of a human fœtus, the genesis of the small number of odontoblasts that is formed in this specimen from confluence of conjugation of pulp-cell (mesoblasts) can be clearly seen. In those places in which no odontoblasts have been formed, single fibrillæ—*i.e.*, preformed den-

FIG. 10.

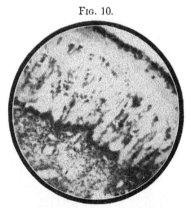

Formation of dentine in the root of a cow's tooth without typical odontoblast layer; stage of conjugation of dentine cells in the dentine and in the pulp; direct transformation of dentine cells into dentine substance.

tine fibres—appear underneath the layer of enamel cells at the margin of the dentine germ.

FIG. 11.

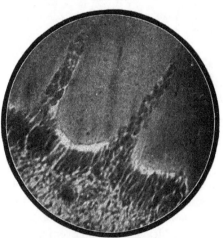

First formation of dentine from the root of a young cow's tooth. Gradual transformation of pulp-cells to odontoblasts and of those to dentinogenous globular masses and trabeculæ. Typical layer of odontoblasts not present.

In a somewhat later stage and after dentine has already been formed, odontoblasts arranged in trabeculæ appear; many of these later odontoblasts, however (as shown in Fig. 8), no longer possess a nucleus, whereas the odontoblasts in Fig. 7 may even possess two or three nuclei.

I believe that I have adduced valid arguments against the existing odontoblast theory by the demonstration of Figs. 1 to 8, for I have been able to show (1) that, at least in the earliest developmental stages of the teeth, an odontoblast originates from several cell units, (2) that during the different periods of tooth formation a multiple layer of odontoblast cells can be demonstrated, (3) that, finally, the external rows of this layer undergo metaplastic trans-

FIG. 12.

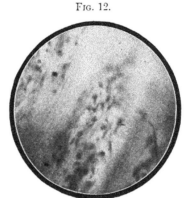

From the same specimen as Fig. 11, higher power. The first formation of a typical layer of odontoblasts disappears at once, owing to the rapid transformation of the latter into the dentine; here those dentine cells that are still in a stage of metaplastic transformation appear enclosed in finished dentine.

formation, so that they disintegrate; consequently I argue that it is impossible for each odontoblast to persist throughout the whole period of tooth formation without being destroyed and subsequently replaced by other cells from which the dentine is ultimately formed.

The innumerable smaller cells that are seen underneath the layer of odontoblasts have been completely ignored by the adherents of the odontoblast theory. The fact, moreover, that the nuclei of the odontoblasts show no karyokinetic figures has been misinterpreted by them. The replacement of the odontoblasts that are destroyed in process of dentine formation does not occur by cell regeneration and karyokynesis of nuclei, but by proliferation of the small underlying pulp-cells that are connected by innumerable protoplasmic anastomoses with the dentine cells.

2. The salient feature of this whole investigation is to show that dentine cells are actualy used up in the process of dentine formation. If it should be possible to demonstrate the presence of transition forms between the different forms of cells that are in process of metaplastic metamorphosis this postulate would be fulfilled. When the formation of dentine proceeds quietly and uniformly, such transition forms are not easy to find; when the formation of dentine, however, proceeds in an irregular manner,—*i.e.,* when " functional irritants influence the formation of dentine,"—

Fig. 13.

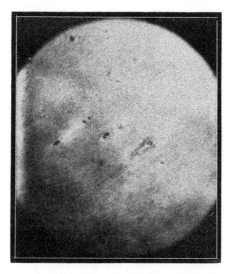

A somewhat broader layer of dentine, with inclosed dentine cells that are partially arranged in rows or groups. Transverse section through the root of a young rabbit.

then it is an easy matter to find such forms of cells. I take the liberty of demonstrating by the following slides what I wish to show; the specimens are taken from the roots of teeth from ruminants, rodents, and fish. I have already, in a separate monograph, described the results of these particular investigations on the formation of dentine in these species.

Figs. 9 and 10 are made from cross-sections through the root of a cow's tooth in its first stage of development. We see a narrow strip of dentine with fenestrations; within the openings of the dentine are seen odontoblasts, some of them still connected with one another by protoplasmic processes; the substance of the majority of the cells is changed, and, owing to " dentinogenous transformation" that is taking place, they appear black. In the narrow odontoblast layer we see pale odontoblasts, and, in addition, some cells that are colored black; in this layer, therefore, we see the same change in the substance of the cells throughout.

In Fig. 10 the layer of odontoblasts is irregular, somewhat

FIG. 14.

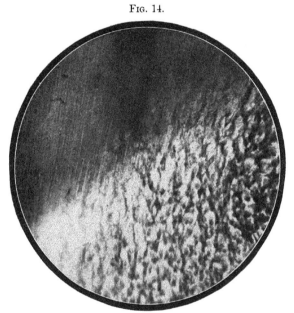

Plugs of pulp remaining in young dentine. They consist of columns of dentine cells that have undergone partial metaplastic change; consisting also in part of small pulp-cells and capillaries.

broader than above, and interrupted in many places by protruding plugs of dentine. The odontoblasts of this layer correspond, in regard to arrangement, form, and substance, to those that are found in the interior of the dentine.

The gradual transition of pulp-cells into the layer of odontoblasts, as well as the transition of the odontoblasts into particles of dentine, can be seen clearly in Figs. 11 and 12; these sections are made from the first dentine appearing in the roots of a cow's

tooth. In Fig. 11 the changes in form that the odontoblasts undergo in the process of dentine formation can be seen particularly

FIG. 15.

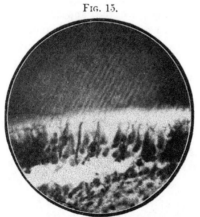

Plug of pulp in the dentine in which the nuclei still appear quite unchanged. From the
tooth of a sheep's fœtus.

well, and in Fig. 12 the arrangement of the pulp-cells and their
gradual transition to odontoblasts is especially clear.

FIG. 16.

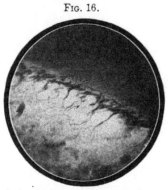

Different cell territories in the dentine of a molar tooth of a human premolar. Fibres
passing from layer of odontoblasts deep in pulp.

In Fig. 13, in which we see that the dentine is broader, the
arrangement in rows, the conjugation, and the changes in the substance of the odontoblasts can be seen on a somewhat larger scale.
In Fig. 14 the dentine contains two plugs consisting of different

kinds of cells; the other margin of these plugs is very pale, and is seen to be undergoing metamorphosis to dentine.

In Fig. 15 a plug of cells within the dentine is shown; here we see the nuclei unchanged, while the protoplasm is beginning to pale. This condition is always seen immediately before the dentinogenous metamorphosis begins.

These plugs that frequently pass through the layer of odonto-blasts and almost penetrate to the cement layer in the dentine may easily create the impression that dentine had been previously formed, had again been absorbed, and had been subsequently re-

FIG. 17.

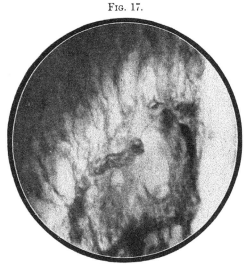

A few perennial cells from the dentine of a molar tooth of a somewhat older rabbit.

placed by pulp-tissue that had penetrated into the spaces created in this way. This view, however, is opposed by very valid arguments. I have studied the peculiar formation under discussion through all developmental stages,—*i.e.,* from the very beginning of tooth for-mation to the completion of root growth,—and I could determine on the basis of thousands of observations that these plugs never penetrate into finished dentine, but are always found before the formation of dentine has begun. The plugs represent masses of pulp that remain behind in certain areas owing to an irregular de-velopment of the dentine; later these plugs are destined to undergo the same metamorphosis as other portions of the pulp that are further advanced in their development. Finally these plugs disappear and the area they occupy is replaced by normal dentine.

Gero Rudas has recently stated that the presence of cells in the dentine is always due to the invasion of leucocytes, and that the development of the pulp is deficient in those places in which incapsulated pulp-cells are found; I am forced, however, to deny the correctness of these statements from my own experience. I believe I have shown that the cells within the dentine do not consist of invading pathologic leucocytes, but of mesodermic cells and dentine cells that have been passively inclosed. Under normal conditions these cells disappear without leaving a trace; only in those cases in which the developmental processes are arrested—as, for instance, by rapid and great destruction of the cutting edges of the teeth from overuse, with resulting atrophy of the pulp—do we see deficient development of dentine in such places.

In the dentine of certain animals, however, we sometimes see single cells, cell groups, and cell territories that probably persist during the life of the animal; they must either persist as living cells that are normal or as decayed cell rudiments. I have been able to find such cells particularly in the teeth of rodents, and most frequently in the molar teeth of rabbits. In Fig 16 such cell territories are shown, and in Fig. 17 single cells inclosed in the dentine of rabbits. We know nothing positive in regard to the significance of those cells.

What we learn from the formation of dentine under the influence of functional irritants is that dentine may be formed without a typic layer of odontoblasts, that the pulp-cells that were heretofore considered to be completely indifferent are directly concerned in this process, and, finally, that the latter are arranged in rows during this developmental process without ever being transformed into typic odontoblasts. The transformation of these cells into dentine may, however, be followed step by step, for it can readily be shown that they as well as the odontoblasts that are enclosed within the dentine are gradually converted into dentine; and this, I argue, proves that in the formation of dentine, dentine cells are used up.

At all events, we may assume positively that no conclusions can be drawn from the fact that the odontoblasts form one layer. In regard to the permanence of the odontoblasts, nor in regard to the continuous disintegration of these cells and the replacement of the destroyed cells by new ones, I am inclined to the belief that the formation of a single layer of odontoblasts constitutes merely a transitory stage in the development of dentine, and a stage, moreover, that need not necessarily be observed in all cases.

3. In connection with the old odontoblast theory, the idea is often expressed that the perennial dentine cells (whose number always remains the same) advanced towards the pulp as well as towards the déntine, and that in process of advancing towards the pulp they displace this tissue; the question is not decided, however, whether or not all the constituents of this displaced pulp undergo atrophy or whether they are merely compressed. In the light of my discovery of the metamorphosis of pulp-cells into dentine cells and of the continuous degeneration of the latter this view is altogether untenable.

Only one explanation seems satisfactory,—namely, that more and more of the pulp becomes included in the process of dentine formation. We must assume that the pulp becomes smaller and smaller, and we do not need to postulate compression nor atrophy of the pulp to explain its gradual shrinkage.

What becomes of the blood-vessels and the nerves in those portions of the pulp that are converted into territories of dentine cells?

I attempted to solve this query many years ago and have made it the subject of a comprehensive investigation. The main results of my studies have been described in a lecture. I found that the blood-vessels undergo atrophy or are converted into intraglobular spaces. I also showed that the nerves, with exception of the axis cylinders, are converted into a hyaline substance that later undergoes calcification, and that the axis cylinders partially atrophy and partially persist. At the same time I demonstrated that these cylinders are very difficult to demonstrate histologically.

One of my arguments in favor of the view that new pulp areas are constantly included in dentine formation is that the histologic structures within and below the odontoblast layer undergo continuous changes. At one time we may see numerous capillaries between the odontoblasts, occasionally even between them and the layer of dentine; in other cases a layer of odontoblasts will be found containing no trace of blood-vessels. Sometimes the pulp immediately below the odontoblasts contains very many cells, and sometimes it contains very few. Frequently a large number of very fine fibres are seen in this zone, constituting what is called Weil's

layer; in other instances this layer will be found to consist of a
finely granular material containing neither cells nor fibres. The
vaso-dentine of fish teeth is a classical example of the continuous
participation of pulp territories in dentine formation without the
agency of odontoblasts.

If we look at the question in this light, the dentine fibres must
need assume an 'altogether different histogenetic relation to the
odontoblasts than has hitherto been postulated; it seems impossible
that the fibres should arise exclusively from the odontoblasts that
are situated at the surface of the pulp, and they must also be im-

Fig. 18.

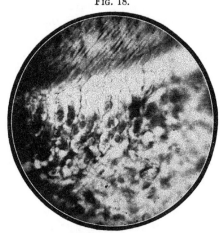

Between the dentine and the odontoblasts is seen a finely granular zone from which the
dentine cells have already disappeared; this zone is traversed by numerous preformed
dentine fibres. Tooth from a young rabbit.

agined to arise in part from pulp-cells situated deeper down in the
pulp; in other words they must be more or less preformed in the
pulp and cannot be said to originate by metaplastic transformation
as a residuum of the dentine cells in the process of dentine formation.

The next figures demonstrate these postulated conditions. In
Fig. 18, made from the molar tooth of a young rabbit, a layer is
seen underneath the young dentine that contains very few cells and
that is traversed by fibres. Here dentinogenous disintegration of
odontoblasts has taken place and the dentine fibres originate from
the deeper cells.

In Fig. 19 made from a longitudinal section through the dentine germ in a sheep's fœtus, numerous fibres will be recognized that pass from the dentine through the multiple layer of odontoblasts, and that in part originate below this layer. I observed that many of these fibres belong to the nervous system, and originate, as will

FIG. 19.

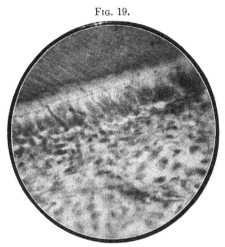

The layer of odontoblasts is traversed by numerous dark fibres that in a great part originate externally to it and that pass into the dentine. Longitudinal section through the dentine germ of a sheep's fœtus.

be seen, from nerve-branches in the pulp that are running a parietal course.

Fig. 20 is made from the same series of cuts, and under a high power shows fibres that run between the multiple layer of odontoblasts; in other words, these fibres pass through the whole layer of the odontoblast cells into the dentine.

Fig. 21 is made from the pulp of a young human premolar. Fibres will be seen passing from the layer of odontoblasts deep down into the pulp; these fibres constitute the so-called layer of Weil.

Sections made from the same series of cuts as Fig. 21 show a spot in Weil's layer under a higher power. Numerous fibrillæ are seen to originate from the circumference of a single capillary; these fibres enter the odontoblast layer. They are very different in appearance; most of them stain like fine connective tissue fibres; some of them are fine tubules that are occasionally found to contain a few red blood-corpuscles; in most cases, however, they are

so fine that blood-corpuscles cannot pass through.   Formerly I
described these tubes as lymphatic channels, but am now inclined

FIG. 20.

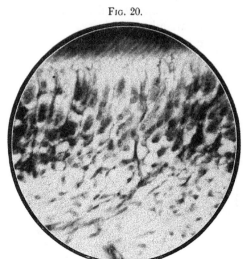

The same as Fig. 19 under a higher power.

to the belief that they are blood-vessels and that they constitute
very fine nutritional or tissue fluid fibres of a variety that has

FIG. 21.

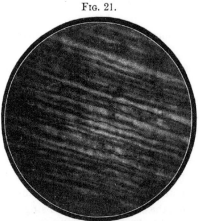

From the longitudinal section of a human premolar.   The entrance of the fibres from Weil's
layer into the layer of odontoblasts is shown.

hitherto never been described in dental tissues. By a special method
of preparation I have been enabled to demonstrate large numbers of

them between the dentine cells, and could also repeatedly demonstrate their presence in dentine.

A large number of these fine channels is shown between the odontoblasts in a molar tooth of a young rabbit. Some of these odontoblasts are in process of dentinogenous disintegration, and in most of them only the nuclei are preserved. These channels, that vary in thickness from one-fourth to one-third the width of a cell nucleus, usually terminate in a knob-like loop.

A very thin capillary in the layer of odontoblasts and another one in a cell group situated in the dentine of a young calf are shown.

I call your attention particularly to these channels and capillaries that pass between the dentine cells, for there is resemblance in regard to distribution and location between these structures and the dentine fibres; in Figs. 20 and 21, both structures are seen to pass side by side through the odontoblast layer and below it, —*i.e.*, in Weil's layer. But I have also been able to show repeatedly that in addition to Tomes's fibres fine channels frequently enter the dentine, the method I employed for demonstrating their presence being either injection of the specimens or special preparation of a series of cuts made from the fœtus of cows, fish, and sheep.

4. The question of the nutrition of dentine can only be solved after the relation existing between Tomes's fibres and the fine channels that I have demonstrated between the odontoblasts is explained.

I believe, however, that I have definitely solved the question of the sensibility of dentine by my demonstration of the entrance of nerves into the dentine. That the sensibility of dentine is not dependent on the presence of odontoblasts in the dentine, as taught by Black, Walkhoff, and other authors, could be demonstrated clinically by the fact that teeth whose pulps were completely decalcified and that contained no more odontoblasts were still highly sensitive. In these cases of general calcification the axis cylinders were not involved in the process and remained intact.

Boll in 1868, Bödecker in 1883, I in 1892, and Romer in 1899 demonstrated the fact that pulp-nerves pass into the layer of odontoblasts. The deviation of nerve-fibres between the odontoblasts and the dentine was observed in 1892 by Retzius, and by Huber in 1899; the entrance of nerves into the dentine I demonstrated in 1892, and Romer in 1899.

In older specimens nothing but pale fibres are seen in those places where nerves enter into the dentine; these fibres, however, are clearly differentiated from the other tissues; this may be seen in an old specimen prepared from a young rabbit's tooth.

In preparations made according to my modification of Mallory's stain, the axis cylinder is clearly different from all other stained tissues; preparations of this character, as will be seen from the following figures, can be preserved for a very long time.

In a specimen made from the dentine germ of a sheep's fœtus a few of the axis cylinders that run towards the centre of the odon-toblast layer between the dentine cells can be clearly recognized; they pass from the parietal sheath of the nerves of the dentine germ, and can be followed through the whole odontoblast layer beyond the boundaries of the dentine.

In one specimen the entrance of nerves into the dentine can be seen still more clearly; one of the axis cylinders is seen to termi-nate in a knob-like ending in the dentine, and another one to terminate in a similar way before reaching the dentine—*i.e.*, in the odontoblast layer.

The course of the nerves in the odontoblast layer varies greatly.

They often traverse the layer in the same direction as the dentine channels and the odontoblasts; in some places they deviate from this direction. Sometimes they form a veritable plexus with their small lateral branches; such a plexus in the odontoblast layer can be seen in specimen. The nerve fibrils *apparently* origi-nate from cells and cell nuclei; if one looks carefully, it will be seen, however, that they are merely close to the cells and really pass alongside of them.

At the point of division of the nerves of the odontoblast layer I have frequently seen one or more spindle-shaped enlargement.

In conclusion, I take the liberty of demonstrating the course of the nerve-fibres within the dentine channels in a cow's tooth. The preparation was made according to Golgi by the sublimate method after the specimen had previously been injected with methylene blue. The fibres of Tomes appear pale; the fibres that I call axis cylinders are darker and frequently form spirals around the dentine fibres; they are situated between the walls of the dentine channels and the fibres of Tomes.

Basing on a series of histologic facts that I have attempted to illustrate to you with the aid of a few photographic slides of some of my specimens, I believe I have demonstrated that the generally accepted odontoblast theory, the theory of dentine formation, and of the sensibility of the dentine are untenable. While I do not dare to substitute a new and complete theory for the old one, I hope, nevertheless, to have contributed a few new facts by my investigations that may form the basis of an odontoblast theory that will satisfy us both in an anatomic and physiologic sense.

REPLY TO DR. E. K. WEDELSTAEDT.

BY M. L. RHEIN, M.D., D.D.S., NEW YORK.

In the January number of the INTERNATIONAL DENTAL JOURNAL there appears an article by Dr. E. K. Wedelstaedt, which is intended as a reply to an article of mine in the September number, entitled " The Technique of Approximal Restorations with Gold in Posterior Teeth."

Dr. Wedelstaedt's article is so replete with errors, that it becomes a difficult matter to reply to the same and preserve the temperate demeanor which only is becoming to a scientific discussion. It is my intention to take up the points that he has raised, and answer them in order, as briefly as possible.

First. He starts in with a general objection to the praise and honor which was given to Marshall H. Webb in the article in question, but fails to reply to the only reason that Webb's name was introduced into the article. It was not my purpose to leave the impression that the method of preparing cavities pursued by Webb, or his method of inserting fillings, was distinctively new with him; but rather that it was a culmination of the practice of many men preceding and contemporary with him.

The main reason for bringing the name of Marshall H. Webb to the foreground in the article in question was to clearly demonstrate by the illustrations taken from his writings, and by his own words, that the principle of extending cavity margins for the prevention of recurrence of decay was well understood and practised by him. This was done because it had become a popular delusion in a certain section of the country that this was an entirely new doctrine evolved by Dr. G. V. Black. The only reply that Dr. Wedelstaedt makes to this point is, that they have stopped talking about extension for prevention in the Northwest.

It is rather a poor way of giving credit to a man who died practically a martyr to the cause of saving teeth. I say advisedly that he died a martyr to the cause, because the last few years of his active life were devoted almost exclusively to giving clinical demonstrations throughout the world, in the method of preparing cavities and properly filling them with gold. He did this at the expense of the necessary comforts for his own family, and in the course of this work contracted a cancer of the colon, which shortly after proved fatal.

In the models prepared by his own hand, and from which the drawings in his work were taken, there can be no question that Webb recognized the value of a flat gingival wall or seat. His students understood this thoroughly, and when Dr. Wedelstaedt says that "Dr. Rhein has at last recognized the value of having fillings properly seated on a flat gingival wall or seat," it is difficult to comprehend the necessity for such a statement, as this has been my practice for over twenty years. The same is true of occlusal anchorage in these cavities.

I regret that the illustrations of my article in the September number of this journal are done so poorly that it is difficult to understand them. This is not my fault. The blame is entirely at the door of the publishers, who made their cuts from actual models with natural teeth, which I turned over to them.

It was not intimated in my paper that Webb's preparation of cavities is precisely that of to-day. It is admitted that there have been important advances made, such as the elimination of retaining points; but the principles remain the same.

Second. The next point which Dr. Wedelstaedt takes up is his objection to finishing the cavo-surface angle with a sand-paper disk. In his well-known dogmatic style, he says, "Tight margins cannot under any circumstances be made against a smooth margin, if gold is the filling-material used." If Dr. Wedelstaedt had ever examined with a strong magnifying lens the ends of enamel-rods polished at their best, it is doubtful whether he would make such a statement. In reply, I would say that I consider it very objectionable to condense gold in the proper manner against the surface of enamel-rods which are necessarily left unsupported, if prepared by chisels, leaving a roughened surface such as he describes.

Furthermore it is denied that there is any tooth-surface at the occlusal portion so smooth that cohesive gold cannot be perfectly adapted to it, so as to make an hermetically sealed joint. His very statement indicates that he is unacquainted with the proper method of inserting cohesive gold so as to make a perfectly homogeneous plug. It might as well be stated here, that it is not possible to produce ideal results in cohesive gold by the use of pellets, cylinders, ropes, or any form except the regular foil or rolled gold. The use of any of these supposed labor-saving preparations, such as pellets or cylinders, is only productive of imperfect condensation and the leaving of air-spaces between the laminæ of the gold, and consequently preventing the accomplishment of what is most essential,—a homogeneous solid plug.

Third. The third and main objection which he finds to my article is the advocacy of an all-cohesive gold filling. The article in the September number was written distinctively for the purpose of bringing out discussion on this point. The cavities under consideration (approximo-occlusal in posterior teeth), when filled, must bear the stress of mastication, which we know varies from one hundred to three hundred pounds pressure.

If it can be proved that the fillings advocated by Dr. Wedelstaedt and his school, which consist of filling the gingival third with non-cohesive gold, will stand the same amount of stress as a perfectly condensed all-cohesive gold filling, there is no need of further argument. That Dr. Wedelstaedt claims such to be the case does not necessarily make it a fact, and part of my object has been to get at the real truth of this question. Dogmatic " say-so's" will not prove the correctness of this assertion on either side. In his article, he repeatedly refers to articles by Black published in 1891 and 1895 in the *Dental Cosmos,* in order to maintain his contention. A careful perusal of perhaps the most scientific articles on this subject that have ever been written—those just referred to— leaves in my mind only one impression. In such places as this it is impossible for us to obtain too great a density of our filling-material, in order to withstand the stress of years of wear.

In making his argument on this subject he mentions the fact that in the *Dental Cosmos* for 1895, commencing with page 749, there is given by Black a list of the specific gravity of different gold fillings. Three of these were made by Black himself. The remainder were made by different operators whose names are not given. The only ones in which a specific gravity above 19.3 was attained (which is the normal specific gravity of cast gold) were the three inserted by Professor Black himself. It appears from Dr. Wedelstaedt's article, that the three fillings inserted by means of the electro-magnetic mallet, and of which the highest specific gravity obtained was 13.2, were made by some one whom he calls an expert in the use of this mallet. From this he forms the conclusion that a filling made of cohesive gold, packed with the electro-magnetic mallet, is incapable of giving us the proper specific gravity.

In order to show that such a conclusion is incorrect, I made a filling out of the mouth under practically all the conditions set forth in my article, in the presence of two other dentists. The cavity was a distal approximate occlusal cavity of a superior molar. After the gingival half was completed, the filling was allowed to soak in water for an hour. The gold was then carefully smeared over with vaseline, so as to give it an opportunity to penetrate into the interstices, if possible. It was then carefully washed with chloroform and alcohol, and the surfaces freshened with a clean fissure bur. The filling was then continued precisely in the same manner as if this interruption had not taken place, and it was impossible, at the completion of the filling, and after the tooth had been cut in half and the filling removed, to tell where the point of union had taken place. Previous to its removal from the tooth, the filling had been polished in the ordinary manner. It was sent to the office of Dr. Ludwig Saarbach, a well-known expert, of this city, who gave as a certificate of its specific gravity, 19.87. When it is considered that this filling was inserted practically as one is placed in the mouth, so far as the amount of time and number of blows is concerned, the difference in the specific gravity obtained and that obtained by the so-called expert referred to by Dr. Wedelstaedt is worthy of notice.

It might be well to call attention to the fact that the highest specific gravity reported by Black was 19.42. If there should be any question as to the correctness of this specific gravity as compared with those stated in Black's article, there is one simple way of arriving at the truth,—and this has been tried before,—by an open competition of the various methods of packing gold.

At a clinic given before the First District Dental Society of the State of New York, in January, 1881, there was such a competition. It is peculiar that the simple expedient of obtaining the specific gravity of each filling was not thought of. Fillings were put in matrices of precisely the same mathematical dimension, and the following results were obtained:

By means of the electro-magnetic mallet, Dr. Webb inserted 9.65 grains.

With the automatic mallet, Dr. Ottolengui inserted 9.4 grains.

With the steel mallet, Dr. E. Parmley Brown inserted 9.25 grains.

With the lead mallet, Dr. Rynear inserted 9.2 grains.

With hand-pressure, Dr. Weld (who practically inaugurated the challenge) inserted 7.8 grains.

Only a similar form of experimentation, where the operators are known, can demonstrate the correctness or incorrectness of my assertion.

Dr. Wedelstaedt questions the ability of any operator to make tight margins with cohesive gold, especially at the gingival portion of a cavity. I might say, in reply, that the man who cannot perform such an operation, after a little practice, and having had the proper teaching, has but little claim to the confidence placed in him by patients who come to him for such work.

The frequent observation of my own fillings inserted in this manner, from the very commencement of my practice in 1881, and the fact that a large majority of them are doing as good service to-day as when they were inserted, is to my mind the strongest refutation of this argument. The whole matter is summed up in the fact that a great many dentists make a difficult operation out of the use of cohesive gold, because they have never been taught how easily it can be manipulated. Instead of being an "intractable material" as Dr. Wedelstaedt would have us believe, it becomes the most docile of agents when properly handled. It is on this account that my critic does not understand how a cohesive gold filling can be brought in a perfectly even surface from the gingival seat to the occlusal anchorage. It is on this account that he does not understand how a properly condensed filling of cohesive gold can be made in sections at different sittings, not only without any bad joint showing, but resulting in one homogeneous whole, and defying the detection of the joints.

Cohesive gold cannot be made into a solid homogeneous plug by means of the blow given by an instrument such as the automatic mallet, or a hand mallet, except at the expense of the most strenuous labor. It becomes, however, one of the easiest of operations under the direction of the electro-magnetic mallet with a current directed from a battery, so that the instrument is capable of giving at least three thousand five hundred blows per minute. By this means, the pieces of gold-foil laid upon the portion of the filling already inserted are not punched into the filling already made, but are carefully ironed into the filling through the aid of the innumerable blows given. It is my contention that with this form of manipulation the highest specific gravity of gold can be attained. It must not be overlooked that in the proper manipulation of cohesive gold a most essential feature is to prevent the gold coming in contact at any time with any foreign substance except carefully polished instruments and the surface of the annealer. Any deviation from this rule will imperil the perfection of the filling and is too frequently the sole cause of failure.

My critic goes to considerable length in taking exception to the plan which I advocated for anchoring my first piece of cohesive gold. He states that in examining three such fillings which have been anchored by this method, he found that the cement used was simply a white powder. He does not say what methods he has used in order to make his examination. I might reply that, in the course of similar examinations, I have found a condition precisely similar to the removal of a porcelain inlay after it has been set,—viz., a portion of the cement adhering to the inner periphery of the cavity, and another portion adhering to the surface of the gold. In other words, that it was impossible to remove the cement in a clean way from either the gold or the tooth surface, which I consider the ideal result to be obtained. I do not deny that this cement is capable of being reduced to a powder similar to the condition it was in before it was made into a cement, but I have never seen it in this pulverized state by simply dislodging the filling from the broken tooth. It might be well to state that the anchorage of a gold filling in this manner produces all the advantages that are claimed from a porcelain inlay that has been cemented into place.

Dr. Wedelstaedt has laid considerable stress in his article on the advantage of measuring the size of his tooth and the cavity in its different relations. He then proceeds to estimate how much non-cohesive gold such an approximate surface will stand and still retain sufficient solidity, from the amount of cohesive gold on the occlusal portion, to withstand the stress of ordinary use. It has never yet been my good fortune to meet with one operator, whose work I have valued, who can find any practical advantage from the system of cavity measurements which has been so extensively taught by Dr. Wedelstaedt.

It appears to me that this millimetre equation is fit to be placed in the same category with the problem of, " Given the age of Mary, how old is Ann?" It is impossible to teach the insertion of gold fillings in these surfaces by any mathematical calculation such as is used in building operations, for the simple reason that we never find two mouths in which exactly similar conditions prevail. If the majority of teeth that presented themselves to us conformed even in an ordinary ratio to the form which we designate as the correct physiological one, the filling of teeth might logically be taught in such a manner. As it is, however, the exceptions to the normal position of teeth are the rule, and it becomes the problem of the dentist in this form of cavity, how to best give to those teeth the most serviceable form of contact point, and one which will best preserve the health of the interproximal space at the gingival angle.

In many of these cases the operator is compelled to perform operations that must be devised entirely for the case in hand, and it is absolutely impossible, under such circumstances, to rely upon any of Wedelstaedt's equations.

In another place Dr. Wedelstaedt speaks of the fact of his seeing failures of fillings made with all-cohesive gold. I might say, with perfect candor, that I have seen the same thing in all-cohesive gold fillings, and at the same time a great many more failures where non-cohesive gold and gold-and-tin fillings have been used in the gingival third. I need not call the attention of any operator who has removed even a single non-cohesive gold filling to the vile odors which emanate from the separated laminæ of the gold which burs out like wet sand.

This sort of observation will not prove that either method of filling teeth cannot be used so that the teeth can be saved permauently. The only question at issue is. Which method properly pursued will best preserve the teeth? In this respect, I might call attention to the fact that if the gold is more solidly condensed, if it is used in a cohesive manner at the gingival third,—supposing that it is correctly placed in position,—it certainly will be better able to withstand the scaling of those places in the years following a supposed good operation by either method.

I have seen fillings, where the gingival third was filled with non-cohesive foil, that have been practically ruined in the scaling of the teeth by the careless instrumentation of the operator.

There are a number of places in Dr. Wedelstaedt's article in which he simply says that the operation advocated in my article cannot be done, and consequently cannot be endorsed. There is nothing to be gained in this kind of talk, nor in answering a criticism like this. If, however, in open contest my critic can demonstrate the falsity of my views, or the superiority of those which he so grandiloquently maintains, I shall be only too pleased to change my venerable form of practice for one that is capable of giving more benefit to my patients.

SUGGESTIONS RELATING TO THE EXAMINATION OF THE TEETH.[1]

BY CHARLES G. PIKE, D.M.D.

CAN any one tell me how one may derive more benefit and pleasure than by gazing upon something that is of special interest to him. For instance, of course you all remember your first visit from home, how carefully and critically you watched everything, and on your return you spent much time in talking and thinking to yourself of the many beautiful and wonderful things which you had seen. How improving, how lasting were those first impressions! I am sure you will never forget them as long as you live.

Now, gentlemen, a number of months—yes, years—have passed since we first travelled or looked over this ground, and in the intervening time it has been our custom to travel, or, better, see it daily. Are we as critical and careful in our observations as we were on our first examination of the object, or whatever it might be? I am afraid we do not pay as marked attention as we should.

Now, do you suppose that there is any one present that has forgotten his first patient, the first examination that he was called upon to make? How carefully, observingly you went about it, not failing to ask many questions, many no doubt entirely uncalled

---

[1] Read before the Harvard Odontological Society, September 24, 1903.

for. In all probability you had taken at least a good half-hour, if not longer, in making your first examination.

How many of us now spend as much time? Would not our diagnosis of a case be more successful not only to ourselves, but to our patients, if before remarking about a filling or the treatment of a certain case we gave it a few moments careful thought? How quickly a patient will question us, and especially if we have made a statement that would have been much better unsaid. In order to make a proper examination, of course the teeth should be thoroughly cleansed, but this may not always be necessary.

A perfect examination, in my opinion, is not an easy thing to make. I do not mean that we are not all capable of doing it properly, but simply that we must give it as much care and attention as any filling that we put in. Time is a very important factor, and should always be considered. How often you will have patients say that they have not been satisfied with the operation or opinions of others, and ask at the same time a careful examination of their teeth.

In making an examination I have always made it a plan to first dry the teeth as much as possible with napkins and rolls and then proceed to examine, beginning at the superior right third molar, or as near it as is possible if such teeth are lacking, exploring with any suitable explorer every surface before passing to the next.

It is especially wise to explore every fissure and groove very carefully, never relying on the eyes for a decision, for often, on exploring in this manner, you will find spots which upon being broken down are found to be quite large and could have been detected in no other way.

After following these directions with each tooth of the superior arch, I then take silk and make as careful an examination as I can of the approximal surfaces. If there is the slightest doubt in my mind about the condition of any of these surfaces I suggest a wedge. I am a great believer in wedges, and know of nothing that can be used, if used with ordinary precautions, with less discomfort to the patient or better advantage to the operator. It seems to me to be the only correct way of examining doubtful approximal surfaces. If there is the least particle of doubt, a small wedge for a few hours will place you on a firm foundation, and that is what we must have in order to do satisfactory work.

Now, the question that some will ask is, Are the patients willing to allow this wedging? In some cases I will say that they will object at first, but after spending a few moments explaining the importance of it they will readily consent, and I am sure that after the first examination they will see for themselves the importance of it and you will never be criticised thereafter.

Oftentimes your patient will get so accustomed to rely upon the wedge for a diagnosis that before making their semiannual or annual visit to you, as the case may be, they will of their own accord insert wedging in doubtful places, so that if there is any trouble it can be detected at once.

In regard to a fee for this work, is there anything we do that requires any more attention on our part? If we take ten or twenty minutes for a small operation on a patient we expect a suitable fee, then why should not we expect the same from a patient after we have made an examination and pronounced the mouth in good condition, if such is the case. It is quite as much an operation as anything we do, and we should certainly receive proper remuneration for it.

Most any chart is suitable for an examination record, but a chart record should certainly be kept of each mouth for reference at any time. It is of special value to the operator in saving time, for by a hasty examination of it, just before the appointment, he can readily see what there is to be done and be ready to begin upon the arrival of the patient. Personally I use them to make notes on in regard to the patient or anything that is of special importance to me.

In closing, gentlemen, let me state that if there are any present who have at times allowed themselves to be lax in this apparently simple operation, I hope from now on they will try and make this one of their ideals and objects in their profession, for in order to attain the height for which we are all striving we must do our best in all things.

There occurred this short article in one of the recent publications of the *Dental Cosmos,* which, with your kind attention and permission, I will quote. Its subject is " Purpose in Life."

" Whoever desires to cultivate his firmness of purpose does well to begin with this leading one: He must have a definite aim, and keep it strictly in view; to it he must steadily direct his efforts and apply his powers. If he does this he will soon acquire a facility in its details which can come in no other way, and his interest in it will increase, for we always like to do that which we can do well. Of course, whether or not he will actually attain to that on which he sets his mind must depend upon the aim itself.

"He may aspire to be a great artist or statesman or lawyer or architect, and never be able to reach the goal, but his persistence will enable him to come as near the mark as his powers will allow, which is all that any man can do; whereas, with tenfold the ability, but with no steadfast purpose, he would have fallen far short of the place he now occupies.

"Success in its best sense is not always found in attaining that for which we plan; but rather in making the best that can be made of ourselves, doing as well and rising as high as our powers will allow. As the poet Young has well said,—

> "'Thy purpose firm is equal to the deed.
> Who does the best his circumstance allows,
> Does well, acts nobly; angels could no more.'"

ORTHODONTIC FACIAL ORTHOMORPHIA — IMPORTANCE OF DIFFERENTIATION IN CASES OF APPARENT MANDIBULAR PROTRUSION.[1]

BY WILLIAM ERNEST WALKER, D.D.S., M.D., NEW ORLEANS.

QUITE a little has been written on the etiology and treatment of cases presenting the appearance of protrusion of the mandible, the "chin-cap" treatment being recommended in young subjects and the removal of sections from each side of the mandible in older patients, and of late much has been written regarding the technic of this latter operation.

In a recent article Dr. E. H. Angle mentions a case in which this operation was successfully done in St. Louis,[2] and tells of a failure having been made in New Orleans.[3] I have heard rumors

---

[1] Read at the annual session of the American Medical Association, Section on Stomatology.

[2] Dental Cosmos, April, 1903.

[3] Items of Interest, April, 1903.

8

in New Orleans concerning this failure, but have never seen the case.

Much has been written about treatment and a little about etiology, but apparently very little thought has been given to diagnosis, and the object of this brief paper is to emphasize the importance of a correct diagnosis on which to base an intelligent prescription.

It appears to have been taken for granted that the case which has the appearance to the surgeon of being a case of mandibular protrusion must necessarily be such, but I think that by presenting a case illustrating the erroneousness of that assumption, I can make it evident that this is not a fact.

From boyhood this patient was in the hands of a prominent dentist, who more than once was asked if anything could be done to remedy the defect; the invariable reply being " No, except in case the patient be willing to undergo a surgical operation for the removal of a section from each side of the mandible." The patient, at the age of nineteen, called on me, and my first impression was, as his brother had previously told me, that his lower jaw was very prominent.

Study of the case, however, convinced me that it was very much less a case of mandibular protrusion and very much more a case of arrest of the superior maxillæ.

Without explaining the diagnosis to the patient, he was allowed to return to his dentist, to whom he stated that Dr. Walker had told him that his case was remediable without a surgical operation, and again the dentist expressed as his opinion that nothing could be done for him except the operation previously mentioned, and that if Dr. Walker could otherwise remedy the defect, and if the patient had confidence, a trial might be made.

I mention these details to emphasize the perfect satisfaction the dentist manifested in his own diagnosis and prescription, notwithstanding its erroneousness, and to thus emphasize the necessity for the word of caution I am uttering, in order that errors in diagnosis may be avoided, for, on the diagnosis the treatment depends, which makes for success or failure.

The patient has been taking a rest for some months, waiting for the alveolar process to redevelop around the teeth in their new position, which has now taken place and we are about to carry the upper teeth a step farther. This waiting was considered advisable in order not to carry the teeth too far away from the bone, and because it has been found that if these periods of rest be given, the teeth can be moved great distances, the alveolar process developing around the teeth in their new position just as it did originally, and as it does after fractures, provided that the teeth are held still.

We know that in some pathologic conditions in adult life there is a great difference in the ability of the alveolar process to reproduce itself, but the movements of the teeth in alternating periods of activity and rest so closely resemble physiologic processes that Nature assists us by placing energetic osteoblasts at our service.

In the present case, the space made by the moving forward of the bicuspids and oral teeth has been closed by the moving forward of the second molars, assisted by the developing of the third molars, for which room has thus been made.

The next step will be to apply an apparatus which I am now constructing and which will have the effect of moving the maxillary teeth forward, using the chin and forehead as anchorage. This apparatus will somewhat resemble a baseball mask, but will have to be worn only during the night, the molars affording anchorage to retain during the day what we have gained during the night.

I hope by limiting myself to this one phase of the subject to so focus your attention on the subject of differentiation as to give it sufficient emphasis to attract the attention of the profession to its importance.

PYORRHŒA ALVEOLARIS.[1]

BY FRANK R. MAYER, D.D.S., WORCESTER, MASS.

HAVING been requested to present this paper to you, which I read at the Central District Dental Society, I immediately felt that the paper in its original entirety was too incomplete, the subject having been handled from a point starting from the supposed and almost unmistakable diagnosis familiar to the average dentist also treating the subject, omitting much that might have been said, because of a previous understanding of the Society that the reading of papers should require but the short space of five minutes.

Hence you can see that my paper, unless exceeding the allotted five minutes, must be incomplete.

I have treated this subject pathologically from what many consider its secondary cause,—namely, salivary calculus, having ignored the primary causes, constitutional disturbances, blood impoverishments, and serumal deposits, which I fear many like myself are uncertain whether to consider a prominent manifestation worthy our first consideration, or, to take its place, a possible cause which we in our uncertainty cannot lose sight of. It is left to the dentist, whose profession entitles him to the highest respect, to deserve such respect in a befitting manner, and, through a scientific research, to place upon a plane of unmistakable certainty the true cause of this devastating disease, that we may treat the disease unhampered by mistrust or any unsatisfactory previous disposition.

A cure must be effected from our starting-point, which is a proper knowledge of the probable cause, whether hereditary or acquired, from which point we can effect a cure. Often we find this lesion flourishing in patients without a history of rheumatic diathesis, blood impoverishments, or other abnormalities; we have found it in patients presenting characteristics dissimilar in many ways; how then can we discover it, unless by the chemical or analytical treatment of found conditions. There must be but one primary cause for this disease. I have treated the subject in my original paper mostly from a mechanical point of view, leaving the pathological causes which lead to this disease to those men who have scientifically endeavored to unearth the secret. I will now read the original paper as read at the infant society.

I feel that I owe you all an apology in attempting to handle a subject of which there has been so much written, yet one not altogether understood and, until recent years, not satisfactorily treated.

Pyorrhœa alveolaris, I consider, ranks second to none in stubborn defiance and resistance to the skill of the persistent dentist. Perhaps at this point it would be well to revert to history and acquaint ourselves with the origin of this disease, the pathological diagnosis of which we owe to Dr. Riggs; also its name,—Riggs's

---

[1] Read before the Massachusetts Dental Society, Boston, Mass., June 3 and 4, 1903.

disease. Resorting to a more remote past, we find evidence that the disease was treated with more or less success years before the lesion presented itself to Dr. Riggs. I can see no reason why the disease should not bear the name of Riggs, not that he was the first to treat it, but because he made it a distinct lesion, classifying it as necrosed alveolar process. So we understand that the disease called Riggs's disease is a distinctive form, like others, named after persons who first described their characteristics, as Bright's disease, etc.

The disease has been treated with varying success since 1746. The treatment was then divided into two classes,—first, surgical, and second, medical. Among the surgical methods is the extracting of the teeth, thus ending the infection of the disease to other healthy dental articulations. This method was soon considered to be a too severe loss, and other surgical methods followed quickly. Among these was a V-shaped incision corresponding to the shape of the tooth, its summit directed towards the apex of the root, forming a triangular flap; this flap was then removed and a cautery passed over the basic portion, and was then allowed to heal naturally.

American dentists modified this treatment by lancing from the apex towards the neck of the tooth, then cauterizing the under surface of the flap with nitrate of silver and carbolic acid.

Dr. Riggs's surgical method was to scrape the surface of the root of the affected tooth to remove all salivary calculi, and also removing any necrosed bone, then continuing with the cauterizing. Even extreme methods, as replantation, were resorted to where there was elongation of the incisor teeth.

Many medical methods have been used to conquer the disease, such as the use of bichloride solutions, aromatic sulphuric acid, iodide of zinc, iodoform, ether, aristol, caustic potash, carbolic acid, peroxide of hydrogen, nitrate of silver, etc.

The most important therapeutic consideration in this disease is the local treatment, yet we cannot lose sight of the constitutional treatment. The disease generally begins with gingival inflammation, then periostitis or inflammation of the periosteum; when the attack has destroyed the outer crust of the bone the osseous tissue is open for infection.

The first step towards the treatment of this disease is the removal of tartar, also the affected alveolus. The removing of the tartar at first thought seems easy, but upon closer observation we find that what we supposed we had dislodged remains to partly undo what would otherwise have proved a successful step towards complete recovery.

We have the visible and invisible tartar. It is quite an easy matter to remove the visible, but to thoroughly remove the tartar which runs oftentimes to the extreme end of the root is a problem that can only be solved by the dexterous use of appropriate instruments peculiarly adapted for this purpose, such as the several forms of scalers. In my own practice I have two instruments or scalers, one whose cutting edge cuts towards the operator or neck of the tooth, using a drawing motion; the other quite the reverse, its cutting edge acquiring a direct pushing motion towards the apex of the root; this latter instrument, because of its thin edge, obviates the otherwise painful operation of removing the tartar at the extreme end of the root.

After we feel confident of the complete removal of this tartar we often find a slight nodosity, which must be removed or scraped until smooth and well polished, as the least particle of life forms a new alveolar infection. This point I consider the pivot upon which the dentist meets with success or failure.

In spite of the most favorable instruments, the operation is often attended with unbearable pain. I have used with success a local application of cocaine, which, when applied to gum corresponding to and opposite the apex of the root, has rendered that tissue insensible to pain, consequently satisfactory to both operator and patient. Peroxide of hydrogen can be used with success because of its peculiar properties, forcing any particle of loose calculus to the surface, which can then be washed out.

We often find the disease has progressed to the stage where there has been a severe loss or disintegration of the bone, first attacking the periosteum, then the inner structure of the bone, resulting in the death of that organ.

After the use of peroxide of hydrogen I have generally used sulphuric acid to cauterize each gum pocket, but have lately found this to be too strong for the healthy granulation of surrounding tissue, aside from the danger of exposing the dentinal fibrils, resulting in extreme sensitiveness.

You are probably aware of a preparation that has recently appeared for dental use which has been adopted with success in some instances. It is named "Glyco-thymoline." I believe that any antiseptic for oral use should be alkaline in reaction, as the least acidity is dangerous to the teeth and connective tissues. The secretions of the mouth normally are found to be alkaline, and when diseased they become acid; so we need a strong alkaline reaction to produce a normal condition of the secretions.

We must have an antiseptic that is strongly alkaline, one that will not coagulate albumin; it should be a deodorant, non-irritating, and, in fact, should correspond to the natural healthy constituents of normal blood and mouth secretions.

In several patients I have found the following efficacious in arresting the rapid formation of tartar:

<blockquote>
℞ Citrate of lithia, gr. x ;
Glyco-thymoline, ℥iv.
Sig.—Inject deep into the pus-pockets, this treatment to be followed every few days until there are signs of complete restoration to a healthy condition.
</blockquote>

Massaging the gums often increases the capillary circulation, the lack of which is one of the principal causes of this disease. We often meet the disease advanced to the stage when the teeth have become loosened. I have found ligation, in the not too far advanced stage, satisfactory in lessening the danger of increasing the surrounding inflammation, but when the gums have loosened to such an extent as to entirely fail to support the teeth I use a number of bands, either of gold or other suitable metal, made to tightly fit the necks of the teeth well up towards the biting edge. After placing these bands in position I take an impression, removing bands in same, soldering bands together in relative positions, and then replacing with use of cement if found necessary; then proceed with treatment heretofore described.

I might speak of several cases that have come under my observation and for treatment, but would make the paper too long, so will desist.

Reports of Society Meetings.

AMERICAN MEDICAL ASSOCIATION, SECTION ON STOMATOLOGY.

(Continued from Vol. XXIV., page 704.)

DISCUSSION OF DR. CHITTENDEN'S PAPER, " IS THE REALIZATION OF REASONABLE IDEALS IN DENTAL EDUCATION NEAR AT HAND ?"

(For Dr. Chittenden's paper, see Vol. XXIV., page 524.)

Dr Eugene S. Talbot.—There is perhaps no one in the country so well posted on the management of dental colleges as the essayist. He is one of the foremost men who has been looking forward to the future of dentistry, and has done a great deal in the way of legislation. He would have been here at this meeting but for the fact that the Legislature is now in session, and changes are being brought about in the State law in Wisconsin. He wished me to extend his thanks to the Association for its courtesy in having his paper read, and regrets that he could not be here.

There is no doubt but that there is a good deal of underhand work going on in some of our dental colleges. I have in mind a city where there are three or four dental schools from some of which agents are sent out to solicit students, and to whom a percentage of the fees are paid for procuring them. There are many other glaring deficiencies in the methods of obtaining students. I was a little surprised that more was not said along these lines.

I understand that it is the intention of the National Board to bring this subject before their meeting for the purpose of discussing some of these points. I believe that the time has arrived when the Departments of Dentistry connected with universities will have a large influence. Now that the universities have a method for the purpose of uniforming the education in all their departments, and also for the purpose of raising the standard of qualification for admission to these different departments, I believe the time is near at hand when the graduate of dentistry in this country will be on an equal standing with the graduates of other specialties.

Dr. M. H. Fletcher, Cincinnati.—I do not know that I have much to say, except that I am interested in dental education and the higher standard that some of us conceive of being brought about. The author of the paper is more familiar with the progress in dental education than I, but as a member of the State Board of Dental Examiners for five years, it is a matter of great chagrin to me to know that our laws compel the examiners to give such elementary examinations that what I would consider a first course student in a college when I was teaching either dentistry or medicine could pass an examination. There is every reason from my stand-point for extreme effort in raising the standard, and no doubt such men as the essayist and those interested in bringing it about need the co-operation of all good men in this work. I sincerely trust that the day is not far distant when the standard of efficiency may be raised.

Dr. M. L. Rhein, New York.—No one more appreciates the good work that has been done in forwarding dental education in this country than I do that of Dr. Chittenden. It goes without saying how much we are in sympathy with the elevation of the standard of qualifications for admission to a dental educational school. I feel personally that Dr. Chittenden made his paper a little weaker than he intended when he spoke of the smaller colleges being irretrievably hurt by the length of the course, because I feel very much on this subject as was expressed by Dr. Billings, the president of the Association, in his opening address, that the time has come when the smaller educational institutions must go out of existence. There is no use for them at the present time. I would even say that I think the idea of proprietary educational institutions is a mistake. I think this Section should come out flat-footed on the question of men enjoying a salaried position due entirely to the income of the institution with which they are connected. That has invariably been one of the worst features connected with proprietary dental education in this country. If the efforts to raise the standard of dental education is a blow at this sort of institution, it is a blow that is well-merited and in which personally I am in full sympathy, because the sooner they are eradicated and destroyed, the better for the interests of the country at large. How much better it would be if there were fewer institutions in which there was a distinctive salaried position of an amount to enable the proper teacher to be selected, irrespective of the necessity of earning their living by the practice of their profession. It is impossible at the present day for the real professor of any branch in a dental institution to be engaged in the active practice of his calling. His attention to practical dentistry should be confined to the infirmary division of the institution with which he is connected. This is the idea we have to look forward to in dental education. It makes little difference, to my mind, how much we raise the standard, if we fail to accomplish the real results.

There is just one little point of difference that I have with Dr. Chittenden in his paper, that is, the words of criticism that he makes at institutions of character for keeping themselves advertised, as he says, in the eyes of the public, advertising their superiority over the smaller institutions. I hardly believe, if I could talk this matter over with Dr. Chittenden, that he would see this in the light in which he appears to, judging from his paper. To my mind, it is one of the forms that is necessary to use to drive out of existence the inferior institution. It is impracticable in my view to compare any one of our great institutions with an advertising dental parlor; so I think Dr. Chittenden has made rather an unfortunate mistake in a comparison of this kind. These large institutions are constantly before the eyes of the public in the public print. A very necessary form of the education of the young men to-day is the athletic surroundings of the university. There are differences of opinion regarding their value, but at the present time they have the sympathy and the accord of the American people. I myself believe that they play an important part in the welfare of our educational institutions. I believe they do good, and can do harm. Devotion of time to them to the neglect of studies is the same evil which besets every young man in all surroundings of life. A great deal of the advertising of departments of universities is of such a nature as is not directly sought for by these universities. It is worked up by the individual parties, and I personally see no harm in it. I believe this is a sort of competition which will bring out better features from the opposite institutions. I must say that I differ from my friend Dr. Chittenden on that one point.

Mr. T. Constant, Scarborough, York, England.—I have so little knowledge of the condition of education in this country that I am hardly in a position to speak upon the subject. At the same time, speaking generally on the question of education, a subject to which I have given some attention, I think the most necessary thing in considering the educational conditions of any kind is to insist upon a very high standing of preliminary education. The time that is necessary to give to the application of technical knowledge, when the mind is very receptive, as in the case of medicine and surgery, and especially in dentistry, is so largely devoted to the requirements of special knowledge that one's general knowledge is liable to be neglected. I think, therefore, that prior to examinations of special studies one's general education should be as complete as possible. I feel that the fewer educational centres we can have, the better. The facilities for travel now are such that distances are not the consideration they used to be, so that one great objection to having centres of education is removed. I therefore think that great harm is done, and I believe, from my little knowledge, particularly so in this country, by multiplication of centres of education. On the same lines I believe, myself, in the uniform standard of examinations. I think if all the States of America united and had one national standard in examinations to which it became necessary for every student to present himself before being licensed to practise it would be a good thing. He could then succeed in taking the ordinary university degree. License to practise, I believe, should be determined by national examining centres.

Dr. W. E. Walker, New Orleans.—I believe the idea of the formation of great universities with dental departments is the correct one, and that the working out of the plan as it is being done in Harvard is really what it ought to come to; that there should be the unification of preliminary requirements for all the different departments instead of having one for medicine and another for dentistry, the basal studies being taken alike by all, and capped by the special work according to the field a man intends to make his lifework.

The question of preliminary requirements is a very difficult one to handle. Because it was found that when the dean examined the students he was so influenced not only by his desire for the college to grow, but by the forces brought to bear upon him by other teachers, that he would sometimes admit students that ought not to be admitted, it was thought that that would be overcome by the requirement that the dean should no longer examine students for entrance, but that the county superintendent of education should have the matter in hand. The law does not specify whether it shall be the superintendent of the county in which the school is located or in which the student resides. The result is that there is a different standard. We find many boys coming from the country where the standards are low and where the county superintendent will allow himself to be influenced by personal feeling and give him a certificate which he would not have received had he come to the educational centre to be examined by the county superintendent in which the school is located where the standard would be higher. I have an instance in mind in which a student was examined and refused by the examiner of the county in which the school was located, and went home and was passed by the superintendent of the county in which the student resided. There must, therefore, be some change in that direction. Just how it is to be done I do not know. Regarding the universities, if there could be a national body to examine all applicants it would seem to work more satisfactorily than any other means.

A paper entitled "The Vasomotor System of the Pulps," with exhibition of slides, was read by Eugene S. Talbot, M.D., D.D.S., of Chicago.

(For Dr. Talbot's paper, see page 89.)

DISCUSSION.

Dr. M. H. Fletcher, Cincinnati.—There is not much which occurs to me in the way of discussion of this paper except to commend what has been said. The subject of the nerve distribution of the pulp seems to be greatly neglected, and it is a matter of great pleasure to know that it has been taken up by such physicians as Drs. Talbot and Latham, because through these studies one may be able to find out why its tendency is to recede from any attempt at investigation. I do not think the doctor has given any definite theory, except to show us the distribution of the nerves about the vasomotor system. If I have overlooked that point I shall be glad to have the doctor tell me whether his theory shows anything aside from discovering to us the anatomy as it now is. I am certainly very much pleased to have this subject taken up, because it will result to our knowledge.

Mr. Constant, England.—I would like to express my appreciation of Dr. Talbot's very valuable paper. I regret that he did not read the whole of it, because it would be of great interest to me to have learned the later views of American writers on the subject of the vasomotor system. The photographs and micrographs were extremely interesting, and the feature that struck me more particularly was the great continuity of the non-medullated fibres that the photographs showed. It is of particular interest to me, because the work that I have recently been doing in connection with the pulp comes into touch with that work in one or more ways. From clinical reasons I have for some years been under the impression that the so-called odontoblasts have more to do with the vasomotor system than the mesoblasts. They have, in my opinion, very little to do with the formation of dentine, excepting so far as regulating the blood-pressure. They undoubtedly assist, but not in the direct manner in which most English dental anatomists have described.

The paper, therefore, of Dr. Talbot has been of great interest to me, and to have heard that alone I should consider my visit here fully repaid.

Dr. Gilmer.—The subject is not one that I can discuss. I think, however, that we are greatly indebted to Dr. Talbot for this work and the success he has met with. The facts are before us. He shows us what is in the pulp, and I think it is not a matter which we can criticise.

Dr. Eames.—I am much interested in this paper, because I can see how one may take advantage of the idea therein expressed clinically. For instance, there is no place in the body where we can see the control of the nervous system over the tissues as in the nose. I believe that in many inflammatory conditions of the pulp we may control these conditions, as we understand what could influence the general nervous system. I have had a patient say to me, " When I am tired I have a pain in my tooth." I hardly realized at the time what that meant, but I can see now how exhaustion of the nervous system will so influence the control of the blood-supply in that organ that it will be paralyzed in a way so that it will let blood in there and cause pain. I can see also how, in a subacute inflammatory condition, a person whose nervous system has been exhausted may acquire a chronic state of inflammation in the pulp by paralyzing these fibres so that the blood-vessels themselves become permanently stretched. Therefore, I do think that these demonstrations have a clinical value in this respect.

Dr. H. E. Belden.—I feel a good deal like the student who wrote to the physician, asking how he would tell when he had reached pulp. The physician wrote back that the patient would tell him. I have never made any minute study of the anatomy of the pulp, but I can see the good that would arise from it, and I am very glad to have had the pleasure of seeing the paper demonstrated.

Dr. Jules J. Sarrazin, New Orleans.—I have nothing to add to the discussion. I thoroughly appreciate the work done, the magnitude of which is appalling. I agree with the expression that the amount of knowledge given may become of great usefulness in a better understanding of the physiological conditions. The paper presented by Dr. Talbot reveals an enormous amount of thorough research, but in my opinion, we are not yet in position to fully profit by the work. We have to get a greater elucidation of the work and the deductions which may be drawn from that work in order to get the practical application in the fields of pathology.

Dr. Talbot (closing).—In connection with this work, six years ago, it occurred to me that a symposium each year upon the dental pulp would be a valuable contribution. About thirty years ago I realized that there were other conditions that assisted in the decay of the teeth than those that have been brought out by Professor Miller. My studies in degeneracy in this country and in Europe have taught me that in degenerates decay of the teeth takes place much more rapidly than in healthy individuals. The same thing is true in families of four or five children where all but one child is healthy. The teeth of the degenerate child decay much more rapidly than do those of the others. My work for the last thirty years has to a certain extent been along that line. My research work has taken such a great part of my time that I have not been able to prepare papers that would have pleased me to have written. With so much of my work in that direction finished, I am now taking up the study of the dental pulp, or the nervous phenomena in decay of the teeth. We have had views expressed in regard to the pulp, and have been able to find out what has been done in these directions. That is the reason we have invited gentlemen from abroad to read papers or send them to us. They are specialists along certain lines. They have advanced ideas on certain subjects, and while they do not agree with each and every one of us, yet I would just as soon have a paper from a man who has fixed ideas, whether they are correct or not. Such papers create a discussion and the happiest feeling, and assist greatly in elucidating facts. My paper to-day, as I have said, covers work of four years, and Mr. Constant has rather anticipated me in my work that I have on hand, which to my mind will bring out certain points in relation to the teeth as suggested by him and Dr. Eames. I shall present it very soon, and expect to show certain results. It demonstrates conclusively the vasomotor system of the pulp. Had I undertaken this work ten or fifteen years ago, it would have been impossible for me to have shown the pictures I have because the modern stains have developed an idea of the terminal structures of the nervous system which could not have been done years ago.

An exhibition of slides was given, demonstrating the papers of Drs. D. E. Causch, Brighton, England, on " The Development of Hard Tissue in the Pulp;" M. H. Fletcher, of Cincinnati, on " Tolerance of Tissues to Foreign Bodies, with Special Reference to the Pulp and Gums;" Martha Anderson, Moline, on " Notes on Pulp Technic;" Michael Morgenstern, Strassburg, Germany, on " Some Histologic Facts that contradict the Generally Accepted Odontoblast Theory."

Dr. Anderson's paper was read by Dr. Talbot.

(For Dr. Anderson's paper, see Vol. XXIV., page 449; for Dr. Fletcher's paper, see *ibid.*, page 596; for Dr. Morgenstern's paper, see page 161.)

Dr. A. E. Baldwin, of Chicago, Dr. M. H. Fletcher, of Cincinnati, and Dr. W. E. Walker were appointed a Nominating Committee.

Adjourned to Wednesday, May 6, at two P.M.

A paper entitled " Professional Responsibility" was read by Dr. A. E. Baldwin, of Chicago.

(For Dr. Baldwin's paper, see Vol. XXIV., page 673.)

DISCUSSION.

Mr. T. E. Constant, Scarborough, England.—I think that short papers on such practical every-day questions as this raised by Dr. Baldwin are extremely valuable. I agree with him more particularly in his remarks upon the necessity for the care of children's teeth. We as dentists recognize the extreme importance of the care of children's teeth, but I regret to say that in my country, and perhaps also in yours, the majority of the members of the medical profession do not systematically examine the teeth of children placed under their care and, when it is necessary, recommend them to consult a dentist. I am quite sure that if that were done many infantile troubles would be avoided, and by preserving the temporary teeth a great deal of work subsequently done by dentists in the way of regulation of permanent teeth would be rendered unnecessary.

Then, too, there is the point of the troubles dependent upon neglected conditions of the dental organs in adults. When connected with the general hospital I had many opportunities of seeing incipient gastric ulcer. In almost all of these cases the teeth were in very bad condition. In the prehemorrhagic stage of gastric ulcer, patients treated in the general hospital were relieved without any attention to the mouth, but with careful dieting, etc. It is the experience of physicians in England—I have not been able to demonstrate it—that careful repair of dental decay, removal of suppurating roots, and careful attention to the hygiene of the mouth has cured the patients without further medicinal treatment, and that so long as the aseptic condition of the oral cavity was preserved by the patient after leaving the hospital the gastritis has not recurred. It seems, perhaps, a bold thing to say, but in my opinion the majority of cases of severe gastritis in young women is due to defective oral hygiene. I therefore think the point in the paper is well taken.

Dr. Gilmer.—I think it very important that the attention of the members should be directed to this subject. The suggestions of the paper have been sufficiently broad to open up a wide discussion. I feel more and more that we do not get hold of children sufficiently early. As soon as the teeth have erupted we ought to see the children regularly for examinations. We frequently have children brought to us with the teeth decayed to the extent of an uncovered pulp, and with a child of nervous temperament it is no wonder that extractions are made. I therefore insist that the children shall be brought to me, not only to examine for decay, but to see whether the caretaker is giving proper attention to the dental organs and to the mouth. I believe I have in this way saved many more teeth than by filling. Prophylaxis, if intelligently carried out, will do a wonderful amount of good. We should examine not only the dental organs of the patient coming for examination, but every part of the oral cavity. If we do otherwise we are little more than beginners. If the laryngologist examined only for one diseased condition, he would hardly be considered a valuable man to the profession. Not long since, in examining the mouth of a patient, I discovered under the tongue a stone in Wharton's duct. If allowed to go on this might have been the cause of a serious condition.

Dr. Eugene S. Talbot, Chicago.—If there is any one time in the life of the child when oral hygiene should be at its best it is at the time of the eruption of the temporary teeth. In my studies along the line of evolution on which I have written so much it is noted that the face and the jaws and the teeth are changed from generation to generation, and that we can judge to a certain extent of the nationality of an individual by the evolution of the head and face. Therefore, I believe that in these transitory structures the conditions in the mouth, decay of teeth, etc., are very apt to occur. It is at the time of the eruption of the temporary teeth that we have what I have termed the second period of stress. These periods of stress are very much on the same order as the systemic changes every seven years the old people speak of. At this time the dentist has an idea that all diseases of the human body revolve around the teeth, and to a certain extent this is true; but he forgets that the mucous membrane throughout the body is undergoing a great change at this time. Up to this time the child has been taking liquid food, and now the system is preparing itself for harder food, and the cells of the mucous membrane are undergoing a great change. Therefore, as the essayist has stated, the greatest care of the teeth should be taken at this time. I am not in harmony with Weissman regarding the inheritance of acquired defects. I do believe in the inheritance of acquired defects, and have proved the theory. In Mississippi, and I suppose in other parts of the South, and in England, the habit is to extract the first permanent molar, especially if it is decayed. In the South it is customary to extract it on general principles. The reason is that this tooth comes in irregularly, and by its extraction the balance are allowed to come in in normal condition. This particular point is important because of the transitory nature of the jaws; this has a tendency to produce arrest of development. It is therefore a cause of irregularities of the teeth seen in England which is further intensified from generation to generation.

Dr. Curtis.—Mr. Constant's remarks are well taken. I believe that the greater part of the work done by our throat specialists is necessitated by the pathological condition of the teeth.   The children should be brought to the dentist for examination yearly, and he should direct to whom they should be sent for proper treatment of the affections caused by these pathological conditions of the mouth.   I remember quite early in my practice a throat specialist meeting me on the street and saying, " I shall soon have to send you a percentage of my income."   I asked upon what ground he made the statement, and he replied, " You send me more patients in nose and throat work than all the other dentists in the city."   That stimulated me to send more, to be more careful in my examinations of the nose and throat of my patients.   I did not, however, accept a percentage.

I think the extraction of the sixth-year molar is a lazy man's way of avoiding work.   I believe it should never be done except where the child's tooth is abscessed, and in many cases not then. There are, however, conditions, as I said yesterday, in which you have to treat the case individually and according to the conditions of the mouth and of the patient.

Dr. M. L. Rhein.—At such meetings as this, the necessity for men who assume the position of caring for the teeth to realize their responsibility cannot be too strongly urged.   It is my invariable rule to pay absolutely no attention to the suggestions or directions of people coming to me until I have made a thorough examination. I then inform them of what I deem advisable to be done, and if it does not meet their wishes our relations end at that point.   I believe that is the only truly professional line of conduct.   This, I think, differentiates between what we are pleased to call stomatologists and dentists.

Dr. Hans Pilcher, Vienna.—I do not think I have anything to say in this matter.   I am pleased with the suggestions of Dr. Baldwin, and I shall bear them in mind in my practice.

Dr. W. E. Walker, New Orleans.—It occurred to me (if I may discuss the discussion as well as the paper, for I can only commend the paper) that we do not always " see ourselves as others see us."   I did not know that it was the practice of England and the South to sacrifice the first permanent molar.   That this extraction does occur here I am aware, but I judge from articles written on it that this is practised elsewhere.   Here I know it is too common.

In regard to examining the whole mouth instead of looking

simply at the tooth to which attention is directed by the patient, that this practice is not sufficiently common among dentists has been impressed upon me by the surprise of the patient manifested when I have proceeded to examine the whole oral cavity rather than simply the tooth complained of.

Dr. M. L. Rhein.—I thoroughly agree with Dr. Walker that there is as much extraction of the first permanent molar in the East and West as in the South. I do not believe it is confined to one section of the country, and I am pleased to put myself on record as taking the position, the exception proving the rule, that there is no warrant for the removal of the first permanent molar.

Dr. George F. Eames, Boston.—The subject of the essayist's paper is one of the greatest importance. I can conceive of no other that can come before this body being of so great importance as this. It has to deal with three or four items always to be considered in our professional life: (1) The relation of the stomatologist to other specialists in general medicine, or the dentist to the doctor. That is a great subject in itself, and should be ever kept in mind. (2) Another is the relation of the stomatologist to his patients. (3) The relation of the stomatologist to other dentists. (4) The relation of the stomatologist to himself. This subject should be brought to the attention of the general practitioner and to other specialists, that patients may be advised in regard to oral conditions. It should be brought to the attention of the laymen. The subject deals with the relation of the local conditions in the mouth to the general health, and this I consider of the greatest importance, far and away above other considerations.

Dr. Baldwin (closing).—Of course, in a paper of this kind one can do nothing more than touch upon the different subjects. I would especially emphasize what Dr. Gilmer has said in not having patients sufficiently early.

As Dr. Eames has said, there are relations to be recognized. Our object should be to unify all the departments of the healing art in one great whole.

I thank you for the discussion, and realize more than any one the shortcomings of the paper.

A paper by Dr. O. N. Heise, of Cincinnati, entitled " Empyema of the Antrum," was then read.

(For Dr. Heise's paper, see Vol. XXIV., page 608.)

Dr. Gilmer, Chicago.—Mr. Chairman and gentlemen of the Section, I had the pleasure of looking over this paper previous to its reading, and I feel that it is a valuable paper, although the field which it covers is a narrow one. I feel that Dr. Heise has done well in differentiating between a pus sac in the end of the root and true empyema. I do not know whether I could agree with him in the nomenclature, but I think he has done well in the differentiation. We are often defective in diagnosis of the various diseases to which the anatomy is subject. We take, for instance, the condition spoken of here. He calls it cystic empyema; the other, true empyema. It may be that it will be pretty difficult to separate these two, although there is a vast difference. Both of them practically are encysted. We have a root of a tooth which approximates closely to the floor of the antrum, and we have a sac on the end of the root filled with pus. Some years ago this was spoken of as pyogenic membrane. Of course, there is no such thing as pyogenic membrane. There are conditions in which the bone is absorbed and the sac continues to grow, completely filling the cavity. We will have difficulty, therefore, in making a diagnosis. We will say that the patient has all the symptoms perhaps. He has the thinning of the buccal and nasal walls, but there is no appearance of pus. It may be said it is not an encysted maxillary sinus, but to all intents and purposes it is an empyema of the maxillary sinus. An empyema really means a cavity that is completely filled with pus, having no opening. Therefore, the so-called empyema of the maxillary sinus is not an empyema at all. But here we do have an empyema of the maxillary sinus because it is a sac that is filled with pus.

It is difficult to differentiate between the various diseased conditions in the antrum. Regarding the causes of the diseases of the antrum it seems to me that usually they come from only two sources. We may have syphilitic disease of the antrum. This I have seldom seen. The two sources are from the nose, the inflammation extending by the continuity of tissue into the maxillary sinus, and from the roots of the teeth. The root of the tooth is often given as the cause of the trouble when it is not primarily so. We have as a result of a catarrhal condition of the lining of the membrane an inflammation which may cause the death of the live and healthy tooth. You will find the floor of the antrum thinned out, representing the roots of the molar or bicuspid. If you will remove one of these little hillocks (indicating), you will find the merest swell. The mucous membrane overlying becomes inflamed; it may involve the pulp, and the tooth may die. The condition may not be recognized. We have a pyogenic condition at the end of the root which keeps up a slow inflammation and continues the disease of the antrum. Therefore, this trouble is secondary rather than primary. ˙ I believe we have a great deal more of the disease of the antrum since the advent of influenza in this country. We have an irritation of the lining of the antrum causing a stenosis, which in turn causes an excess of fluid, and by infection of that fluid we have an empyema. I find another condition resulting from a pulpless tooth and an antrum not fully antiseptic. We may have a small pus cavity walled off. The inflammation of the lining membrane comes from the continuity of the tissue from the nose, and results in an empyema of the maxillary sinus, which we would not have had we not the inflamed tissue. My experience teaches me that in the case of a root of a tooth in which the pulp is dead extending into the antrum, nothing will cure the condition but the removal of the tooth. If an opening is required I would not make it from the antrum, but from the nose. If the case demands an operation upon the antrum, a broad surgical treatment should be carried out. If I should make the opening just above the membrane of the gum, I would expect to find in people between forty and fifty the bone very thin. I would make the opening sufficiently large to insert my little finger, receiving an impression of the condition. Another reason for opening here (indicating) is that the cheek falls in. An opening here allows also the insertion of an electric lamp into the maxillary sinus and permits a thorough washing out.

It may be that Keil erred in attributing so many cases of the teeth as a cause of disease of the antrum because he did not recognize that here was a secondary cause in the pulp of the tooth having been destroyed. He says that they are the largest factor in etiology. That may be true; not, however, primarily, but secondarily.

It seems to me that we ought almost never use arsenic for the destruction of pulps. The application of cocaine is very much better. There are sometimes accessory or additional openings in the roots of teeth larger than the apical openings, and through these the arsenic may do much harm. I cannot conceive why chloride of zinc or carbolic acid should be used in such cases.

Dr. M. H. Fletcher, Cincinnati.—This subject is one which has interested me very greatly and one upon which I have had a great deal of worry. I have had many cases in which I have blamed myself for not being able to fully understand. I find, however, that my experience is the duplicate of many others. I would like to speak of some of the features of the anatomy spoken of by Dr. Gilmer. In 1891 or 1892 I took occasion to go through the Army Medical Museum to study the anatomy of the antrum, and it turned out, in the examination of fourteen or fifteen hundred antra, that the descriptions by anatomists known to me at that time were erroneous. In other words the anatomy as pictured by Dr. Gilmer and pictured by anatomists was found in twelve skulls out of the fifteen hundred. On the other hand, when we came to the connection of the floor of the tooth with the floor of the antrum, I found in a large percentage of cases that there was no bony covering to many roots of the teeth. Instead of being thin and parchment-like, you will have an opening here, the apex of the tooth coming against the soft tissues of the antrum. That being the case you can easily see the condition spoken of here. I have seen several cases of such perforation and an abscess discharging into the antrum in which healing took place as readily as if there had been an opening by the alveolar process. We all know that on the buccal surfaces many of the roots are perfectly bare of bone, being simply covered by a mucous membrane, and, as I have stated, many cases are so in the antrum. An abscessed tooth coming in contact with the antrum in that way would discharge in the antrum and the pus go in the way of least resistance. Fortunately, the majority discharge into the mouth. It is my experience that pulpless teeth producing antral trouble can be made to heal as readily as though they discharged into the mouth. On the other hand, my recent experience in treating these cases has confirmed me in the belief that diseases of the alveolar process and calcareous deposits are more largely to blame for antral trouble than pulp lesions or the loss of the pulp. It is natural from my reasoning as to pathology that a diseased bone about the tooth can much more readily cause diseased antrum from continuity of tissue than a diseased pulp producing an abscess. If you have necrosed bone about the tooth you must have inflammation extending in every direction, and the bone extends upward, towards the antrum. The extension of dead bone and inflammation is apt to be very great if it has entered to any considerable distance into the alveolar process. It never has been my experience to see a bicuspid that came very near to the floor of the antrum as compared with the molars. I have seen these openings referred to by Dr. Gilmer.

I have talked with Dr. Heise about antral trouble from the live tooth. I fail to see any condition about the tooth with a vital pulp that would cause antral trouble. I can conceive of an exostosis producing some inflammation, but if the pulp is alive I do not see any reason why it should cause antral trouble or produce pus in the antrum.

The use of arsenic is a pet scheme of mine. I have used it about ever since I have been practising, and it is my habit, if I feel that in any way I have been inefficient in opening the root-canals, to insert some arsenic and leave it, expecting it to produce asepsis. I have done this not only a few times, but a great many. I do not, however, use arsenic to any degree in destroying pulps.

Dr. Belden.—In view of the fact that you use arsenic at all, what is your objection to using it in destroying pulps?

Dr. Fletcher.—If we use enough of it to destroy the pulp in a reasonable time, it is sufficient to cause sloughing afterwards. As to the use of zinc and other medicaments that destroy bone, I have seen carbolic acid destroy quite a large area of the alveolar process. On the other hand I never have seen arsenic do it. Arsenic, however, if applied to live tissues, will probably destroy a small zone. It never has in my experience produced a necrosis. It may produce destruction, but that may be compared to traumatic injury. The tissues are dead. They do not continue to die and necrosis ensue. Also, it has been my experience that the tissues will remain sore for months, may be for years, if the application is short of destruction of tissue. There is, however, no septic condition, no necrosis, no pus. The arsenic is so aseptic that it stops that process.

Dr. Gilmer.—Have you not seen the destruction of bone between the teeth from the use of the arsenic?

Dr. Fletcher.—I never have.

Mr. Constant.—I have on three occasions.

Dr. Gilmer.—I have seen it many times.

Dr. Fletcher.—The author has distinguished between the cystic condition and that of empyema. I think I have to stretch my imagination quite a little bit to think a tooth would produce that trouble. I would think such trouble more like adenitis than a pus cavity.

Mr. Constant, Scarborough, England.—I would speak of two points; first, with regard to the etiology. As a student I was much impressed with the importance ·of the tooth in the causation of empyema of the antrum. It is my experience that the longer one is in practice the less one feels inclined to suspect the tooth as the cause of empyema of the antrum. In my own experience it has been very exceptional to be able to find a case in which disease of the antrum could be definitely traced to the tooth.

In regard to what Dr. Gilmer says of the difficulty in distinguishing between secondary trouble in the tooth after the empyema,—that is, in determining cause and effect,—I am quite sure that in many cases of so-called empyema, put down as due to abscess connected with the tooth, is putting the cart before the horse. I can recall two cases in which empyema of the antrum was supposed to be due to trouble in the first molar. When the first molar was removed, it was found possible to evacuate the pus, and that was taken as proof that the tooth caused the trouble. I could not convince myself that the tooth was the cause of the trouble. I think the fact that the apices actually went into the antrum made it easy to get the discharge in that way. On that point I quite agree with Dr. Fletcher that it is far more common to find the apices of teeth bare within the antrum than to find them covered. A great number which I have examined in England show that.

The other point is the distinction drawn between so-called cystic conditions within the antrum and pus in the antral cavity. In one case, in connection with the second bicuspid, such a condition was present. When the second bicuspid roots were removed there was a very copious discharge of aqua-sanious fluid which kept discharging. The antrum must have been quite filled with it. The sac gradually contracted and healed in less than three weeks, and there was no further trouble.

Dr. M. L. Rhein.—I feel convinced, from a careful study of this subject, that too often a mistake in etiology is made in these cases, and that the cases in which the tooth is the primary etiological factor are very very rare. The tooth becomes involved through pathological conditions between the end of the root and the antrum, and is too often given the blame. I think it is wise to emphasize this point.

Dr. Fletcher.—I think Dr. Talbot and I found that the molar tooth could produce this trouble in about five per cent.

Dr. A. E. Baldwin.—I am a firm believer that arsenic can seldom if ever affect the tissues beyond the pulp of the tooth. Dr. Gilmer has referred to the septum being lost by the careless application of the arsenic in the particles getting down between the teeth.

Dr. Gilmer.—I spoke of the particles on the sides of the root which I· have found and been able to pick off.

Dr. Baldwin.—Years ago I suspected the same thing, and I made several examinations in this way: In a central incision I would make application to the pulp of the tooth, and after a sufficient time I took out the pulp. I then took several sections of the pulp, but could find no evidence of the arsenic in the several parts. I do not think, therefore, that the pulp could convey the arsenic to the adjacent tissues. I think a great deal of the injury is done by the careless application of the arsenic and the ease with which it gets outside of the tooth, causing the destruction of bone and soft structures.

Dr. Curtis.—The anatomical features have been beautifully brought out. I would just like to say that I think there are very few diseases of the antrum of a primary nature. I think the large majority of diseases of the antrum are due to affections of the teeth. Some reasons for slow results in treatment are on account of a tuberculous condition. I think the paper is particularly valuable in the matter of differential diagnosis. The cystic conditions usually found in the antrum I believe are largely due to alveolar abscess, to septic conditions of the pulp, or of the canal. I have seen some cystic tumors where there was very extended absorption of the bone, and where the periosteum of the antrum was so crowded to the opening at the nares that there was actually no antrum left. This was one of the most serious cases of antrum affection that I have seen.

(To be continued.)

Editorial.

REPLY TO HARVARD'S CORRECTION.

Upon another page, under the heading of " Correction from Harvard," is a communication from Dr. Eugene H. Smith, Dean of Harvard Dental School, in which he takes exception to a certain paragraph in the editorial in the February number of this journal, under the general title, " Will Dental Colleges reverse their Decision?" He especially finds subject for criticism in the third paragraph of said editorial, in which there was a mere statement of fact, as understood by the writer, in regard to what the editor pleased to call " Harvard's application."

In order that this may be understood it is necessary to quote from the paragraph in question. It is there stated, " Rumors were rife that this session [Faculties' Association at Asheville, N. C.] would witness a change of opinion and possibly an effort might be made to rescind the former action [four years' course]. The vote, however, on the *Harvard application,* refusing permission for that school to remain at three years, seemed to settle all fears in that direction, in the minds of those present, as to the stability of the four years' course."

The criticism that Dean Smith makes is, that " Harvard did not make application for permission to keep to the three years' course. Harvard simply stated her position and the reasons therefor." If this were the sole reason for the presence of the delegates from Harvard at the Asheville meeting, why, may it be asked, was it required that two representatives from that university should be sent a long journey when this could as well, and perhaps better, be stated by letter? It would seem from this acknowledgment, that the time spent at the Association of Faculties was more than wasted, and it would also seem that Harvard had decided in advance not to accept the four-year rule, no matter what might be the ultimate action of the organization. This portion of the Dean's letter admits of no other construction.

The members of the Faculties' Association did not, however,

so regard it, and they considered that Harvard *did* make an application to be permitted to continue the three years' course. Both her delegates were strenuous in their statements that the entrance requirements, with a nine months' session, were in advance of other schools in membership, and should entitle Harvard to some consideration.. The discussion occupied much time and the delegates from Harvard were energetic in their efforts to impress the members with the importance to the profession, and to Harvard, of these requirements. They failed, however, to make the matter clear that these were far in advance of many departments of universities connected with the Association, and possibly others. They did succeed, however, in convincing the members that Harvard proposed to advance the entrance to the Dental Department, in 1904, to the A.B. degree. Upon this understanding a committee was appointed to consider the entire question. This committee, according to Dean Smith, " failed utterly to understand the scope of our entrance requirements and reported accordingly." In view of this rather serious charge of incompetency, it may be well to state here who were appointed upon this committee. The President named Dr. J. D. Patterson, Kansas City Dental College; Dr. G. V. Black, North Western University, Chicago; Dr. H. P. Carlton, University of California; Dr. D. Stubblefield, Dental Department of Vanderbilt University, and James Truman, Chairman, University of Pennsylvania.

This committee met several times and fully considered the subject matter as stated by the delegates from Harvard. They were unanimous in the opinion that Harvard had proposed to advance the entrance requirements to the A.B. degree, and that it was expected to have this in full force by the year 1904. In view of this the committee were also decided in the opinion that this marked advance in dental education demanded peculiar consideration at the hands of the Association, and accordingly a report was prepared for presentation to the main body substantially as follows:

That in view of the fact that Harvard proposed to advance the entrance requirements, as stated, permission be granted said school to continue at three years, and further, that any other school in membership with the Association equally willing to advance to the same standard be granted a similar concession. When the Chairman presented this report, the delegates from Harvard immediately announced that they had not been understood. That

Harvard had no expectation of advancing the entrance requirements to the A.B. degree immediately, or the following year, but hoped in the course of time to reach that desirable position. That which they claimed may be best understood by quoting the remarks of Dean Smith, as officially reported in the proceedings, and which is deemed to be substantially correct.

The Dean said, "I regret that the committee has misunderstood our position in stating that the requirement is to be the A.B. degree. I have tried to make it clear that it is not our purpose, at this time, to require the A.B. degree. We state in our Catalogue that the requirements for admission will be as follows: Candidates for admission holding the degree of A.B. from any reputable college, are admitted without examination; all other candidates must qualify from the following list of studies amounting to sixteen points. (These were not given in report.) I will simply say, that, beginning in 1904, we will require the same examinations for students entering the dental school as for entering the collegiate department of Harvard College, the same in quality, but not in quantity. Now, you must bear in mind that the requirements for entrance to Harvard College differ, in this respect, from the entrance examinations of any other university in the country: that they do not accept certificates from any preparatory school. The candidate must stand an examination."

This statement of the Dean created a sensation. It was contrary to the understanding of the members of the committee, as well as that of the entire body. The report of the committee was, therefore, at once recommitted for further consideration. The committee, on reassembling, were left but one course to pursue, and, while unanimous in their decision, they reluctantly felt forced to report the following:

"WHEREAS, Your committee on the Harvard matter, in obedience to the direction of the Association, has reconsidered the question, and concluded that the advance proposed by the Dental Department of Harvard University, as now understood, does not warrant, at present, any reduction in the length of the course established by the Association. Therefore, be it

"*Resolved,* That the Association cannot, under the rules, consider that Harvard is entitled to less time than other schools having an equal standard of admission, with the exception, it may be, of Analytical Chemistry and Physics."

This was adopted, and at a later period in the Session the resignation of Harvard was handed in and accepted.

The assertion of the Dean, that no school in the Association demanded as much in their entrance requirements, was only true in a minor sense. Examination of the announcements of several colleges indicate very clearly that the Dean was not fully informed as to the requirements of certain schools, and, while there is a difference, it is not sufficiently marked as to place Harvard as an exceptional department. The requirements of three schools, including Harvard, each having a course of nine months, is subjoined.

REQUIREMENTS OF HARVARD DENTAL SCHOOL.

The 16 counts previously alluded to are as follows: English, 4; Physics, 2; Latin, 4; or, French, 2, and English and American History, 2; or, French, 2, and Greek and Roman History, 2; or, German, 2, and English and American History, 2; or, German, 2, and Greek and Roman History, 2. Theoretical and Descriptive (Inorganic) Chemistry and Qualitative Analysis, 4. In addition, the candidate will be obliged to offer either Algebra (2), Plane Geometry (2), or any two of the following: Solid Geometry (1), Botany (1) Zoölogy (1), Anatomy, Physiology, and Hygiene (1), Wood Working (1), Blacksmithing (1), Chipping, Filing, and Fitting (1), Machine Tool-Work (1).

The examination in English is nearly identical with that for the Department of Dentistry, University of Pennsylvania.

UNIVERSITY OF MICHIGAN, COLLEGE OF DENTAL SURGERY.

For 1903–04 the requirements are

English. An essay of not less than five hundred words, correct in spelling, etc.

History. Myers's General History, or an equivalent, and McLaughlin's History of American Nation.

Mathematics. *Arithmetic:* Fundamental Rules, Fractions (common and decimal), Denominate Numbers, Percentage, Proportion, Involution and Evolution, and the Metric System of Weights and Measures. *Algebra:* Fundamental Rules, Fractions, Equations of the First Degree, containing two or more unknown quantities. *Geometry:* Plane Geometry. *Trigonometry:* Plane Trigonometry.

Physics. An amount represented by Avery's Natural Philosophy or Carhart and Chute's Elements of Physics.

Chemistry. General Inorganic, such as is given in Freer's or in Remsen's Elementary Chemistry.

Latin. Jones's first Latin Book, or Harkness's Latin Reader, or an equivalent amount in any other text-book, and four books of Cæsar. One year's work in German or French may be substituted for the second year of Latin.

The applicant must offer two of the following subjects: Botany, Zoölogy, Physical Geography, and Physiology.

UNIVERSITY OF PENNSYLVANIA, DEPARTMENT OF DENTISTRY, FOR 1894-95.

English. This is practically the same as Harvard.

History. (*a*) American History, with the elements of Civil Government. (*b*) General History, including Greek, Roman, and English History.

Mathematics. (*a*) *Algebra:* Fundamental operations; factors; common divisors and multiples; fractions; equations of the first degree, with one or more unknown quantities; quadratic equations; the binomial theorem. (*b*) *Plane Geometry:* as in Wentworth or Philips and Fisher.

Physics. As in Carhart and Chute or Gage's Elements.

Chemistry. As in Remsen's Elementary Course in Chemistry, or Arey's Elementary Chemistry, will be accepted in lieu of Physics.

Latin. (1) A thorough knowledge of elementary grammar. (2) Cæsar, or an equivalent course in German, French, or Spanish.

The Chemistry demanded by Harvard is part of the first-year course in this department.

A comparative examination of the requirements of these three schools give about the following in counts:

Harvard.		Pennsylvania.		Michigan.	
English	4	English	4	English	2
Physics	2	Physics	2	History	2
Inorganic Chemistry.	4	History	2	Physics	2
Latin	4	Latin	2	Chemistry	2
Electives	2	Algebra	2	Latin	2
		Geometry	2	Science	2
	16		14		12

These quotations certainly do not bear out the broad assertion of Dean Smith that those who have decided upon the longest term will have entered upon a "*desultory* course of four years for students insufficiently trained for a professional education." That word "desultory" has an unpleasant sound used in this connection. Our critic may have a modified meaning connected with it, but to some of us it is defined as unmethodical, unsystematic, unconnected, irregular, etc. When applied to institutions having the training of large numbers of young men, it means that the education they offer is in large degree worthless. Does Dean Smith really believe this? The writer has had a somewhat extended acquaintance with dental educational institutions for half a century, but that experience would not enable him to decide upon the effectiveness of the teaching in any school outside of the one he is regularly connected with year in and year out. He must, therefore, regard the use of the word desultory as either a slip of the pen or an unwarranted reflection on the dental colleges of the country outside of Harvard.

While it is true that the Dental Department of the University of Pennsylvania accepts diplomas of High Schools in lieu of examinations for matriculation, it must be remembered that every diploma, so presented, is passed over to the examiner appointed by the State Board of Education, and his judgment is final in regard to its value. This is not reached through a cursory examination and upon its face value, but according to the curriculum and known standing of the school. In other words, said diploma must represent a standard equal to that demanded by the University for entrance to her department. The State examiners' endorsement must, therefore, accompany every diploma before acceptance. If the applicant presents without such a diploma, the same State officer is required to make a careful examination based on the requirements for entrance to the University. The same course is pursued with all other schools in Pennsylvania, the only exception being that he follows in others the standard required by the National Association of Dental Faculties. This plan seems to the writer, to have many advantages, and avoids the charge of partiality which may be made where the examination is held in the University. It certainly has the merit that all are treated alike and that without fear or favor. The gentleman conducting these examinations is held in proper estimation not only for his general culture, but also for his wide range of information regarding the schools of the country.

It may be well to add that the reference of diplomas and examinations to this gentleman by the University of Pennsylvania is a voluntary act and made out of respect and in obedience to the laws of the National Association of Dental Faculties.

It may seem to some that the reply to the criticism of Dean Smith is given more space than is warranted, but it must be remembered that the action of Harvard, whether intended as an application for the permission of the Faculties' Association to remain at three years, or a mere statement of this school's position, has had a very injurious effect upon dental education, as a whole. This is not supposed to have been the intention, for, undoubtedly, Harvard felt that there was more than sufficient strength embodied there to stand alone, and the delegates did not, at the time, regard their action as influencing other colleges to lower their standard or that of the Faculties. It must, however, be recognized that Harvard is one of the leading dental schools of the United States, and any action taken by its governing body necessarily exercises a wide influence. The course pursued by an influential member of a community for good or ill must always be counted upon to produce a marked effect, and what is true of the individual is increasingly true of large and influential educational institutions. The moral force of the world is made strong for good or otherwise in proportion as these influences move in one direction or the other.

It is very clear to the writer that had not Harvard withdrawn, upon the plea stated, there would have been no attempt made at Buffalo, at the special meeting, to return to three years. The National Association of Dental Examiners helped along this work by their resolution passed at Asheville (INTERNATIONAL DENTAL JOURNAL, Vol. XXIV., page 905), but it is not supposed that the delegates from Harvard were aware of the action of this body, but the resolution of the Examiners as adopted was a serious blow to dental education in the United States. When a university as well sustained as Harvard should refuse to advance, it is very natural that the schools in the Association not well financially supported should be anxious to have the same privilege. It is, therefore, beyond controversy that the example of Harvard has made it very difficult to maintain the standard established by the Association of Faculties. If, however, Harvard is satisfied that the course adopted is the best for that institution, it must be left to work out the problem alone; but in doing this the officials of that department are not justified in charging lack of thoroughness upon other schools, who maintain that no undergraduate can be taught all that pertains to dentistry in three years. By dentistry is meant the collateral branches pertaining to medicine and those directly connected with its practical work. If Harvard can accomplish this in three years of nine months, congratulations are in order, but the consensus of opinion among the most advanced dental educators is, that this is impossible with the present curriculum.

Domestic Correspondence.

CORRECTION FROM HARVARD.

To the Editor:

Sir,—Will you kindly publish this letter and by so doing correct an error in your editorial entitled, " Will Dental Colleges reverse their Decision?" In this editorial, which appeared in the February issue of the International Dental Journal, you are made to say,—

" The vote, however, on the Harvard application refusing permission for that school to remain at three years, etc."

Harvard did not make application for permission to keep to the three years' course. Harvard simply stated her position, and the reason therefor, hoping that the Association of Dental Faculties might see the wisdom of first materially advancing the entrance requirements, and bringing all schools to three years of nine months each, before entering upon a desultory course of four years for students insufficiently trained for a professional education. The committee, of which you were chairman, appointed by the Association, failed utterly to understand the scope of our entrance requirements, and reported accordingly, and the resignation of the Harvard Dental School followed.

Very truly yours,

Eugene H. Smith.

Obituary.

RESOLUTIONS OF RESPECT TO DR. JONATHAN TAFT.

Whereas, It has pleased the Divine Ruler to call into eternal rest Jonathan Taft, who passed the portals of the great unknown October 15, 1903, after a long and vigorous career of usefulness in the profession; and

Whereas, This Society especially feels his demise from the fact that one-half of the members constituting this body have re-

9

ceived a large portion of their early dental knowledge and training directly from his lips; and we further recognize that he was unique in his power to impress upon the pupils who sat under his instruction sound principles of ethics and practice. He was great in his goodness, a characteristic which stands as a shining light for others to see and follow in his footsteps; therefore, be it

Resolved, That the Odontological Society of Chicago hereby testifies to the loss experienced by the profession in the death of Dr. Taft, and extends sympathy to the family in their bereavement; also

Resolved, That these resolutions be spread upon the records of this Society, and that a copy be forwarded to the dental journals for publication.

(Signed) J. G. Reid,
L. L. Davis,
J. W. Wassall.

Adopted January 12, 1904.

Miscellany.

The Abuse of the Gold Cap.—One of the evils—growing evils, we may say—which needs persistent words of condemnation and censure is the abuse of the gold cap. Its easy adaptation renders it a too common product of "Dental Parlors," also of offices that have a professional standing but are sadly deficient in what is artistic.

It is almost never permissible to cover any of the ten anterior teeth, particularly of our lady patients, with one of these glaring abominations. It is a pitiful acknowledgment of inefficiency on the part of the operator who makes such use of them.

What is more distressing than the sight of a few gold caps to mar the smile and weaken the features of a beautiful and cultured woman? And yet this is a sight not infrequently met with. This disfigurement is conspicuous oftentimes with public speakers and persons whose taste should rebel against anything so unsightly.

In this day of porcelain art, when nature can be so closely imitated as to almost defy detection, such inartistic displays of dentistry have no excuse for being. One can scarcely attend a convention without encountering among the exhibitors from one to five outfits, all "superior methods" of swaging seamless gold crowns. The spirit of commercialism is here taking precedence over the artistic.

We are taught, and we should practise, the "art" of dentistry. And this means the restoration and repair of lost and injured members in such a manner that the casual glance will detect as little as possible of the inharmonious or artificial.—N. A. STANLEY, D.M.D., New Bedford, Mass.

GRIND LOWER TEETH RATHER THAN FORCE DOWN.—Dr. J. N. Farrar says it is better to grind off the front lower teeth when too long rather than to attempt to crowd them down into their sockets. He grinds a little at a time at intervals of several weeks.

REDUCTION OF TENDENCY TO HEMORRHAGE.—Dr. C. Edward Wallis reports that ten grains of calcium chloride administered internally three times a day for a week previous to extracting reduces very materially the tendency to hemorrhage in patients who exhibit a predisposition to excessive hemorrhage.—*Dental Digest.*

TO REMOVE OXIDE FROM GERMAN SILVER.—Dr. V. E. Barnes, in the *Dental Summary,* suggests hydrochloric acid, full strength, used cold, to remove oxide from German silver regulating applianecs.

ADRENALIN: A NEW HÆMOSTATIC.—This comparatively new drug is recommended for controlling hemorrhage in tooth extraction for patients with the hemorrhagic diathesis. Immediately before the operation a few drops injected into the gum around the tooth makes the extraction practically bloodless. It is also recommended as a preventive of the annoying hemorrhage attending the preparation of teeth or roots for crowning, and preparing for filling cavities which extend below the gum margin.—*Dental Cosmos,* May, 1903, page 399.

Current News.

BILL REGULATING DENTAL PRACTICE IN THE DISTRICT OF COLUMBIA.

[THROUGH the courtesy of Hon. William H. Wiley, of New Jersey, and Hon. A. A. Wiley, of Alabama, we are enabled to lay before the readers of the INTERNATIONAL the passage of an amendment that may have wide-spread influence upon State legislation in this direction. The bill as passed finally and approved by the President is herewith subjoined.—ED.]

An Act To amend an Act entitled " An Act for the regulation of the practice of dentistry in the District of Columbia, and for the protection of the people from empiricism in relation thereto," approved June sixth, eighteen hundred and ninety-two.

Be it enacted by the Senate and House of Representatives of the United States of America in Congress assembled, That the Act of Congress entitled " An Act for the regulation of the practice of dentistry in the District of Columbia, and for the protection of the people from empiricism in relation thereto," approved June sixth, eighteen hundred and ninety-two, be, and the same is hereby, amended by striking out all of the proviso in section three of said Act and inserting in lieu thereof the following: *"Provided,* That the board of dental examiners may issue a license to practice to any dentist who shall have been in legal practice for a period of five years or more, upon the certificate of the board of dental examiners of the State or Territory in which he practised, certifying his competency and moral character, and upon the payment of the certification fee without examination as to his qualifications."

Approved. February 5, 1904.

MINNESOTA STATE DENTAL ASSOCIATION.

THE twenty-first annual meeting of the Minnesota State Dental Association will be held in St. Paul, June 16, 17, and 18, 1904.

GEO. S. TODD,
Secretary.

NATIONAL ASSOCIATION OF DENTAL EXAMINERS.

THE National Association of Dental Examiners will hold their annual meeting in the Coliseum building, corner Thirteenth and Olive Streets, St. Louis, Mo., on the 25th, 26th, and 27th of August, beginning promptly at ten A.M. Telephone and telegraph offices in the building. Hotel accommodations will be secured for the members.

CHAS. A. MEEKER,
Secretary and Treasurer.

NEW JERSEY STATE DENTAL SOCIETY.

THE New Jersey State Dental Society will hold its annual convention in the Auditorium at Asbury Park, July 21, 22, and 23 next. The Exhibit Committee are prepared to allot space to exhibitors. Make application to the Chairman,

DR. W. G. CHASE.

MINNESOTA STATE BOARD OF DENTAL EXAMINERS.

THE Minnesota State Board of Dental Examiners will meet, for the purpose of examining applicants for license, April 5, 6, and 7, 1904. No application received after twelve M., April 5.

Meeting held at Dental Department of State University at Minneapolis.

C. H. ROBINSON,
Secretary and Treasurer.

AMERICAN DENTAL SOCIETY OF EUROPE.

THE next annual meeting of the American Dental Society of Europe will be held at the Hamburger Hof, Hamburg, Germany, April 1 to 4, 1904.

DR. CHARLES J. MONK,
Hon. Secretary.

DENTAL BOARD OF NEW SOUTH WALES.

I, THE undersigned, hereby notify that the following persons were the successful candidates at the recent election of the Dental Board of New South Wales, held on the eighteenth day of December, 1903:

Medical Practitioners.—Sir James Graham, K.B., M.D.; Arthur Palmer, M.B., F.R.C.S.

Dentists.—Henry Peach, D.D.S., Cornelius Charles Marshall, Charles Hall, Charles George Hodgson.

And I hereby declare the said Sir James Graham, Arthur Palmer, Henry Peach, Cornelius Charles Marshall, Charles Hall, and Charles George Hodgson to be duly elected as members of the Dental Board of New South Wales.

Witness my hand at Sydney this nineteenth day of December, 1903.

HORACE TAYLOR, J.P.,
Returning Officer.

IOWA STATE DENTAL SOCIETY.

THE forty-second annual meeting of the Iowa State Dental Society will be held at Des Moines, Tuesday, Wednesday, and Thursday, May 3, 4, and 5, 1904.

W. R. CLACK, *President,*
Clear Lake, Iowa.

C. W. BRUNNER, *Secretary,*
Toledo, Iowa.

FRATERNAL DENTAL SOCIETY OF ST. LOUIS.

The Fraternal Dental Society of St. Louis meets every third Tuesday evening, at eight o'clock, at the Lindell Hotel. Following are the officers for 1904:

President, Edward Everett Haverstick; Vice-President, W. E. Brown; Secretary, E. P. Dameron; Treasurer, Sam. T. Bassett.

Executive Committee.—B. L. Thorpe, W. L. Whipple, Geo. A. Mathae.

READING DENTAL SOCIETY.

A MEETING of the Reading Dental Society was held February 4, 1904. Dr. Walter H. Neall was the guest of honor, and read a paper on "Food and Health from a Dental Stand-Point."

The following officers were elected: President, W. H. Scholl; Vice-President, Charles Grim; Treasurer, Elwood Tate; Secretary, C. R. Scholl.

Executive Committee.—George Schlegal, E. M. Bohn, L. E. Tate.

C. R. SCHOLL,
Secretary.

SOUTHERN DENTAL SOCIETY OF NEW JERSEY.

AT the annual meeting of the Southern Dental Society of New Jersey, held January 20, 1904, in Camden, the following officers were elected:

President, Alphonso Irwin; Vice-President, W. A. Jacquette; Treasurer, Mary A. Morrison; Recording Secretary, Stanley Ironside; Corresponding Secretary, C. Ironside; Librarian, J. G. Halsey.

Executive Committee.—W. W. Crate, J. G. Halsey, Charles P. Tuttle, E. E. Brown, O. E. Peck.

Membership Committee.—Alphonso Irwin, W. H. Gelston, W. A. Jacquette.

W. W. CRATE,
Chairman Executive Committee.

NEW HAVEN DENTAL ASSOCIATION OF CONNECTICUT.

The annual convention of the New Haven Dental Association will be held March 15 and 16, at Harmonie Hall, New Haven, Conn.

This promises to be the largest meeting ever held in the East, a large number of clinics and one of the finest exhibits ever shown.

Essays by the following distinguished members of the dental
and medical profession: Drs. R. Ottolengui, New York; Henry C.
Boenning, Philadelphia; G. Lenox Curtiss, New York; Herbert
L. Wheeler, New York; R. A. McDonnell and Wm. H. Metcalf,
New Haven; J. Wesley Shaw, Springfield. A large clinic from
residents of New York, New Jersey, Philadelphia, Massachusetts,
and Connecticut, and two surgical clinics, provided suitable cases
are presented. The business meeting will be dispensed with,
thereby allowing ample time to the thorough discussion of all
papers.

It will amply repay all to attend this convention, and enable
those who have never had an opportunity to visit the Elm City,
with the privilege of the freedom of Yale University and the
campus.

The Arrangement Committee have been especially active, having
arranged for a banquet on the evening of the first day, and in addition are arranging with the Northeast Passenger Association for a
one and a third rate on the certificate plan, provided one hundred
tickets are sold for seventy-five cents or over. (Secure certificate
when purchasing ticket.)

An invitation is extended to all ethical practitioners to join
with us, and take active part in our meeting.

FREDERICK H. BROWN, *President.*
E. FRANK COREY, *Secretary.*

NEW HAVEN CONN., February 8, 1904.

PENNSYLVANIA ASSOCIATION OF DENTAL SURGEONS.

THE fifty-seventh annual meeting of the Pennsylvania Association of Dental Surgeons was held at the Continental Hotel, Philadelphia, on Tuesday evening, October 10, 1903. After the reading
and discussion of papers the following officers were elected for the
ensuing year: President, Wilbur F. Litch; Vice-President, M. I.
Schamberg; Secretary, J. Clarence Salvas; Treasurer and Librarian, Wm. H. Trueman.

J. CLARENCE SALVAS,
Secretary.

THE

International Dental Journal.

VOL. XXV.   APRIL, 1904.   No. 4.

Original Communications.[1]

THE DIATORIC TOOTH IN BRIDGE-WORK.[2]

BY R. M. SANGER, D.D.S., EAST ORANGE, N. J.

THAT crown- and bridge-work has come to stay no one will question, but that it has not reached perfection from either a hygienic or æsthetic stand-point is obvious to all of us. To the dentist who is worthy of that name a gold crown on any of the anterior teeth is a source of humiliation, and even the second bicuspid is covered with gold only when there is nothing more feasible. In fact, the bold display of gold crowns is rapidly becoming the sign manual of the dental parlor and the fakir, and I hope and believe that the time is not far distant when the self-respecting public, as well as the self-respecting professional man, recognizing the fact that a display of gold in the mouth is indicative of the parvenu and the shoddy, will cause a demand for some other and more æsthetic means of restoring their broken-down teeth to a condition not only of usefulness but of ornamentation. It is true that single crowns

---

[1] The editor and publishers are not responsible for the views of authors of papers published in this department, nor for any claim to novelty, or otherwise, that may be made by them. No papers will be received for this department that have appeared in any other journal published in the country.

[2] Read before the Academy of Stomatology, Philadelphia, November 24, 1903.

for the anterior teeth have reached a high state of perfection, and
in the Logan, the Richmond, the Darby, and the half-collar crowns
we have at our disposal methods of restoring those teeth which are
almost ideal, but when perfectly sound anterior teeth are to be used
as anchorage piers for bridges, the methods at our disposal for
utilizing and at the same time preserving those teeth intact are
somewhat faulty. The open-faced or window crowns so commonly
used for this purpose are not only very unsightly, but in the majority of cases prove to be a delusion and a snare, their early failure
usually being accompanied by a woful amount of destruction of
tooth-substance, compelling the final loss of the natural crown and
the construction of the pier on entirely different and more radical
principles. The Carmichael and the Marshall systems offer a less
conspicuous and possibly more effective method of retention, and if
they prove to be all that they promise they will certainly be a welcome addition to our outfit, but their introduction is of so recent
a date that we can only hope that time will prove them to be all that
we desire.

Dr. F. L. Marshall, of Boston, describes his method, which he
calls a staple crown, about as follows: With an enamel fissure bur
cut grooves in the mesial and distal surfaces of the tooth just back
of the contour, as deep as the fissure bur, then connect these grooves
across the tooth by the use of an enamel bur, making this groove
as deep as the other two. If the articulation is very close, grind
off enough to allow for the thickness of the gold. Then knife-edge
your tooth from the cross groove to the edge, as you would an artificial tooth before backing. Next select a piece of platino-iridium
or 22-carat gold wire, a trifle smaller than the fissure bur, bend a
right angle on the end long enough to fit one approximal groove,
take the distance across the tooth between the grooves and bend
another right angle in the wire, thus forming the staple (Fig. 1),

FIG. 1.

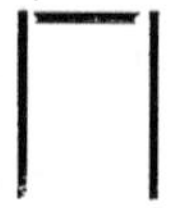

which gives the crown its name. Cut the ends of the staple the
proper length to fit the grooves and allow the cross-section to be
flush with the palatine surface of the tooth. A piece of pure gold
is selected, a little larger than the crown, and one side of the staple

is held against it, at right angles, with a pair of pliers, and it is caught with a little 22-carat solder. It is then placed in position on the tooth in the mouth and the gold burnished down to fit the lingual portion of the tooth and the approximal surfaces sufficiently anterior to the staple to allow of burnishing. Remove carefully and solder the staple to the crown around its entire length. Now replace the crown in the mouth and burnish carefully to place, trimming off all unnecessary gold. When a perfect adaptation is obtained, the piece is carefully removed and the outside is over-flowed with solder to give rigidity; the entire free edge, however, to about the width of one thirty-second of an inch is kept free from solder to admit of burnishing when the final placing is done and before the cement is hard.

The Carmichael method, as I understand it, is about the same as the foregoing, except that the gold is burnished into the groove instead of using the staple.

In my own practice I have had frequent recourse to an old, but, because of its more heroic nature, less commonly used method than either of the above, with much satisfaction both to my patient and myself,—that is, the immediate anæsthetizing and removal of the pulp and the swaging or burnishing of a piece of gold to the palatine surface of the tooth, passing a platino-iridium pin through it and soldering, giving a pier as shown in Fig. 2, *a* and *b*. This

Fig. 2.

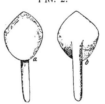

admits of the covering of the minimum amount of tooth-substance with gold and at the same time gives the maximum amount of strength to the pier. If an adjustable bridge is to be made, a platinum tube is used in place of the pin, and the pin, which is attached to the bridge, telescopes into the tube. In the earlier days the necessity for the administration of a general anæsthetic (gas in my practice) for the immediate removal of the pulp painlessly, was ofttimes a serious objection to the patient and to some oper-ators, but with the introduction of cocaine and adrenalin chloride, the painless removal of the pulp by pressure anæsthesia has become

such an easy and certain operation that I do not hesitate to do it
whenever such an operation is indicated. believing that the subsequent results fully warrant a procedure which at first glance may
seem very radical.

Next to the unsightly piers of your bridges are the solid gold
cusps of the bicuspid and molar dummies, and it was to a method
of overcoming this difficulty that I wished especially to call your
attention to-night. By the use of the diatoric tooth instead of porcelain facings you can construct a bridge which is more æsthetic
in appearance. simpler in construction, has greater strength. and is
more readily repaired in case of fracture.

Using a bicuspid diatoric tooth for purposes of illustration. the
procedure is as follows: The teeth are carefully selected to fit the
case with as little grinding as may be necessary. The form in
which they are made. with a long curve on the inner surface (Fig.
3. *a* and *b*), permits the cervico-lingual surface to fit the curve of

FIG. 3.

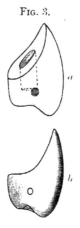

the average ridge with little or no grinding, but if any grinding
is necessary. it should be done on the base of the tooth rather than
on the morsal surface. A piece of pure gold plate about 32 gauge
is cut to a size sufficient to cover the base of the tooth and project
over the sides about one-eighth of an inch. This is laid on the
base of the tooth and burnished to fit as nearly as possible, the
edges being turned up all around to form a cup-like shape. A
metal ring which will fit in a crown swager of the style shown in
Fig. 4 is filled with hot modelling composition and the morsal surface of the diatoric tooth is pressed into it to a sufficient depth to

hold it firmly (Fig. 5), and the whole plunged into cold water to harden the composition. (I procured my metal rings by cutting a small bicycle pump in sections). With the piece of gold in position on the embedded tooth, they are placed in the swager and covered

Fig. 4.

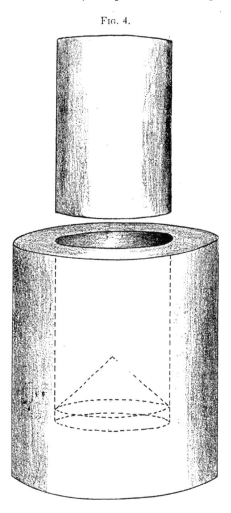

with cornmeal or some equally yielding substance, and swaged down until the gold cup fits the tooth accurately. Upon removal the gold is trimmed to the desired height around the edges, always allowing it to extend well up to the little holes on the approximal

sides of the tooth, and then with a ball burnisher it is burnished
into the central depression in the base of the tooth. The gold will
be perforated when burnishing it into this hole, but the burnishing
should be continued until the metal accurately fits the margins. It
is then filled about one-third full with gold-foil, or a coil of pure

FIG. 5.

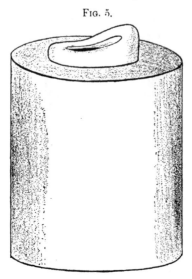

gold plate is placed in the cavity and burnished to fit. The gold cup
is then removed from the tooth and the balance of the hole is filled
with 20-carat solder until it is flush. This gives you a gold cup and
pin which closely fits the diatoric tooth, holding it so firmly that it

FIG. 6.   FIG. 7.   FIG. 8

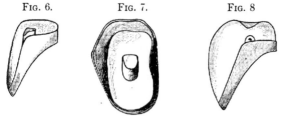

would almost keep its place without cementing. Fig 6 gives a side
view of the cup and pin, Fig. 7 gives a front view of the same, and
Fig. 8 shows the tooth in position in the gold cup. With the teeth
in the cups, but not fastened, they are assembled on the cast and
waxed to each other and to the piers on the lingual side. The
assembled piece is then carefully placed in the mouth, and any

error in the occlusion is corrected by allowing the patient to bite the teeth to place. The diatoric teeth are then removed from the cups, and the piers and cups are taken from the mouth in an impression of terra-plastica or some suitable investing material. This gives you the pieces invested and ready to solder at the approximal surfaces. For additional strength a piece of gold plate is laid across the lingual aspect from pier to pier and the whole overflowed with solder. When this is done the work is allowed to cool slightly, and

FIG. 9.

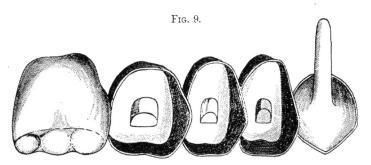

it is then plunged into cold water, which disintegrates the investing material and allows the work to come away clean and without injury to the fine edges. The polishing should be done with the porcelain teeth in position to prevent possible injury to the fine edges of the gold cups, but they should not be fastened permanently in the cups until everything is completed and ready for the mouth, thus avoiding dirty joints. (Fig. 9 shows the work ready for the final cementing of the diatoric dummies.) The teeth may be permanently fastened in the cups with oxyphosphate of zinc, guttapercha, after the method devised by Dr. George Evans, and which I have found very satisfactory, or by the use of powdered sulphur, after the manner of attaching English tube-teeth to gold plates. In case of the fracture of one of these dummies, the repair can be quickly and easily done in the mouth, as the diatoric teeth are readily duplicated, but the danger of fracture is very remote, as the porcelain is at no time subjected to heat, and you have the full thickness of the tooth incased in gold to withstand the force of mastication. As I intimated at the beginning of this description, this method gives you a maximum degree of strength, a minimum display of gold, and an occlusion which is well-nigh perfect, and I am sure that the æsthetic appearance of a bridge constructed in this way will appeal to you all.

THE DEVELOPMENT OF HARD TISSUE IN THE PULP
OF HUMAN TEETH.

BY DOUGLAS E. CAUSH, L.D.S., ENGLAND.

OF the functions performed by the various organs of the body there are few, if any, more interesting or have the power of producing more varied results than that of the tooth-pulp.

In health it is the benefactor of the surrounding hard tissue; in disease, the medium whereby we are warned of the mischief that is going on. Among the varied functions of this organ may be placed the power of developing "secondary dentine."

FIG. 1.

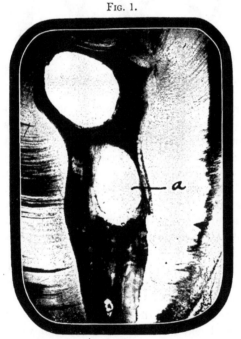

a, pulp-nodule showing structureless character of secondary dentine.

Nature in many cases endeavors to overcome the evil produced by the destroying microbe, by forming a layer of fresh tissue between the soft, sensitive pulp and the dentine that is being broken down by decay. The same protective measure also occurs in those cases where erosion has commenced its destructive work.

as well as in many other instances where disintegration of the hard tissue has been produced by the various known causes. In all these examples the newly formed hard tissue is known as secondary dentine, the development of which we desire to consider in this paper.

On the examination of teeth, we find we may have new tissue more or less continuously developed from the pulp, until the tooth is lost either by disease or as a result of old age; in other cases the new tissue may be developed without any apparent cause, and the development may be either continuous or spasmodic, until the whole of the pulp-chamber becomes filled with this new tissue.

FIG. 2.

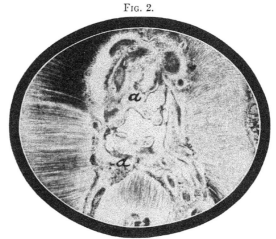

a. osteodentine.

Again we may find it in the pulp itself more or less surrounded by pulp-tissue in the form of pulp-nodules, and as Professor Jos. Arkövy has designated certain growths. "Odontoma interum liberum."

In any and all of these cases the new tissue is spoken of as secondary dentine; it will thus be seen that there is a variety of tissue grouped under the head of secondary dentine, ranging from the comparatively structureless tissue as seen in the pulp-nodule (Fig. 1) to that of the complicated character known as osteo-dentine (Fig. 2).

It may enable us to better understand the development of this tissue if we divide it into classes. We shall therefore consider, first, normal secondary dentine; second, dentine of repair; third, pulp-nodules; and lastly, a form of secondary dentine found in teeth where pyorrhœa alveolaris has been pronounced.

In the first class we shall include all tissue produced apparently without any cause, the whole of the pulp and surrounding tissue being healthy at the time of the deposition of the tissue; a good example of such may be frequently found in those teeth perfectly free from diseases such as decay or erosion, nor have the teeth been worn down by attrition, yet on examination they are found to have their pulp-chambers partially or entirely filled with new tissue. This tissue may be very varied in its microscopic appearance, from that of an almost structureless character to the more complicated, containing lacunæ-like spaces and frequently an innumerable number of tubuli (Fig. 3); the tissue is usually

FIG. 3.

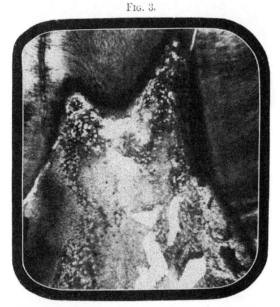

Pulp-chamber superior bicuspid, formation of secondary dentine.

found in the twelve anterior teeth, but perhaps more frequently in the lower incisors and canines; there is, as a rule, no inconvenience produced by its development, and its presence is only detected on examining the tooth after extraction.

It would appear to be Nature's way of reducing the size of the pulp-chamber, and is much more pronounced in those who have passed age. It is rarely found in the pulp-canals; the deposition commences usually at or near the apex of the pulp-chamber, gradually working downward towards the point where the chamber is united to the pulp-canal; even when the tubuli are in large numbers they rarely assimilate with those tubuli previously formed, hence it is not at all difficult to define the line of demarcation between the two tissues. This line is usually very pronounced,

FIG. 4.

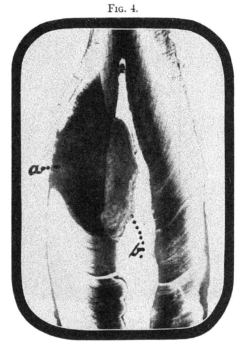

Secondary dentine under decay: *a,* decay; *b.* secondary dentine.

owing to the fact that some time has elapsed between the calcification of the old tissue and the commencement of the deposition of the new, and, as a consequence, the first layer laid down usually appears structureless and often followed by a number of irregular spaces very similar in character to the inter-granular layer of the dentine; and then, if the deposition is continued, tubuli are regularly formed. If, on the other hand, from any cause the deposition is interrupted, we have a mass of mixed tissue, structureless, lacunæ-like spaces, and tubuli, all mixed together.

The development of this tissue is as follows: After the dentine has become perfectly calcified in a healthy tooth, fresh formative material is brought to the pulp by the blood; this, passing to the outer layer of the pulp by capillaries, is taken up by the layer of globular or semi-globular cells surrounding the odontoblasts (Figs. 4, 5, 6, 7, 8), and these cells become eventually calcified. As this calcification takes place the odontoblasts are restricted in size by compression and the odontoblast cells forced inward towards the

FIG. 5.

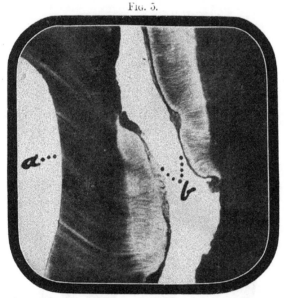

Section of superior canine worn away at the sides by a metal band on artificial tooth plate; though the tooth is worn away by attrition, the deposition assimilates that found in eroded teeth: *a*, portion of tooth worn away by band; *b*, deposition of secondary dentine.

centre of the pulp, the constricted portion forming the tubuli; if the deposition is slow, the outer mass becomes very solid, and, as a consequence, structureless with few tubuli; if, on the other hand, it is rapid, some of the cells do not calcify, and lacunæ-like spaces are thus formed with their canaliculi produced as minute spaces between the calcified cells. As this process goes on new cells are formed by cell division. If during the process of calcification any dense tissue is met, such as the walls of the blood-vessels (arteries or veins), the cells surround this dense tissue, and, calcifying around them, form the circular openings so frequently seen in the sections of this tissue. often carrying by pressure the odontoblasts with them, and thus tubuli are seen surrounding the openings; if, on the other hand, no dense substance is met, the calcification goes on continuously until the whole of the pulp-chamber is filled with new tissue, thus producing the variations found in this tissue.

The cause of all this may be—probably is—the slight irritation —" so slight that the patient is unconscious of it"—produced in the pulp by the constant use of the teeth.

Fig. 6.

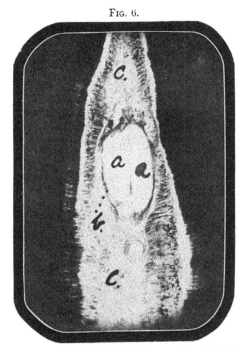

Pulp-nodule surrounded by hard and soft tissue: *a*, pulp-nodule: *b*, soft tissue: *c*, hard tissue. For nodule surrounded by soft tissue see Fig. 1.

The second class, and by far the most numerous, spoken of as dentine of repair, may be divided as follows, the pulp-nodule being produced from quite a different cause,—" irritation produced in the pulp itself:" 1, that found in teeth with eroded surfaces; 2, found in teeth that are decayed: 3, found in teeth worn down by attrition and mastication.

On the microscopic examination of the teeth placed in Section 1, " teeth with eroded surfaces" (Fig. 9), we have found in

ery tooth examined that there has been a deposition of secondary
dentine. This new tissue assimilates that of normal dentine more
than in those of the other sections; the line of demarcation is
more pronounced following the area of the eroded surface: it is
much more clearly formed, and certainly more restricted in its
development, having, as a rule, tubuli assimilating with the tubuli
of the dentine, and apparently there is little or no break in their
continuity: at the same time there appears to have been a marked

FIG. 7.

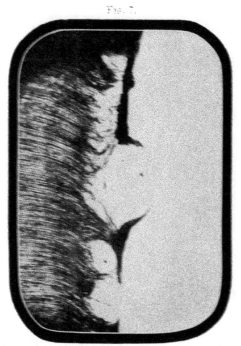

Section of tooth showing exposure of normal dentine, with tubuli curved or endproduced

change in the contour of the tubuli of the original dentine. Immediately under the eroded surface we find the tubuli of the
original dentine very difficult, if not impossible, to stain: it appears
as if these tubuli had been filled with some deposit from the outer
surface of the tooth that prevents them from performing their
usual functions. The function of the secondary dentine is to
prevent any acute irritation passing from the eroded surface to the
pulp itself: owing to the restricted area of its development, it

would appear as if the deposition was caused by the slight local irritation produced in the earlier stages of the disease of erosion.

The development of secondary dentine in the second section is, so far as my examination goes, much more rare, and is found only in those cases where the decay has gone on slowly (Fig. 10) and the irritation to the pulp-tissue has been as a consequence slight and continuous but extending over a long period, differing from the former in microscopic structure. It varies very much in

Fig. 8.

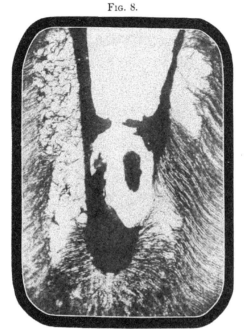

Nodule at apex of root-canal. in this position causes great pain.
The dense tissue almost surrounding nodule is pulp.

structure as well as in the area of its deposition. The earlier deposited tissue does not, as a rule, contain any tubuli, but a number of lacunæ with canaliculi; as the tissue increases in thickness it assumes more the character of normal dentine, and a number of tubuli are developed; it usually spreads over a much larger area than that of the secondary dentine in eroded teeth, and does not terminate in such a pronounced or irregular manner. It would lead one to suppose that the irritation to the pulp-tissue had been much more general; it is still an attempt by Nature to protect the pulp from the results of the diseased condition of the tooth produced by the action of the spreading of the decay. In the form of secondary dentine, placed in the third division, that produced by attrition or mastication (Figs. 11 and 12), we have the teeth worn down oftentimes in extreme cases until the original pulp-chamber has become exposed. The teeth usually affected by attrition are the six front ones of both upper and lower jaw; those worn down by mastication, the bicuspids and molars. In either case

FIG. 9.

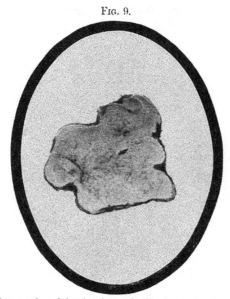

Section of pulp-nodule taken from pulp-chamber of superior molar.

the result is the same. The tissue is usually quite structureless at the commencement of the deposition, passing from that through either of the other forms until we have a mass of dense tissue all fused together and entirely filling the pulp-chamber, so dense that, in extreme cases, even if the original pulp-chamber has been exposed, there is little or no discomfort to the patient. This tissue is more like the tissue previously referred to as normal secondary dentine than that of any of the others. In all these cases the method of development has been the same, and the cause that of irritation in one form or another, but in *all* cases the exciting cause has been from the outside,—*i.e.,* from that portion of the tooth above the gum line.

In the development of the pulp-nodule we have a pronounced deposit of secondary dentine either in the pulp-chamber or the pulp-canals, sometimes in both, but, unlike the deposit in the previous sections, the nodule is always formed as a result of irritation *in the pulp itself.*

FIG. 10.

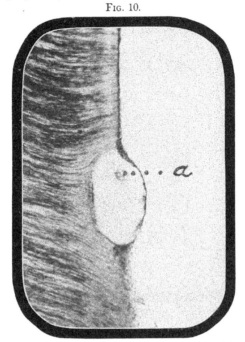

Pulp-nodule showing what I believe to be the origin of nodule at *a*

On examining a tooth there is nothing in the external appearance to suggest the existence of even the smallest of pulp-stones, nor can we take into consideration as a factor the age or sex of patients in the development of this tissue, as these nodules are to be found in the teeth of patients in their teens as well as in those of advanced age, and in many cases producing as much pain in the youngest as in those of old age. The result of my examinations tends to show that the position of the nodule is usually the cause of the pain produced.

In external appearance the nodules vary from a small, more or

less globular, or oval, structure to that of any size or shape, controlled only by the size of that portion of the canal or chamber in
which they are found. Thus we have them from a minute point
to those entirely filling the pulp-chamber, and in teeth of two or
more roots it is not unusual to find them not only filling the pulp-
chamber, but with spines of hard tissue passing into the various
canals, and thus producing the most irregular-shaped nodules.

FIG. 11.

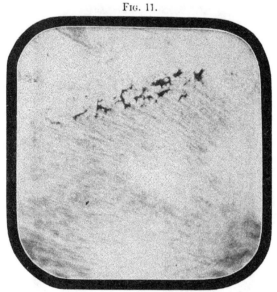

Interglobular spaces in dentine as seen in teeth affected by pyorrhœa alveolaris.
Note the globular character of the dentine.

Their position is almost as varied as their outline, for, as I have
already said, we may find them in the pulp-canals and pulp-
chambers, quite free from the surrounding dentine (Fig. 13), or
we may find them attached to the sides of the pulp-canals and
quite surrounded by the dentine. It is not the largest of these
that cause the greatest amount of pain, as the pain is produced
by the position, and not by the size of the nodule; thus a small
nodule near the apex of the canal will probably produce pain by
the constriction of the pulp and, as a consequence, pressure upon
the nerves, whilst a nodule much larger in size (unless there is
pressure produced upon the nerves) may almost entirely fill the

pulp-chamber without producing any discomfort. Though their size, shape, and position may vary very much, such is not the case with regard to their microscopic structure. All the nodules I have examined have a somewhat similar structure when viewed by the microscope. We have usually in the centre, or somewhere near the centre, of the developed tissue a space, more or less pronounced, and it is at this point that the nodule has its origin; it grows outwardly, and radiating from this point there are

FIG. 12.

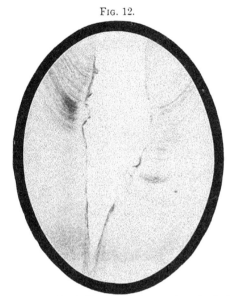

Absorption of dentine in teeth having pyorrhœa alveolaris.

usually a number of more or less concentric rings caused by additional layers of calcified tissue; it is in this way a nodule increases in size. This may continue until two or more nodules touch each other and become united into one, thus forming a compound nodule large and irregular in shape. Its structure. as thus seen, is quite different from either ordinary or secondary dentine. We may sometimes find a few isolated irregular tubuli, but rarely do we find any tubuli approaching the character of those seen in secondary dentine. This may be accounted for by the fact that its origin is generally some distance from the odonto-blastic layer, and the nodule is developed from a different layer

of cells from that of secondary dentine. Its position would imply
that no odontoblasts had taken part in its development, and, if
this is so, a very interesting question arises as to how these tubuli,
if they are tubuli, are produced.

The origin of the development of the nodule is some irritation
in the pulp itself, and I believe the primary object of the nodule is
to cover up, by calcification, some substance that has been the cause
of irritation in the pulp-tissue. Its structure as well as its mode
of development would lend itself to this supposition, for under the

FIG. 13.

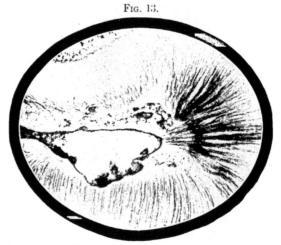

Absorption of pulp-canal in teeth exostosed. Many of these excavations are filled with
secondary tissue cemental in character and similar to the tissue found outside the
cementum.

microscope we have a structure similar in appearance and, I believe,
identical in its mode of development to that of the pearl found in
the oyster, the origin of the pearl being a foreign body found in
the mantle of the mollusc. As it is impossible for the oyster to get
rid of this foreign body by absorption, it builds around the cause
of irritation that which is known to us as the pearl. So in the
development of the pulp-nodule the same has occurred. Nature
has found in that delicate and complicated structure, the pulp,
something it cannot get rid of, something it cannot absorb. The
irritation produced by this something causes the pulp to endeavor
to get rid of it; as, however, it cannot absorb it, there is nothing
for it to do but to encyst it.

If this is the true origin of the pulp-nodule. we ought to be able to find in some pulps. as a result of microscopic examination. the exciting cause, and this exciting cause is. I believe. to be found in either a dead cell or cells. or perhaps a few blood-corpuscles that have by some means escaped from their ordinary course. by the rupture either of one of the capillaries or small blood-vessels abounding in the pulp: such an accident may occur by a sudden shock to the tooth. or. again. the corpuscles may be found out of their place as a result of the breaking down of some of the smaller arteries, veins. or even the capillaries. by disease such as the pulp is exposed to.

I think the former method is the one that usually causes the development of pulp-nodules in our younger patients. whilst undoubtedly the changes in the pulp lend themselves to the development of these nodules as age advances. We will suppose. from either of the above. or some similar cause. that such a change has taken place in the pulp. and as a result there will be irritation of a more or less pronounced character in this tissue produced by what has become a foreign body: there are no lymphatics for the reabsorption of this body. and it does not require a very great stretch of the imagination to trace the growth of the pulp-nodule on the lines laid down. The course followed would. I believe. be somewhat as follows:

The irritation produced by the foreign body causes an increased activity in the blood-vessels surrounding the cause of the irritation, and. as a necessary consequence. an increase of formative material brought to hand. This material is taken out of the blood by the surrounding cells. and it becomes a very simple matter for these cells to cover up the cause of the irritation by a deposition of hard tissue. This probably occurs as follows: the increased blood-supply, produced by the irritation. causes immediate activity in the cells surrounding the cause of irritation. and the result of the activity is to produce a number of new cells. The pressure produced by this increase in the number of cells again increases the blood-supply, and after a time the cells deposit a hard tissue in the same manner as the cementum is produced in exostosis.

As the deposition takes place in very small quantities. and probably very slowly. we have a more or less perfectly calcified and. as a consequence. homogeneous deposition. This accounts for the structureless character of the nodule.

Again, we sometimes have a larger mass more rapidly formed, and perhaps nearer, or even including some of the odontoblasts in the newly forming mass. We shall then have variations in the structure, consisting of lacunæ with canaliculi, irregular spaces, and a few markings like the tubuli of dentine. As the calcification of these cells continues, we shall have an increase in the size of the nodule; in some cases this increase causes a further irritation of the surrounding pulp-tissue, and thus a constant supply of fresh formative material is brought to the cells. The increase of size eventually produces pressure upon the nerves of the pulp and, as a consequence, frequently the most acute pain is experienced; this is the course, I believe, of the pulp-nodule when surrounded by pulp-tissue.

There is yet another class of nodule; though previously mentioned, it may be interesting to briefly follow its history. I refer to those nodules attached to the dentine. We may also, if we are fairly successful in our search, find them not only attached at one side, but entirely surrounded by dentine, and that at some little distance from the pulp-canal; wherever I have found these they have always been near the apex of the root and embedded in the last formed dentine; and this, I think, gives the key to the explanation of the position in which the nodules are found.

At the time the cutting edge of the tooth is passing through the gums the apex of the root is in an uncalcified condition, and with a new tooth in this position it is much more subject to a shock than it will be after it is fully erupted; as a consequence, we have a nodule formed in precisely the same manner as those formed in the pulp-tissue, with the exception that those found in the pulp-tissue are always formed after the calcification of the dentine has taken place, whilst the latter class are formed prior to the calcification of the tooth, and when first formed are surrounded by uncalcified dentine. Any careful examination of a tooth with nodules in this position will fully illustrate my meaning, as the tubuli of the dentine will be found to be bent around the nodule, proving the nodule must have been formed prior to the calcification of the dentine. If it had been otherwise, and the dentine had been absorbed to make a space for the nodule, we should then have found the tubuli ending abruptly at or near the margin of the nodule, but this is not the case.

This will also account for the nodules found in the pulp-canals but attached to the dentine, and here, I believe, the development has been the same as in nodules surrounded by dentine.

The last of the forms of secondary dentine we wish to draw your attention to is to be found in the pulp-chambers and pulp-canals of teeth having been removed owing to the pronounced action of " pyorrhœa alveolaris." In all the teeth examined (about one hundred) the original dentine has been of very poor structure, containing a large number of interglobular spaces, the dentine, generally, badly calcified, and more or less absorption of the cementum and sometimes the dentine at the apex of the root. In the pulp itself the first thing that attracts our attention is the absorption of a portion of the original dentine forming the pulp-chamber and canal, probably the result of acute inflammation prior to the development of the secondary dentine. The new tissue is very varied in character, and apparently consists of a mixture of tissue similar in structure to that found in the previous cases, with the addition of a very large number of isolated globular secondary dentine wherever there is a piece of pulp-tissue; so that the whole of the pulp-chamber canals are more or less filled with either secondary dentine, as previously described, or an innumerable number of these globular bodies, generally isolated but sometimes though very rarely found fused together. I have noticed similar excavations in the pulp-canals of teeth that are exostosed, but with this difference: the cavities in the latter case are frequently filled with secondary tissue like the additional layer of cemental tissue on the outside; in the case of pyorrhœa alveolaris, the excavations are not filled with any special tissue.

All the microscopic slides used for illustrating this paper are hard sections ground down, as I believe decalcification in any form is liable to alter the conditions of the tissue under examination.

DENTIGEROUS CYSTS.[1]

BY CHARLES GREENE CUMSTON, M.D., BOSTON, MASS.

In considering the subject of dentigerous cysts, a few remarks on the pathology of the condition may not be out of place, as the literature is rather scarce relative to the condition under consideration. The first important work on the subject was published in 1872 from the pen of the well-known Parisian dentist, Magitot. After a careful study of all material he had at hand, Magitot gave a systematic classification of dental cysts, and at the same time he took their etiology into consideration.

As most of the writers who have studied this question since Magitot's paper appeared have concurred in most of the statements therein found, it would seem proper to consider his paper a little in detail. Magitot considered every cystic production lined with a membrane and situated in the interior of the jaws as a maxillary cyst. These cysts usually contain fluid contents varying in nature from one case to another; they may be thin and fluid or, on the other hand, quite thick and pasty. Every cystic production arising spontaneously in the maxilla usually originates from a tooth. Magitot also believed that if a foreign body penetrated the jaw a cyst could form around it. and this fact has been proved by a case long ago published by Maisonneuve.

Cysts developing spontaneously he termed progenous cysts, and, in contrast to these, those developing around a foreign body he termed perigenous cysts. To these two forms which develop in the bone substance he adds a third type, to which he applied the name of neogenous cysts, which develop outside the osseous tissue.

Magitot subdivided follicular cysts into embryoplastic, odontoplastic, and corona-forming-period cysts according to the time of their development, and he again subdivides them according to the nature of their contents into serous, colloid, and caseous cysts.

By the classification given, it is readily seen how Magitot accounts for the formation of progenous cysts. From some influence he believes that the enamel may perish in different stages of development by either resorption or by maceration. The dental sac then

---

[1] Read by invitation before the Harvard Odontological Society, October 29. 1903.

slowly develops by a proliferation of its structures. The contents found in embryoplastic cysts will be composed of shapeless embryonal dental elements, in those of the odontoplastic cysts more or less regularly developed tooth elements will be present, while in cysts arising during a later period of dental development coronal structures should be present.

Magitot believed that neogenous cysts arise in the periosteum of the root, and he supposes that this membrane undergoes development by proliferation of its cellular structures and thus forms a cystic sac. The primary causative factor is an obliteration of the canal of the root due to an inflammatory thickening of the periosteum following infection from the canal of the root or by formation of a denticle in the pulp. The epithelial lining of these cysts is derived from a marked proliferation of the connective tissue cells.

Although Magitot unquestionably did much to enlighten us on the question, he could not reconcile his theory with facts,—namely, that the epithelium could arise as if by regeneration from the connective tissue elements. It was naturally most important to discover the true origin of the epithelium which is exclusively found in neogenous cysts when it has not become destroyed by a suppurative process of the contents of the cyst.

In 1885 appeared a paper by Malassez, and it is to him we are indebted for discovering in the maxillæ of embryos in different stages of development that during the period of the formation of the teeth there takes place, besides the physiological proliferation of the epithelium for the formation of the dental follicle from the embryonal enamel, other proliferative processes, arising both from the organon adamantinæ and from the mucous membrane. These epithelial masses are in structure exactly like the enamel organ, arranged around the root of the tooth in various manners. They are also found present in normal lower jaws of adults, and he came to the conclusion that these epithelial masses persist not only during the period of dentition, but are normally present during adult life. He asserted that not only the neogenous cysts of Magitot, but also every other neoplasm having an epithelial character developing in the jaw, especially multilocular cystomata and cystadenomata of the maxilla, originate from these masses of cells which he terms paradental epithelial débris.

The conclusions arrived at by Malassez were examined and found correct by other investigators. Von Brunn, especially, has given a satisfactory explanation, basing his assertion on the writings of Hartwig, published in 1874, and he shows how the epithelial masses, pre-existing around the root of the tooth, become constricted by the fetal enamel organ, and from its connective tissue with the epithelium of the buccal mucous membrane. If Malassez's theory relative to the origin of periodontal cysts from the paradental cell agglomeration is correct, these cysts should occasionally be met with in their early stages, and, in point of fact, Witzell published a paper on cysts of the roots of the teeth in 1896, in which he fully describes them and gives a satisfactory explanation for the development of periodontal cysts. He points out that one occasionally finds tumors varying in size from the head of a pin to a pea in extracted teeth, especially when they are the seat of caries. These neoplasms are sometimes spherical in shape, at others egg-shaped, varying in their connection with the roots, sometimes being near and sometimes being distant, while occasionally they are pedunculated.

On section these small, grayish-white bodies will be found composed of one or more cavities containing serous contents. Microscopically the external layer of these minute growths is composed of a rough connective tissue, then by a layer of tissue abounding in blood-vessels and leucocytes, while the cavities are lined with epithelium. The larger cystic cavities show a more evenly distributed epithelial layer, while in the smaller ones the thickness of the lining epithelium varies considerably.

We consequently are here dealing with a miniature cyst which on account of its diminutive size has never given rise to symptoms. The microscopical examination of well-developed cysts exactly corresponds with these small pathologic productions described by Witzel.

In the first case of dental cyst that I have to report, the lining membrane consisted of several layers of flattened epithelium, and outside of this was a connective tissue layer measuring about 1½ millimetres in thickness. Outside of this connective tissue layer was found another of connective tissue in which nuclei were easily distinguished. The history of the patient was briefly as follows: She was a well-built girl of twenty-five, who had always enjoyed good health. About three years ago she noticed for the first time a small bunch under the left nostril. This small growth gave rise to no pain and grew slowly, and continued to do so until, at the time of the patient coming under observation. the left nasolabial fold had completely disappeared, while a tumor about the size of a large walnut was found immediately underneath the labionasal fold. The skin covering the growth was movable, while the left nostril was pushed upward. By palpation, fluctuation could be detected.

Under ether narcosis the growth was incised, giving issue to a transparent serum. The opening was enlarged, and it was then found that a cavity existed between the nasal cavity and the antrum of Highmore, into which the apex of the root of a small incisor was found protruding. After extraction of the tooth and the removal of a corresponding part of the alveolar process, the cavity was plugged with gauze and the skin incision united by wire sutures. These were removed on the fifth day, and the patient was discharged well in three weeks.

It is easy to understand why we have a flattened epithelium in large cysts, while in the smaller ones cubic epithelium is present because it is well known with what ease epithelial cells adapt themselves to the amount of pressure brought to bear on them. In all the cases of dentigerous cysts which have come under our observation, the microscope has revealed practically the same histological structure, but in some instances the epithelial layers were so thick that the lining membrane of the cyst was readily peeled out from the cavity. Such was the condition found in the two following cases:

A healthy boy ten years of age had had what was called by the mother a swollen cheek for over three years. The swelling had apparently never given rise to any pain. It had slowly increased until at the time the boy came under observation the deformity was very marked. By palpation, a tumor the consistency of bone was found in the anterior aspect of the right superior maxillary bone. The nasal cavities were normal. Under ether an incision was made over the most promintent part of the growth, the gum was stripped back, and the bone opened with the chisel. This led into a large cavity lined by a whitish membrane, which was easily stripped off and removed. The cavity contained a light-yellow serum, but no evidence of any tooth could be found within it. On account of the large size of the cavity, which might be estimated that of a small hen's egg, it was deemed more prudent to obtain drainage through the nose, so a communication was made with the right nostril and a drainage-tube inserted. In terminating the operation, a portion of the anterior wall of the jaws was removed so that the cavity might contract more rapidly. Drainage was continued for a week, after which time the wound was found to be granulating nicely, and the patient was discharged cured at the end of four weeks.

The next case was a man thirty-seven years old, who for about eighteen months had noticed the presence of a tumor situated in the neighborhood of the left wisdom-tooth. The swelling was hard and had slowly increased in size. By examination an oval tumor was found situated in the neighborhood of the wisdom-tooth on the left-hand side, and might have measured in size that of a large English walnut. Under ether the last molar on the left was removed, and it was then found that we were dealing with a rather thick-walled cyst of the jaw. The cavity was split open with the chisel, and by exploration it was found to communicate with the antrum of High-more. It was lined with a thick, whitish membrane, which was easily removed by blunt dissection. Drainage was obtained by making an opening into the nasal cavity, and a rubber tube was inserted, the cystic cavity being plugged with gauze. No evidence of a rudimentary tooth could be detected within the cavity. The liquid contents consisted of a thick, light-yellow serum.

Now, if we assume that these periodontal cysts are produced by an irritative process arising from the paradental epithelial débris of Malassez, and that the cavities increase in size on account of an increase of their fluid contents, we have all the conditions found in cysts of long standing explained. A cyst will naturally grow in the direction of the least resistance, and since the root of the tooth is firmly lodged in the alveolar process by its periosteum, the bone, being less resistant, gives way to the pressure. On account of the pressure on the surrounding structures produced by the growing cysts, the vessels and nerve supplying the tooth and periosteum of the root undergo pressure atrophy and resorption. Thus may be explained the absence of periosteum covering the root and the apices projecting into the cavity of the cyst, although their presence is by no means constant.

The perigenous cysts of Magitot can be explained by a foreign body directly in contact with, or in the neighborhood of, the so-called epithelial streaks of Brunn. This produces a constant irritation, which finally causes a proliferation of the latter, and to this type those cysts, in which fully developed teeth are found present, belong in all probability.

It is easily conceivable that a tooth which did not make its exit from the jaw from faulty position or some other similar circumstance becomes enclosed in the maxilla and at length plays the part of a foreign body, causing the epithelial streak to proliferate. It would appear that such cysts are generally considered under the head of follicular cysts, but under these circumstances it is difficult to explain the presence of fluid. But if we adopt Malassez's theory, it will be found to explain the formation of these cysts very well. One such case has come under my notice, the history of which is briefly as follows:

A woman sixty-four years old had had all her lower teeth removed several years ago. About twenty months before coming under observation a swelling made its appearance on the angle of the right jaw. The tumor gradually increased in size, so that when the patient was first seen it was as large as an egg. Later a certain amount of pain had been felt in the growth, and the latter had become quite tense and the patient complained of much annoyance from a throbbing sensation more or less constantly present. Under ether an incision was made through the skin over the most prominent part of the growth, and while peeling off the periosteum of the ascending ramus of the lower jaw a cystic cavity was opened, giving issue to a considerable quantity of malodorous pus. The cavity was at once enlarged, and by digital exploration the root of a tooth was found protruding into it. The root was extracted, and the cavity was thoroughly curetted and drained. The patient made an excellent recovery, although drainage was necessary for over three weeks on account of a more or less abundant discharge of pus, but she eventually recovered without a fistula.

If a tooth develops normally, it is evident that it can never become entirely enclosed within a cyst, but its root may be contained within the cavity, and this is what is found in the larger number of cases. Most of the text-books on surgery are very deficient in explaining the pathology of these cysts, and even commit gruesome errors in their statements. It is an unimpeachable fact that one tissue can only reproduce itself, and consequently epithelium can only be derived from epithelium : and it is also well known that the lining membrane of these cysts is always epithelial and never composed of granulation tissue. Now Malassez's theory explains satisfactorily the absence of the periosteal covering of the dental roots protruding into these cysts, but the cause giving rise to the pro-

liferation of the epithelial streak of Brunn and to the formation
of a periodontal cyst is not so easily demonstrated. Without any
question an inflammation of the membrane of the root may be the
starting-point of this process, and many cases unquestionably do
originate in this way. In such cases caries of the tooth, inflammation or gangrene of the pulp must have preceded, but if the
root of a perfectly normal tooth is found protruding into a cystic
cavity, and where there is a complete absence of all signs of a
periodontitis, or if no trace of tooth is found within the cavity of
these cysts, such as has been observed. we consequently must admit
that there are other causative factors existing. It is possible that
traumatism may be the starting-point of some of these cysts, because the lower jaw is particularly well placed to receive external
injuries, and it is a well-established fact that retained teeth may
be the cause of periodontal cysts. But it is also well demonstrated
that a perfectly normal tooth may be the etiological factor when
such a tooth is deviated from its normal position, an example of
which will be found in the following case:

A boy seventeen and a half years of age had always been fairly
well excepting for the ordinary ailments of childhood. For the
past eighteen months he had suffered more or less intensely from
toothache. About five months ago he first noticed a slowly growing tumor on the left side of his cheek. The growth did not give
rise to any pain. Examination showed that the tumor extended
from the left nostril underneath the malar bone. The skin covering the growth was not reddened, and was found freely movable
over the tumor. The teeth were in extremely bad condition. The
left upper canine appeared healthy, but it pointed directly backward in an oblique direction. At this point the superior maxilla
presents a swelling extending from the labial to the palatinal
aspect. Crepitation could be elicited on pressure. Under ether an
incision was made over the tumor, attacking it from inside the
mouth, and when the cavity of the cyst was opened a large amount
of thick, ill-smelling serum made its exit. The opening into the
cyst was enlarged, the cavity being found lined with a smooth,
glossy membrane. The apex of the root of the canine tooth was
found protruding into the cystic cavity, and was extracted. The
alveolar edge was chiselled away and the cavity packed with gauze
and drained. The patient made a rapid and uneventful recovery.
Examination of the tooth extracted showed that the apex of the
root was bare of its periosteum.

On the other hand, the retention of developed teeth does not necessarily produce the formation of a cyst, as has been proved by several cases reported in literature. In one case reported by Hildebrand, that of a boy during his second dentition, he removed from the upper and lower jaws over two hundred perfectly developed teeth without any evidence of cystic formation around any of them.

It would also appear that the period of dentition may also play an important part in the etiology of periodontal cysts, and this should not seem surprising, because at that time processes of resorption and regeneration are taking place everywhere in the maxillæ. Now, during such a time of active metabolism there is no reason why an increased activity may not be present in the epithelial streak of Brunn.

In many cases periodontal cysts do make their début during the period of the second dentition, but in other cases the cysts begin to develop long before this period, as has been proved by certain cases reported in the literature. The second case narrated in this paper in all probability enters into this class, because evidently the cystic formation commenced at an early time in the dental development, and, in point of fact. microscopical examination showed a picture closely resembling an embryonal dentinal sac. This type of cyst may always be suspected if the tooth corresponding to it is absent, and this is an important point to be noticed in making a diagnosis. It may also occur that although the entire set of teeth is intact, a supernumerary tooth follicle may undergo cystic transformation, but such instances must be very rare. The cause of the cystic transformation is as yet unknown.

It may not be out of place to refer, in a few words, to a certain class of tumor which perhaps in reality does not strictly belong to the subject of this paper, but whose histological nature and origin is closely allied to that of periodontal cysts. The tumors to which I refer are usually encountered in the lower jaw near its angle. They suddenly begin to develop after they have been present for a number of years in a latent state, so to speak, and when they commence to increase in size they do so very markedly. Traumatism is usually the cause of their sudden increase in size and growth. After they have attained a certain size they present symptoms of cysts,—namely, fluctuation and parchment crepitation. These cysts have been treated by incision, curettage, and drainage, which has rarely been the means of curing them, and in most instances an extensive resection of the jaw has been necessary.

These cysts have been described by a number of surgeons. Some of them have been multilocular, while others were unilocular. Microscopically they are found composed of small cavities or canals, the inner wall of which is lined with an epithelium of the cylindrical, cubic, or polygonal type, while in the larger cysts it is flattened. Malassez believes that these cysts also originate from the paradental epithelial débris, but the reasons why in one case a simple periodontal cyst should develop, while in others cystomata or cystadenomata arise, is as yet insufficiently explained, but a large number of authorities agree that the original epithelial cells of periodontal cysts originate from the enamel organ, while the other types of cysts take their origin from the buccal mucous membrane.

As I have already stated, the development of dentigerous cysts is caused by the increase of the fluid contents, which is evidently constantly secreted by the lining membrane of the cysts, and the development of the growth naturally extends in the direction of least resistance. The bony structures of the jaw enveloping the cyst become thinner and thinner until finally they entirely disappear by pressure atrophy, and then the cyst assumes a soft consistency. If the cyst continues to grow, the soft parts covering it become thin, and finally the cyst ruptures and its fluid contents are evacuated spontaneously. This, however, rarely happens, because operative interference is usually undertaken before a marked development has been reached. I have had one case of this description, which I will here briefly report:

A man aged thirty-two years had complained of an inflammation of the buccal mucosa covering the root of the first molar on the left side about eighteen months before coming under observation, and at the same time he noticed a swelling appearing under the left nostril. A few weeks later the tumor opened spontaneously and a considerable amount of pus escaped. On examination a fistula was found near the root of the left first molar, and the patient stated that the swelling would increase in size and then give exit to quite an amount of pus, after which it would decrease. The pus was always discharged through the fistula. When the tumor would increase in size on account of the collection of pus within it, it gave rise to a certain amount of pain. In other respects the patient was entirely well. The skin over the tumor was movable and not reddened. An incision was made over the tumor, including the fistulous opening, which gave exit to a yellowish fetid pus. The anterior wall of the alveolar process was resected, and then a cavity lined with a membrane was exposed. The cyst sac was carefully dissected out and the cavity packed with gauze. This was removed in three days and the patient was discharged well in eighteen days.

The fluid contents of these cysts are usually serous, and it is only after secondary infection of the cyst has taken place that the liquid becomes purulent. Infection can occur very easily from the buccal cavity or from the remains of teeth within the cyst. In those cases where decayed roots protrude into the cystic cavity, infection may also arise from the canal of the root.

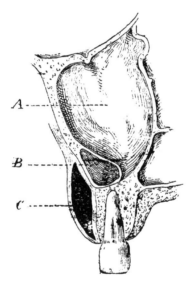

A, empyema of sinus; *B*, dentigerous cyst; *C*, dental abscess.

Regarding the diagnosis of dentigerous cysts it may be said that when the growth has reached a certain size but little difficulty will be experienced. We will here find a circumscribed unilateral swelling of the bone giving rise to a parchment crepitation and a fluctuation. If there is any doubt, an exploratory puncture will in most instances give issue to a serous fluid. In the early stages of the process, when the swelling of the bone is of small dimensions and the tumor hard to the feel, the diagnosis is less easy, because in this condition the cyst resembles any circumscribed tumor of the

11

jaw. The absence of pain during the entire progress of the growth will aid one in making a differential diagnosis. Dentigerous cysts might be mistaken for cystomata, but it should be remembered that the latter class of growth pertains almost exclusively to the lower jaw. Suppurating dentigerous cysts may simulate an alveolar abscess, but if the topography of the parts be remembered an erroneous diagnosis can hardly be made, and the accompanying illustration, taken from the excellent " Manuel de Diagnostic chirurgical," by Duplay, shows extremely well the relationship between the various forms of fluid collections occurring in the upper jaw.

If the cyst should burst into the antrum of Highmore, a primary empyema of this cavity will arise, and, *vice versa,* an infected cyst of the superior maxillary opening on the outside might easily simulate an empyema of the antrum if the cystic sac protrudes into the cavity, completely filling it.

The prognosis of dentigerous cysts is in every respect benign. The only serious complication that might arise would be when a cyst of the lower jaw becomes infected, because the danger then would be that the pus might extend and infect secondarily one of the large veins of the neck; but this is only a supposition of my own, for I must confess that I have been unable to find any such instance recorded.

The treatment of these cysts is simple. They should never be punctured unless for diagnostic purposes, and after this, when the diagnosis has been made, operation should be immediately undertaken. In undertaking the surgical cure of these cysts it is absolutely necessary to remove all vestige of the lining membrane, otherwise a relapse is practically certain to arise. In order to do this, the cavity should be freely exposed by a large opening, and the curette, scissors, and, if necessary, the thermo-cautery should be freely used, because if any epithelial cells remain within the cavity they can regenerate and cause recurrence.

After the cavity has been thoroughly cleared of its lining membrane it should be plugged with gauze for a few days, so that the epithelium of the buccal mucous membrane and the granulations arising within the cystic cavity unite, so that the latter becomes filled and only leaves a slight trace behind it.

If any tooth or root is found protruding into the cyst, it should be removed. In large cysts it may be necessary to drain through the floor of the nose, as was done in one or two cases here reported.

When dealing with these cysts developed in the lower jaw, it is oftentimes impossible to reach the tumor by way of the buccal cavity, and it must be attacked through a cutaneous incision. In this case it is indicated to remove as much of the lining membrane of the cyst as possible, and to accomplish this a sufficient resection of the outer shell of bone should be done.

THE EARLIER PRACTICE OF DENTISTRY IN HAWAII.

BY DR. J. M. WHITNEY, HONOLULU.

Mr. President and Gentlemen of the Dental Association of Hawaii,—At this close of the pleasant relationship we have sustained during the past year, I wish to express my appreciation of the honor conferred upon me, in electing me the first president of this Association. I thank you for the kind assistance you have rendered, and am glad of the unanimity with which we have worked, and the sense of good fellowship which from the first we have enjoyed. I think, for our first year, we have reason to congratulate ourselves upon what has been accomplished. Besides becoming fully organized, we have had two excellent papers, with a full discussion of them. I feel sure the coming year will witness an even more active growth. Let us labor earnestly to induce all our members living in Honolulu to attend all our meetings, and try to make them feel that the success of the Association rests upon all alike.

As your oldest member, who has practised our profession upon these islands much the longest time, I have thought that a hasty review of some things I have seen and done may be interesting to you, my younger brothers.

At the time of my graduation from the Pennsylvania College of Dental Surgery, in 1868, there had been but about six hundred dental students who had previously graduated, and so we felt that practically the world lay before us.

In partnership with a friend and classmate, I had prepared and expected to make some city of France my future home. But unexpected occurrences prompted, and I was obliged to look for another field. While still undecided where to locate, an earnest invitation came to a friend of mine to come to Honolulu, as there was no dentist here at the time. My friend did not care to accept, and turned the invitation over to me. As soon as we could make our arrangements my wife and I were married and started upon what seemed a very long wedding-journey in August, 1869.

The Union Pacific Railroad had been opened less than a month when we crossed the continent. After leaving Omaha we found ourselves in a wild country indeed. Faro and other gambling games were at many stations placed by the side of the cars to catch the unwary, and in every car was a conspicuous notice: "Passengers are warned against playing three card monte or other games of chance with strangers. You will surely be robbed if you do."

In San Francisco I was strongly urged to stop or go to Oakland, where at that time there was not a dentist! But we continued our way, and reached Honolulu September 12, 1869, and received an immediate and hearty welcome. Dr. Mott-Smith, after a long and most successful practice, had given up the dental profession, and gone into government employ under the king, Kamehameha V. Much of Dr. Smith's practice fell to me, and, considering that his knowledge had been gathered many years before from one dental office, much of it was very commendable. He evidently knew little about the treatment of teeth with devitalized pulps, but his soft-gold fillings were above the average of his day, and his mechanical work was excellent. But the best thing he did for his people was strongly impressing them with the value of their teeth, and the necessity of frequent and continued watching and caring for them. The result was that when I came with more modern knowledge and methods, I found them eager to know the best methods of saving their own and their children's teeth. I think I am safe in saying that no man ever had quite so pleasant a practice as was mine in those early days. We all know that delightful sensation when we feel we have the full confidence of our patient, and are at full liberty to go forward and do what under the circumstances we consider the very best to be done, without consulting or considering cost. This was in the main my experience, and I enjoyed it to the full.

Allow me to tell you that I brought, in the way of preparation, to my field of work eighteen months instruction by one of the best operators I ever knew, and two years in a dental college, with two full courses in anatomy in Jefferson Medical College, Philadelphia. The germ theory of decay of teeth was, of course, then unknown. The chemical theory was then universally received. Cohesive gold had but recently been introduced, and all students were trained in the use of soft gold and tin, a legacy I have valued above price. The use of the rubber dam had not been introduced into the college curriculum, and all our longest and most difficult operations had to be performed with napkins without the use of the siphon. The careful work we had to do in this line was not lost to future usefulness.

I had brought some rubber dam with me, but it deteriorated so rapidly in this climate that I was generally unable to use it. We had no rubber dam clamps then, which increased the difficulty. I noticed among my Hawaiian patients who were awa users, that their mouths were excessively dry, and it occurred to me that I might make use of the awa to reach places before inaccessible. So in some cases where the rubber dam could not be held, and the mouth was very moist, I tried the experiment of having the patient chew a little awa for fifteen or twenty minutes before I began to operate. In most cases this was successful. However, very soon the rubber dam clamp was introduced, and the awa was of no further use.

We had been taught the destruction of the pulp and the treatment of pulp-canals, filling them with gold or gutta-percha, but as the germ theory was then unknown, much that we did was empirical. Nothing was then taught about pyorrhœa alveolaris, though I soon found thorough cleansing of the teeth and roots and treatment with oxychloride of zinc very helpful. About two years after commencing my practice here Dr. Riggs, of Hartford, Conn., wrote his first articles for the *Dental Cosmos* upon his treatment of this disease, and from that time to the present the mode of treatment has changed but little. Some two years after his writings appeared I had the privilege of spending a day with Dr. Riggs in his office, and through his courtesy and kindness I gathered much that has since been of great value. The present methods of crowning and bridge-work were unknown in our college work, and it must be within the memory of many of you present when they were first brought clearly before the profession.

The first dental machine was invented by a Dr. Green. He lived in Milwaukee, Wis., if my memory serves me right. This was pneumatic, and the burs and drills screwed into the hand-piece. I possessed the fourth one that crossed the Rocky Mountains, and found it of very great help. After some two or three years that was superseded by the present machine invented by Dr. Morrison, of St. Louis, which was the same as the one now in use excepting the great improvement given it by the steel cable, an invention of Mr. A. H. Kennedy, brother of Mrs. W. A. Bowen of this city, a young man who lived in a town adjoining the one in which I spent my boyhood. I well remember the interest excited among the boys of my town when it was told that young Kennedy had invented a machine for conveying power, which was first used for shearing sheep, and many went to see it work, but I did not happen to be among the number. He sold his patent to S. S. White for the small sum of three thousand dollars, and probably he made a million on it, as there is hardly any place where power is to be transferred where it is not used. Of course this put the Morrison machine in much the same place as the Morrison had put the Green machine.

Through the training of my preceptor, whose superior I never saw in filling with gold, and my teaching in the dental college under Dr. James Truman, I became deeply impressed with the superiority of gold for the filling of teeth above every and all substitutes. From the first to the present, with very few exceptions, unless the question of expense prevented, it has been used, and my thirty-five years' experience has more than proved to my mind that, without regard to age except in the anterior teeth of the young, especially of Hawaiians, gold for durability and cheapness in the end far outranks any and all other material. Rarely a week or day passes that I do not see gold fillings in occlusal or approximate surfaces that have been doing perfect service for ten, twenty, thirty, or more years. Fillings of recent date, made with all the instruction given by such men as Dr. Black and a host of other gold workers, should prove much superior to those of early days. Some years ago, before preparing a paper for the California State Dental Association on the value of gold for fillings, I put my ledger into the hands of a professional book-keeper, in order to eliminate the personal element, and he chose the first twenty-one names that I had had upon my books for twenty-one years, followed each filling through the twenty-one years, and in summing up the results found but five per cent. had required refilling within that time. Oxyphosphate was then unknown to the profession at large if at all. Oxychlorate was known but rarely used. As it was then made it was of small value.

Silver alloys have been greatly improved since I began practice. Arrington's was probably as good as any, but then as now they proved a very uncertain material upon which to rely. We were carefully trained in regard to cleanliness of all instruments to be used in the mouth, though without our present knowledge of germs and their influence. I may say, however, that in nearly forty years of life in a dental office, under all the many conditions I have seen, I have never met a single case that showed that disease had been communicated by dental instruments in the hand of a regular dentist. I do not mention this to detract from the great importance of the most scrupulous care with our instruments, but to show that there is less danger than some would have us believe who write scare articles for our journals. We cannot be too careful, but to make capital by working upon the fears of our timid patients in this direction is not only unprofessional, but has in it all the elements of the charlatan. Do unto others as you would be done by, use upon others any instrument or appliance that you would be willing under the same conditions to have used upon yourselves, is to me a good and safe rule, and make no show about it.

I used to battle with my preceptor about his wholesale extraction of teeth, but he was but following the peculiar conditions of the times. Vulcanizable rubber had then just been discovered. Gold and silver plate, with their difficult working and expense, had up to this time held back the untrained and ignorant from entering the dental profession. There was no law regulating the practice of dentistry. Any one by paying a hundred or two dollars could go into a dental office, in a couple of weeks learn to make a set of teeth on rubber base, and the week after hang out his sign as a dentist. The people, then as now, expecting to get something for nothing, would flock to his rooms. He knew nothing but to drag out their teeth and put in their place his miserable substitute for as miserable a pittance, and thus began the great destruction of the people's teeth and the beginning of the sad condition we see to-day in the mouths of their children. For I think it is the testimony of every observant dentist, that he has never seen in the mouth of a descendant a normal condition of the teeth, whose mother has before his birth lost her full upper or lower set or both.

When I first came to my practice in Honolulu it was the custom for the physicians to give instructions to the dentist what to do. This I resented with considerable spirit, for, as I said to them, " I have spent as many years in preparing for my specialty as you did for your general practice, and under as severe discipline, .and it is but common sense that I should know more about it than you do who did not probably give it an hour of time in your full course." I had so much of this to contend with that I resolved to see for myself the foundation upon which they built their sense of such superior knowledge. I at once put every spare moment into study for a medical course, and, returning to Ohio, matriculated and graduated from one of the best medical schools in that State. I have to state that in the six months' course but a part of one hour lecture was given to the special diseases of the teeth and mouth. Doubtless that same school would now do much better by its graduates. It is needless to say that when I returned with my medical degree, I never heard further from my medical *confrères,* but was allowed to save teeth that I thought best to preserve without their contention.

The whole subject of antiseptic mouth-washes has grown up since my graduation—I am not quite sure but to the serious injury of the mouth and teeth. There is no question about the great care which should be given to cleansing the teeth as thoroughly as possible with brush and silk, using, if necessary, a carefully prepared tooth-powder once a day at night. But to be constantly washing the mouth at all times of the day with strong, pungent aseptic mouth-washes seems to me to weaken and put to sleep nature, which, left to herself, would prepare her battalions, and with her guards ever out would seek the most vulnerable points of her enemies, and thus be able to fight them much more successfully than would be done by foreign help.

I cannot close this reminiscent paper without saying something about our profession, and the inheritance with which you younger men have entered. After I had returned from service in our Civil War, and had decided to study dentistry, several of my influential friends were greatly opposed to it, and said, " You are too much of a man to go into that miserable charlatan kind of work. It is no place for you; you can find a better calling." I mention this simply to show the feeling existing at that time against the profession. And can it be said to have quite disappeared at the present time? After my graduation I went to visit a dear old friend whose life was among the upper classes. Her daughter told her I had graduated a doctor. They did not dare tell her I was to be a dentist, for it would greatly shock her and cause her to commiserate me instead of congratulating me as she did. To the day of her death she thought of me as a physician, and was happy in the thought. The first instance was in Ohio, the second in Vermont, so you see the same feeling prevailed east and west. Physicians would not recognize our title of D.D.S., and if they called us doctor it was with much the same spirit as they might give the title to an apothecary. In a measure we deserved some of the opprobrium, for many graduated were without much if any preparatory study, and thus were at great disadvantage with their much more highly cultured brothers, and the great majority gave themselves the title of doctor, and of course such could have no standing with the regulars.

But to you young men this is ancient history. You find yourselves in a learned profession with your degree recognized by the International Medical Association, the highest authority, as on a par with the degree of M.D. You have reason to feel but little of that slight which the older members had to carry. We to-day ought to give thanks and reverence to those who so bravely and persistently fought our battles before legislatures and courts and the more trying and cynical great meetings of scientific and medical men, and greater still by their true lives and great usefulness before the people. We cannot stop more than to mention the names of Dr. Harris, Dr. Taft, Dr. Tucker, Dr. Atkinson, and Dr. Barrett, great men of our profession who have passed on before. And the host of such names as Dr. Truman and Dr. Brophy and Dr. Black and Dr. Harlan and Dr. Kirk and Dr. Johnson, who are still in the great work of bringing our profession to the forefront. It is no mere boast to say that our profession does more than any or all others in assuring comfort and happiness to mankind. Therefore let us take great pride in it, and be loyal to its highest ideals. Let us feel by our true lives and earnest work that we are the peers of any who call upon us for our services, and let us see to it that no man nor class of men shall exceed us in honest, earnest and intelligent endeavors to minister to the well-being of our fellows.

PYORRHŒA ALVEOLARIS.

BY DR. B. F. ARRINGTON, GOLDSBORO, N. C.

This may to many seem to be almost a threadbare subject, but it is not, and it must and will be discussed in the interest of humanity until a reasonable, practical, and definite line of treatment that will cure shall be established and accepted by the profession, and in dental colleges proclaimed to students as orthodox and reliable, and students shall be taught that the disease, when uncomplicated, is amenable to a simple, practical line of treatment, and is speedily curable, and that there is no need for all the *big noise* some are making about extreme features of the disease and difficulty in effecting cure.

I have for several years past been impressed with the idea that some men in the profession when writing about and discussing this very prevalent disease, especially some of those professing to make a specialty of the treatment, were in effort making a mountain of a very small hill. Upon reflection, since attending the meeting of the National Dental Association at Asheville, and more recently reading a most ably written, but extravagant paper on the subject, by a prominent dentist of Chicago, and published in the *Dental Summary,* June and July issues, 1903, I am more forcibly impressed with the fact, and can plainly see, as many do, that there has been much buncombe indulged by some, with a very great amount of unnecessary extravagant talk about the disease, and largely magnified difficulty of treatment. The extreme features in practice so conspicuously proclaimed and indulged by that class of practitioners, singly or as a whole, have not evidenced any marked ability as practical practitioners, especially as pertains to this disease.

During the meeting of the National some very extravagant and out of place " spread-eagle" utterances were indulged in in relation to treatment of the disease by dentists who were seemingly disposed to impress listeners with the idea that they certainly knew it all, and held the subject definitely in hand, and could dispense treatment successfully beyond a question of doubt, and that the disease was something wonderful to treat, and was the disease of all diseases difficult to treat, and that so and so, especially the use of sharp scalers in the hands of experts, were requisites for success.

One dentist of some prominence, much heard, ventured to say that he did not know to what to attribute his success in the removal of deposits and his successful treatment of the disease, unless it was his peculiar sensitiveness of touch in the use of scalers; and similar expressions, evidently designed to convey the impression that treatment was extremely difficult, and but few men were equal to the task. Others talked on the same line with marked extravagance of expression, and as much out of place considering the occasion, but were not quite so flippant and harmful in effect. Some have boasted of their high charges for treating the disease, mentioning bills rendered and paid, for hundreds of dollars, thousands, for treating a single case. Unquestionably feeling (false assumption) that they were moving on a high plane, as was the case (pitiable) with some men in the profession several decades back, who were addicted to boasting on public occasions of their high charges, fifty or a hundred dollars for a single gold filling. Not much to their credit in the face of the fact that there were numbers of dentists all around them that could and were probably inserting fillings, daily, as perfect, possibly, for less than one-tenth the amount. But so it is, and long has been, a weak, corrupting, and demoralizing feature in practice, but possibly, very probably, will continue to prevail until the profession in open meeting condemns such unprofessional conduct, and demands clean expression, clean action, and no trick and trade or humbuggery in dental practice, and put a stop to the existing crying shame that is so unbecoming and hurtful to the status and dignity of dentistry.

Some harangues at the National meeting were listened to with considerable feeling of disgust by many present, and with much desire and hope that a different order of things may soon prevail, and the National will be national truly, in work, dignity, and elevation. Some men of distinguished prominence in the profession are accountable, to a large extent, for much of the prevailing extreme and unreasonable opinions now entertained concerning pyorrhœa alveolaris as a disease, and the want of an established, correct line of treatment.

Many have written and talked entertainingly on the subject, but few wide of the mark for successful treatment. I will, in connection with the paper in the *Summary* above mentioned, enumerate some of the extravagant sayings and false teachings on the subject that have tended to confuse and mislead rather than enlighten and establish correct views and a curative line of treatment.

A recent writer has said, " This disease is peculiar, in that it is often found in mouths the care of which has been rigidly looked after. . . . As a rule, if the pulp is removed at the first evidence of developing pyorrhœa, the disease is arrested." He mentions the use of solvents, and advises the " use of cauterants of such strength that it is requisite to protect the mouth; also to use a soft rubber brush after treatment." All of which evidences plainly his utter ignorance of the disease uncomplicated, and his inability to treat successfully.

A dentist of decided ability, and regarded by those competent to measure professional merit as a first class practitioner, has said, in discussing a paper pertaining to treatment of pyorrhœa, " that in one instance, after several years treatment of a case and failure to cure, he cut off the natural crown and substituted an artificial crown, and cure followed." Truly wonderful! why should he have conceived such an idea? No explanation offered, and it is presumable that none could be given. Another dentist in Chicago, quite as prominent, has said,—

" I do not remove deposits at first sitting, but obtain a sample of patient's urine and examine it, and immediately request patient to drink from eight to twelve glasses of water daily." He further advises to " lance the gums if much inflamed," and he ventures the utterance that " modern dentistry is producing more pyorrhœa than any other cause." And then, to cap the climax and make absurd more absurd, he says, " Since nature tolerates lime deposits in all parts of the body, it would seem immaterial whether the deposits are removed from the roots or not. . . . Nature takes care of all such deposits." He also advises, " in place of instruments for removal of deposits, the use of a dissolving fluid, especially when the disease is extensive." He does not name the fluid, possibly an unfortunate oversight that may yet be remedied, but I think it questionable.

Some dentists, embracing some of the ablest men in the profession, contend that " extraction is the only means of cure." Strong men on some lines, doubtless, but as pertains to treatment of pyorrhœa, weak theory and condemnable practice. Others advise to " sink bars in the crowns, and to drill holes in the teeth when loose and ligature to hold firm." And another has said,

"Treat with cautery and burn it out as you would a fistula." Some say "the disease is confined exclusively to middle life, and is always found in connection with good teeth, exempt from decay." Truly a beautiful display of ignorance concerning the disease. Such is inexcusable for dentists of experience and prominence, but so it is, and there is much of it.

One dentist, quite notable, advises "that patients shall smear the ends of two or three fingers with vaseline and menthol and rub the gums surrounding all the teeth for five minutes twice daily." Presumably, very large mouths and small fingers. Whether this treatment is for several days only, or during life, is not stated.

Some contend that when the alveolar process has wasted half or two-thirds, exposing roots of teeth, with gums festooned and flapped to the depth of alveolar waste, they can, by a certain (not explained) line of treatment, "restore the process to original proportions to necks of teeth, and establish normal attachment of gum tissue to the cementum." If such were possible, what cause for rejoicing! but it is not possible. There is no reason why any one shall be deceived about such a result. To carefully watch the treatment is all that is requisite to establish facts that will be convincing. Another dentist somewhat prominent, but very impractical and sensational, says, "When teeth are very loose, the first consideration shall be the devitalization of the pulps." Most absurd and very misleading. Then comes another, quite his equal in radical extreme, in treatment, one who has written and talked much about the disease, and says, "Treatment consists in patient's drinking eight or nine glasses of water each day, in brushing the gums with a stiff brush to make them bleed, and the employment of proper mouth-washes." A shot far from the mark for one so notably prominent as a teacher, and a treater of this disease, but nothing but irrational or extreme on this line need be surprising, since so many of much prominence, and some of little prominence, have so wildly side-tracked and drifted along with a wild craze on the subject, and are making guess-work the foundation basis of theory and practice.

Some advise to "lay open the gum over each tooth, and to cauterize the surface of the flaps with nitrate of silver and carbolic acid." Then follows advice of others to "cut away the lateral flaps and apply the hot iron (galvano-cautery) over the cut surface of all the affected teeth in one or several days." Others say,

" Scrape away the cementum, also the alveolar process, and to get at it successfully cut through the gum, then close with sutures."

Can anything in line of treatment be more unreasonable, the nature of the disease considered? But so it is. Some one anxious for notoriety will bleat out something as a new feature in treatment, whether in accord with reason and sound judgment or no, and the bleating is taken up by apists, and so goes, passing down the line with loud acclaim based on ignorance. A conspicuous dentist of California, rather sensational and not very practical, advises to " pass silk thread through the gums, both external and internal spaces on each side of the teeth, and to ligate the gums in contact with the teeth."

For what purpose not stated, and no one can imagine. Yet he has his followers to endorse and herald such a feature in practice as requisite and important, and the craze goes on.

Dr. M. has recommended " cauterization of the pockets with pure chromic acid, the use of chlorate of potash, scarification of the gums, leeches, and purgative mineral water." Another of much reputation suggests " partial destruction of the gum forming the alveolar pockets, followed with bichloride solution." Another, in New York, of considerable notoriety, but quite as impractical for successful treatment as the distinguished Californian, has advised " to fill the pockets with paste composed of two-thirds caustic potash and one-third crystallized carbolic acid." Pretty severe treatment for any disease short of cancer; but some will argue that it is from a New York dentist of note, and must be good practice.

Others advise the use of " pure sulphuric acid, full strength, to burn out pockets and decalcify the cementum." This is heroic out of reason, and must do more harm than good.

The " wearing of copper plates and bands for a year, and to be continued longer if necessary," was advised and practised by a New York dentist, one of the most notable and conspicuous men that have ever joined the ranks of the dental profession, but no favorable report was ever made of such coppery treatment, and none could reasonably be expected.

A dentist now prominent in New York insists " that pyorrhœa alveolaris is always caused by syphilis, and he treats accordingly. Such may be the lamentable condition of New York patients, but it is questionable, and when so treated we can easily guess the result. Now comes a fancy delicate feature in dental surgery that almost tempts a smile. Dr. H., of Chicago, advises, when there is much receding of the gum, to "make an incision in the gum a little below the border and insert crystals of iodide of zinc; this irritates the gum, pushing it up on the tooth where it adheres." When the doctor can produce positive evidence of *such adhesion,* then will be time to credit and sanction such practice, not before. One small practical fact is of more intrinsic value in practice than a thousand fine-spun fancy theories. Give us facts foundationed upon results obtained; that is what we want.

Some are recorded as advocates of "lactic, trichloracetic, and sulphuric acids as solvents of pyorrhœa deposits," and profess to obtain satisfactory results. Such is deception. The deposits cannot be dissolved or even softened in the mouth by any acid, liquid, paste, or powder known to dentists or chemists without serious detriment to soft tissues. Some advise "hot baths, cold baths, Turkish baths, life on sea-shore, sea-bathing, resort to mountain sections, open-air exercise, and heroic exercise as essential for cure of the disease."

If this be true, there is but little chance for cure of the poor as a class, who are most afflicted with the disease. They are ignored entirely. Such treatment may be admissible and may help to cure sometimes, but certainly it is, to say the least, entirely out of the reach of the masses. Others contend that "perfect occlusion is requisite for successful treatment," and they shorten teeth and rearrange accordingly, and then fail of desired results.

One Chicago dentist advises: "If a three months' course of treatment does not affect a cure, let the patient go for a month; then give a second trial of same vigorous treatment for another three months." Most unreasonable. A true case of pyorrhœa alveolaris (Riggs's disease), or *interstitial gingivitis,* if disposed to so call it, a true typical case, uncomplicated, can be as successfully treated in from three to four weeks as in three months or three years. The thing requisite is to do the work thoroughly in removal of deposits, and treat mildly.

Dr. P., of Philadelphia, a superior man and a splendid dentist, has said, "The disease commences at the apex of the roots," and he sticks to it, right or wrong, in the face of much convincing argument and evidence to the contrary. Such, however, is human nature, and now and then will crop out and display conspicuously, whether for good or evil.

Most dentists who have written about and discussed treatment of this disease have advocated use of sharp scalers, and herein lies the failure of successful treatment. Some say, " Curette the cementum, and cut or scrape away the edge of the alveolar process." Possibly, but few greater blunders pertaining to treatment of the disease have ever been perpetrated.

Now we approach the zenith of all treatment that has ever been proposed, possibly the most unreasonable, extreme, and unjustifiable as a whole, that ever has or ever will be perpetrated in civilized communities. The doctor in question writes considerably, and most extravagantly, on the subject. Too much of it to relate in full; it would be overtaxing. I will quote only a brief clipping from a dental journal. Just a little of such will suffice to enlighten or disgust. He says, " Rinse the mouth with permanganate of potash solution, one-half grain to ounce of water. Touch the gums with carbolic acid, and inject five per cent. solution eucaine; then carry down quickly, from gum margin to alveolar process, a three-edged flexible lancet, passing it around the teeth, severing gum entirely from teeth. With scraper or chisel scrape away the diseased pericementum, the external layer of the cementum, and the diseased portion of the process. Success depends upon the thoroughness with which this is done, and it requires skill and practice. Wash out the pocket, and with cotton wrapped on a broach protect the mouth and carry to the bottom of the pocket sulphuric acid full strength. Wipe away oozing blood, and repeat, holding the acid in contact until the root surface is decalcified. Rinse mouth with soda solution, and prescribe as mouth-wash permanganate of potash one-quarter grain to ounce of water, used hourly until gum heals. A dose of Epsom salt daily for three weeks, also sarsaparilla and potassium iodide three times a day. Devitalize the pulp in all cases presenting in advanced stages. In very advanced cases cut off crowns just above gum level. After root treatment, crown, and solder crowns together if several."

If this treatment fails to cure, most probable; but should it kill, who would be surprised?

In my humble opinon, just so long as dental journals will consent to accept and publish papers taxing the profession with so much of such conglomerate, impractical treatment as above mentioned, we cannot reasonably hope that the disease will be better comprehended or more successfully treated than at present. It is but seldom we read a paper pertaining to the disease that is reasonable, conservative, and practical. Hence the much leading astray that has prevailed.

Pyorrhœa alveolaris is a very common disease, possibly of more frequent occurrence, in many sections of country, than any disease known to man. It is easily recognized, and can be easily treated, with good results following if rightly treated on a plain practical basis of local procedure, provided there is not syphilitic complication, as specified by a New York dentist. In treatment of the disease there can be no justification for severe or prolonged treatment, nor for excessive charges for treatment. Maltreatment and overcharging for same is censurable and condemnable.

The thing requisite for success in treatment is the *thorough removal of deposits* from the roots of teeth,. thorough as thorough can be practically, no guesswork about it. This accomplished, the requisite following treatment of soft tissues is simple and easy, and cure speedily follows in a large percentage of cases.

In the removal of deposits it is all important to avoid, as far as possible, injury of the soft tissues, the cementum, and alveolar process. Hence the necessity for use of *smooth-edge scalers.*

The time limit for cure of a typical case, pus discharging and teeth loose in sockets, does not exceed from three to four weeks, seldom more than three, and a large majority of cases presenting for consultation or treatment can be successfully treated in less time than two weeks.

One sitting for removal of deposits is all that is requisite in most cases, and is best for patients. The removal of deposits with smooth scalers is much more expeditious than with sharp ones. But few remedies (two or three), campho-phenique chiefly, for the healing of gums and restoration to a healthy state, will accomplish as much or more than dozens, as advised by some.

The use of toothpick and tooth-bursh after meals daily, after the removal of deposits and treatment, is important for effective cure and to prevent return of the disease. Patients must follow instructions as to use of tooth-brush if they wish to preserve and enjoy the blessing of a healthy mouth, teeth and gums especially.

I hold that any member of the profession can do, in the treatment of this disease and the accomplishment of results, just what any other member can, accepting the fact that the disease is local and is curable, and he will not try to do too much after successful removal of deposits, and will discard from mind all thought of impractical papers and discussions, and false teaching on the subject.

From experience in practice, and watchful observation of results following treatment, I feel justified in saying that any practical dentist of fair comprehension, can, in a few hours' observation of the use of smooth scalers in the removal of deposits, be able to manipulate such instruments effectively, and will fully realize in a limited period of time that the deposits can be removed more quickly and more thoroughly than with sharp scalers, and will feel satisfied that successful treatment of the disease is possible with the whole profession, if desired, and all can treat and cure if they will. And that all this extravagant sensational talk and writing about the disease, and the difficulty of treatment and cure, is unnecessary and unauthorized, and cannot be sustained by facts demonstrated through a correct line of practice or otherwise.

Shall sensational writing be longer indulged? Is there need for it? Can good come of it? are questions that present themselves for thoughtful consideration.

Let us work on right lines for good results, that the public may be more favorably impressed and definitely realize the fact that we can, as a whole, treat successfully for relief. The idea that a disease of so small compass, never extending to greater extent than the length of the roots of teeth, so easily reached and so easily treated, should be such a stumbling block to the profession as it has been, and baffled the best skill in dental ranks for these many years, half a century or more, does not speak well for the advance of the profession, and it is surprising and humiliating. It is not that the disease is so difficult to treat that has caused failure of general success in treatment, but the much false theory and teaching as to etiology and treatment that has been heralded through papers and discussions on the subject.

May we not reasonably hope that the day is not far distant when the profession will know more about this disease and better how to treat it than at present, more humanely and practical, requiring less time and fewer remedies with better results?

In conclusion, I feel that I cannot do better for the profession and the public than to advise old and young practitioners to procure if possible, and read carefully, a paper, " Pyorrhœa Alveolaris," written by Dr. Henri Letord, of Orlando, Fla., published in

Dental Hints, May issue, 1903, which, as a whole, so far as it goes, is the best paper I have ever read pertaining to this disease. Practice based upon such a foundation of theory as he has laid down could but promise good results, and would do away completely with all this big craze so long indulged concerning cause and treatment of the disease.

When the principles of prophylaxis shall be more generally understood, and shall be taught in dental colleges (not on extreme lines), and the practice of prophylactic treatment for purification and health of mouths shall be more universally indulged than at present, there will, proportionately, be less of pyorrhœa alveolaris to treat, and less of tooth decay and other abnormal features in the mouth, and there would be unquestionably a better state of general health.

The possibility of satisfactory results will justify the expenditure of time, trouble, and expense requisite in experimenting for truth and conviction that will be realized through watchful observation of results.

APPARENT TRIPLES: THEIR IMPORTANCE IN DENTAL PRACTICE.[1]

BY DR. F. MILTON SMITH, NEW YORK.

" He that is faithful in that which is least is faithful also in much." More than nineteen centuries have passed since these words came from the lips of the Great Teacher, and from that time to the present, in forms almost without number, the truth has been restated.

In no field is this teaching more clearly demonstrated than in our work. Were it not for the fact that many of our " craft" who have passed to " that bourne whence no traveller returns" realized the force of this truth, we to-day would not meet with the measure of success we do.

If I speak to-night to any young man who is not willing to give the utmost attention to any detail that may in any way

---

[1] Read before the American Academy of Dental Science, Boston, Mass., March 2, 1904.

effect the accomplishing of the work he may have in hand, I would urge him not to waste his time trying to build up a dental practice, but immediately get a position as trolley-car motorman or conductor. While there is plenty of room for young men who are determined to succeed, and are willing to pay " the price thereof," there is, indeed, only just standing-room for the young man who considers details beneath his notice.

How familiar to our thought is the story of the battle lost through the want of a horseshoe-nail, yet how many there are who are willing to pay almost any price to succeed, but will pass by that great stepping-stone to success,—namely, attention to details, with scarcely a thought.

One has but to read the average article in the dental journal to be persuaded that this lack of attention to detail is not confined to the mere boys in the profession.

In a recent issue of a dental journal there were two articles by good men. After very careful reading both were thrown aside as worthless, because in each article an important detail was missing.

Apparent trifles are exceedingly important in their bearing upon the comfort or discomfort of the patient; and to the lack of appreciation of their importance may be charged the loss of the good opinions of many patients.

All other things being equal, any genteel patient will select the dentist whose office and surroundings are pleasing.

While a man of skill and integrity will sometimes gather around him a good practice, even if his office and reception-room are not such as might be expected, he would nevertheless attract more people if the surroundings were pleasant.

When a patient enters the office of one practitioner he is pleasantly impressed. There is a place for everything and everything is in its place. In another everything is confusion. The one has a flower or two on the mantel. The other has everything else in creation but a flower or two. In the one case the operator is strictly neat and clean in his personal appearance. There is about him neither the odor of pipe, cigarette, beer, nor onions. He cares for his own mouth and teeth and employs a good dentist: therefore his breath is not loaded with the odors of pyorrhœa or abscessed teeth. In fact, he studies to keep himself absolutely free from odors, with the possible exception of a faint suggestion of cashmere bouquet soap with which he washes his hands very often. In the other the reverse is true.

In the one case the operator opens a drawer of his cabinet, whence he takes a towel or napkin which is immaculately clean. If the other opens a drawer there is revealed in its recesses two or three extracted teeth, some broken pieces of wax with which the floss is waxed, a broken hand-piece, some old scratched mirrors, and a miscellaneous assortment of other things too numerous to mention.

In the latter case the operator may have a machine on his table conspicuously marked "Sterilizer," and make a pretence at antiseptic work, but the aforesaid drawer is silent yet forcible evidence to the contrary.

It was my privilege on one occasion to visit a friend who made quite a pretence at things aseptic. In order to demonstrate to me his methods, he opened his aseptic napkin-box, then moistening his finger with his tongue, after the fashion of a trolley-car conductor when separating slips, picked up one of the napkins.

He then demonstrated to me his method of rolling absorbent paper points for root drying, pursuing the same course as to moistening the fingers, so that the paper would roll well. He said after they were rolled they were sterilized. I think that was right; they needed it.

In another case a dentist, who is also a great preacher of antiseptic methods, requested me to wash my hands before examining the mouth of a patient whom he was kind enough to let me see; yet he was so busy superintending my proper sterilization that he forgot to change the napkin on which he was constantly wiping the mouth-mirror, although he changed patients four times while I was present.

As to the apparent trifles which affect the comfort of the patient. The careful man sees to it that the chair is adjusted to the comfort of his patient as well as to his own convenience. A few minutes carefully spent in this seemingly unimportant detail will pay large interest on the investment. The patient will almost invariably thank you to make an application of some cooling emollient to the lips, if they are at all dry or have a tendency to crack.

The rubber dam, if applied before excavating, will save much valuable time, though there may be room for question as to whether the average patient would not prefer to have its application delayed until the last moment. When ready to apply it there is room to demonstrate your ability to do things carefully. It will pay almost always to make six holes through the rubber and surround that number of teeth.

I think the average dentist should have the dam applied to his own teeth by some careless man at least once a week. He would then use care in applying it for others. Ordinarily there should be no pain and very little discomfort through its application. In the cold weather if you will place the clamp in the forceps and then hold the clamp over your Bunsen burner just long enough to warm it, your patient will bless you. If, in carrying your ligature between the teeth, you are careful not to let it strike the gum suddenly, your patient will appreciate it. If you are about to fill an ordinary cavity, it is absolutely cruel to ligate several teeth, carrying the ligature up above the natural gum line.

When preparing a cavity it is not necessary to have it so dry that the tears will course down the patient's cheeks because of the pain caused by the dryness and low temperature of the room, as compared with the body. A pledget of cotton dipped in carbolic acid and passed through the lamp flame, then to the cavity, will change the expression on the face as if my magic. If applied cold the patient will dread it as much as the pain you seek to control. If, when applying the dam clamp, you fold two little pieces of muslin and lay them between the clamp and cheek, your patient will appreciate it.

If you are filling a large sensitive cavity with amalgam, it will lessen the discomfort greatly if you will warm your plugger or burnisher each time you use either of them. If it is a gold filling you have made, you will find much less complaint from your patient during the finishing if your bur is run into a bit of beeswax and your disk against a piece of soap or coated with vaseline before use.

A corundum point is much less annoying if coated with vaseline instead of water, and answers as well when used on metal.

When you are ready to remove the dam your patient will leave you in a happier frame of mind if you do not jam the clamp down unnecessarily on the already sore gum, nor remove it so suddenly that every particle of blood shall seem all at once to be trying to get to the gingival margin. Having removed the clamp and dam in the most approved method, your patient will be exceedingly grateful to you if you will thoroughly spray the gums with an antiseptic, or syringe carefully with warm water and antiseptic. In order to have this water always at the right temperature you need a small Bunsen gas-burner with a rack to hold a glass of water over it, placing between the flame and the glass a piece of asbestos mat. If you do not have something of this kind, one of two things will occur,—either you will torture your patient by throwing cold water into a sensitive tooth or else you will waste an enormous amount of time between the warm water faucet and your chair. As to the various methods of relieving the sensitivity, each operator will have his pet method. Your essayist finds that the cases differ materially as to their responsiveness to drugs. Besides the many in common use, I find the plan recently suggested by Dr. L. C. Bryan, of Basel, Switzerland, to be very useful in many cases.

In a communication through The New York Institute of Stomatology he suggests a pledget of cotton saturated with carbolic acid, which, after being placed in the cavity, is touched with a metal point which is heated sufficiently so that when applied to the moist cotton a vapor is produced. This repeated several times works beautifully in many cases.

Lack of time forbids my recounting more of the apparent trifles, and they are almost without number, which affect the comfort of the patient. I will therefore call attention to some which have to do with the quality of the service we render our patients.

Why is it that the magnificent gold filling in the distal face of a certain bicuspid tooth has failed?

The one in the mesial face of the adjoining tooth still is doing service, although five years longer in place. The former filling bears evidence of having been made by a clever mechanic, yet has not saved the tooth. The reason for failure is that the operator considered that a blow from an automatic mallet upon a piece of cohesive gold, driven directly against the cervical wall, was a trifle not to be reckoned on. His neighbor who placed the other filling in position considered it wise to see to it that, previous to any blow being struck by a mallet, he had first placed a large mass of non-cohesive gold against the cervical wall. He may have also thought that suggestion a valuable one (first made public, I think, by Dr. S. G. Perry, of New York City) which consists in placing a very large piece of non-cohesive gold in the cavity, following with a large ball of bibulous paper, which paper is packed with a large pointed plugger, carrying before it the soft gold. The paper then being removed, the gold is found safely carried to the floor of the cavity without being punctured or cut through with the plugger point. It is then with smaller points very carefully condensed without the mallet. After making two or three layers thus, the cohesive gold may be malleted *ad libitum.*

Many a young man has wondered why his filling did not finish up like the filling of some excellent operator whose work he has admired. If you see him tell him that it is not that his ideal operator is so much more skilful than he. It is because he got tired out too soon and failed to appreciate that all that was needed to make his filling finish perfectly was two or three large pieces of gold, covering the whole surface of the filling like a blanket carefully laid on with a broad, flat, almost smooth-face plugger; this to be followed by a very small point with which the surface is condensed.

Tell him also, for his encouragement, that his ideal operator has not skill enough to put a perfect filling in the cavity where he failed yesterday, with no more room than he had. It is not that his ideal is so much more expert as a mechanic. It is that he knows that to fill the cavity perfectly he must have room, and without it he will not attempt the task.

Who has not seen the disreputable-looking gold-band porcelain crown, showing more gold than porcelain? It is the simple result of lack of attention to details (apparent trifles). First, the gum was not crowded up on the labial side when the root was ground away, therefore it could not be ground above the natural gum line without injuring the gum. Second, the root was not so reduced in diameter at the exposed portion as to make it possible to so fit a band that it would hug the root snugly under the gum. Third, the band was not cut off even with the already too long root. Fourth, a thirty-guage piece of gold was used to cover the root instead of forty. Fifth, the porcelain did not fit perfectly against the cap. Result, a frightful disfigurement. Why has the patient found it less useful than ornamental? Another trifle. Care was not taken that it should be sufficiently wide at the swell portion so that it would crowd closely between the adjoining teeth when set. Had this been done it would have been comfortable.

Some one says, " I get along well with the operative side, but my plate work is not successful. The plate I put in yesterday would not stay up until I sprinkled it with gum tragacanth." Of course it wouldn't. You were too hurried, and concluded to let a compound impression do when it should have been a plaster one. " Yes, but the one I put in the day before did not stay up, and it was made from a plaster impression." The reason for its failure was that you did not make a groove in the impression across the roof of the mouth, so that the extreme back edge of the plate would surely go up to place; or maybe you did not take time to notice that the hard palate is very hard in the centre of that mouth, and the hardness reaches almost to the alveolar ridge in front. A very large piece of thin air-chamber metal should have been carefully placed on the model, covering the hard territory before packing the rubber. It is more than likely you did not wait for the flask to cool thoroughly before opening; therefore there was a slight drawing away from the centre. Again you have treated as apparent trifles the valuable suggestions which have appeared from time to time in the journals. In other words, the majority of your failures are the results of neglecting details.

Not the least among the apparent trifles is the habit of wasting time which prevails among dentists.

If one's fee is six dollars per hour, his minutes are worth just ten cents each. Imagine a poor man sitting on a cracker barrel in a country store throwing a ten-cent piece out of the window every minute, and you have a forcible illustration of the dentist whose fee is six dollars per hour and upward, when he wastes his time. I am not familiar with your habits in this town, but in the one whence I came many dentists have no time to read the dental journals, yet they will squander more time every day in reading the details of the latest social scandal, murder trial, or other trash than would suffice to read any one of the dental journals. Were the average man to be impressed with the fact that half an hour spent each day in this useless reading would in the course of a year run away with eighteen days of eight hours each, he would, I think, put his time to better use. Many of this class would not think they could possibly take a three weeks' vacation.

Since the dentist must, with his own brain and hand, do almost everything that is done in his office, it is of the utmost importance that he shall make every minute count for its full value. He must certainly, as soon as he can possibly afford it, employ some one to do the little things about the office. It is the habit of some excellent practitioners to take time for which they are charging their patients ten or twelve dollars an hour, and use that time in folding, rolling, and cutting gold, rolling up paper pellets, and such like work, when a girl for five dollars a week can do it as well.

A little thing worth attention is the time lost between patients. It is absolutely impossible to tell just how long a given operation will take; therefore it is best to make appointments for one hour, one and a half, or two hours each, always saying to the patient that the next sitting will be for one of these stated periods. If the appointment is made over the telephone or by mail, a most excellent way is to mail to the patient a duplicate slip, each part of which contains the date, hour, and time reserved. One is retained by the patient, and the other, which contains the words, " Mrs. ——— accepts the appointment," is returned by mail. This plan obviates the embarrassment of having a vacant chair for an hour unexpectedly. It also impresses the patient with the value of our time.

For suggestions in this direction I am greatly indebted to my present associate and friend, Dr. George S. Allan.

The appointment having been made for, say, one and one-half hours, it is well at once to proceed with the preparation of a cavity or other piece of work that can surely be done in that time. This will usually leave a few minutes before the next patient. These minutes can almost invariably be used to benefit to the patient in removing calculus or in polishing the teeth. At the next sitting the same course is pursued, so that by the time we have the fillings all made we have the teeth cleaned and polished or so nearly finished that we can judge very closely as to how much time will be required for its accomplishment.

Had we spent two hours at the first sitting in cleansing and polishing, we could not conscientiously have made all our appointments come out evenly.

By this method we have practically saved the time required for this work, which is no small item.

Another waste of time is caused by the practice of permitting lady patients to remove their hats and wraps in the operating-room. This needs no further comment other than to say that ten minutes lost at each change of patients means, if repeated six times in a day, just one hour out of your working day.

Lest I weary you, I will thus abruptly close, leaving you to think out the many, many apparent trifles which hitherto you have overlooked, hoping that you, as well as I, may have indelibly stamped upon our minds and hearts the value of time as conceived by one who says,—

> " Across the years I fly on tireless wing;
> No rest I ever know; on, on I go,
> Nor stay my ordered flight for friend or foe.
> Once past I never shall return to bring
> Again my gifts so often spurned, for, lo,
> Each moment is a bridge that's burned.
> I know no haste, yet in my flight outspeed the light,
> While out of seconds ageless cycles grow.
> Who knows my name and freely will
> Bestow on me his best of hand, and heart and mind,
> I'll give him true success and clearly show
> The secret of my power to bless mankind;
> He me enjoys who me employs aright.
> My name is Now. Lay hold with all thy might."

Reviews of Dental Literature.

SOMNOFORME.[1] By W. H. Gilmour, L.D.S. (Eng.).

Dr. Rolland, Dean of the Dental School of Bordeaux, in his capacity of Professor of Anæsthesia, not feeling satisfied with the anæsthetics in general use for dental purposes, made up his mind to try, if possible, to formulate or discover an anæsthetic that would be more idealistic from a dental point of view.

He first of all resolved his problem under three headings or rules,—viz.:

1. In order that anæsthesia should be produced, the tension of the anæsthetic vapor should be superior to that of oxygen and to replace it in a certain quantity in the blood.

2. That the more a vapor or gas is volatile the greater in con-

---

[1] Paper read before the Liverpool District Odontological Society, March 17, 1903.

sequence will be its tension and the more easy its substitution for oxygen.

3. That the ideal anæsthetic would be one that approaches most nearly the conditions of absorption and elimination of oxygen in the blood.

Since most anæsthetics are administered by the respiratory organs, he therefore calculated the amount of air-space in the lungs, tabulating the amount of air taken in by an ordinary inspiration, the amount of residual, complimentary, and reserve air, and, in order to arrive at the necessary volume of anæsthetic vapor for each dose, he then calculated the tension of oxygen in the lungs and determined two further rules for the absorption of his ideal anæsthetic,—viz.:

That the greater the tension of a gas in the pulmonary vesicules, the more easily will be its absorption.

That the volatility of a gas determining its pressure, it follows that the more volatile a gas, the greater the rapidity of its absorption by the blood.

The lungs being the means of entry of the air or a vapor into the system, the blood is the distributer through its red corpuscles.

The amount of blood in the human system was then calculated, and the length of time it took to complete the cardiac circle was determined,—viz., twenty-five minutes or, more simply, thirty minutes. In other words a red blood-corpuscle would occupy thirty minutes from the time it left the heart to return to it again.

Knowing further that oxygen is only active in the arterial blood and passive in the pulmonary, it follows by simple division that oxygen is only active during fifteen minutes.

The ideal anæsthetic, therefore, being absorbed under the same conditions as oxygen, ought or will produce its effect in fifteen minutes; again it follows that if the doses are not renewed the anæsthetic ought to eliminate itself, measure by measure, as the red corpuscles return to contact with oxygen or air. It is in this manner that Dr. Rolland states that somnoforme acts.

Somnoforme is the name given to the mixture composed of chloride of ethyl, sixty per cent.; chloride of methyl, thirty-five per cent.; and chloride of ethyl, five per cent.

As to the action of an anæsthetic on the nervous system very little is known, but Dr. Rolland states that somnoforme excites the great sympathetic, producing increased cardiac contraction and arterial tension, proved by sphygmographic tracings of his own radial artery during anæsthesia, but as to how this takes place he does not know, but hopes some day to be able to find the key.

Somnoforme is sprayed into a funnel-shaped mask (formed out of a handkerchief with a sheet of parchment paper placed between the folds [1]) which is placed over the respiratory passages, care being taken to allow of no admission of air or escape of vapor.

Signs of Anæsthesia.—The patient must be requested to keep the eyes open during administration. When anæsthesia is about complete the eyelids will fall or the eyeballs become fixed.

The patient may also be asked to hold up the left arm, which will in time either assume a fixed or cataleptic position or fall to the side relaxed.

The patient briefly and rapidly passes through the following stages: Subconsciousness, noticing things that are going on, hearing words, sensible to touch and pain; analgesic condition, insensible to pain; anæsthesia absolute. The stages are naturally varied by the idiosyncrasies of the patient.

Whilst reflexes may be present one can still operate. With a dose of five cubic centimetres of the drug, fifty seconds to five minutes anæsthesia can be produced.

The patients recover in slightly modified ways, which can soon be learnt, the complete recovery being usually preceded by several deep inspirations. To prolong the anæsthesia it is simply necessary to replace the mask with another dose from time to time on the patient showing signs of recovery.

Clinical Observations.—Dr. Bailey and myself have administered somnoforme to one hundred patients at the Dental Hospital, giving an average length for administration from one dose (five cubic centimetres) of thirty-eight seconds, and an average length of fifty-one and one-sixth seconds complete anæsthesia.

In my own cases the average length of administration was thirty-nine and one-half seconds, giving fifty-five and one-sixth seconds anæsthesia. Our best results are as follows: fifteen seconds giving fifty seconds anæsthesia; twenty seconds giving one minute; twenty-seven seconds giving one minute twenty seconds; thirty seconds giving one minute thirty seconds; fifty seconds giving one

---

[1] Dr. Field Robinson, of Bordeaux, has since brought out an ideal mask which insures more accurate and uniform results.

minute forty seconds; thirty-five seconds giving two minutes five seconds.

These statistics, like all others, may or may not be very reliable as a guide; roughly speaking, I should say twenty-five to thirty seconds for administration giving an average duration of anæsthesia from fifty to sixty seconds.

Most of the cases are recorded from hospital patients, and we all know what peculiar creatures they are; one never obtains the same satisfactory results with them. Apart from the fact that they discuss the gruesome details whilst collected together in the waiting-room, recipients worthy or otherwise of the benefits of a charity are never thoroughly responsive, having an ingrained conviction that they are always being experimented upon, consequently retaining very little confidence in the operation inducing extreme nervousness.

In private practice most of these adverse conditions are absent, the results therefore being much more satisfactory.

For the single dose (five cubic centimetres) administrations we selected only those cases were it was necessary to extract a few teeth; the average number of teeth and roots extracted being from four to five.

In one case only have we failed to extract a tooth, and he was a pensioned-off soldier from South Africa, of alcoholic habits, extremely strong and excitable, although even to him we had a week previously administered the drug with success.

In a great number of our single dose administrations, seven teeth were extracted, our greatest number being thirteen.

Our average would, undoubtedly, have been greater had we been more courageous in our primary cases, and had the faith in the anæsthetic which we ultimately acquired.

We had a very fair number of male patients, all giving equally as satisfactory results as the females. One patient only refused to take the anæsthetic after commencing the administration, and she ripped the mask off her face, her reason being that she thought we were giving her chloroform, and as she had been a waitress in a dentist's house, and in the habit of attending to patients during the administration of anæsthetics, she was consequently more nervous.

Difficulty was experienced in administering the drug to the highly nervous, and also the alcoholic patients, though certainly not so great as with other anæsthetics, owing probably to the greater rapidity of anæsthetization. There was a marked quietness shown by nearly all patients during anæsthesia, particularly when compared to that of nitrous oxide. In most cases there was no period of excitation, and in all cases a complete absence of jactitation and stertor, very little if any change of color taking place, and then only by obstruction to breathing, sometimes by the blood in the pharynx, or by depression of the lower jaw when extracting lower teeth.

The breathing after one or two nervous inspirations (and this can be checked by asking the patient to swallow) becomes quiet and regular, resembling the normal breathing during sleep. We have remarked a particularly advantageous condition of analgesia which allows of the operation being continued until within a second or so of complete recovery, no patient ever showing signs of that condition of hypersensitiveness so often observed just before recovery from nitrous oxide anæsthesia. None of the patients showed any signs of retching or vomiting. The tongue retained its natural size throughout, and never abnormally interfered with the extraction of lower roots or teeth, another distinct advantage over nitrous oxide.

The bleeding was much the same as would occur after an extraction under normal conditions without an anæsthetic.

Signs of Anæsthesia.—We have not found the drooping of the eyelid or the fixity of the eye to be so prevalent a sign as suggested by Dr. Rolland, or even when present so accurate as the rigid or cataleptic position of the upheld arm or its other condition of relaxation. One most prevalent sign has been the cataleptic condition (this I may say in no way interferes with the operator) ; it is also with patients in this condition that our best results have been obtained. The conjunctival reflex was not always lost in commencing, and in no case have we lost the corneal. The other reflexes we have not yet been able to ascertain through want of the necessary time and opportunity to test. The pulse in most cases at the commencement is rapid on account of the patient's either expressed or hidden nervousness. It, however, in a short time assumes a regular, full, strong beat, which persists during the whole period of anæsthesia. In several cases I was conscious of a slight lowering of the pulse after the first or second inspiration, due, I imagine, to the probable shock from the cold volatile vapor. The breathing also assumed a very regular type, so much so that Dr.

Bailey thought he could take it as a definite sign of complete anæsthesia.

The recovery of all the patients was very rapid, the patient recovering his or her normal condition at once, and being able within
a second or two to walk away without signs of giddiness and without help.

In one case only was there any sign of collapse, and she explained afterwards that she was subject to frequent fainting attacks.

With the exception of the last patient we have had only two
who complained of any after-effects, and then only for a few seconds. In one case the patient complained of earache, and the other
of headache. Against this, again, I had one patient in private practice who complained of violent headache before administration, and
who, on recovering from anæsthesia, was delighted to find that her
headache had disappeared as well as her teeth.

We have lately prolonged the anæsthesia by replacing the mask
(into which a second dose has been sprayed) on the patient showing signs of recovering, and in this way the patient has remained
anæsthetized during a period of three and one-half and three and
one-quarter minutes, allowing one minute thirty seconds and two
minutes for operating, and during which time all the roots and
teeth of the upper jaw were extracted.

In these prolonged cases the recovery is not quite so rapid as in
the single dose cases, being more in the nature of the recovery from
the major anæsthetics, though certainly more rapid.

One patient alone showed signs of collapse, probably due to the
great number of teeth extracted.

I feel certain that with more courage in prolonging the anæsthesia the whole of the mouth could be cleared of teeth and the patient thoroughly recovered in probably less than five minutes from
the commencement of administration, allowing the patient to leave
the operating-room in less than ten minutes. I need hardly point
out what a boon this would be.

Dr. Rolland has maintained complete anæsthesia for an operation lasting one hour, and has himself been anæsthetized over one
hundred times, and on one occasion was kept under its influence
for twenty-five minutes whilst observations were recorded.

The question most naturally occurring to all is whether somnoforme possesses dangers like chloroform, etc. In answer to this

Dr. Rolland states that if you deprive any patient of the essential amount of oxygen necessary to life any anæsthetic will produce death. If somnoforme is properly administered, death should not ensue, its great safety lying in the fact of its rapid elimination.

Another question is likely to be asked by many dentists,—Is it possible for a dentist to both administer somnoforme and operate himself, as many do with nitrous oxide?

Yes! I have done so for experiment, but only in one-dose cases. I do not think it advisable with this or any other anæsthetic. It is the work of the anæsthetist to look after the patient, and the operator to devote himself entirely to operating; the object should be to allow the patient to recover in as short a time as possible.

In conjunction with Professor Sherrington, University College, somnoforme was administered to several animals, giving much the same results as observed in the human subject. The analgesic condition was extremely well marked and tested. A marked progressive effect was noticed in some of the animals.

It was proved by an experiment that death would supervene if the mask was held on the face too long, whether from intoxication of the drug or asphyxia we are unable to prove. Respiration was arrested first, the heart continuing to beat for many seconds afterwards.

After almost five minutes from the time the respirations of a cat ceased (heart still beating), it was brought round to perfect health by artificial respiration.

As compared with other anæsthetics, the most remarkable feature was undoubtedly the rapid anæsthetization and the subsequent rapid recovery.—*The Dental Record.*

Reports of Society Meetings.

ACADEMY OF STOMATOLOGY.

A REGULAR meeting of the Academy of Stomatology of Philadelphia was held at the rooms of the Academy, 1731 Chestnut Street, on the evening of Tuesday, November 24, 1903, the President, Dr. L. Foster Jack, in the chair.

12

A paper was read by Dr. R. M. Sanger, of East Orange, N. J., entitled "The Diatoric Tooth in Bridge-Work."

(For Dr. Sanger's paper, see page 233.)

(For Dr. Sanger's paper, see page 233.)

DISCUSSION.

Dr. H. Roberts.—I have been very much interested in the doctor's method, which seems to cover ground very improperly covered heretofore. One of the greatest objections I have had to bridge-work is that the occlusal surface had to be of gold; otherwise, one is liable to have a broken surface very difficult to repair. I am heartily in sympathy with the essayist in regard to devitalizing an anterior tooth instead of putting a jacket on it, which I think is almost as bad as a full gold crown,—as the cement will wash out underneath. The method of covering the palatine surface in conjunction with a pin in the root furnishes a good support for an anterior bridge. Adjusting the caps by means of wax is very simple, and you can get a better adjustment in that way than by a cast. There are some few cases where I think a gold crown on a front tooth the only thing to be used with safety, although, as a rule, I condemn its use in this position.

Dr. P. B. McCullough.—I would like to ask Dr. Sanger how, in uniting the tooth with the gold, he prevents the sulphur taking fire.

Dr. Sanger.—The sulphur is on the inside of the cap and the flame on the other side, so that the flame does not touch the sulphur. Of course, one must be careful not to overheat it.

Dr. C. R. Jefferis.—In replacing the porcelain, would the doctor use oxyphosphate?

Dr. Sanger.—I would repair with oxyphosphate. There is no difficulty in holding these teeth with it, as the amount of exposed surface is very small. The action of the saliva on the oxyphosphate would be slight.

Dr. A. W. Jarmon.—I am in accord with the system and the cornmeal method of swaging. The ordinary facing with the pins bent can be held in position on an ordinary bridge with oxyphosphate. This is better than simply to have the pin bent.

Dr. E. C. Kirk.—I had opportunity in 1901 to see a great deal of this diatoric work in the office of Dr. John Girdwood, of Edinburgh, who wrote a paper on it which he presented to the Columbian College in 1893. Since the advent of modern crown- and bridge-work he has been developing this particular crown to that class of work. I examined a great many cases in his office in which the diatoric tooth was used, and I can testify to the utility of the work. A number had been in use from six to ten years, and were doing good service. All the advantages that Dr. Sanger has claimed for this class of operation were fully exemplified by the cases I saw.

The question has been raised as to the value of the sulphur cement. Much depends upon the accuracy with which the sulphur is used, and all the joining should be carefully done. Close adaptation requires but a small amount of sulphur to bring about union. The method is a very old one. The point which Dr. Sanger brought out, which seems to be an improvement upon the method advocated by Dr. Girdwood, is his swaging the base of the plate. Dr. Girdwood has done that by grinding, which takes more time and is not so accurate. I am very glad to see the diatoric tooth taking root, as it were, in America, because it is a very valuable tooth and adjustable to a great many conditions, and the results obtained are artistic.

Dr. H. C. Register.—I am pleased with Dr. Sanger's method of using the diatoric tooth. It is an advance in the right direction, —anticipating a possible breakage and restoration of a crown without disturbing the base support.

The principle Dr. Sanger has given us is about the same as that I have used in my practice. I commenced bridge-work, I suppose, nearly twenty years ago, and one of the first objects sought was to make it of such a character that in case of accident a crown could be easily replaced. I am still experimenting. The teeth I have handed to Dr. Sanger shows the *evolution* of my experimentation, ultimately discontinuing the use of a pin tooth for one pinless, using instead of pins a grooved staple formed around the approximal and gingival surface, thus forming a cup or cups by the staple and backing; these united at their approximo-occlusal portion, leaving the necks or base spaced, so that the tongue movements can sluice that portion, form the base. The articulated teeth are taken out and the metal portion finished to a perfect contour. I believe this crown is *universal in its* adaptation for every kind and position of prosthetic work,— bridge-, crown-, or plate,—which is easily replaced in case of accident without in any way moving the fixture. If a break happens after the piece has been set, the remaining portion of porcelain is taken out and a new crown slipped into the cup and cemented to place. Teeth of this character have been used with but rare breakage for eighteen years. The field is open to a more natural form and artistic arrangement of bridge- and crown-work, in which, in case of accident, the crowns can be replaced with little or no trouble. Either of these crowns meet the condition. I called the attention of the profession to this crown in its crude development many years ago. I spoke then of having a small saddle and of restricting the saddle to the tooth itself. While this is a helpful support, it also gives conciousness of the tactile faculty. I have found it clean, and it reproduces the contour line. The enunciation is better and the whole mouth restoration complete. The principal involved in these two kinds of tooth-crowns is much the same, with the favor of strength, I think, being on the side of a tooth being dove-tailed into its base.

Its use will be limited to the real artist; the " dental jeweller" wants something easier.

Dr. J. H. Gaskill.—Since the primary object seems to be to prevent the appearance of gold, I would like to ask Dr. Sanger why he has gold at the neck of the tooth?

Dr. Sanger.—I feared that in the downward pressure the pin might not sustain the weight; but I believe the lower part of that cap is not necessary. In practice the teeth are set so well up on the gum that the gold is not in evidence. I have not as yet found a bridge where it was a serious objection. (Replying to a member.) I have not been troubled with discoloration. I find that the life of the tooth is longer than if covered with a cap of any kind which would subsequently induce decay. My experience with open-faced crowns has been disastrous. Leakage occurs without loosening, and by the time the patient finds it out, the entire palatine surface of that tooth is decayed and you lose the entire crown. That is more liable than when a pin is made and when a minimum amount of gold is used. .I think the Carmichael and the Marshall systems would come under the head of open-faced crowns; yet the systems are so recent I would hesitate about putting myself on record as condemning either of them before another trial. They are as yet practically new.

Dr. Register.—This tooth that I have shows there is no necessity of running the gold on the labial side.

Dr. James Truman.—I have not much to say about crowning

or diatoric teeth; but, I want to add my observation of the fact that we seem to be approaching a period of more artistic dentistry than I have seen in the past. Therefore it is with peculiar gratification that I listened to Dr. Sanger speak of his application of diatoric teeth, and especially of his mode of attaching them by means of sulphur. I used it many years ago in fastening the old tube-teeth upon plates, and I have never yet found any teeth which you could possibly separate without melting the sulphur. It is better than oxyphosphate.

In my reading of the dental work advocated throughout the country I find that there is a tendency to the belief that pulps can be destroyed indiscriminately without any harm to the teeth. I think it is time that a warning should be sent out that this is an error. The statement has been made by some high in authority that the tooth is just as good after the pulp has been destroyed, that it is simply a formative organ, and therefore the sooner gotten rid of the better. If there ever was a wrong idea promulgated, it seems to me that is one. You cannot destroy the pulp without destroying a large portion of the vitality of the tooth and rendering it more liable to the influences which must subsequently act. I do not want to discuss the subject, but I think this discussion should not go out without some protest against the destruction of pulps as practised by the great majority of dentists. I do not speak of Dr. Sanger's custom. He is probably justified in his practice, but there are many who destroy pulps where it is not necessary.

Dr. Sanger (closing).—I seem to have occupied the floor about four-fifths of the time already, though I want to thank you for the reception you have given the paper. I want to thank Dr. Truman for disabusing your minds of the idea that might have been engendered that I believe in the indiscriminate destruction of pulps. I do not think that at any time I said that, and certainly I do not practise it. I only said that when it was indicated as a desirable course, then I would pursue the method described as pressure anæsthesia. Certainly no one recognizes more than I do the intrinsic value of the pulp. I believe most heartily that any living body is better than one that is half dead.

After some discussion on Incidents of Practice, the meeting adjourned.

OTTO E. INGLIS,
Editor Academy of Stomatology.

Editorial.

THE GOLDEN ANNIVERSARY BANQUET.

This banquet, in honor of the surviving members of the Class of 1854, took place at the Hotel Bellevue, Philadelphia, February 27, 1904, and has now passed into history, as all things earthly must do, but it is thought that those who participated in it will not, as yet, consign it to oblivion, but will continue to remember it as one of the most interesting experiences of their lives. This seems to have been the general consensus of opinion of those present.

It is reasonable to ask why such should have been the feeling over a banquet, good as that proved itself to be. It was not the menu, for the average man may be fond of eating and drinking, but these pall and are not uncommon experiences. It was not the men who represented the early training in dentistry, for these, worthy as they may have been, simply recalled one period in educational development. It was not the men who were present from many parts of the country, brilliant as they made this occasion; but the real sentiment that animated that gathering and gave it its joyous character was deeper and more impressive than any or all of these, for, it seemed to the writer, that each one present felt that, in celebrating the passage of fifty years, there was a feeling that the most trying period in dentistry had been surmounted and that the dental profession had come out of it all triumphant.

Fifty years ago dentistry, in the estimation of the world, was only one remove from charlatanry. It was making brave efforts to hold a proper place in professional circles. It attempted local and national organizations, but with only moderate success. Its educational institutions were few in number and young in experience. The teaching was excellent and laid the foundation for a broader culture. Everything in dentistry fifty years ago was in the formative period, and no man then had prescience sufficient to even anticipate the progress of the future. It was that future realized, more than the men who represented it, that made this occasion something to be remembered and one in which the experiences of the past and the hopes of the future were all concentrated. The men came from various sections, not only to act as hosts to the five honored, but, so to speak, to break the bread that represented the promised land which, if not yet quite reached, was in sight, and the years of trial, anxiety, and continuous effort were all comprehended to their fullest extent. The pioneer days were practically ended, the ground had been cleared and the fields prepared for the harvest of the future; nor was it difficult to read the results to be secured, through this past, in that future. The prophetic thought is based on that fifty years of intelligent practice; fifty years of educational effort; fifty years of concentrated thought. The fruitage in the next fifty years must progressively bear an intimate relation to the soil from which it sprang.

The banquet was pre-eminently a family gathering. Men from New England shook hands with men of the South, men of the East gloried in the growth of the West, and the home group felt they were honored by the presence of men, of many sections, who represented the highest in dentistry.

Thus the present met the past, and the glories of the latter paled in the brilliant successes of the former. Speeches were made, for a banquet can have no prestige without this formality, but this, through the delightful and tactful management of Professor Darby, was carried through most successfully. It was throughout an ovation, not wholly to men, but to the profession.

When we contemplate the progress of the past fifty years, not alone in our special line of work, but in all that has marked an advance in science and art in the world at large, the mind is lost in the confusion of new and startling discoveries. Things to-day important, and yet so common that they are regarded by the present generation as though they had always been, were then not only unknown, but were not even a desideratum in the world's life. Civilization has lived in that half-century as it has lived in no former period, and it is, therefore, not surprising that dentistry received its largest growth through an influence that pervaded the entire mentality of the period.

When the young men have passed through a similar half-century of work and in a similar celebration, the question may appropriately be asked, What progress has been made since 1904? It is to be hoped that the answer will be returned that, in comparison, the dentistry of 1904 bears no relation to that of 1954 in its ability to meet all the requirements of a scientific profession. We are very prone to think much further progress in dentistry is impossible, but so thought we all when the spring of 1854 saw the graduating class of the Philadelphia College of Dental Surgery launched upon a sea of professional troubles.

The dentists of Philadelphia have reason to thank those of the country at large for their interest and co-operation in making this not simply a banquet, but a mark in the passage of time from which to date other steps in the advancing years. Without this aid the banquet would have lost its best and most inspiring feature.

The men especially honored upon this memorable occasion, were the surviving members of the Class of 1854. As far as known, but five remain:

Louis Jack, D.D.S.	W. Storer How, D.D.S.
C. Newlin Peirce, D.D.S.	Eri W. Haines, D.D.S.
James Truman, D.D.S., LL.D.	

The committee in charge deserve special mention, for through their earnest and energetic efforts the success of the banquet is mainly due.

Edwin T. Darby, M.D., D.D.S.	G. L. S. Jameson, D.D.S.
Edward C. Kirk, D.D.S., Sc.D.	J. D. Thomas, D.D.S.
R. Hamill D. Swing, D.D.S.	Wilbur F. Litch, M.D., D.D.S.
Albert N. Gaylord, D.D.S.	H. C. Register, M.D., D.D.S.
Earl C. Rice, D.D.S.	William H. Trueman, D.D.S.
I. N. Broomell, D.D.S.	Robert Huey, D.D.S.
J. T. Lippincott, D.D.S.	William L. J. Griffin, D.D.S.
L. Foster Jack, M.D., D.D.S.	J. Clarence Salvas, D.D.S.
D. N. McQuillen, D.D.S.	

The class that graduated in 1854 from the Philadelphia College of Dental Surgery was as follows:

William Calvert, Pennsylvania.
Horton Bailey, Pennsylvania.
Firman Coar, Pennsylvania.
Alexander G. Coffin, Massachusetts.
E. H. Cogburn, Mississippi.
Benjamin Cohen, Germany.
Samuel W. Frazer, Pennsylvania.
William Gorges, Pennsylvania.
Eri W. Haines, Delaware.

W. Storer How, Maine.
Louis Jack, Pennsylvania.
Bernard T. Laughlin, Pennsylvania.
C. Newlin Peirce, Pennsylvania.
Isaiah Price, Pennsylvania.
David Roberts, Pennsylvania.
John M. Rothrock, North Carolina.
John R. Rubencame, Pennsylvania.
Thomas H. Shaw, Alabama.
James Truman, Pennsylvania.

The Toasts of the evening were upon the following:

"Welcome," Dr. Wilbur F. Litch.
"Class of '54," Dr. James Truman.
"Our College Days," Dr. Louis Jack, Dr. C. N. Peirce, Dr. W. Storer How, Dr. Eri W. Haines.
"The Mother of Colleges," Dr. B. Holly Smith.
"The Veterans of New England," Dr. L. D. Shepard.
"The Pioneers of Dentistry in New York," Dr. S. G. Perry.
"The Ohio College of Dental Surgery," Dr. H. A. Smith.

Those present at the banquet were the following:

Robin H. Adair, Ga.
Geo. Emery Adams, N. J.
Fred'k Amend, Jr., Pa.
W. Y. B. Ames, Ill.
E. H. Angle, Mo.
Frank L. Bassett, Pa.
E. A. Bogue, N. Y.
Chas. F. Bonsall, Pa.
W. A. Borden, Pa.
C. M. Bordner, Pa.
Albert P. Brubaker, Pa.
S. P. Cameron, Pa.
William Carr, N. Y.
J. N. Crouse, Ill.
M. H. Cryer, Pa.
M. B. Culver, Pa.
E. T. Darby, Pa.
Geo. D. B. Darby, Pa.

L. W. Darlington, Pa.
John F. Dowsley, Mass.
J. E. Dunwoody, Pa.
J. Endelman, F., Pa.
J. N. Farrar, N. Y.
L. Ashley Faught, Pa.
Frank D. Gardiner, Pa.
A. N. Gaylord, Pa.
E. S. Gaylord, Conn.
Cyrus M. Gingrich. Md.
Clarence J. Grieves, Md.
S. H. Guilford, Pa.
Joseph, Head, Pa.
D. M. Hitch, Pa.
R. H. Hofheinz, N. Y.
F. Holland, Ga.
Robert Huey, Pa.
George E. Hunt, Ind.

Charles S. Jack, Pa.
L. Foster Jack, Pa.
V. H. Jackson, N. Y.
G. L. S. Jameson, Pa.
C. R. Jefferis, Del.
G. F. Jernigan, N. Y.
Victor S. Jones, Pa.
E. I. Keffer, Pa.
E. C. Kirk, Pa.
Edward P. Kramer, Pa.
C. V. Kratzer, Pa.
Louis C. LeRoy, N. Y.
J. A. Libbey, Pa.
J. Edw. Line, N. Y.
E. G. Link, N. Y.
J. T. Lippincott, Pa.
Wilbur F. Litch, Pa.
J. Bond Littig, N. Y.
H. B. McFadden, Pa.
Charles McManus, Conn.
James McManus, Conn.
D. N. McQuillen, Pa.
Louis Meisburger, N. Y.
Geo. G. Milliken, Pa.
Walter H. Neall, Pa.
J. J. Nelson, Pa.
Joseph W. Noble, China.
R. H. Nones, Pa.
A. W. Orr, Pa.
Fred. A. Peeso, Pa.
S.·G. Perry, N. Y.
Chas. E. Pike, Pa.
Chas. M. Porter, Pa.

William J. Potter, Pa.
H. C. Register, Pa.
Ralph B. Reitz, N. Y.
Hugo Rettich, N. Y.
M. L. Rhein, N. Y.
Howard E. Roberts, Pa.
J. Clarence Salvas, Pa.
M. I. Schamburg, Pa.
J. H. Schlinkmann, Md.
Howard S. Seip, Pa.
L. D. Shepard, Mass.
N. T. Shields, N. Y.
B. Holly Smith, Md.
Eugene H. Smith, Mass.
G. Marshall Smith, Md.
H. A. Smith, Ohio.
Thos. C. Stellwagen, Pa.
C. S. Stockton, N. J.
Clinton W. Strang, Conn.
R. H. D. Swing, Pa.
W. H. Taylor, Pa.
Ambler Tees, Pa.
John D. Thomas, Pa.
Burton Lee Thorpe, Mo.
William H. Trueman, Pa.
Chas. R. Turner, Pa.
F. T. Van Woert, N. Y.
Geo. W. Warren, Pa.
S. C. G. Watkins, N. J.
William C. Wilson, Pa.
James M. Winner, Del.
J. A. Woodward, Pa.
H. Newton Young, Pa.

The Faculty of the Philadelphia College of Dental Surgery was composed of the following:

Elisha Townsend, M.D., D.D.S., Professor of Operative Dentistry and Dean.

J. D. White, M.D., D.D.S., Professor of Anatomy and Physiology.

Ely Parry, M.D., D.D.S., Professor of Chemistry, Materia Medica, and Special Therapeutics.

Robert Arthur, D.D.S., Professor of the Principles of Dental Surgery.

T. L. Buckingham, M.D., Professor of Mechanical Dentistry.

D. B. Whipple, M.D., Demonstrator of Surgical and Mechanical Dentistry.

This College completed only four sessions, during which time there were sixty-three regular graduates. Among these should be named Dr. James E. Garretson and Dr. J. Foster Flagg. The faculty of the College withdrew, owing to a disagreement with the Board of Trustees, the latter conferring honorary degrees in opposition to the wishes of the faculty. The latter, on withdrawing, organized the Pennsylvania College of Dental Surgery, and the Philadelphia College of Dental Surgery ceased to exist.

Thus closes the history of this banquet and, in part, the history of the Philadelphia College of Dental Surgery. We may give utterance to a sigh of mournful regret that our companions of 1854 are not with us to mark the developments of time and experience, but such is ever the struggle,—the great battle of life. Civilization is based on continued change, life to death, death to life. The departure of the old, the incoming of new vitality. Let us be thankful that a few remain to glory with their fellows in the progress of their loved profession.

Bibliography.

A COMPEND OF DENTAL PATHOLOGY AND DENTAL MEDICINE. Containing the most noteworthy points upon the subjects of interest to dental students. By Geo. W. Warren, A.M., D.D.S., Professor of Principles and Practice of Operative Dentistry, Pennsylvania College of Dental Surgery, Philadelphia. Fourth edition. Illustrated. P. Blakiston's Son & Co., Philadelphia.

When a compend has reached a fourth edition, it demonstrates conclusively that it has met a need existing in undergraduate study. There have been many improvements in this small volume since it was reviewed in an earlier edition in this journal, and, for brief statements, the chapter on Development of the Teeth, and the following sub-chapters, on the Structure and Anatomy of the Teeth, are well condensed, principally from Broomell and Peirce.

It seems to the writer that it is impossible to consider, in the space usually given to subjects in compends, the important topics connected with dental pathology and therapeutics, hence criticism must be left for more elaborate productions. This, however, must be said of it, that the author has been measurably successful in managing his pathology so far as he has gone. In his efforts to condense he has omitted much that should have been noticed, and has not detailed treatment sufficiently to make it valuable to the average student. Forty-five small pages is the limit of Dental Pathology. This is followed by " Dental Medicine," to which seventy-three pages are devoted. An Appendix on " Emergencies" close the book. For a pocket reference the book has a special value to students, but if it is desired to know the subjects thoroughly, more extensive works must be consulted.

ORGANIC AND PHYSIOLOGIC CHEMISTRY. A Manual for Students and Practitioners. By Alexius McGlannan, M.D., Associate Professor of Physiologic Chemistry, Instructor in Clinical Laboratory, College of Physicians and Surgeons, Baltimore, Md. Series edited by V. C. Pedersen, A.M., M.D. Illustrated. Lea Brothers & Co., Philadelphia and New York.

The author says of his work in this manual, that " The purpose . . . is to select from the immense mass of knowledge accumulated in its department such facts as are of essential importance to medical students and practitioners, and to present them in a style facilitating comprehension and recollection."

To give a general idea of this manual and its comprehensive treatment of subjects, the contents, under general heads, in Part I., Organic Chemistry, is given. Chapter 1. General Principles. 2. The Constitution, Decomposition, and Classification of Organic Compounds. 3. The Hydrocarbons. 4. The Alcohols. 5. The Aldehydes. 6. The Organic Acids. 7. The Polybasic and Hydroxy Acids. 8. The Ethers, Esters, Fats, Oils. 9. Nitrogen in Organic Compounds. 10. The Carbohydrates. 11. The Benzene or Aromatic Series. 12. Benzene Derivatives containing Nitrogen. 13. The Proteins. 14. The Methods for Quantitative Analysis.

This is followed by Physiologic Chemistry in seven chapters, followed by an Appendix on Physical and Chemical data, Weights and Measures, Metric and Apothecaries' System Equivalents, etc. Similar to the others of the Pedersen Series, this manual is quite superior to books that ordinarily are published under that name, and are proportionably valuable to the student as a pocket reference.

Domestic Correspondence.

REPLY FROM "TRINITY UNIVERSITY," TORONTO.

To the Editor:

Sir,—I am happy to be able to assure you that the fears expressed in your editorial entitled " Novel Method in conferring Degrees," which appeared in the February issue of the International Dental Journal, have no foundation whatever in the true facts of the case. As it seems evident from your article that you have been misinformed in several important points, I hope you will allow me to lay the facts before you.

A careful study of the curriculum prescribed by Trinity University, Toronto, for the degree of Doctor of Dental Surgery, and the regulations in connection with the same, all of which I enclose herewith, will, I feel sure, lead you to recognize that the knowledge required to obtain a D.D.S. from this University is equal to that required by the most advanced dental institutions on this continent. Such, at least, was the intention of those who constructed the curriculum, and their purpose was as far removed as possible from the taint of commercialism. In further evidence of this I might mention that the University not only demands proof of thoroughly sound theoretical knowledge and practical ability, but also requires that a candidate, in order to hold a Trinity D.D.S., must pledge himself to observe the ethical side of his professional life. This is shown by the following declaration, which must be subscribed by all candidates before receiving the degree:

" All candidates who successfully pass the Final Examination for the Degree of D.D.S. will be required to subscribe to the following declaration before receiving their Diploma:

" I, ..., do solemnly promise that so long as I hold the Diploma of the University of Trinity College, or remain on the rolls as a Graduate in Dentistry, I will not resort to any advertising of a kind that may be adjudged by the said University to be unprofessional, nor will I be guilty of any other practices deemed by them unbecoming to my profession or calculated to bring discredit upon the University.

" And I hereby agree that if, in the opinion of the said University, I shall at any time be shown to have violated this undertaking in any way, I will, if the said University shall so decree, surrender my Diploma and Degree and all rights whatsoever that I may be in the enjoyment of as a graduate of the said University, and will consent to my name being struck off the rolls."

As to the special regulation which apparently led to the writing of the editorial, I am convinced that all that is needed to entirely do away with the objection urged against it is that the facts should be clearly and fully understood. The regulation reads as follows:

" All legally qualified practitioners of Dental Surgery of Great Britain or of any portion of the British Empire will be admitted to the Final Examination without passing further matriculation, and without further attendance on lectures."

Now it must be allowed that this special privilege, whether or not it be deemed a wise one, does not make the degree easy to obtain, nor does it call for a low standard of knowledge on the part of the candidate. The qualification of which the candidate must furnish proof in order to be admitted to the Final Examination, is that he has been licensed by the government of his own country for the practice of dental surgery, and that that country be a part of the British Empire. As a matter of fact all parts of the empire, with only one or two minor exceptions, require regular apprenticeship and a college course in order that a candidate may obtain his license to practise. If in the vast extent of the British Empire there are one or two exceptions to this rule, still it must be admitted, even then, that a candidate from such a district will need to devote himself to a very thorough course of private study, or else spend some considerable time in a dental college in attendance on lectures, before being able to pass the examination prescribed by Trinity University. Indeed, so strict has this examination always been, and so high is the estimation in which it is held among the profession, that only one candidate (and be came from Great Britain itself) has as yet ventured to present himself for examination without previous attendance at college lectures.

The editorial says, " One of the singular conditions demanded in conferring this degree is to be found in the fact that the recipient is not to make use of it in the Dominion of Canada, but it is available only in the other portions of the colonial possessions of Great Britain." How this idea could have arisen I am at a loss to understand. It is an entirely mistaken one, and I know of no ground whatever which could properly have given rise to such a report. As a matter of fact, the University confers, as one would naturally expect, more degrees upon residents of our own Dominion than upon those who come here from other parts of the empire and from abroad, and the degree is freely used and held in high esteem in Toronto itself, throughout the Province of Ontario, and in other parts of the Dominion.

If I am not trespassing too much upon your space, I might refer briefly to one or two other points of lesser importance. Your editorial seems to have confused the universities, which have the power to grant D.D.S. degrees, with the Royal College of Dental Surgeons, which is the body authorized to confer the L.D.S. There is, however, no necessary connection between this college and the several universities, and, as a matter of fact, none whatever between it and Trinity University, although it is in this college that nearly all candidates for university examinations in dentistry in Canada receive their teaching. The College maintains a high standard of work, and in order to obtain the L.D.S., which it alone is authorized to confer in this Province, the candidates not only must have attended four full winter sessions at the College, but also must have been articled to a dentist for three and a half years. It will be seen, therefore, that there is a double misapprehension underlying the implied statement of your editorial that the schools of the Dominion of Canada offer an easy pathway to the D.D.S. degree. For, in the first place, such schools or colleges have no power to confer academic degrees, and in the second place the license which they do confer is hedged about by a thorough and prolonged course of training and by examinations of a high standard.

It may perhaps be well that I should take this opportunity of stating that inasmuch as Trinity University has recently entered into a Federation Agreement with the University of Toronto, the curriculum of the former institution, which I am sending to you herewith, will give place, on and after the first day of October next, to that of the University of Toronto. Consequently, the regulation as to exemptions allowed to regularly qualified practitioners of dental surgery within the British Empire will then cease to be operative, except for candidates previously enrolled, there being no similar provision in the regulations of the University of Toronto. Therefore, even if there were anything to object to in such a provision, it would quickly cease to be a matter of practical concern, by reason of the Federation to which I have referred.

Robert J. Reade, M.A., D.D.S.,
Secretary Board of Dental Studies, Trinity University.

CORRECTION OF STENOGRAPHER'S REPORTS.

To the Editor:

Sir,—I have just seen in the International Dental Journal the discussion on Dr. Heise's paper, " Empyema of the Antrum," read at the meeting of the American Medical Association, and am humiliated with the report of my part of the discussion. Parts of the report are so bad as to be uninteligible. In some instances words, parts of sentences, and whole sentences are omitted; which spoils the sense; in others the stenographer's report, which was very bad, has been edited so as to make me say things I did not say. A few of the errors I note.

Line 5, page 212, should read pus sack *on* the end of root, not pus sack *in* the root.

Line 9, page 212, should read to which the *antrum* is subject, not to which the *anatomy* is subject.

Line 33, page 212, I am made to say that I have *seldom* seen syphilis of the antrum. What I said was that I had *never* seen syphilis of the antrum.

Lines 12, 13, 14, page 213, as they stand are without meaning.

Lines 20, 21, page 213, I am made to say, if an opening is required, I would not make it from the *antrum,* but from the *nose.* What I said was, if only drainage was needed I would make the opening from the *nose,* but if curettement was necessary I should make an opening from the *buccal wall* of the cavity.

Line 23, 24, page 213, should read at the *duplication* of the mucous membrane and the gum, not just *above* the membrane of the gum.

Lines 27, 28, page 213, Another reason for opening here is that the *cheek falls* in, should read, because if the opening is made through the buccal wall the cheek *falls over the opening* and in a large measure prevents food from getting into the cavity, etc., etc.

In justice to myself and Dr. Heise, I request that this communication appear in the April number of the JOURNAL, and that with it you publish my part of the discussion as it apppeared in the January number of the *Journal of the American Medical Association,* page 25, a copy of which is enclosed. I regret that a copy of the stenographers report from which your report was made had not been, as was that of the *Journal of the American Medical Association,* sent me for correction. In this correcting I made no changes except to correct the stenographers errors and condense the matter in a few instances.

By kindly complying with the above request you will greatly oblige,

THOS. L. GILMER.

[Our Correspondent is in error in supposing changes were made by the editor of this journal in the discussion referred to in the foregoing communication. The report was received at this office from the official stenographer of the Section on Stomatology, American Medical Association, and supposed to be practically correct, the editor having no means of determining this question except through the very uncertain method of sending proofs of the discussion to e ·h one taking part. This the INTERNATIONAL cannot undertak , unless it is specially requested.

A fair exa tion of the errors noted, while annoying, are not so far ou i the way but that any intelligent reader could make the corrections. Our correspondent does not allow for this. Every speaker is subject to these minor errors in reports.

The stenographer receives the blame when it more often is the fault of the speaker. Some get accustomed to these errors, others do not.—ED.]

CORRECTION OF ARTICLE IN MARCH NUMBER.

I desire to enter a protest against what will be, to many, misleading regarding Dr. Riggs's methods and treatment. On page 197, March issue of this journal, the writer states: " Dr. Riggs's surgical method was to scrape the surface of the root of the affected tooth to remove all salivary calculi, and also removing any necrosed bone."

Thus far the writer has stated the exact truth regarding Dr. Riggs's operation. Had he stopped here—but he adds: " then continuing with the cauterizing. Even extreme methods, as replantation, were resorted to where there was elongation of the incisor teeth."

This last part is entirely contrary to Dr. Riggs's practice or teachings. Dr. Riggs condemned cauterizing or excision of the festoons severely, as well as replantation. Dr. Riggs did not believe in therapeutics of any kind in connection with his treatment, depending wholly on the thoroughness of his operation; but occasionally, when patients felt they must have some wash, he would tell them, in apparent disgust, " Use a little tincture of myrrh, then."

L. C. TAYLOR.

Obituary.

DR. OTIS AVERY.[1]

DIED, Monday, February 22, 1904, Dr. Otis Avery.

Dr. Avery was born in Bridgewater, Oneida County, N. Y., August 19, 1808. At the time of his death he had nearly completed his ninety-sixth year, and continued to practice his profession until his ninety-fourth year. At that time he was regarded as the oldest living dental practitioner in the United States, and this was undoubtedly true, certainly as far as practice was concerned.

Dr. Avery was one of the remarkable men of the last century. He was a many-sided man, and this versatility, in some degree, prevented his obtaining a deserved national reputation in the profession of his choice. A writer briefly sums up his life-work in the order of acquirement: " Silversmith, watchmaker, dental surgeon, inventor, statesman, philosopher, judge, and one of the most remarkable men of genius of the century."

" The paternal grandfather of the deceased was born at Groton, Conn., and served all through the Revolutionary War, after which conflict he engaged in teaching, and lived to be nearly a century old. The father of the subject of this sketch was also born at Groton, but removed to Oneida, where he was identified with its very earliest settlement. He was a silversmith and watchmaker, and taught his son the trade.

" At the age of fifteen our subject left home and worked for awhile as a journeyman at Waterville, N. Y., and three years afterwards removed to Cochecton, where he served as clerk in a store for his brother John and afterwards opened there a jewelry and repair shop. While at that place he became a captain of a military company. In 1827 he came to Bethany, where he established a shop, and from that place removed to New Berlin, N. Y., where he continued his vocation. While there he decided to become a dentist, and, going to New York City, passed two years with Dr. D. C.

---

[1] The INTERNATIONAL is indebted to Judge George S. Purdy, of Honesdale, for valuable papers connected with Dr. Avery's life.

Ambler, a prominent dentist, who on December 6, 1833, gave to Dr.
Avery probably the first certificate ever issued to a dentist in this
country, as at that time there were no dental schools or dental supply houses in America. During the next four years Dr. Avery prae-
tised his profession over a large area of country, one of his fields
being between Honesdale and Ithaca, N. Y. In 1839 he located at
Bethany, where for ten years he spent the summer, going to Columbia, S. C., every winter. Subsequently he opened an office in
New York City, but finally gave up the practice there and in 1850
settled permanently at Honesdale. His skill and prominence in the
profession were largely the result of his genius, self-education, and
constant research. Besides pursuing his profession he gave attention to invention, and the year he settled here patented a sewing-
machine, which he sold to a company and as its agent visited
Europe and sold the patent to parties in London and also to Emperor Louis Napoleon in behalf of the French government. In
1851 he received from Prince Albert, President of the Royal Commission having in charge an exhibition of the works of industry
of all nations, a medal for superior dentistry, and a similar medal
the following year from the agricultural society of the State of
New York."

In 1850 Dr. Avery removed to Honesdale, Pa. In 1855 he was
sent to the State Legislature, where he served one term. He was
appointed one of the associate judges of Wayne County in 1871,
and in 1877 was re-elected by an overwhelming vote; but at the
end of his second term he declined further service. It is probably
the first and only instance on record of a judge descending voluntarily from the bench to practice dentistry, or of a dentist being
elevated to that position.

An interesting fact in Dr. Avery's life was his riding on the
" Stourbridge Lion," the first locomotive seen in this country. This
was on August 8, 1829. " We," he writes, " were determined to see
what we could of the thing, and went up to where it stood. The
man in charge was just emptying the fire from under the boiler
and quenching it with water. We stepped upon the platform and I
asked him if he could not start it so that we might see how it worked.
He let on the steam and ran it about the middle of the river. I
told him that would do, and he reversed it and ran it onto the land."
It is difficult to realize the fact that one lifetime has witnessed the
development, from that single imported locomotive, to the great

railroad interests dominating this country. It vividly brings to mind the progress made in the nineteenth century.

In one of the last letters of Dr. Avery written to the editor of the INTERNATIONAL, August 18, 1903, he stated that he was interested in an editorial article entitled "Avoid the Road to the Poor-House," and further wrote: "Your valuable suggestions ought to be put in operation, for it is a conceded fact that ten or a dozen years in dental occupation unfit a man for any other business, and there should be some means provided to protect him from the sharpers, especially that abomination the 'pious fraud.'"

No one could fail to appreciate the high character of this man when brought in personal contact with him. He lived quietly and unostentatiously, yet, while largely isolated from the active work of his profession, he contributed much to maintain its dignified character and honorable position among the callings of men. A writer sums up the character of Judge Avery briefly, but very truthfully, as the present writer of this sketch knew him.

"He was always conspicuous for independent thought, positive convictions, unflinching courage, and spotless integrity; and those characteristics were abundantly displayed in the discharge of his official duties. He was not content to accept the current tradition relative to the position of a lay judge, and to pose as a mere judicial figure-head. On the contrary, his official career was marked by the active, intelligent, and conscientious discharge of its duties, and his influence was largely felt in the administration of justice."

At his death he was connected with the First Presbyterian Church at Honesdale.

He was twice married, first, April 19, 1829, to Louisa Hoel, of Bethany. She died in 1853. He subsequently married, in 1855, Mary Agnes Addoms, of New York, daughter of Richard Clark, a former merchant of that city.

The services were held at his home, Park Street, Honesdale, the final interment taking place at New Dorp, on Staten Island.

Current News.

NEW JERSEY STATE BOARD OF REGISTRATION AND EXAMINATION IN DENTISTRY.

THE New Jersey State Board of Registration and Examination in Dentistry will hold its next examination in the theoretical branches in the Assembly-room of the State-House at Trenton, N. J., on the 5th, 6th, and 7th of July, sessions beginning promptly at nine A.M.

The practical work done in Newark. All applications must be in the hands of the Secretary ten days prior to the examination.

For information regarding the examination, apply to the Secretary, 29 Fulton Street, Newark, N. J.

CHARLES A. MEEKER,
Secretary and Treasurer.

KENTUCKY STATE DENTAL ASSOCIATION.

THE coming annual meeting of the Kentucky State Dental Association promises a dental convention of unusual interest; to be held in Louisville May 17, 18, and 19, 1904.

Members of the profession are extended a hearty welcome.

W. M. RANDALL,
Secretary.

MASONIC BUILDING, LOUISVILLE, KY.

MONTANA STATE DENTAL SOCIETY.

THE first annual meeting of the Montana State Dental Society was held in Helena, Mont., February 22 and 23, 1904, and the following officers were elected for the coming year: President, Dr. W.

H. Barth, Great Falls; First Vice-President, Dr. J. D. Sutphen, Helena; Second Vice-President, Dr. Joseph Oettinger, Missoula; Secretary, Dr. George E. Longeway, Great Falls; Treasurer, Dr. W. M. Billings, Helena.

The second annual meeting will be held in Butte, Mont., February 20 and 21, 1905.

GEORGE E. LONGEWAY,
Secretary.

CENTRAL DENTAL ASSOCIATION OF NORTHERN NEW JERSEY.

AT the annual meeting of the Central Dental Association of Northern New Jersey, held at Newark, February 15, 1904, the folowing officers were elected:

President, C. S. Stockton, Newark; Vice-President, T. Starr Dunning, Paterson; Secretary, H. Parker Marshall, Newark; Treasurer, C. A. Meeker, Newark.

Executive Committee.—R. S. Sanger, East Orange, Chairman; W. Moore Gould, Newark, Secretary; N. M. Chitterling, Bloomfield; Frank L. Manning, Red Bank; Frederick W. Stevens, Newark.

FREDERICK W. STEVENS,
Secretary.

ILLINOIS STATE DENTAL SOCIETY.

THE fortieth annual meeting of the Illinois State Dental Society will be held at Peoria, Tuesday, Wednesday, and Thursday, May 10, 11, and 12, 1904. A splendid programme, including attractive and unusually interesting features, is under course of preparation. The usual fare of one and one-third—certificate plan—will be obtained on all roads in the State and from St. Louis. Remember the date. All reputable practitioners cordially invited.

HART J. GOSLEE,
Secretary.

FIRST DISTRICT DENTAL SOCIETY OF NEW YORK.

THE following officers have been elected for 1904:

President, Dr. Henry D. Hatch; Vice-President, Dr. Arthur L. Swift; Secretary, Dr. Benj. C. Nash; Treasurer, Dr. James W. Taylor; Librarian, Dr. F. L. Stanton.

Executive Committee.—Dr. Wm. C. Deane, Dr. F. L. Fossume, Dr. Wm. Carr, Chairman.

Clinic Committee.—Dr. W. D. Tracy, Dr. Ralph B. Reitz, Dr. S. L. Goldsmith, Chairman.

B. C. NASH,
Secretary.

THE

International Dental Journal.

| VOL. XXV. | MAY, 1904. | No. 5. |

Original Communications.[1]

IMPACTED TEETH: THEIR DIAGNOSIS, LIBERATION, AND EXTRACTION.[2]

BY M. H. CRYER, M.D., D.D.S.

THIS subject has been selected because of the wide diversity of opinion concerning the proper procedure in cases of impaction. The views which will be presented are based entirely on personal observations. While the conclusions to which these observations have led differ radically from those of many others in this field of work, the writer wishes to disclaim at the outset any intention or desire to criticise opposing views. He has no sympathy with the spirit which condemns without reservation methods based on experience, merely because they do not agree with one's own.

IMPACTED TEETH.

The term "impacted teeth" is generally used to designate a permanent tooth which has failed either wholly or partially to erupt. It is also sometimes employed to indicate the retarded eruption of a deciduous tooth.

---

[1] The editor and publishers are not responsible for the views of authors of papers published in this department, nor for any claim to novelty, or otherwise, that may be made by them. No papers will be received for this department that have appeared in any other journal published in the country.

[2] Read before the Academy of Stomatology, December 21, 1903.

Deciduous teeth, when impacted, are usually held in their developing capsule, which is covered by a dense fibrous gum tissue, the thickening being claimed by some observers to be due to the deposit of intercellular substance; by others to cell enlargement; by still others to the non-exfoliation of the older layers of the cells. Whatever may cause this tissue to become thickened and more dense is a problem which may be left to the pathologist.

In order to more clearly understand the anatomy and position of the teeth and their roots, a few illustrations will be introduced which the writer thinks may well be termed "Typical Anatomy."

Fig. 1 is a lateral view of a typical skull showing the teeth in relation with one another in an almost ideal position and occlusion.

FIG. 1.

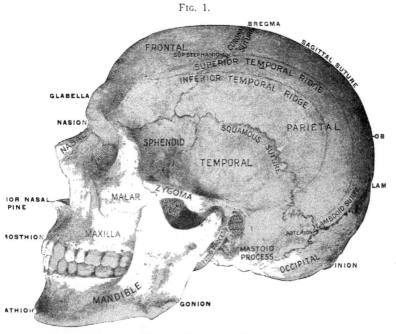

Side view of a typical skull.

It is evident that there has been but little interference with the nutrition of either jaw or the teeth of this subject from the beginning of their development to the death of the subject. A little study of this illustration shows why, except in rare cases, the lower second molar should not be extracted in order to remove an impacted lower third molar. If the lower third molar be extracted only, the upper third molar is left without an antagonizing tooth; but if the lower second and third molars are both removed, the upper second and third molars have no antagonizing teeth.

Fig. 2 shows a jaw from which the external plates of the alveolar process have been removed, together with part of the

FIG. 2.

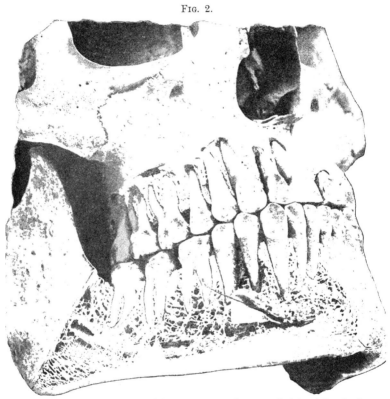

Antero-lateral view of upper and lower jaws, with the external plates of the alveolar process and some of the cancellated tissue removed.

cancellated tissue. The extraction of teeth from a jaw of this character would be comparatively easy, as the tissue is yielding and the tooth could be easily loosened and lifted out.

The writer so far has failed to find impacted teeth in jaws the cancellated tissue of which was in the typical condition shown in this illustration. One reason of this is that in jaws of this character, where there has been no interference with nutrition, the other teeth move forward to give proper room, as they are not held back by the cancellated tissue becoming dense and adherent to the cortical portion of the bone.

Fig. 3 is made from a section of the skull of a child about six years of age. The external plates of the alveolar process of the

FIG. 3.

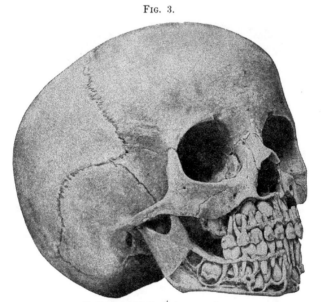

Skull of a child about six years of age.

upper and lower jaws have been removed, exposing the deciduous teeth with their roots and developing permanent teeth, except the lower third molar and the upper first, second, and third molars. Parents of children often ask why teeth come in irregularly. Looking at this picture, in which the teeth are in normal position for a child of this age, one might rather ask, How do they ever get into their normal position at adult age? From experience alone it is known that these teeth will assume their normal positions, provided there is no interference with normal nutrition and no undue pressure from adjacent tissue. On the other hand, the least variation from normality in these respects will cause disarrangement of the teeth, the irregularity ranging from a slightly deflected incisor to an inverted molar, as shown in Fig. 12.

ORDER OF IMPACTION.

The experience of the writer has been that the frequency of impacted teeth is as follows: First, the lower third molar; second, the upper canine; third, the upper third molar; fourth, the upper central incisor; fifth, the lower second premolar; sixth, the upper second premolar; seventh, the lower canine. The first and second groups of this classification will, without doubt, be accepted by all familiar with the subject under discussion. There are in the museum of the Dental Department of the University of Pennsylvania specimens as follows: Ten impacted lower third molars; nine impacted upper canines, two of which are in one jaw; two impacted upper third molars, both in the same jaw; two impacted central incisors; two impacted lower second premolars.

Examination of Fig. 3 makes apparent reasons for this order of impaction. It will be seen that the germ of the lower second molar is well back and partly within the ramus of the jaw. The germ of the lower third molar is still further upward and backward. As these teeth are developed and the jaw grows, the teeth and the cancellated tissue pass forward between the U-shaped cortical bone. If this sliding forward and downward of the tooth be interfered with by reason of inflammatory phenomena within the substance of the jaw, causing the cancellated and cortical portions to become adherent, the already erupted teeth will be prevented from yielding slightly to the eruptive force of the moving molar, and there will be no room for this tooth to slide into its proper position. The lower portion of the capsule is more liable to become retarded or fixed than the upper: consequently, in such a case the upper portion or crown of the tooth is carried forward and downward, causing it in many cases to take a horizontal position. In some instances it is turned directly upside down, as seen in Fig. 12.

If the position of the germ of the upper canine tooth be examined, it will be found at a higher level and deeper in the bone than the other teeth. The first premolar is erupted about three years before the canine, and often closes in towards the lateral, erupted five years previously, especially if the deciduous canine has been lost early. Under ordinary circumstances the canine will be forced into a fairly typical position, but if any inflammatory condition of the jaw has been manifested the bone may become firm and the canine more or less impacted. Similar conditions can be predicted of nearly all impacted teeth.

Occasionally supernumerary teeth may cause impaction. Fig. 4 shows a number of supernumerary teeth in the place which should

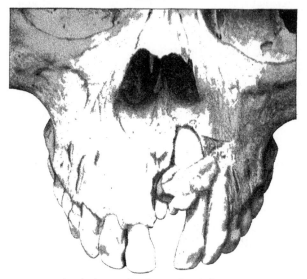

An odontoma and an impacted central incisor.

be occupied by a non-erupted left central. After the supernumerary teeth and a small portion of bone were removed, the true central tooth was located between the plates of bone forming the floor of the nose and the roof of the mouth.

Dr. Robert Huey, a member of this society, had a patient who had a similar impacted central incisor. Situated in front of it were some thirty-five small supernumerary teeth, which were removed, leaving the impacted tooth in its abnormal position, after which Dr. Huey succeeded in getting it into its proper place.

The case affords a good example of one of the methods by which the liberation of impacted teeth is accomplished. The writer has often found that where hard, dense bone prevented teeth from erupting into their proper position, upon the removal of this obstruction the teeth have passed into place, in some cases without mechanical aid, though usually this aid had to be extended.

THE REASON FOR THE LIBERATION OR EXTRACTION OF THE DE-
CIDUOUS OR PERMANENT TEETH.

When a deciduous tooth is held beneath strong fibrous layers of gum tissue its growing roots extend in the direction of the blood- and nerve-supply, and their sharp edges cause irritation of the parts and through reflex action bring about various troubles. In such cases the crowns of these teeth must be set free. There is but one surgical operation justifiable,—*i.e.,* to cut the gum tissue in such a manner—varying somewhat in detail according to the shape of each tooth—as to liberate them from their prison. A deciduous tooth should be extracted when it is preventing a permanent tooth from taking its proper place. The non-performance of these duties at the proper time has more or less influence upon the position of the permanent teeth in adult life.

Permanent impacted teeth should, as a rule, be either liberated or extracted. When the impacted tooth can be brought into useful position through the extraction of supernumerary teeth, as in the case of Dr. Huey's patient, or by the removal of other causes impeding its eruption, the necessary steps for its liberation should be undertaken, whether the tooth be an incisor, canine, premolar, or molar. If left impacted, these teeth are liable to prevent the proper nourishment of other teeth, as shown in Figs. 9 and 15. They are also liable to interfere with healthy nutrition of the surrounding tissue as well. They may press upon the branches of the fifth pair of nerves, producing neuralgia, not only in the local region but in remote parts, and through reflex action they may cause various disturbances in and about the head and face. They are liable to bring about inflammatory conditions of this region, produce cellulitis in the tissues of the mouth, neck, throat, and the temporo-mandibular articulation, interfere with deglutition, etc. Then, again, parts of the roots may penetrate into the maxillary sinus or into the nasal chambers, as shown in Figs. 10 and 12, under which conditions, if they become devitalized, they are liable to infect these cavities.

INSTRUMENTS USED IN DIAGNOSIS AND EXTRACTING.

Fig. 5 gives an idea of some of the instruments used by the writer in diagnosing, liberating, and extracting impacted teeth. A shows the general shape of the excavator used as an exploring

Fig. 5.

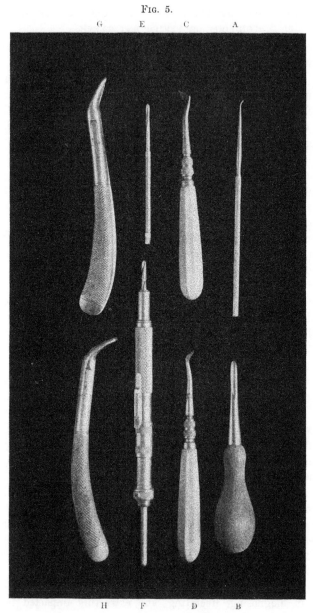

Instruments used in diagnosing and extracting impacted teeth

instrument. Small portions of bone may even be cut away with it until the crown is reached, and by a little manipulation the general direction of the crown and root could be usually diagnosed. B is a universal elevator. The blade is concavo-convex, and is long and sharp at the point. Its principal use is to loosen or dislodge a tooth by passing the thin blade between it and the adjoining tooth or between the tooth and the bone, with the concave portion next to the tooth. C and D are right and left elevators, which are especially useful in removing a root. E is a spiral osteotome used both as a drill and to cut bone laterally, or even to cut a portion of the tooth away. It is also used in removing bone which holds the tooth in a false position or prevents its removal. F is a surgical hand-piece. Both the osteotome and the handpiece are made very strong. The osteotome cuts with great rapidity when driven at full speed by the surgical engine. G is one of the most useful forceps the writer has used for extracting either upper or lower impacted teeth. H is a small forceps, similar to G, but used only for the lower teeth.

Many writers are very arbitrary in recommending instruments and methods of procedure. The instruments here shown are those which have been used by the writer for a long time, but he would not wish to criticise those who do not use them. Every man should use the tools he can handle best. The writer's method of diagnosing impacted teeth and their positions may also differ from that of others. Each man has his own way of doing these things, and he should do them in the way by which he can accomplish the best results.

THE RADIOGRAPH AS AN AID IN DIAGNOSING THE POSITION OF IMPACTED TEETH.

The X-ray pictures have been of great service in locating foreign substances in various parts of the body, many of which could not have been located and removed without this assistance. Soon after the discovery of the X-ray for making skiagraphs of the human body, the writer gave considerable attention to the utility of skiagraphing the blood-vessels of the face for the study of their anatomy, also of impacted teeth as an assistance in diagnosis. In 1896 he wrote the following for the first edition of "The American System of Operative Dentistry:" "The diagnosis of unerupted teeth occupying abnormal positions has been greatly facilitated by

special application of the newly discovered skiagraphic method."
As a means of diagnosing the true position of impacted teeth, the
method has not so far given the writer quite the same satisfaction
as it does in general surgery. The position of an obscure impacted
tooth renders it very difficult to get a good picture of the tooth
with its anatomical relations to the neighboring structures; the
cancellated tissue often becomes very dense from the same cause
to which the impaction is due,—*i.e.,* malnutrition. Often only
a slight shadow of the tooth shows in the picture. Even when a
good shadow is obtained it is rather difficult to judge of the
depth of the tooth in the bone. In other parts of the body
pictures at right angles to each other can more readily be taken,
so that if the foreign substance is indicated in both pictures the
locality is much more easily established.

Great improvement has been made, however, in the past few
years in obtaining radiographs of the jaws, and as this improvement advances the X-ray will doubtless become a more important
aid in diagnosis.

After having seen some most beautiful stereoscopic radiographs,
last July, in Europe, showing the internal anatomy of the brain-
case, the writer thought that by making stereoscopic radiographs
of the face, not only could the shape and size of various pneumatic sinuses and cells be diagnosed, but a much better idea of
the position of impacted teeth could be given.

Through the kindness of Drs. Kassabian, Leonard, and Pancoast, of Philadelphia, the writer is enabled to show several skiagraphic pictures.

Fig. 6 is made from a radiograph taken by Dr. Pancoast. The
permanent canine is missing from the arch. The patient did not
lose the deciduous canine until after twenty years of age. Soon
after the loss of the tooth a "bridge" was adjusted by being
attached to the lateral and first premolar. This appliance is shown
fairly well in the illustration; one can also see that the root-
canal filling of the first premolar extends a little above the pin
of the artificial tooth. The pulp-chamber and canal are also
quite well shown in the second premolar. The permanent canine
is distinctly visible in the picture, which also indicates that a
portion of the crown is on the palatal side of the lateral incisor.
Having carefully examined the patient's mouth before the picture
was taken, the writer was able to make the same diagnosis as to

the position of the tooth. It is possible that this tooth can be brought into position. Much, however, will depend upon the condition of the bone and the root. If the bone has become more than normally dense, and if the root has thickened or has curved,—the picture faintly indicates these conditions, especially the latter, —then it will be difficult to bring the tooth into position. At the time when this tooth should have made its appearance in the arch, a proper search made with an exploring instrument and the X-ray, and the removal of the deciduous tooth and whatever bone was holding it, would have permitted the tooth to advance, more than likely without other mechanical aid than guidance into its proper

FIG. 6.

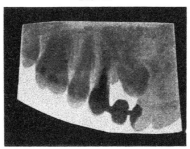

Radiograph showing impacted canine tooth.

position. It is very interesting to note that the root of the first premolar is slightly curved backward. The second premolar is sensitive to percussion, which leads to suspicion that the impacted canine is interfering with the surrounding tissue.

ILLUSTRATIONS OF IMPACTED TEETH.

The various illustrations which follow have been selected to afford a good idea of the variable positions in which impacted teeth are found. They are taken from specimens in the museum of the Dental Department of the University of Pennsylvania.

Fig. 7 is made from a specimen owned by Professor James Truman. It shows a rather common form of impacted canine. In the living subject the diagnosis in this case would have been comparatively easy. In the first place, as the canine tooth would not have been found in the arch, the enlargement of the alveolar process over the impacted tooth would have indicated its position without much difficulty.

Occasionally there are cases of impaction of the canine and other teeth which do not produce external enlargements of the bone or gum tissue. The writer's experience has taught him that when the canine tooth is missing from the arch and it has not been extracted, the tooth lies somewhere within the jaw, though this is not always the case with the third molars and lateral incisors.

The writer has just had a patient about thirty-five years of age, from whose arch the two upper second premolars were missing, and who claims that he has not had them extracted. As he was suffering from neuralgia in the anterior portion of the maxillæ,

Fig. 7.   Fig. 8.

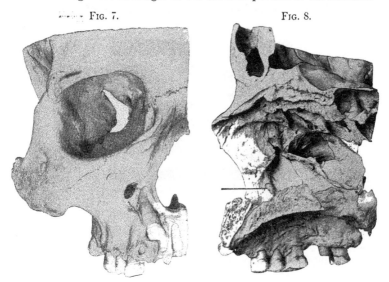

An impacted canine tooth, with the apex of the roots in the nasal fossa.

the writer thought that these teeth were impacted somewhere within the jaw, but careful exploration with instruments and radiographs taken at various angles and by different skiagraphers, failed to show any evidence of the missing teeth. The failure of these methods of examination leads the writer to believe that the teeth in question have never developed.

Fig. 8 is made from the nasal surface of the same specimen as is Fig. 7. It will be observed that the point of the root of the impacted canine is exposed on the outer wall of the nasal chamber. If this tooth should become diseased and an abscess form around the point of the root, the abscess would break into the nasal chamber.

Fig. 9 shows an impacted canine. It would be more difficult to diagnose the true position of this tooth than of those shown in

FIG. 9.

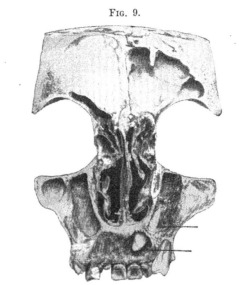

Impacted canine tooth.

FIG. 10.

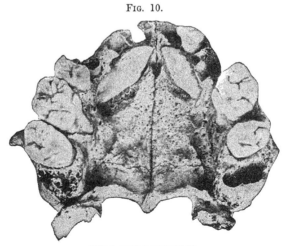

Two impacted canine teeth.

Figs. 7 and 8. The crown would be easily located, as it was in the cadaver, even before the tissue dried, but the root, being em-

Original Communications.

bedded in the anterior wall of the antrum, would be difficult to locate.

Among numerous cases referred to the writer, was one sent to him by the late Professor Harrison Allen, who had been unsuccessfully treating the nose, and thought the teeth might possibly have something to do with the trouble. The crown of an impacted canine was easily located. The bone of the roof of the mouth had become hard and dense and adherent to the tooth. After removing the soft tissue and a portion of the bone, a fairly good hold could be taken of the crown, but the tooth could not be removed without danger of fracture. Fearing that damage might

FIG. 11.

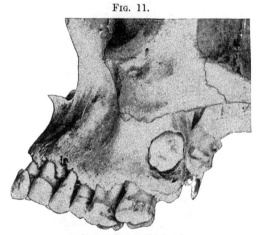

An impacted upper third molar.

be done to the roof of the mouth, a small osteotome was attached to the surgical engine. The point was passed into the bone near the tooth, and as the osteotome would cut sidewise as well as penetrate, it was carried around the greater portion of the tooth until it could be loosened and removed. Afterwards treatment was comparatively easy, and the nasal trouble was easily cured.

Fig. 10 shows two impacted canine teeth. Their malposition caused the loss of the right second premolar, also the loss of the left first and second premolars. These teeth are in a rather common position for impacted canine teeth, though it is very unusual to have two in the same mouth. Their existence and position could easily have been diagnosed by an exploring instrument.

Fig. 11 shows an impacted upper third molar. A similar condition was found on the opposite side of the skull. In this case it would tax the powers of the radiographer to make a picture from the living subject which would reveal the true position of a tooth and roots when thus impacted.

The extraction of this tooth would be most difficult. When the mouth is thrown open the upper portion of the ramus of the jaw comes forward and interferes with the surgical work. The writer thus far has extracted all similar teeth that have been sent to him, leaving the second molar *in situ*. But they were not in so difficult a region as those shown in this picture. If teeth in similar positions do not interfere with the action of the mandible, or are not likely to produce a disturbance, such as abscesses or neu-

FIG. 12.

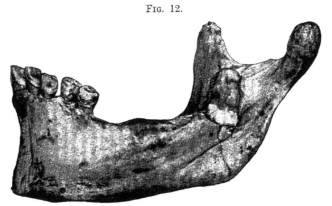

An impacted lower third molar.

ralgia, the writer would be inclined to let them remain in the jaw. But if they gave trouble, then they should be removed with as little injury to the surrounding tissue as possible. In rare cases it might be best to extract the second molar in order to reach the offending tooth, though every reasonable endeavor should be made to extract the third molar without disturbing the second.

Fig. 12 shows an impacted lower third molar turned completely upside down. Teeth of this character may give no trouble for years, or even be unsuspected, when, for some cause unknown, there may ensue a general inflammation of the surrounding tissue which might prevent proper movement of the mandible, interfere with deglutition, produce abscesses, neuralgia, etc. If such conditions should manifest themselves, and no other reasons could be found for this disturbance, then an impacted lower third molar should be suspected and a proper search made for it with the X-ray. The writer has diagnosed teeth in similar positions with proper exploring instruments, and, after finding them, has removed them with the aid of the surgical engine and forceps.

Fig. 13 shows a side view of two impacted lower third molars, the bone having been removed in order to expose the roots. It will be noticed that the anterior cusps are pressing against the concavity of the distal surface of the second molar. This condition makes these teeth most difficult to extract. The following plan

FIG. 13.

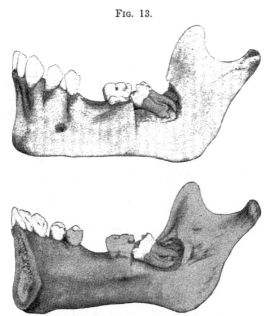

Side view of two impacted lower third molars.

has been adopted in a few cases: With a thin carborundum disk the anterior cusp has been cut away, then with an elevator the teeth have been turned out of their sockets. Occasionally these cusps are very deep down, as shown in Fig. 15, and are covered with gum tissue and situated below the level of the upper margin of the alveolar process, which makes it very difficult to cut off that part of the molar which is wedged in and against the second molar.

Fig. 14 is an interesting case of an impacted lower third molar, its position being on the inner side of the jaw, resting immediately upon the inferior dental nerves and vessels. It also rests partly below the line of the floor of the mouth and in close relation to the mylohyoid nerves and vessels. In extracting great care should be taken not to wound these.

Fig. 15 gives two views of an impacted lower third molar. A shows it in position, while B shows the tooth turned out of its socket. Part of the distal root of the second molar has been resorbed, exposing the root-canal, which more than likely caused pain and eventually the devitalization of the pulp. As the roots of the teeth are pressing in the region of the inferior dental nerve, it is possible that the function of the nerve was interfered with, which would probably cause neuralgia.

FIG. 14.

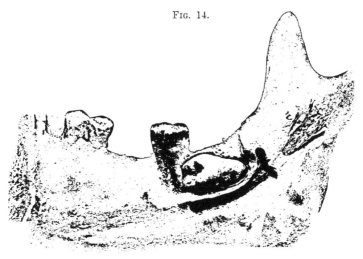

An impacted lower third molar.

An impacted tooth in this region would be somewhat difficult to diagnose, unless all the conditions are carefully studied, especially its position and relation to the second molar and surrounding tissues. In order to diagnose the tooth and its position all facts should be considered, such as the history, and the condition of the other teeth, especially those on the same side of the jaw. The patient, no doubt, would have had certain symptoms of disturbances. These facts should be ascertained, also the time of decay of the second molar, whether the third molar had been extracted, etc. A radiograph should be taken, as it would assist in confirming the diagnosis by other means that a tooth was impacted in this region. In examining the teeth in the lower jaw

all were found to be in position except the lower third molar, which
was not in view. When the patient was living he doubtless suf-

Fig. 15.

A

B

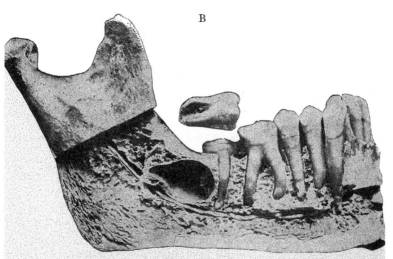

Two views of impacted lower third molar.

fered from neuralgia. The history of the case would have led
one accustomed to close observation to suspect an impacted lower
third molar. With the proper-shaped excavator, similar to that
shown in Fig. 5, the sharp point could have been passed down

through the gum tissue, immediately back of the second molar, to the enamel of the impacted tooth, a substance which cannot be mistaken by a trained dentist. There would be no difficulty in this, because the bony tissue would be porous, as it is in the specimen from which the illustration is taken. Sufficient bone could then be removed to give a general idea of the location of the tooth. The removal would be most difficult, as the entire tooth is so far down in the jaw, and the crown is well locked under and within the second molar. It would be possible with the surgical engine to remove the overlying bone until the tooth could be extracted. When a tooth is to be extracted it should be done with as little damage to the surrounding tissue as possible, and the extraction of another tooth, such as the second molar, in order to dislodge the third molar, should, if possible, be avoided.

In a living case like that shown in Fig. 15, if the patient were in distress, the writer would consider it good surgery to extract the second molar and allow the third molar to move forward, when it would more than likely be possible to remove the tooth without injury to that portion of the jaw. If the specimen be examined, it will be found that the bone on the lingual surface of the tooth is a mere shell, and that the bone below the tooth is so frail that it would fracture clear through if much pressure were put upon it. It is, in fact, so thin that the specimen has been broken through handling. Knowing the condition of this particular specimen, and having seen numerous fractures through the extraction of the lower third molar, the writer has been very cautious in such matters. He thus far has been fortunate in not having fractured a jaw, but he has seen cases of fractured jaws by thoroughly careful and competent surgeons.

As illustrating this caution regarding the extraction of the second molar under such circumstances, the writer remembers only one case where it seemed necessary to extract this tooth in order to relieve a disturbance caused by an impacted third molar. The late Professor Goodman, one of Philadelphia's well-known surgeons, called at the writer's office and asked him to come at once and bring his extracting instruments, as he had a patient on the verge of collapse. Upon examination a swelling was found near the angle of the jaw. The patient could open the mouth only a little way, and deglutition and respiration were difficult. In examining the parts with an excavator an impacted lower third molar was found. There was little time to be lost in relieving the patient, therefore the small lower forceps, G, shown in Fig. 5, were passed backward along the buccal cavity of the mouth, the inner beak passing between the upper and lower teeth until the lower second molar was reached, which was grasped in the beaks and extracted.

Two of the following illustrations are from X-ray pictures.

Fig. 16 is from a beautiful radiograph made by Dr. Kassabian. It shows two impacted lower third molars, which partly coincides

Fig. 16.

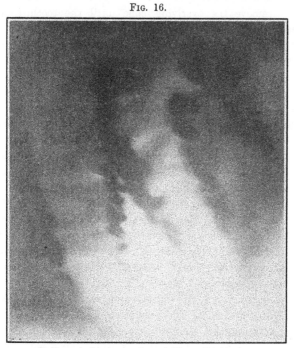

Radiograph showing two impacted lower third molars.

with the diagnosis made previously with the excavator. The history of the case is, that part of the crown of the left third molar has been broken away in an endeavor to extract the tooth, leaving the pulp exposed. The radiograph shows that the crown was deformed, also that the anterior cusp was apparently interlocked under the second molar. By careful examination with an excavator it was found that both of the anterior cusps were so far down in the tissues that the disk could not be used to remove them.

The patient being etherized, a mouth-gag was placed in position and a portion of the soft tissue removed with a small knife. The revolving spiral osteotome was placed within the broken crown or into the pulp-chamber, cutting almost through the balance of the crown. By passing the point of the osteotome under the crown and between it and the bone, a space was made partially in the tooth and partially in the bone, which allowed the point of the elevator B to pass between the tooth and the jaw.

The writer now seldom uses the forceps to remove a tooth after loosening it with the elevator. In using the elevator on the left side, as in this case, it is operated with the right hand, the surgeon standing on the left side of the patient. The left forefinger is placed in the mouth by the lingual side of the tooth and the thumb is placed on the buccal side of the first and second molars. This gives steadiness to the jaw and lessens the risk of slipping. As the tooth is raised from its socket the finger is placed so as to bring the tooth out of the mouth. If the tooth to be removed is on the right side, the elevator should be used with the left hand if possible (the surgeon standing on the right side). If the operator must use the elevator with his right hand, he should, however, manage to guard and steady the parts with his left hand.

FIG. 17.

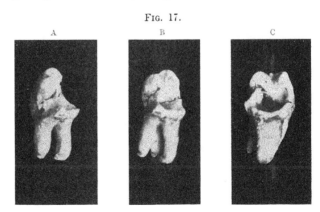

A   B   C

Fig. 17 is made from three photographs of the tooth after extraction. A shows the outer or buccal side and its roots, in about the same position as when in the jaw. The distal cusps were broken away in a former endeavor to extract it. The greater portion of the crown was cut away with the surgical engine. On the side of the tooth there is a groove extending backward, downward, and inward, cut by the osteotome. It was along this groove that the elevator was forced under the tooth, causing the slight portion of the crown that remained to fracture. In B the tooth is turned slightly outward, in order to show three roots and the line of fracture which liberated the tooth. In C the tooth is turned upon its buccal surface, showing the two anterior cusps which were locked under the distal surface of the second molar.

Fig. 18 is from a good radiograph made by Dr. Leonard. The patient had some neuralgic trouble within the ear, and after having

FIG. 18.

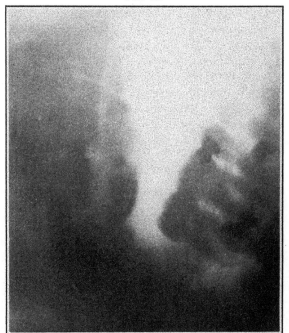

Radiograph showing impacted upper third molar.

excluded several supposed causes, the teeth were suspected, as the upper first and second molars appeared to be sensitive, and this radiograph was taken. When one becomes accustomed to examining X-ray pictures, it is not difficult to detect a shadow of the crown of a tooth in the region where the upper third molar might be impacted, but one can get only a slight idea as to the depth of its occluding surface. No idea whatever is possible as to whether it is on an occluding line with the other teeth,—*i.e.,* whether it is near the buccal surface of the alveolar ridge or on the lingual surface. The roots of the tooth, their number, shapes, and positions, are not shown in the radiograph. All of this practical surgical diagnosis has to be learned by other means. In this case a careful exploration was made with an excavator, and the position of the crown was partially located. After the tissue covering the crown of the tooth had been cut away the tooth was grasped with the small forceps, G, shown in Fig. 5. The firmness of the tooth indicated that the roots were crooked and held by bone harder than normal. By carrying the handle of the forceps in the line of least resistance, which was outward, backward, and upward, the roots were unlocked from under the over-calcified bone.

Fig. 19 is made from four photographs of the tooth after extraction. A shows the anterior surface. B shows the distal sur-

FIG. 19.

A   B   C   D

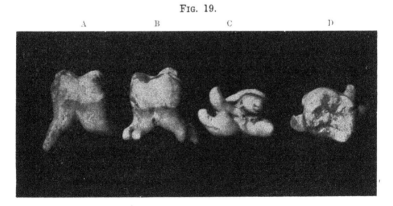

face, with the hook-like form of the buccal roots. C shows the upper surface, or the root end of the tooth, with the four roots spread outward, approaching a horizontal direction, and D shows the occluding or grinding surface, with the points of the roots extending outward. It will be noticed that this tooth is quite a different object from that shown in the skiagraph. It may be interesting to know that the ear has improved since the extraction, and at the same time the other molars appear to have lost their sensitiveness, indicating that the tooth was interfering with the nerve supplying these teeth.

TREATMENT OF PROTRUDING AND RECEDING JAWS BY THE USE OF THE INTERMAXILLARY ELAS-TICS.[1]

BY DR. H. A. BAKER, BOSTON, MASS.

To my mind, of all the authors who have written upon the subject of Orthodontia, no one has given the term irregularities of the teeth so correct a definition as Edward H. Angle when he defined the term as malocclusion, for wherever you find irregular teeth you will find malocclusion. With perfect occlusion you will invariably find regular teeth.

Not only do I give him the credit of giving the most correct definition, but I also believe he has given to the profession the best appliance for its correction, although he disclaims the originality of it, his only claim being a modification of an old method.

I consider that this appliance can be adapted to the correction of a greater number of classes of malocclusion than any other one method. When the appliance is properly handled, better results can be obtained in the least possible time and with less discomfort to the patient.

The arches can be expanded or contracted, protrusion or recession of the jaws corrected, bringing into line in- and outstanding teeth, correcting lack of anterior occlusion by elongation of the teeth, and by the same means bringing into position partially erupted teeth; also rotation in all its forms and combinations can be accomplished to advantage with it, which practically covers all varieties of malocclusion.

A feature that I want to especially emphasize, and want all to appreciate, is that all of these deformities can be corrected at the same time, and, what is more, during the time that other appliances are correcting one. Take, for example, a case where the arch has to be expanded and there are crowded teeth, which generally occurs with contracted arches. The arch can be expanded in as short a time as any other device can accomplish the object; and while this is going on the twisted teeth can be rotated as readily as with a specific appliance for that purpose.

I hope I have made myself clear on this point, for, as I have above stated, it is an important feature.

[1] Read before The New York Institute of Stomatology, January 6, 1903.

FIG. 1.

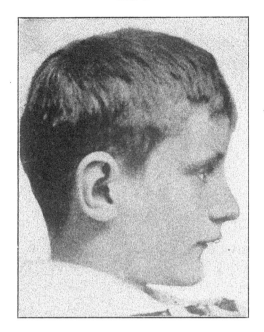

FIG. 2.

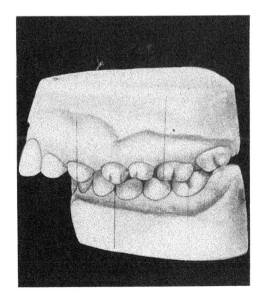

FIG. 3.

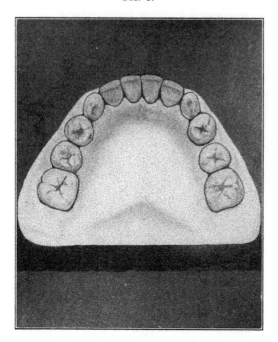

FIG. 4.

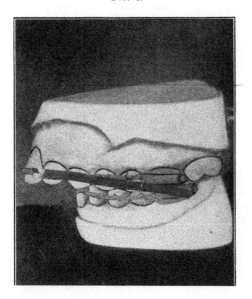

Another advantage of this appliance and its modifications is the great amount of resistance that can be obtained, not only from the anchor teeth, but from all the teeth of the jaw which can be brought to bear on those that are to be moved, thus diminishing the danger of displacing or tipping the anchor teeth, which is apt to occur unless the operator is very skilful. I wish to go a step farther and say that the teeth of the opposite jaw from which the appliance is fixed will serve as resistance by the principle of inclined plane, a force that is of great importance in regulating, both to help or retard the work, according to whether the operator uses the force to work with him or ignores it, in which case it is very liable to work against him, and he wonders why he fails. Still another advantage is that if one or more of the teeth need more force applied, simply ligate them firmer or oftener than the others, or, if they are moving too rapidly, reverse the process and give them rest; thus the appliance is well under control.

One more feature is that after the deformity has been corrected, but the occlusion is not as good as desired (I refer especially to the bicuspid and molar region), by still keeping the appliance on enough freedom can be allowed the teeth for them to settle, so to speak, into position and adjust themselves. By keeping it on still longer it makes a very good temporary retainer. I have found that this is of great value in producing good occlusion.

We will endeavor to show how it is especially adapted to correct the class of cases that come under the title of this paper,—namely, protruding and receding jaws, which affect the expression of the face more than any other class. To be successful in correcting them, one should always have an ideal in mind and endeavor to approach it.

As we all very well know, the common device for correcting protrusion is the head-cap and the bit, which in the first place is very unsightly as well as uncomfortable; and secondly, my experience is that the patients object to it more than any other device connected with orthodontia. Because so many patients refuse to undergo the treatment with such an appliance, I have given the above question considerable study.

My youngest son was afflicted with a very pronounced case of protrusion and recession of the jaws, for which I studied out a course of treatment which I thought would be effective.

I brought my study model before the American Academy of

Dental Science and explained my method, after which I proceeded as I explained and carried the case through without a false step, if you will permit me to say so. I believe the illustrations will prove this to be true.

CASE I.—When my youngest son was an infant of six weeks conditions were such that we were obliged to bring him up by artificial means, and he acquired the habit, so common among children, of keeping the rubber nipple in his mouth almost constantly. As a result, the gentle pressure of the soft rubber caused the deformity in his delicate jaws before being discovered, and after his permanent teeth had been erupted presented the appearance as shown in Fig. 1. Carefully considering the case, I decided to wait until just before the lower twelfth-year molars erupted, as shown in Figs. 2 and 3.

While studying these models, by sliding the lower jaw forward so that the sixth-year molars would be in a normal occlusion I found that with a very little spreading of the arches and slightly retracting the upper incisors I would get proper occlusion. By close observation we notice the deformity is confined to more of a recession of the lower jaw than protrusion of the upper. As the correction requires very little tooth movement and considerable forward bodily motion of the lower jaw, it was a great problem to me what force to apply to produce this result. I studied the case long and carefully, and it occurred to me that by using the Angle appliances in combination with elastic pressure applied in such a way as to obtain what we might call reciprocal anchorage, that is, to retract the superior incisors and at the same time bring the lower jaw forward to its normal position, we could obtain the desired results. To apply this theory I attached a moderately heavy elastic to each side of the lower appliance by slipping them over the ends of the tubes of the anchor bands, stretching them forward, and fastening to the superior expansion arch between the cuspids and laterals, as shown in Fig. 4. (Being a case that I could constantly watch I decided to make the trial.) I took my models before the American Academy of Dental Science and explained my method of procedure, requesting it to be put on record as a new device for correcting protruding and receding jaws. I commenced the case in the spring of 1893. I was astonished with the result. In two months' time the teeth were occluding in a normal position; but for fear that they might

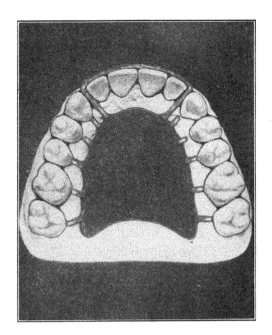

Fig. 6.

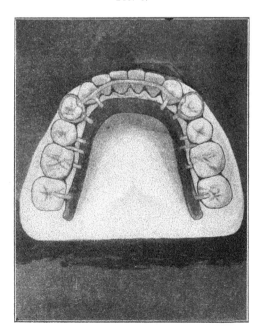

FIG. 7.

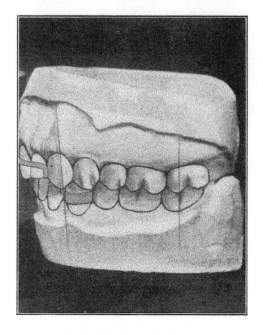

FIG. 8.

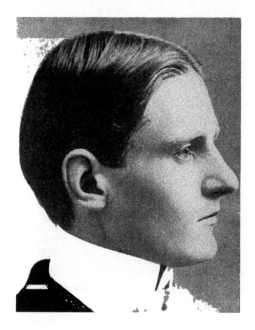

FIG. 9.

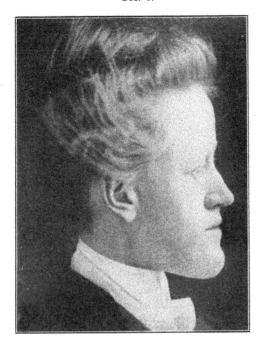

FIG. 10.

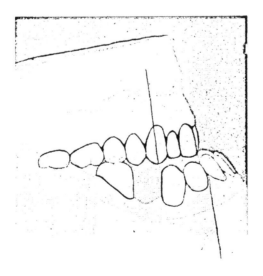

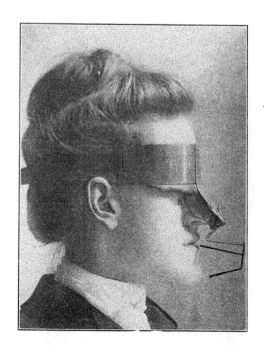

FIG. 12.

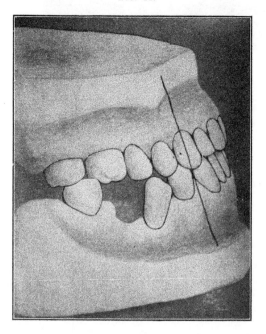

return to their former position, I reduced the size and strength of the elastics and kept them in that way several months longer, and by so doing they settled into perfect occlusion.

The next step was to retain them. My experience with rubber retaining plates festooned around the teeth was so unsatisfactory that I thought out a method of retaining which I hoped would be more satisfactory. By considering carefully Fig. 5 we get a good idea of the superior retainer. The features of this device are, first, the extreme small amount of contact between the retainer and the enamel of the teeth, therefore improving the sanitary conditions which reduces the liability of causing decay to a minimum. The second feature of advantage is the amount of freedom that is allowed the teeth, permitting them to settle into proper occlusion, as well as the range of adjustment that is allowed by the alterations of the metallic spurs.

The retainer consists of a vulcanite suction-plate covering enough of the vault to insure its stability. From the plate radiate platinized gold spurs bearing at a single point against the cuspids. bicuspids, and molars. The incisors are held in their intended position by a wire of the same material passing around their labial surfaces and entering the palatal surface of the plate by being adjusted between the laterals and cuspids, care being taken not to interfere with the occlusion, either by the striking of the lower teeth or by separating the cuspid and lateral.

The lower retainer was made on the same general principle as the superior, excepting that suction was out of the question for holding the appliance in place. For this purpose I arranged a snap device similar to those used in coin-purses. We see in Fig. 6 that the first bicuspids are banded, and to these bands solder was flowed to thicken them, into which deep notches were filed for the purpose of holding spurs projecting from the plate. These spurs snap into the notches in the same manner that the snap fastener of a coin-purse works. The plate is further prevented from sinking into the soft tissue of the floor of the mouth by uprights from the heel of the plate hooking over into the crevices of the molars. To prevent backward movement of the plate spurs were extended from it on either side, resting on the mesial surface of the sixth-year molars. It is readily seen that both of these retainers can be removed by the patient for cleansing purposes, which I consider a great feature.

14

Fig. 7 shows occlusion after the retainers were adjusted. Fig. 8 shows the patient a few years later after the retainers were removed.

CASE II.—Miss ——, aged between twenty-six and thirty, an extreme case of prognathism, as shown in Fig. 9. Fig. 10 shows model of case before beginning treatment, with the rear part of the lower model cut away to show the upper molars, which otherwise would have been concealed. This case is characterized by the extreme backward slant of the lower incisors so prevalent among cases of this class. There has been considerable controversy among the profession regarding the changes that take place during the treatment of a case of this description by means of the intermaxillary elastics, some holding that the change produced was due to tooth movement alone, while others were of the opinion that the results were obtained by the bodily retraction of the lower jaw itself. In order to settle the matter, in my own mind at least, I constructed a device at the suggestion of my son, Dr. Lawrence W. Baker, to record whatever changes took place. The construction and principle of the apparatus can be readily understood by studying Fig. 11, which shows the "recorder" in position. It consists of a metallic skeleton framework on a base of modelling compound covering the bony protuberances of the forehead and nose. to which indicators are attached to measure the relative movement of both teeth and jaw, the upper indicator measuring the tooth movement of the lower jaw and the lower one the movement of the jaw itself. It can be readily seen that this apparatus could be accurately placed in exact position at the various stages as the work progressed.

Fig. 12 shows the model of the completed case. It will be noticed that the six anterior teeth were carried forward to their normal position. It was proved by the indicator that the jaw was retracted by actual measurement one-quarter of an inch more than the teeth. This proved to me, beyond a question of doubt, that the lower jaw was retracted independently of the teeth.

Fig. 13 gives the change produced in the facial expression. The series of photographs illustrating the case shows clearly the importance of working for and getting the normal relations between the two jaws, and, furthermore, that the direction of the teeth and the proper modelling of the alveolar process all have their effect in producing harmony in the facial expression. The

FIG. 13.

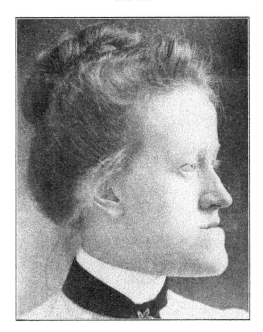

FIG. 14.

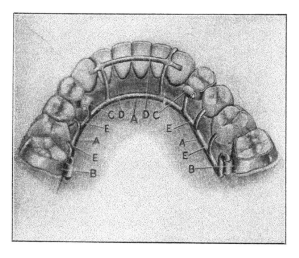

method of retention employed in this case was based on the same principle that we have already considered in the first case,—that is, the retainers were constructed on the single contact point theory. However, they differed from the first, inasmuch as those were of a combination of vulcanite and metal, while these are entirely metallic. as shown in Fig. 14, giving the principle of construction much better than I can describe. I might, however, add that the anchor bands are of 22-carat gold, while the wirework is of platinized gold. The appliance is so made that it can be removed by springing the horizontal uprights out of the half-tubes attached to the bicuspid bands by the operator for adjustment and for cleansing purposes. I have treated many similar cases since adopting this method. but have shown to you the two extremes. which I trust has proved its efficiency.

THE THERAPEUTIC USE OF THE X-RAY IN THE ORAL CAVITY.[1]

BY GEORGE F. EAMES, BOSTON, MASS.

The remarkably good results which have been recently achieved by means of the X-ray as a therapeutic agent are astonishing. The X-ray itself was accidentally discovered, as was also its chemical and therapeutic effect; its good results, therefore, are all the more surprising. The history of the discovery of the Röntgen ray, its wonderful penetrating power, and its use in photographing tissues and substances hidden from the ordinary sight are too well known to need further comment, but some attention to the nature of this wonderful electrical force. the means by which it is produced, and the methods of its application for the purpose of obtaining a therapeutic result have a claim to recognition in connection with the subject under consideration.

The X-ray is known chiefly by the phenomenon which accompanies it. as no one has yet been able to define it. Many scientists have, however, advanced theories with the object of explaining its nature and character. Many agree that it is a form of transverse

---

[1] Read before the American Medical Association, Section on Stomatology, New Orleans, May 5 to 8, 1903.

ethereal vibration, and formed in a series with sunlight and what is known as the Becquerel rays, the ethereal vibration being less in the case of ordinary light, more irregular in the Becquerel rays, and still more irregular in the X-rays.

Dr. H. P. Pratt, who has given this subject much attention, considers the X-ray as an electric current of a very high potential, which makes its circuit from the inner surface of the tube outward, perpendicularly to the surface, then radiates in straight lines until the potential falls, when the rays return to complete the circuit by the terminals. During the passage of the rays through the walls of the tube, through the atmosphere and into the body, it is accompanied by a liberation of oxygen from the body, as well as from the surrounding atmosphere. One of the most important agents in the application of the X-rays is the Crookes tube; indeed, the greater part of the technique and much of the therapeutic effect depends upon the proper handling of the tubes. The tubes themselves are usually designated as hard and soft, or, what is the same thing, high and low vacuum tubes. The condition which determines whether a tube is hard or soft is the number of molecules of residual gas in the tube; this fixes the degree of the vacuum and, consequently, the condition of the tube as to whether it is hard or soft. An X-ray tube when acted upon by the electric current has been compared to a Leyden jar: it discharges in one direction, the outer surface of the tube becomes electro-positive, and the inner surface electro-negative. The usual method of producing the Röntgen ray by means of a Crookes tube consists in furnishing electricity to it by means of a static machine,[1] or by the street current through a Rhumkorrf coil, the terminals of which are connected with a Crookes tube.

The cathodal and anodal poles are connected, the molecules of residual gas within the tube furnishing the medium through which the current is established. When the current is thus passing, these molecules of gas within the tube are driven with great force against its inner surface, and the point of contact locates the origin of the Röntgen ray.

The following ideas regarding the production of the X-ray, by

---

[1] Dr. William B. Snow advises the static machine for exciting the electric current. This should have ten revolving plates thirty to thirty-four inches in diameter. While coils are often capable of exciting high tubes, it is perilous to both coil and tubes.

Dr. H. P. Pratt, are quite pertinent to our subject. " Every molecule of gas striking the inner surface of the tube causes one or more lines of magnetic force to be thrown out at right angles to the surface of the tube. The distance to which these lines of force are projected, or, in other words, the limit of the penetrating power of the ray, depends entirely upon the potential of the tube, and this in turn depends on the force of the impact of the individual molecules of residual gas. The higher the vacuum, the less the number of molecules of residual gas in the tube; the greater the free path, the higher the potential, the greater the penetrating power. All substances through which the X-rays pass form part of the X-ray circuit. The X-ray circuit is the same as any other electrical current. It has its return forming an endless chain of molecules, arranged in series. . . . The light which is emitted from the tubes is the result of decomposition of the molecules in the atmosphere around and inside the tube. This light is not the X-ray current; the X-ray force is purely electrical and invisible.

" The softer the tube, the greater are the number of lines of force thrown out and the stronger the current which increases decomposition, but the penetrating power is decreased. We are dependent entirely upon the number of lines of force projected from the tube to bring about ionization of the tissues. Ionization means changes in the elementary structures and increase in metabolism.

" We need to have the greatest possible number of these lines of force within a given space for our best therapeutic work. This is only possible with a low or soft tube."

Having considered the nature and character of this electrical force, it becomes especially interesting to investigate the action which it has upon the various tissues of the body. Dr. Pratt suggests that " the magnetic force from the X-ray passes directly into the affected tissues. Electrolysis results, the chemical decomposition liberates oxygen, which unites with the free oxygen of the body and makes ozone. Ozone will kill every bacterium the human body possesses. The X-ray does not destroy germ life by direct action any more than does the sun's rays; the bactericidal effect of both are due to ionization, or electrolysis. Factors to be considered in X-raying are, 1, potential of the ray; 2, the resistance of the tissues to the ray; 3, the resulting intensity of the radiation. The first only is under control and is governed entirely upon conditions in the tube, which are constantly varying, but which, by corresponding changes in the current energizing the tube, the spark-gap, etc., may be made approximately constant." Experience in X-ray work has shown that for therapeutic effect, a low, or soft tube should be used, and the current increased according to the result which it is desired to obtain. The harder the tube the less the number of lines of force thrown out, and consequently the weaker the X-ray current, and the less the decomposition, but the greater the penetrating power. While it is true that the X-ray improperly or incautiously applied will certainly burn the tissues, and that the burns are very painful and serious, it is, nevertheless, of rare occurrence with the careful and experienced operator, who, being mindful of the great difference in susceptibility of patients, adapts the current, the tube, the time of exposure, and the distance of the tube from the body to the conditions he finds in his patient. He will take other precautions, such as the interposition of a celluloid screen between the patient and the tube; this prevents the germs in the air between the patient and the tube from being driven into the body. From the foregoing we may summarize the following marked characteristics of the X-ray when applied to the human body.

1. The power of penetrating deeply into the tissues.

2. Its great germicidal power.

3. The power of destroying diseased tissues with the result of new tissue being formed.

These wonderful properties of the Röntgen ray, and many others of which we know, and probably others of which we do not know, have, in actual practice, worked marvellous results, as we have ourselves seen, and as the published records have shown during the past year. It is reported that at least one hundred different diseases have yielded to the X-ray, the most notable, perhaps, being those coming under the head of malignant growths. These often occur in the mouth, and should interest the dentist. The effect of the X-ray on malignant growths is summarized by Dr. Morton as follows:

1. Relief from excruciating pain.

2. Reduction in size of new growths.

3. The establishment of the process of repair.

4. Removal of odor if present.

5. Cessation of discharge.

6. Softening and disintegration of lymphatic nodes.

7. Disappearance of lymphatic enlargements not submitted to treatment and often quite distant.

8. Removal of the cachetic color.

9. Improvement in the general health.

10. Cure, up to date, of a certain number of malignant growths.

The changes above enumerated are further described by Dr. M. F. Wheatland, who suggests that the X-ray vibrations acting on the cancer cells tend to stimulate many to maturity, at the same time breaking down the weaker ones, which are absorbed by the lymphatics and enter the circulation, producing the autointoxication so frequently observed, the number of cells reaching maturity and those undergoing destruction depending upon the intensity of the reaction established. At the same time changes take place in the small blood-vessels, their coats become thickened, narrowing their caliber, thereby reducing their blood-supply and aiding the return of the circulation to the normal.

Regarding the application of the X-ray to the mouth, the possibilities of its therapeutic effect may have a wide range. Already it has shown a marked influence over neuralgia and in the control of hemorrhage.

In the various forms of benign and malignant growths, provided they can be reached by the X-ray, we may expect the same good results that have been attained in other parts of the body. It is reported, and it has been my experience also, that the beneficent results of the X-ray are not confined alone to the part to which application is made, but that remote parts of the body also come within the range of its influence; indeed, it is often remarked by the patients that their general condition is improved, and that they have a feeling of well-being after an application of the X-ray. The report that there is an increased discharge of uric acid during this treatment seems, from the examinations which I have made, to be true. It is my belief that the application of the Röntgen ray may be effectual in the treatment of that stubborn and obscure condition generally termed pyorrhœa alveolaris, but of this I am not yet ready to report.

I am indebted to Dr. George R. Southwick, of Boston, for the privilege of reporting the following case:

F. H. B., aged forty-five, was troubled, about six months ago, with pain in the left side of the upper jaw, which was located in some of the teeth of that side. Some attention was given the teeth, and as the pain was not then constant or severe, further attention was then delayed. The pain in the jaw continuing, the patient sought advice from his physician, who suggested that he was trou-. bled with "canker," and provided him with an antiseptic wash; but the use of this failed to relieve his condition, and recently, on account of the severity of the pain and looseness of the teeth on the affected side, he sought the advice of a surgeon, who, when he saw the case, suspected malignant trouble, and extracted the teeth on that side. He then sent the patient to Dr. Southwick, who kindly asked me to see the case and make suggestions as to an appliance for the mouth, through which the X-ray might be applied, a positive diagnosis of epithelioma having previously been made.

Finally, after several modifications, a shield was constructed which properly protected the healthy tissues and allowed the ray to reach the diseased part.

This consisted of sheet lead fourteen inches square, in the centre of which was fitted and soldered a mouth-piece which projected into the mouth as far back as the tuberosity of the jaw, closed at the end, but on the side towards the affected part a piece was cut out in order to allow the ray to pass through the opening thus made, and into the diseased tissues. (Fig. 1.) The condition

Fig. 1.

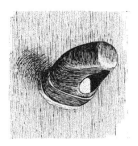

of the part at the beginning of treatment showed some loss of tissue, white patches and inflammatory conditions, and a spreading to the cheek and to the centre of the palatine vault. The treatment consisted in using a direct current of one hundred and ten volts from the street, reduced to one and a half ampères, approximately, before going to a twenty-inch coil, of a Ruhmkorff pattern. From the terminals of this coil a soft Crookes tube of twenty centimetres was used, about twelve inches from the face for about nine minutes, the face and other parts being protected by the shield.

The patient was treated in this way twice a week, and after two visits a marked improvement was shown. A further application of the X-ray was applied to the outside of the face with the object of reaching the facial nerve and controlling the neuralgia. This was effective in lessening the pain, and the good results in this direction have been progressive. The patient has, at this writing, received eight treatments, and the improvement in the mouth continues. All traces of the disease, however, have not yet been removed, and a prognosis must be withheld until a later date.

SPALDING'S PORCELAIN JACKET CROWN.[1]

. BY HENRY W. GILLETT, D.M.D., NEW YORK.

FOLLOWING the suggestion of Dr. C. H. Land for a porcelain jacket crown, Dr. Edward B. Spalding, of Detroit, has worked out a different technique for a crown, which is so artistic in final result, and so fascinating in the precision of the different steps of its development, that it arouses immediate interest wherever shown.

Most of you are probably familiar with the article by Dr. Land in the *Dental Cosmos* for August, 1903, on "Porcelain Dental Art," in which he figures a porcelain crown similar to the one I will show you to-night.

Dr. Spalding wishes to give credit to Dr. Land for the original suggestion of such a crown. The development of the technique of the crown I am to show you is entirely Dr. Spalding's work, and seems to me a distinct advance over Dr. Land's.

In order to describe intelligibly Dr. Spalding's procedure, we will assume that we are dealing with a deformed superior cuspid tooth, with either living or dead pulp, but with such defects of development as to call for treatment of some kind. The first step is to take a wire measurement of the circumference of the tooth at the gum margin. The second is to give the crown of the tooth a conical shape from the gum margin to the occlusal end, to give

---

[1] Read before The New York Institute of Stomatology, January 5, 1904.

.it a distinct shoulder at or just under the gum margin, and to shorten it. This Dr. Spalding accomplishes with rather thin three-quarter-inch disks of carborundum for the broad surfaces, and finishes with small inverted cone carborundum points, mounted for both hand-pieces, at the angles resulting from the use of the larger disk.·

The third step is to cut a piece of matrix platinum in the shape of a trapezoid, with its base line the same length as the wire measurement in the first step.

Fourth, unite the edges of this piece with a minimum quantity of pure gold, forming a truncated cone-shape. Slip this over the tooth, making sure that its edge goes above the shoulder left at the gum margin, and with the dentimeter twist a soft wire ligature around the matrix just below the shoulder, and with suitable pliers begin to draw the surplus platinum to the mesial and distal sides in two flattened wings, and also over the end of the tooth. Clip off most of the surplus at the end, leaving a little for a handle till the fitting is nearly done, and fold over the surplus at the sides, cutting off part of it first if there is much excess. Burnish the matrix accurately and smoothly to the tooth. Dr. Spalding uses for this work a bone instrument, of which I have made a rough imitation for your inspection. It is a valuable instrument, and my use of it convinces me that a bone or ivory burnisher will be very helpful in inlay matrix formation. The feel of the bone instrument as it passes over the platinum is a distinct relief as compared with the drag of a steel instrument.

Fifth, select a rubber tooth (Dr. Spalding uses at present Consolidated teeth) of suitable color and shape, and with carborundum stones cut it to the shape of the sample facing shown. Note that the tip is hollowed out and the shoulder and enamel surface of the palatal side of the tip is left intact. This is accomplished by using the same small carborundum stone used for finishing the shaping of the tooth. This shoulder is a very important aid in the further work.

Sixth, wax this to the matrix, with latter in correct position on the tooth, using gutta-percha and wax mixture; remove carefully; grip with suitable pliers, one jaw of which passes inside the matrix and the other engages a corresponding point on the labial surface of the facing. Remove the wax and place " block body" on one side near the tip and jar it carefully through till it

364 *Original Communications.*

appears on the other side, then build it round the top of the cone
and, setting on end in the furnace, fuse the body. It is essential
that the body for this first bake be kept away from the shoulder
in the matrix. This block body Dr. Spalding makes by grinding
up in the mortar pinless teeth of the same make as the facing he
uses.

Seventh, place the piece in position on the tooth and carefully
perfect the fit of the matrix at the shoulder.

Eighth, apply body, carve, and fuse to finish.

Ninth, remove the matrix and set in suitable cement.

Dr. Spalding is able to report use of these crowns only since
last April,—about nine months. This is, of course, too short a
period to enable us to define their permanent place in our resources
for such work, but his report for that time is favorable without
exception. He has had no breakages yet. He has the matter so
thoroughly worked out, and is so conservative in his own estimate
of it, that the fact that he continues to think well of the method
is sufficient evidence that it has value.

For molars, Dr. Spalding builds up the entire crown with
block body.

A possible objection to these crowns over live pulps is the
difficulty of getting access to the pulp in case pulpitis develops
after the application of the crown.

HOME MANUFACTURE OF FORMALDEHYDE FOR
STERILIZING PURPOSES.[1]

BY DR. H. L. WHEELER, NEW YORK.

THE particular use of formaldehyde that I shall mention in
this paper is in connection with the sterilizing of instruments.
Ever since I have boiled my instruments to make them aseptic I
have been looking for a suitable means to produce the same result,
and at the same time avoid some of the evil effects of boiling water
upon steel and wood, ivory, celluloid, etc. The advent of formaldehyde, or, more accurately, formic aldehyde, as a powerful germ

---

[1] Read before The New York Institute of Stomatology, January 5, 1904.

destroyer seemed to offer the needed substance; and my object in coming before you this evening is to suggest to you an easy way to manufacture this powerful germicidal gas. Formaldehyde (CH_2O) is produced by dry distillation of calcium formate or by the oxidation of methyl alcohol. It is a gas, and is readily absorbed by water, so that a forty per cent. solution is upon the market under the proprietary name of Formalin. For instrument and room disinfection it is prepared either by some dehydrating agent like calcium chloride, or by lamps for burning wood alcohol.

My experience with several of these specially constructed and patented lamps for this purpose having been decidedly unsatisfactory, and an attempt to get the patentee in one case to strive to remedy the difficulty having proved futile, I set about to find something that could be used steadily and regularly without failure in a short period of time. So far as I know, all the lamps sold for this purpose depend upon a platinized asbestos for the agent that will become incandescent and produce the oxidizing process which breaks up the wood alcohol into formic aldehyde ($CH_2O + H_2O$). This platinized asbestos is made by a secret process, and can be purchased by the ounce from any chemical supply house, but it has not proved lasting in the lamps I have used. To remedy its annoying tendency to fail when needed, I adopted the plan, after some experimenting, of taking a small piece of sponge platinum cut thin and holding it just above the wick of any ordinary alcohol lamp by any contrivance one may wish to construct. Light the wick and heat the platinum to incandescence; then extinguish the flame of the lamp and the metal will retain a dull glow and continue to produce formaldehyde as long as there is alcohol in the lamp. I simply bend a piece of German silver wire the desired shape for holding my sponge platinum in place, as is shown by the lamp I will pass around. I have also found that the ordinary lamp used under a chafing-dish, which is filled with asbestos covered with wire netting, works admirably for this purpose, only you must first, after lighting the lamp, hold the piece of metal up where it will become thoroughly heated, then extinguish the flame and drop the platinum upon the wire netting, and you will produce the gas. These lamps can be used in any suitable inclosure, as an oven of tin or copper, a tin box, or a chafing-dish, cutting a hole through the bottom large enough for the burner of the lamp to extend inside the receptacle; and the instruments can be placed in any way desired within the inclosure. The amount of formaldehyde manufactured in a given time depends upon the area of the piece of platinum and the size of the wick. I do not know if this suggestion has ever been published before; if so, I have not seen it, and I give it to you in detail that you may not be prohibited from using it by a patent; for patents seem to be becoming more and more an injury, and are threatening to entirely erase what ethics we possess. It is my desire to call attention to the advantages of publishing, as a matter of record, without securing a patent, those ideas, mechanical and otherwise, which we think may be of advantage to the profession and, through the profession, to humanity.

In order to do this I shall call attention to some examples which will necessitate showing conversely how we have suffered from patents, largely due to a lack of reasonable foresight and a proper regard for ethical standards upon our part. Almost with' one accord we subscribe to the funds of the Dental Protective Association to prevent our being mulcted by the Tooth-Crown Company, and yet as an organized body of men we have taken not one step to prevent the same evil coming upon us in the future in the only way it could be prevented,—viz., to promptly deny standing in any of our societies to any member of our profession who becomes so forgetful of his duties as a professional man as to acquire a patent on any implement or material to be used by the profession. We have courted a recurrence of the difficulty by an apparent approval of those who obtain patents, as is evidenced by observing what a large proportion of men invited to appear before our societies are there for the precise purpose of calling attention to some device which they have patented. From a purely financial point of view this policy of encouraging patents and at the same time raising large sums to fight them is such a lack of intelligent self-interest that I cannot conceive of a body of men of less than ordinary ability who would do these things as a plain business proposition. Note how large sums of the Dental Protective Association were spent in fighting the patents on the Donaldson broach, —in the interest of a rival supply house, unless I am misinformed, —and, after proving invalid a patent that had nearly expired, we are still paying the original price of two dollars and fifty cents per dozen for the genuine Donaldson broaches because those made to imitate them are of such a quality that they in no way compete with the original. Place beside this the decrease in the price of dental burs. Dr. William Rollins, of Boston, published a cut of the so-called "revelation" bur, or a similar one, in the *Archives of Dentistry,* January, 1885. He had previous to this tried to persuade a well-known dental supply house to manufacture this bur, but without success; later they were patented by this supply house, and they began their manufacture. Subsequently a rival house began the making of the same bur, and in the attempt to get an injunction upon this latter house the patent was proved invalid, because Dr. Rollins had published a description of the bur prior to the granting of the patent. The ultimate result was we were able to obtain burs at one dollar per dozen which before had cost two dollars and twenty-five cents, all due to one man having the foresight to publish his device without covering it with letters patent; and it did not cost the profession thousands upon thousands of dollars to prove the patent invalid.

I notice, in a late appeal for more funds from the members of the Dental Protective Association, it is stated that we have been protected from paying royalty on inlays by this Association. The author of this statement must be misinformed, or he lacks information; and that it will probably pass as authoritative indicates what a lack of knowledge there appears to be among the members of our calling, due, no doubt, to our habit of being fed pap by the supply houses through their faithful organs the dental journals published by them. It is a matter of record that Dr. Rollins described various methods for making metal moulds for porcelain fillings in a paper read before the Boston Society for the Advancement of Oral Science in June, 1880, while porcelain inlays ground to fit the cavity were used by Dr. Volck and his method published in the *American Journal of Dental Science* for July, 1857. In view of these published records, is it not obvious that patents taken out by Dr. Land in 1887 upon certain methods could not have required any great amount of time or expense to have proved them invalid? I am minded also of the case of the cervical clamp devised by Dr. Woodward and suppressed because a supply house claimed it was an infringement on an instrument already manufactured by them; although this latter instrument is greatly inferior to Dr. Woodward's. Were members of our profession to refuse to take out patents, and to carefully publish for

record their inventions, the supply houses could not use a patent
on an inferior device as a club to suppress superior instruments
in which, in many instances, there is a grave doubt if there be
any infringement whatever. The organized corporation has the
advantage, as they mostly retain an attorney by the year, part of
whose duties is to protect the corporation by shutting off all implements possible that would compete with their own product;
and every time a member of our profession takes out a patent
and sells it to a manufacturer he is increasing the difficulty of
every member of the profession to obtain instruments suited to his
individual taste and necessities.

PERPLEXITIES IN CONNECTION WITH EXTRACTION OF TEETH.[1]

BY HENRY W. GILLETT, D.M.D.

THE matter of which I wish to speak first will perhaps seem
to you a barren one to present before this society. Certain perplexities of my own in connection with the extraction of teeth have
led me to speak of them, with the hope that I, at least, may get
some benefit from your comments. I am not going to open the
subject of when to extract, but will assume that most of us occasionally feel it necessary to advise the extraction of an impacted
wisdom-tooth, or to insist upon the removal of useless foul and
decaying roots. I also assume that most of us prefer that these
operations should be performed by an " extracting specialist."

This is, at least, a fair statement of my own position, and I
am confident that in the main it agrees with the practice of many
of you.

My own experience in sending difficult cases of extraction to so-
called extracting specialists has been unsatisfactory, in that they
have always returned to me with what has seemed to me an unreasonable amount of inflammation and irritation of the parts adjacent to the operative field. Having spent much of my professional life in a small city where extracting specialists were· not

---

[1] Read before The New York Institute of Stomatology, January 5, 1904.

accessible, I have found it necessary to do some such operations myself. The very marked difference in the sequelæ of cases where the mouth has been thoroughly sprayed immediately before and after the operation with some sterilizing agent, preferably a peroxide of hydrogen solution, as compared with similar cases where this course has not been followed, has forced itself so strongly upon my attention that I now consider such spraying an essential preliminary to the extraction of teeth. Similar spraying after the operation seems to me desirable but possibly less necessary.

The means for preventing the pain of the operation itself have been developed till it makes tooth extraction almost too attractive to the possessor of painful but still salvable teeth, but in many cases the frequently more serious suffering which follows operations in a septic field seems to be taken as a necessary evil, and no effort is made to prevent it.

It would seem as if, in many cases, the only precautions taken by the operator were to ascertain with certainty which tooth its possessor wishes to part with, and to give his anæsthetic so as to avoid pain while the operation is in actual progress.

Personally, I feel that this ruthless tearing away of an organ with little or no regard for the welfare of adjacent tissues is much too common to do us credit. What surgeon would endorse even the smallest cutting operation in any other portion of the human anatomy, when it was surrounded by removable calcular deposits, swarming with all kinds of bacteria, and bathed in fluid bearing pyogenic organisms from adjacent pus-pockets, without preliminary efforts at cleaning and sterilizing the operative field. Yet in this twentieth century this is what many self-styled " Oral Surgeons" are doing.

I realize that some of you will say it is practically impossible to sterilize the mouth. This is undoubtedly true. It is also undoubtedly true that the mouth bacteria may be so thoroughly subjugated in a few minutes as to result in great practical benefit to the patient undergoing operations at that point.

This statement has been preliminary to presenting for your consideration the question whether this society, in view of the importance to its members of knowing that their patients are to receive satisfactory attention with due regard to the progress of surgical knowledge, may assume the duty of appointing a committee to formulate the general rules which seem desirable to observe in such operations, and shall (either with or without preliminary report to the society, as may be deemed best) call to the attention of such local practitioners as advertise themselves as extracting specialists the formulated rules, and, upon invitation by such practitioners, inspect their operating-rooms with a view to reporting to the society the names of those who are found equipped for the carrying out of these rules. This at first thought may seem inquisitorial, but when it is remembered that these practitioners appeal to us for their patronage, and that there is often laxness in the essentials for common cleanliness, not to mention the requirements of aseptism in their establishments, it seems to me a warrantable inquiry, and one which those extracting specialists who realize its value to them will hasten to meet in such manner as to insure the approval of the committee.

Reviews of Dental Literature.

THE DANGERS OF GELATIN INJECTIONS.—Since gelatin injections were first recommended for the control of severe hemorrhages in various organs, and for the treatment of aortic aneurism, they have been used quite extensively. Much has been said in favor of this method, but several deaths have resulted. The fatal results were due to such complications as septic thrombosis, phlegmons, malignant œdema, and particularly to tetanus.

Several communications have recently appeared which again strongly emphasize the dangers connected with the subcutaneous injection of gelatin. Chauffard reported a fatal case of tetanus following a gelatin injection, and states that seventeen similar cases have previously been placed on record. Dieulafoy a few weeks later reports another instance of fatal tetanus developing after a gelatin injection given to control a severe tubercular hæmoptysis, and he adds four more cases not included in Chauffard's statistics, bringing the total number of such deaths to twenty-three.

Quite an elaborate study on the dangers and ·the therapeutic value of gelatin injection has just been published by Doerfler, who has twice lost patients from tetanus following subcutaneous application of gelatin. In one instance the method was resorted to to control a severe postpartum hemorrhage, in the other case to stop a tubercular hæmoptysis.

It is now well known that tetanus following gelatin injections is almost universally due to the introduction of tetanus spores with the gelatin in which they were contained. Levy and Bruns obtained bacilli from eight out of thirteen samples of gelatin examined. It was formerly believed that the spores of the tetanus bacillus are killed by an exposure during eight minutes to streaming steam at 100° C., but the authors quoted have shown that even after thirty minutes' exposure some tetanus spores survive, and only after thirty-three minutes were all samples of infected gelatin so exposed found absolutely free from tetanus germs. According to Forster and Brehmer larger masses of gelatin must be exposed forty minutes to a temperature of 100° to 120° C., and this after a preliminary warming, before all tetanus spores are killed. Many of those who have used gelatin injections have not been aware that it is necessary to so extend the period of sterilization.

In quite a number of fatal cases of tetanus following gelatin injections it was subsequently demonstrated that the gelatin used contained tetanus bacilli or spores. In other cases the sterilized gelatin left was found free from living tetanus spores. We understand now that the sterilization was insufficient, and while it may have made one part of the gelatin free from tetanus spores, it left them alive in other portions.

Doerfler states that prolonged and energetic sterilization does not at all interfere with the therapeutic value of gelatin, and that if indeed sterile it is absolutely void of any danger. He concedes that the great hopes placed in gelatin injections in the treatment of aortic aneurism have not been realized, but that it has done excellent service in tubercular hæmoptysis, or pulmonary hemorrhage from other causes, in intestinal, renal, vesical, and uterine hemorrhages, in hæmophilia, and in melena neonatorum.—*Journal of the American Medical Association,* July 4, 1903.

Reports of Society Meetings.

THE NEW YORK INSTITUTE OF STOMATOLOGY.

A MEETING of the Institute was held at the " Chelsea," No. 222 West Twenty-third Street, New York, on Tuesday, January 6, 1903, the President, Dr. J. Morgan Howe, in the chair.

The minutes of the previous meeting were read and approved.

On account of the lateness of the hour, the communications on theory and practice were omitted. Dr. H. A. Baker, of Boston, Mass., read a paper entitled " Treatment of Protruding and Receding Jaws by the Use of the Intermaxillary Elastics."

(For Dr. Baker's paper, see page 344.)

DISCUSSION.

Dr. C. F. Allen said that, in considering the beautiful work we have seen to-day, as the result of Dr. Baker's methods, it is very hard to differentiate and say how much credit belongs to Dr. Baker, and how much to Dr. Angle. Both of the gentlemen have been working along similar lines; that is, Dr. Baker uses the expansion arch connected with bands fastened to the back teeth as advocated and practised by Dr. Angle, and he in no way antagonizes Dr. Angle's methods or apparatus; *per contra,* Dr. Baker has given us his system of intermaxillary elastics, and these are used in connection with the expansion arch as well by Dr. Angle as by Dr. Baker.

The reciprocal action of these intermaxillary elastics designed by Dr. Baker is perfect; there is absolutely no waste force, and those difficult cases of protruding upper jaws which have been to us all such a serious problem are now made comparatively easy, and the time necessary to bring about the reduction of this malocclusion is easily lessened from fifty to seventy-five per cent. All praise to Dr. Baker! It almost starts a new epoch in orthodontia.

There was present this afternoon at the informal exhibition of patients at Dr. Kimball's office a distinguished member of our profession who has probably done more of this kind of work than any of us. I refer to Dr. Kingsley, and he, looking at the patient

I had in hand, and praising greatly the quick and beautiful results attained by Dr. Baker's methods, said to me, "*Now keep them there.*" He knew what he was saying, and his adjuration to me was born of large experience; and here again comes in the beauty of this intermaxillary combination,—it makes in many ways an ideal retaining device, and it is with its aid that I hope to keep these teeth and these jaws in their proper position.

Dr. E. A. Bogue said that between Dr. Angle and Dr. Baker we were learning a great deal about regulating. Dr. Allan spoke of the "angle appliance." Dr. Bogue's impression was that this went back as far as the "Kingsley appliance," and maybe still farther back. Dr. Allan also mentioned the serious problem of retaining teeth. Dr. Bogue was pleased to hear again from Dr. Baker, regarding his son's case, that owing to lack of time he had been unable to make a retaining appliance, and so left the regulating fixture in place, which made the best possible retaining appliance.

Dr. Bogue said that Dr. Baker did not refer to malocclusion with anything like the emphasis that he might have done. Because upon that point retention depended very largely. The teeth get out of position for various reasons, but when once replaced, the cusps of the occluding teeth would hold them in place. When both arches have been regulated, if the lower teeth are properly retained, we need not bother about the upper ones, if the occlusion is right.

Dr. Bogue believed that regulating should be commenced as soon as the permanent first molars were sufficiently developed to hold an appliance.

Dr. Baker had shown us a case where he had stated that the chin, by actual measurement, was a quarter of an inch farther back after he had finished with it. Dr. Bogue thought if he would consider the relation of the molars and bicuspids, upper and lower, before and after the regulating, and then take into consideration the nature of the hinge of the inferior maxilla, this apparent retraction of the chin would be accounted for. The lower jaw had really been dropped and the chin was consequently retracted. The work Dr. Baker was engaged in was intensely interesting, and it was work that claimed all that was best in a man.

Dr. N. W. Kingsley spoke of seeing at Dr. Kimball's office a case treated by Dr. Allan, according to Dr. Baker's method, and said that he had never seen so ingenious an appliance for this purpose. Dr. Kingsley had regulated many similar cases in past years, but by entirely different methods; this plan of Dr. Baker's was so much more simple and quite as effective, that Dr. Kingsley said that he envied Dr. Baker the credit for having invented it.

Dr. Kingsley added that his greatest satisfaction at this time was, that the question of jumping the bite seemed to have been universally accepted and settled. He believed that he was the first person who ever adopted and carried out that principle of correcting malocclusion of the jaws, and that the term originated with him. That twenty-five years or more ago he had corrected a case in a very brief space of time, and was exhibiting models of the result at a meeting of the Odontological Society. Some one asked how it was done, and Dr. Kingsley answered, on the spur of the moment, that he "jumped the bite." The phrase was taken up, the method discussed, and the facts disputed for many years, notably by Dr. Talbot, of Chicago. Therefore all the gentlemen could appreciate the pleasure it gave him to see that the principles had not only been accepted, but the method of accomplishing it improved upon by Dr. Baker.

Dr. Ashley Faught would like to ask Dr. Baker a little more explicitly regarding the bands he used, and also as to the guide of tension and pressure. Dr. Faught used what are known as election bands, although he had some a little larger in circumference and a little thinner made for him by the Goodyear Rubber Co. His guide of tension was what pressure could be comfortably stood by the patient.

Dr. Geo. S. Allan would like to ask Dr. Baker or Dr. Kingsley to more clearly define just what changes take place in this so-called "jumping the bite."

Dr. Kingsley did not believe any one could tell.

Dr. C. F. Allen said, in relation to this question, that Dr. McBride delivered a paper before the Association of American Dentists. in Europe, upon this subject. He thinks there is a change in the articulation. In a letter that Dr. Allen had recently received from Dr. McBride. he stated that he was going to make some experiments upon monkeys and then kill the monkeys, with a view to obtaining information upon this subject.

Dr. Baker. in closing. said that he had been criticised many times for regulating teeth too fast. but he thought that when we know just where we are going to move them, the teeth could not be moved too rapidly. The teeth always gave a timely warning if it were necessary to relieve the pressure. The fact that he made no false steps would account for some of the rapidity with which he completed the work. Two months was the rule in cases of anterior protrusion.

Dr. Bogue seemed to think he did not put stress enough upon the bad effects of extraction. Dr. Baker thought the cases calling for extraction were very rare, indeed, if they ever occurred. He believed that in fifteen years he had not extracted a tooth for regulating purposes.

It was a point of great satisfaction to him that Dr. Kingsley could be present, and he was much gratified at his favorable criticisms. The profession were greatly indebted to Dr. Kingsley.

It was moved and seconded that a vote of thanks be extended to Dr. Baker for his excellent paper and his kindness in demonstrating this subject so carefully. The thanks of the Institute were also extended to Dr. Baker's patient.

At the afternoon clinic the following case was presented by Dr. C. F. Allen:

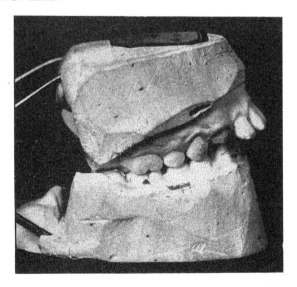

Master W. H., aged eleven years, a case of protruding upper incisors with receding lower jaw; lower front teeth elongated and impinging on palatal surface of upper jaw.

Treated solely from within the mouth with intermaxillary elastics, as suggested by Dr. Baker, of Boston.

First elastics put on November 14, and case practically finished December 20, the protruding upper teeth in proper position, the anterior lower teeth shortened in their sockets and in proper relation with the upper teeth; both jaws in proper occlusion.

Present fixture used for the correction of the malocclusion will probably be the only retaining device used.

Adjourned.

THE annual meeting of The New York Institute of Stomatology was held on Tuesday evening, December 1, 1903, and the following officers were elected for 1904:

President, A. H. Brockway; Vice-President, C. O. Kimball; Recording Secretary, H. L. Wheeler; Corresponding Secretary, J. B. Locherty; Treasurer, J. A. Bishop; Editor, F. L. Bogue; Curator, S. H. McNaughton.

Executive Committee.—S. E. Davenport, Chairman, C. F. Allen, F. Milton Smith.

A REGULAR meeting of The New York Institute of Stomatology was held at the " Chelsea," No. 222 West Twenty-third Street, New York, on Tuesday evening, January 5, 1904, the President, Dr. Brockway, in the chair.

The minutes of the last regular meeting and of the annual meeting were read and approved.

Under the head of " Practical Talks on Interesting Subjects," Dr. S. F. Howland discussed the subject of sensitive necks of teeth.

Dr. Howland stated that we frequently found at the neck of a tooth extreme sensitiveness, which condition was very annoying to both patient and operator. Not very much had ever been said upon this subject except the advocation of nitrate of silver. This seemed to be objectionable, because it discolored the teeth. Dr. Howland stated that he had used with great success tannic acid, which was the active principle of all vegetable astringents. His method was to place a drop or two of glycerin on a slab and mix it with tannic acid. He then sharpened a stick to a flat blunt point, and after drying the sensitive point to be treated he applied the mixture and with the stick rubbed very gently at first, gradually increasing the pressure until finally he was able to rub the tooth as hard as he wished without any pain whatever. One application was usually sufficient. Although a remedy was seldom found that would never fail, Dr. Howland could not remember an instancee where this method had failed to give relief. In reply to a question of Dr. F. Milton Smith, as to how long this relief was expected to last, Dr. Howland had never noted a recurrence of the sensitiveness. He not only used it to reduce this sensitiveness where there was no real decay of the tooth-structure, but he also used it as an obtundent in the same way.

In reply to a question from Dr. S. E. Davenport as to whether this pressure with the stick was necessary, Dr. Howland had never tried it any other way, as it had seemed very effective when rubbed with the stick.

Under the same head, Dr. T. W. Onderdonk stated that he had several things which he wished to present. First, a set of scalers (Fig. 1), which were no more nor less than heavy enamel chisels, one right, one left, and one direct, all curved, with concave cutting edges which act very much as half-round scrapers do in scraping the mast of a boat.

Second, a compromise dental engine arm, which consists of a duplex spring (Fig. 1), with which most cable engines are equipped, a hand-piece attached to one end, and a small pulley wheel to the other (*c*). This is attached to the forearm of any all-cord engine at *cd,* giving all the freedom of the cable engine, together with the direct revolution of the all-cord engine, without the disagreeable features of either.

Third, an electric crown heater (Fig. 2, *a*), an instrument, as its name implies, for softening the gutta-percha cement of crowns and bridges so attached, when their removal is desired. It is a curved strip of metal with some high-heat gutta-percha on the inner surface, attached to one end of the electric tool holder. To use it, bend the metal so that it will pass over the crown to be removed, turn on the current, and in a few seconds the crown can be taken off.

Fourth, Dr. Onderdonk stated that he considered the following general features essential for an ideal matrix. The matrix should grasp the tooth tightly at the cervical margin and at the same time restoring the natural contour. It should be easily adjusted and not interfere with the introduction of the filling, not easily displaced but removable at will, permitting the examination of the filling as it progresses, and be returned to its original position.

He then presented a band dentometer, contour matrix and holder. The apparatus consisted of two parts, band and holder.

FIG. 1.

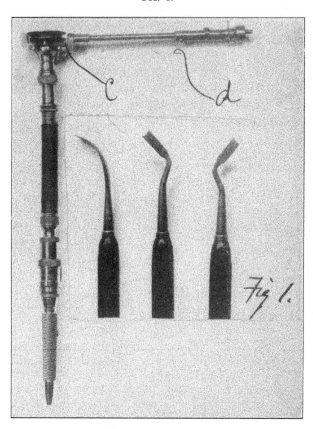

The bands (Fig. 2, *b, c*) are cut from strips of very thin metal, either brass or German silver, two inches long and the width the case requires. For a dentometer the bands are cut straight (Fig. 2, *b*). For a matrix the bands are cut curved, the greater the curve the larger the contour (Fig. 2, *c*). The holder consists of three parts. The movable jaw, or vice, the fixed jaw, or holder, and the rotary handle. The movable jaw (Fig. 2, *d*) is of brass about one and a half inches long and three-eighths of an inch in diameter, with a hole through the centre for the introduction of the fixed jaw and a slot for the bands to enter.

The fixed jaw, or holder (Fig. 2, *e*), is about three inches long and one-eighth of an inch in diameter, with a screw thread cut

FIG. 2.

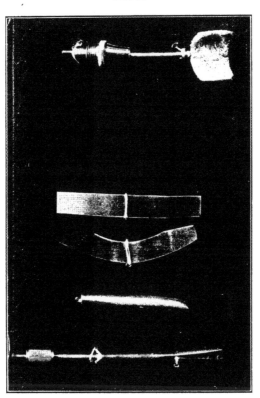

almost the entire length; on one end is the grip, which is very much like a small pair of tape pliers, containing two pins which grasp the metal bands. The rotary handle (Fig. 2, *f*) is about the same diameter as the movable holder, and is from one-half to three-quarters of an inch in length; this turns on the screw thread of the fixed jaw.

Dr. S. E. Davenport thought that Dr. Onderdonk was getting

himself into trouble, as those who were not fortunate enough to sit near to him during these demonstrations would be besieging him at his office, where, as Dr. Davenport had found recently, Dr. Onderdonk was able to explain the many advantages of the appliances in even a better manner than he had done to-night.

Dr. Davenport would like to ask, in the case of a combination gold and amalgam stopping such as Dr. Onderdonk mentioned, where the gold was applied before the amalgam had crystallized, whether Dr. Onderdonk depended upon separate anchorage for the gold, or did he expect a union between the gold and amalgam sufficient to hold the gold? Dr. Davenport said he would also like to know what gold and what amalgam Dr. Onderdonk used.

Dr. Onderdonk stated that it was not his intention to enter into the discussion of the technique of filling teeth, and he merely had mentioned this method to bring out the value of his appliance. His preference was to fill the amalgam portion at one sitting and the gold afterwards, when the amalgam was hard. But if for any reason it was impracticable, the gold could be introduced at once. In either case he treated the gold filling exactly as if it, the amalgam, were tooth-structure. He used Fellowship alloy and Moss fibre gold usually, annealing it in the electric furnace. If the amalgam had not set, he used the first pieces of gold small, forcing them into the amalgam. In certain cavities in bicuspids it was his custom always to use amalgam with the gold. In these cases he preferred the amalgam soft, forcing the gold into it.

Regarding the central that he mentioned, which he filled with amalgam posteriorly, Dr. Onderdonk stated that in giving the operation in detail of course he would use a lining of cement next the anterior enamel, to prevent discoloration. He considered this method good practice in certain cases, rather than to resort to a crown. He never crowned a central tooth if he could avoid it.

Dr. Chas. O. Kimball, regarding various devices, wished to speak first of Dr. Onderdonk's appliance. He had had a couple made some time ago in accordance with Dr. Onderdonk's plans, but he found upon examination that they were not like these. These were much better. He found them exceedingly useful instruments. They were of great value in inserting a composition filling where considerable pressure was desired. Such a matrix could be removed without placing any strain on the filling. He had used them frequently in the amalgam and cement stoppings.

Dr. Kimball also spoke of a trifling little device which he had found almost invaluable. Many of those present used for polishing teeth the little soft rubber cups. If their experience had been like his, they had been found very satisfactory for that purpose, as by this appliance it was possible to polish under the free margin of the gum. This was important in order to polish the teeth thoroughly. These little rubber disks will curve and work up under the margin of the gum on the rounded surfaces of the teeth that are accessible with this instrument. Dr. Kimball had found this difficulty: in a wet mouth the saliva would work back and get into the hand-piece, so that it required to be frequently taken apart and cleaned. It had occurred to him some time ago that this could be obviated by reversing one of the cup-shaped disks and placing it on the shank of the instrument. This worked very well, but with the curious result that when it was revolving the slightest touch would cause it to work right away from the hand-piece and up to the point of the instrument. At first he had cut a groove on the shank and slipped the disk into that, but that had not proved quite strong enough, although it was an improvement. Recently he had soldered, with soft solder, a ring of wire on the shank. This worked perfectly.

Dr. Kimball called attention to the hickory sticks for holding the gum back in cervical operations. He had mentioned this method two years previously. Since that time he had been using another device of the same nature. Instead of the hickory he used a piece of thin steel cut and shaped to fit the individual case and then soldered with soft solder to a broken instrument. This could be cut carefully to fit the curve of the tooth and the gum, holding back the gum with the least possible pain.

Dr. Kimball also presented a very useful instrument for polishing fillings, particularly in concave surfaces that could not be reached with the strips or disks. It consisted of a long instrument, thin and flat at each end, one end charged with corundum, held to the instrument with shellac, and the other end carrying a small piece of Lake Superior stone held in the same manner.

Dr. Gillett, referring to the instrument mentioned by Dr. Kimball for holding the gum back, thought that in many instances an instrument not so long, and that could be held by placing the finger on the end of it, was of great advantage. Also, instead of having the end broad and flat, it was sometimes desirable to have it terminate in points, even a single point being oftentimes desirable.

Dr. F. Milton Smith wished to disclaim originality regarding the gold inlays credited to him by Dr. Onderdonk. As he had previously stated, the method was brought to his attention first by Dr. Rheinhold, of this city. Dr. Dwight Smith, of this city, had also given him some valuable ideas. His own work in this direction was the result of the combined ideas of these two gentlemen and others, with perhaps a trifle of ingenuity on his own part. His friend Dr. Rheinhold stated to him that Dr. Andrews, of New York City, first called his attention to these tips. As Dr. Smith remembered it, the specimen in the cast passed around, *combining* the abraded surface repair and the two approximal surface restorations, was first suggested by Dr. Dwight Smith.

Dr. Kimball stated, relative to the union between gold and amalgam that he had occasion, many years ago, to repair an old amalgam filling with gold. He had done this with no thought of a union between the two, but had prepared a natural retention for the gold. Some time after, the tooth had broken and the whole filling came out. He was surprised to find that although the amalgam filling had been inserted many years before the gold, the two had become firmly united, so that they could be separated with great difficulty.

Dr. Gillett had great faith in these combinations, and used the gold and amalgam fillings to a large extent in favorable cavities. It was his practice always to pack the gold directly on the fresh amalgam, believing that he got a better filling thereby than by doing the operation in two sittings.

Dr. S. E. Davenport thought Dr. Gillett's remarks proved that Dr. Dwight Clapp's influence in New York City was very strong still, and he was very glad of it.

Dr. J. Morgan Howe called attention to a paper by Professor R. H. Thurston, of Cornell University, on " Scientific Research," published in *Science,* September 12, 1902, in which he stated that the late Roberto Austin, an English metallurgist, had placed lead and gold in contact, " and later found that the molecules of gold had started off on a journey independently, into the lead, some of them reaching a distance from their original positions of two inches in as many years." Dr. Howe thought this item worth recording in this connection as throwing some light on the peculiar results observed in combining gold with tin, and gold with amalgam, in fillings.

Dr. H. L. Wheeler read a short paper entitled " Home Manufacture of Formaldehyde for Sterilizing Purposes."

(For Dr. Wheeler's paper, see page 364.)

Dr. Henry W. Gillett read a short paper on " Perplexities in Connection with Extraction of Teeth."

(For Dr. Gillett's paper, see page 368.)

Dr. Swift stated that he had been using this method of sterilization for some time in the form of the Low sterilizer. It had given great satisfaction. The apparatus was manufactured by the Buffalo Dental Manufacturing Company. The sterilizing agent was produced by a cone of sponge platinum fitted over the alcohol lamp. The shape of the instrument was very satisfactory.

Dr. Gillett agreed with Dr. Swift regarding the Low sterilizer. He thought it a very satisfactory apparatus, although he could see no reason why the one devised by Dr. Wheeler would not be of value. Regarding the other part of the paper, Dr. Wheeler argues that the dental profession has suffered greatly from dental patents; *ergo,* there should be no dental patents. Great injury had resulted from the misuse of drugs, but for that reason it would hardly be wise to give up drugs entirely. It would seem that Dr. Wheeler's statement, that the result of patent litigation was always in favor of the organized corporation, was one of the best possible arguments in favor of Dr. Crouse's organization, which Dr. Wheeler is refusing to support. By doing this he was refusing to take the one essential step to make effective the opposition to *unjust* dental patents. It was the unfair dental patents that were objectionable, and it was time now for the profession to rally and make effective the means of opposing these unjust patents. The opportunity should be taken advantage of promptly, lest it be lost.

Dr. Wheeler stated that he was acquainted with the Low sterilizer, but that the cone, instead of being sponge platinum as stated, was really made of platinized asbestos, and required frequent renewal.

Dr. H. W. Gillett read a paper entitled " Spalding's Porcelain Jacket Crown."

(For Dr. Gillett's paper, see page 362.)

Dr. McNaughton presented to the museum of the Institute some curios in the way of teeth carved from ivory, and the superior maxilla of a "sheep's-head" fish. These were donated by Dr. Nash.

A vote of thanks was extended to Dr. Nash for his kindness in presenting these interesting specimens to the Institute.

Dr. Fossume presented an engine attachment for carrying wooden points, used in cleansing and polishing teeth.

Adjourned.

FRED. L. BOGUE, M.D., D.D.S.
Editor The New York Institute of Stomatology.

AMERICAN MEDICAL ASSOCIATION, SECTION ON STOMATOLOGY.

(Concluded from page 217.)

FOURTH SESSION.

THE meeting was called to order at 2.10 P.M., with Dr. M. H. Fletcher, of Cincinnati, in the Chair.

DISCUSSION ON DR. WILLIAM E. WALKER'S PAPER ON "ORTHODONTIC FACIAL ORTHOMORPHIA."

(For Dr. Walker's paper, see page 193.)

Dr. Eugene S. Talbot.—It is very necessary that we should understand the etiology in order to treat these cases successfully. It is unfortunate that in this country the majority of the men treating these cases are mechanics, not pretending to know anything about the etiology. Indeed, one of the best men in the country in this line of work, says he does not care for the etiology, that it is enough for him to be able to treat the conditions. I was surprised and pleased when I went into Dr. Walker's office to find that he grasped the essential idea. It requires a great deal of time and study to understand the manner in which these conditions are produced, and in order to study this one particular phase we must go back to the time of Aristotle. Aristotle laid down the law of economy of growth, whereby the structure or organ is lost for the benefit of the organism as a whole. All students in evolution have based their work on that law. I know of no better work on this subject than "From the Greeks to Darwin." This law of economy of growth is illustrated in many structures, but those of the face, jaws, and teeth are the most important to us. They are being lost for the benefit of the brain. That is the reason we have so much decay in the teeth. That is the reason the jaws grow smaller and the teeth, while they do not grow smaller, work in harmony with this arrest of development. Because of this arrest of development of the jaws and because the great diameter of the teeth is larger than the jaws, we have this arrest of development and irregularities. In the evolution of man we also have atavism, so that in these patients which we call neurasthenic and which I call degenerates, where there is an arrest of development, there is also frequently excessive development. These are beautifully illustrated in two pictures which I shall give to you. One is of Judas. If the painter lived at the present time he could not have portrayed a better representation of a degenerate than he has done. The second picture is that of Charles V. of Spain. Those of you familiar with the history will recall that Charles V. suffered with indigestion all his life; that he could not eat, and that he kept ten cooks preparing food for him. Two hundred years after his death a photograph was taken of his skeleton in the coffin, showing this type of face. With the mouth closed the lower jaw shut above the upper. In other words, the upper teeth closed inside the lower jaw. We had no Walkers at that time, and therefore he could not have his teeth regulated. The lower jaw is a movable organ, and because of this it is frequently more fully developed when the upper jaw, which is attached to the bones of the skull, becomes arrested in development, and hence we have this marked deformity. It is possible that the lower jaw in some cases will be excessively developed and there atavism enters. If such cases are taken at the age of thirteen when the alveolar process is in construction there is a possibility of moving these teeth and having the alveolar process remain with them. If the correction is made at the age of twenty to twenty-four, there is more motion, producing inflammation in the alveolar process and preventing its restoration. Therefore, I question how far we, as operators, are justified in correcting irregularities of the teeth. Every patient coming to us like this little one referred to is a degenerate, having an unstable nervous system. When we undertake to regulate these teeth we put a pressure upon the nervous system of that child which is a very serious matter. I have known many cases laid up from one to three years in bed from nervous prostration as a result of dentists

15

regulating these teeth and not knowing when they were producing neurasthenics. I do not believe that the ordinary dentist should undertake to treat these cases, but one who is medically educated and who is familiar with the general nervous system. I shall look with great interest and pleasure for the results in these cases Dr. Walker has in hand, and which he is so well able to treat.

Mr. T. E. Constant.—I should like to congratulate Dr. Walker upon the method he has pursued in the correction of the deformity, and I can quite concur with him in what he says with regard to the necessity of studying his cases. Very often in the condition where the upper incisor teeth apear to protrude we find that a study of the etiology results in showing a still greater deformity. In many cases diagnosed as superior protrusion the condition is really one of inferior retrusion. This is admirably represented in one case, and I am sorry the patient is not here.

I quite disagree with Dr. Talbot in what he says regarding the moving of the teeth. I think there is no reason, if a good bite is obtained after the teeth have been removed, why the result should not be permanent. The only thing I fear is that it would be extremely difficult to obtain a bite that would be permanent. That will depend entirely upon the condition with which the teeth occlude when the case is finished.

Dr. M. H. Fletcher.—I have nothing to say except in commendation of the essayist from the stand-point he takes, which would indicate his ability to cope with the case. I fully concur with Dr. Talbot in his condemnation of the efforts of incompetent men to do this work. Personally, I have had three cases sent to me in a state of collapse almost from ineffectual efforts of men who apparently understand nothing about the work or had no conception of the stress to the patient. The cases resulted in an absolute failure and a good wholesome fear on the part of the patient of everybody who would undertake the work. These cases have made me a little more timid in my own efforts. The position of the patient and the varying conditions of health, also the surroundings at home have great bearing upon these cases. I see that the child has absolute co-operation and encouragement of the home people. I have had several cases in which there was a tendency to make light of and poke fun at the patient. I absolutely demand that such things shall stop. Otherwise I give up the case. I am to have the absolute co-operation of every one of the family, and I find that better progress is made in this way. The child must have normal recreation. My plan is never to proceed with any painful measure until restoration of the nervous system is complete. As Dr. Talbot has said, it is a pleasure to see these cases presented by Dr. Walker, who is able to carry them to a successful end.

Dr. H. E. Belden, New Orleans.—I agree with Dr. Talbot that the operation carried on in adult life does not always meet with success, especially where a good deal of motion is acquired. I had a case of a young lady whose teeth protruded a great deal. I brought the teeth back to their place, but she has to wear a band to this day. I agree also with Mr. Constant that if the occlusion is good we are more apt to have a successful issue. We see many bridges which, because of inaccurate occlusion, patients are unable to wear.

Dr. Walker.—Showing how little the treatment interfered with this man's nervous condition, I may remark that he took during the treatment two years' course of law in one year and graduated. He has not yet secured occlusion. This we hope to obtain later. The patient tells us that he had not much pain, a little at the first. The bands worn were always stationary.

Dr. M. L. Rhein.—I was very much pleased to hear the remarks of Dr. Talbot in the discussion of this subject. His words almost exactly expressed my views. I think it fortunate that he should have brought out this point of criticism against men doing work of this nature strictly from a mechanical point without regard to the etiological factors at work. In this country of ours it is unfortunate that a certain class of men get a pseudo sort of dental education, with some mechanical dexterity, and appear before the public as advertised specialists on orthodontia. Personally I am a believer in the specialty of stomatology as a specialty of medicine, but I am opposed to any further subdivision of the work. I believe that the stomatologist should have the entire care of the individual mouth under his charge, and if the distinctive and individual portions of the work are to be divided up for the better method of execution, it all ought to remain under his personal supervision. There are a few exceptions, men who have the proper education back of their ability to handle the work. The amount of damage that is done by men improperly qualified is very great. It is my opinion that work cannot be commenced too early in these cases of irregularity. The same principle is brought out here as in the work of Lorenz. The softer the bones are when we handle them, the more easily are they moulded and the better are the results. I have attempted a number of corrections after the age of twenty, and the results have never come up to my hope. It seems almost impossible to get occlusion that is what might be called self-locking. I do not wish to decry the work that can be done at a certain age, but to say that the best results are obtained in the early work. I have at present two patients, one of the age of eight and the other of nine. There was much question in the mind of the parent whether to have work commenced at the time, and the opinion of a number of men was sought. A large number of the profession have the idea that work should be delayed until all the permanent teeth are erupted.

I take exception to the view that the permanent apparatus is less painful than the temporary. There is more than one way of applying one apparatus. I know of no apparatus that will work so painlessly, so easily, so rapidly without the patient paying attention to it as that devised by Dr. Ottolengui. It has only recently been described by him, although it has been in use for some time. I agree that if the work upon the bones cannot be done without giving pain and causing nervous tension, there is a mistake somewhere, and that much harm will be done the child under such conditions. These patients come to my office sometimes as often as four times a week without any evidence of nervous depression. I claim that that is an absolute necessity if the work is to be done at the early age in which the best results can be obtained.

Dr. Walker (closing).—I feel very much pleased with the way in which the presentation has been received, but I must disagree on some of the points. Dr. Talbot, for instance, I think made a reflection upon the effect of this work upon neurasthenics. The child referred to is a most decided neurasthenic, but since I have been working upon her teeth her health has been manifestly improved daily. As the treatment continued, her mental, physical, and nervous condition became better. I think this has been partly due to the self-control I have caused her to exert. Heretofore, the least disturbance would cause her to cry.

The Chairman has stated that the work should be practically painless. He is undoubtedly right in that. The old way of regulating by movable appliances did cause a great deal of pain and damage to the nervous system. With the fixed appliance, however, the soreness does not ensue. I have used Jackson's appliance for some time. It is the one to use when the teeth are coming in. If the teeth are in place the fixed apparatus is better because a greater force is required than can be secured with the Jackson appliance without producing soreness. I agree with the Chairman that the work should be done while the teeth are coming in.

I think no one system should be adhered to, but that the good of all should be selected for the case to which it is adapted. We should undoubtedly avoid producing pain on account of the injury to the nervous system. In cases in which not much pressure or a great degree of speed is needed I feel that a movable apparatus is the one to employ.

Mr. Constant is correct in saying that many cases of inferior retrusion are diagnosed as superior protrusion and so treated and the patients disfigured.

In regard to specialization, I do not by any means think that a man should practice orthodontia without previous general practice, but I think more will be accomplished by a man taking up a specialty after a number of years spent in general practice, and then working in sympathy with the general practitioner.

A paper was read by Dr. George F. Eames, of Boston, entitled "The Therapeutic Use of the X-Ray in the Oral Cavity."

(For Dr. Eames's paper, see page 356.)

(For Dr. Eames's paper, see page 356.)

DISCUSSION.

Dr. Eugene S. Talbot.—I can say very little on this subject, because I have had no experience in this line. I have heard that Dr. Price, of Cleveland, is doing some remarkable work in interstitial gingivitis with this apparatus. From what the essayist has said, and from what I have heard from others, I see no reason why this should not do splendid work in this disease. It has not been tried long enough to give any definite results. It is barely possible that, because of the situation of the tissues inside the mouth, satisfactory results have not been obtained. I regret very much that I am not familiar with the subject and able to discuss it. I would like to ask Dr. Eames if the elimination of the oxygen is comparable to the effect produced in the two poles. I remember a demonstration that was made with a piece of meat in which the coagulation of albumin was made at the cathode pole. Do I understand that the action here is similar to that? From what does it eliminate the oxygen.

Dr. Eames.—The oxygen is liberated from the air which is contained in the tissues and whatever may be surrounding the tissues. It goes right through and decomposes everything with which it comes in contact.

Dr. Fletcher.—I suppose the rays can be seen coming out the other side, if examined with the fluoroscope?

Dr. Eames.—It penetrates the tissues depending upon the tube. The low vacuum or soft tube has greater power for destruction of tissues, but it does not penetrate so far. With surface conditions the soft tube is desirable, because it does greater work. In a growth in the stomach we would have to have a tube of higher power and the quality of the electricity changed greatly.

Dr. Fletcher.—In this case, do you have to use a soft tube?

Dr. Eames.—Yes, that penetrates deeply enough. The distance in the mouth does not count because we hold the tube near the face, so that practically a place in the mouth is on the surface.

Dr. W. E. Walker, New Orleans.—I have had no experience with the X-ray in therapeutic work. Dr. Woodward, of this city, tells me that he has secured very satisfactory results in Riggs's disease with the X-ray.

Dr. Fletcher.—Did he couple it with any other treatment?

Dr. Walker.—What I have told you is as much as he told me.

Dr. Hans Pilcher, Vienna.—I would like to ask Dr. Eames if there is any possibility of the X-ray having any influence upon calcareous pericementitis if it is not removed?

Dr. Eames (closing).—There is very little for me to say beyond what is contained in the paper. I might say, in addition to this paper, that the sun's rays have been utilized in a therapeutic way, and those who have used the actinic rays, so-called, from the sun have in a very simple and inexpensive manner achieved results in many cases similar to that in the use of the X-ray. It only waits for a trial to see whether the rays of the sun may be utilized in the mouth. The use of the sun's rays, of course, is limited to the time when the sun shines. That alone would indicate an opening for some one to utilize the rays for the therapeutic treatment of disease.

A paper entitled " Methods of controlling Hemorrhage of the Oral Cavity" was read by Dr. H. T. Belden, of New Orleans. (For Dr. Belden's paper, see Vol. XXIV., page 502.)

DISCUSSION.

Dr. M. L. Rhein.—The use of adrenalin in dentistry and its advantage should be known to all of us. I simply echo its value as an important part of our pharmacopœia in dental work.

Dr. George F. Eames.—I have used the extract of the suprarenal glands and the various preparations made from it for some time, and I can only say that my experience with it has been very satisfactory. It is the most wonderful drug in the control of hemorrhage I have ever used. In some cases it does not seem to act, but these cases are so rare that they may be classed as cases of idiosyncrasy or peculiar unsusceptibility to the drug. I think Dr. Belden is correct in saying that it probably does enhance the effect of cocaine, but that alone it is not an anæsthetic.

The peculiar diathesis of a patient should be considered and the greatest caution used in the preparation of the patient for an operation which is apt to cause hemorrhage.

Dr. M. L. Rhein.—I do not agree with Drs. Belden and Eames in their views concerning the anæsthetic properties of adrenalin. I believe that we as stomatologists demand a much more profound anæsthesia than the laryngologist in his work. I do not believe it is possible to obtain profound anæsthesia—that is, local anæsthesia—with the chloride of adrenalin. Used in the nose or the eye, a certain amount of anæsthesia is unquestionably obtained, but the fact that it is not complete anæsthesia I think blinds us to the anæsthetic properties that it does possess. I think this anæsthetic property is produced mechanically by the contraction of the capillaries expelling the nerve-cells from the fibrillæ. The fact that we are not satisfied with its obtunding effect is not proof that it has not a certain amount of anæsthetic property.

The papers of Dr. Richard Grady, of Baltimore, upon " The Dentist in the United States Navy," and of Dr. Alice N. Steeves, of Boston, upon " Medical and Dental Libraries," were read by title.

Editorial.

THE REPLY OF "TRINITY UNIVERSITY."

THE INTERNATIONAL of April contained a "Reply from 'Trinity University,' Toronto," Canada, in answer to a charge made in the February number that this University was graduating men, with the degree of Doctor of Dental Surgery, upon examination. This reply from the pen of the Secretary of the Board of Dental Studies, Trinity University, does not seem to the writer to meet satisfactorily the issue as presented.

The main question is, Does the Trinity University grant the dental degree upon an examination? While this is not denied, it is met in a way that leaves the reader to infer that lectures are the all-important method of training in dentistry. The Secretary says, " A careful study of the curriculum . . . will, I feel sure, lead you to recognize that the knowledge required to obtain a D.D.S. from this University is equal to that required by the most advanced dental institutions on this continent." This very broad statement needs confirmation, and the published curriculum should show it if it exists.

The following quotations are made from the " Extract from the University Calendar" giving " the regulations governing the degree of D.D.S." After stating terms of admission, the candidate " must pass three University examinations, called the First, Second, and Third Examinations in Dentistry."

" Before admission to the First Examination he must have attended, in some dental college, recognized by this University, one course of lectures on the following subjects: Chemistry, Anatomy, Histology, Bacteriology, Comparative Dental Anatomy, Technique, Metallurgy." The subjects of the first examination are then given in detail.

For the Second Examination the candidate must have attended " lectures on the following subjects: Operative Dentistry, Prosthetic Dentistry, Anatomy, Physiology, Chemistry, Medicine and Surgery, Materia Medica." It will be interesting to practical men to know the extent of the examination in Operative Dentistry. It comprises " Development of the teeth, clinical history and pathology of caries, pulpitis, pericementitis, and alveolar abscess, the composition and preparation of materials for filling teeth." Subsequently it is stated that "Candidates will be required to satisfy the examiners in Practical Dentistry as to Operative and Prosthetic work, crown- and bridge-work and Orthodontia, either by practical work done under their supervision or by certificate from a recognized dental college."

The Third, or Final, Examination covers about all the subjects enumerated in the First and Second Examinations. The following concludes this matter: "Candidates who present certificates of having passed the First and Second Year Examinations, in some recognized dental college or university, will be admitted to third year standing." Farther on we find the following remarkable paragraph, heretofore quoted in original article. *" All legally qualified* practitioners of dental surgery of Great Britain, or of any portion of the British Empire, *will be admitted to the Final Examination without passing further matriculation and without further attendance on lectures."* (Italics ours.)

It must be evident from these quotations that the assertion that the "knowledge required to obtain a D.D.S. from this University [Trinity] is equal to that required by the most advanced dental institutions on this continent" is only true in theory. Nothing practical is taught, and certificates as to proficiency in practical matters are accepted. The writer is forced to the conviction that this school is not only *not* equal to others on this continent, but is *not a dental school in any sense and is not deserving of that title.*

The Secretary tries very hard to modify the language of the paragraph quoted, and seems to think it "does not make the degree easy to obtain, nor does it call for a low standard of knowledge on the part of the candidates." He acknowledges that "The qualification of which the candidates must furnish proof in order to be admitted to the Final Examination, is that he has been licensed by the government of his own country for the practice of dental surgery, and that that country be a part of the British Empire." Then he proceeds to state, "As a matter of fact all parts of the empire, with only one or two minor exceptions, require regular apprenticeship and a College Course in order that a candidate may obtain his license to practise." Exactly where the "minor exceptions" are to be found he is careful not to mention. Attention was called in our original statement to one portion of the British Empire, and by no means an inconsiderable portion,—that of New Zealand,—where no dental college exists and where a state examination is alone required. If we are not mistaken, there are already at Trinity, or in the neighborhood preparing for the final examination, a candidate or candidates from that country, who will, doubtless, be given the D.D.S. under the ruling stated. The writer is not familiar with the status of affairs in South Africa relating to dental training, but the inference may be drawn that the acquisition of this portion of the empire has been too recent to establish any positive methods in dental training beyond the so-called apprenticeship system.

The secretary lays special stress upon the fact that the candidate, upon receiving the degree of D.D.S., must promise not to resort to any unethical methods, and if at any time it can be shown that he has violated this promise " in any way," he agrees, upon demand, to surrender his diploma and have his name stricken from the rolls.

This seems to require an unbounded faith in human nature, but from experience the writer is of the opinion that the promise will be found to be hardly worth the time expended in exacting it from the candidate.

The writer holds that this method of conferring degrees is wrong in principle and worse in practice. It is a reiteration of the old idea, that no matter where a person has secured his knowledge, he is entitled to present the evidence in order to secure a degree. This, in theory, seems absolutely just and right; but in practice it had been found to be the chief promotor of all the fraudulent diploma traffic of this and other countries. The word examination may mean much or little, depending on who makes it and how it is made.

The secretary wonders how the writer came to the idea that the recipient (of this degree) is not to make use of it in the Dominion of Canada. It is due to " Trinity" to say that it is not responsible for this portion of the original charge. The secretary will find, on page 10 of the Announcements of the Royal College of Dental Surgery, a paragraph containing the following words. This was quoted in the February number, but must have been overlooked. It is repeated here: " Students of dentistry *not desiring to qualify for practice in the Province of Ontario,* by obtaining the L.D.S., of the R.C.D.S. of Ontario, may avail themselves of all the privileges of the School of Dentistry of the R.C.D.S., and proceed to the degree of Doctor of Dental Surgery, either in

the University of Toronto, or in Trinity University, or compliance
with the requirements of their Curriculum in Dentistry." (Italics
ours.) In plain English this means, to the writer's comprehension,
that the degree of D.D.S., as granted by "Trinity," does not
qualify for practice in Ontario. If this be not the correct interpretation, then it is time the scribe who prepared the Announcement of the Royal College of Dental Surgeons should change the
construction of the sentence, for the writer is not alone in his
interpretation.

The secretary acknowledges that after the first day of October
next the Trinity University will be united with the University of
Toronto and "exemptions allowed to regularly qualified practitioners of dental surgery within the British Empire will then cease
to be operative," and we tender our congratulations that a definite
period has been fixed when this very objectionable method will
come to an end with our good neighbors over the border.

Domestic Correspondence.

FIRST DISTRICT DENTAL SOCIETY OF NEW YORK.

To THE EDITOR:

SIR,—In the April number of the INTERNATIONAL, at page
320, appears a notice of election of officers of the First District
Dental Society of New York, under my name as Secretary.

Will you kindly inform me who is responsible for the notice?
I did not send it or authorize it, and it is incorrect, as it is in
advance of the annual meeting, which will not be held until the
12th inst. It is quite likely that some one will criticise this premature action, and I want to be in a position to place the responsibility where it belongs.

B. C. NASH,
Secretary.

[We regret that it is not possible to comply with the reasonable
wish of our correspondent. Copy of this character is not preserved.
When these notices are received they are supposed to be authorized,
and are published as sent.—ED.]

Miscellany.

LOCAL ANALGESIA BY ADRENALIN-EUCAINE.—Barker (*Lancet,*
July 25, 1903) *naïvely* remarks that this method of abolishing
pain has, with little doubt, a future before it. He states that he
believes, now that the principles which underlie it are well understood, it will be widely employed. Full credit is given to Corning
for his admirable work in this direction, and attention is called to
.the fact that because of the rapid absorption of the injected material no operation lasting more than twenty minutes can be performed without a constant reinfiltration of the tissues and nerves.

Beta-eucaine he notes is less toxic than cocaine; both these
drugs have the following drawbacks: (1) The difficulty of in-
jecting directly through the nerve-trunk and through the skin;
(2) the need of employing a large quantity of the solution of
1 to 500 to thoroughly anæsthetize a region supplied by several
nerve-trunks.

It is well known that anything which retards or diminishes the
circulation of the blood in a part infiltrated with an analgesic
agent enhances the potency of the latter. This fact suggested the
possibility of increasing the local anæsthetic effect of eucaine by
the injection of adrenalin, which would necessarily diminish the
stream of blood in the part. It was noted that after a lapse of
about twenty minutes the part thus injected with the combined
drugs was quite blanched and wholly insensitive to pain, and that
this loss of feeling lasted on an average about two hours. Barker
has been so well satisfied with the result of his first test that he
has employed the combination for several months, and with results
far superior to those produced by the eucaine alone. His method
of preparing the solution is as follows: To one hundred cubic
centimetres of boiled sterile water 0.2 gramme of beta-eucaine and
0.8 gramme of sodium chloride are added; thereafter eighteen
minims of adrenalin chloride (Parke, Davis & Co.) are dropped
from the stoppered bottle in which this drug comes into the eucaine
solution. If the bottle be corked at once, it will not spoil. This
makes a solution of 1 to 500 eucaine and 1 to 100,000 of adrenalin
chloride.

There were no instances of secondary hemorrhage, though a number of operations, such as those for the radical cure of hernia, were successfully performed.—*Therapeutic Gazette.*

Current News.

PENNSYLVANIA STATE BOARD OF DENTAL EXAMINERS.

THE Board of Dental Examiners of Pennsylvania will conduct examinations simultaneously in Philadelphia and Pittsburg, June 8 to 11, 1904. Applicants for examination and license must address the Hon. C. N. Schaeffer, Secretary Dental Council, Harrisburg, Pa., for papers or any further information.

NATIONAL ASSOCIATION OF DENTAL FACULTIES.

THE next annual meeting of the National Association of Dental Faculties will convene at 10 A. M., June 9, 1904, in Washington, D. C. The Executive Committee will be in session the afternoon of June 8 to consider such matters as may be brought before it. Arrangements are being made with the railroads for one and one-third fare on the certificate plan. The hotel as headquarters, together with the railroad rates, will be announced later by circular letters to the colleges.

H. B. TILESTON, *Chairman.*
S. W. FOSTER, *Secretary.*

SOUTH DAKOTA STATE BOARD OF DENTAL EXAMINERS.

THE South Dakota State Board of Dental Examiners will hold its next regular session for the examination of applicants for license, at Aberdeen, South Dakota, June 9, beginning at 1.30 P.M. All applicants will be required to insert at least two gold fillings, and such other work as the Board may require. Besides the regular operating instruments each candidate is required to bring a bridge of not less than four teeth, including one Richmond crown and one molar shell crown, invested ready for soldering. Application must be made to the secretary at least one week before examination takes place.

G. W. COLLINS,
Secretary.

PROGRAMME OF THE AMERICAN MEDICAL ASSO-
CIATION, SECTION ON STOMATOLOGY.

(Atlantic City, N. J., June 7 to 10, 1904.)

1. "The Value of Symmetry in the Development of Professional Character and Education" (Chairman's Address), George F. Eames, Boston, Mass.

2. "The Evolution of Standards in Dental Education," Charles Chittenden, Madison, Wis.

3. "Phases of Dental Education," A. E. Baldwin, Chicago, Ill.

4. "Dental Education: A Retrospective and Prospective View," John S. Marshall San Francisco, Cal.

5. "Neoplasm of the Tooth-Pulp," Vida A. Latham, Chicago, Ill.

6. "Vital Principles in Adult Pulp," R. R. Andrews, Cambridge, Mass.

7. "Degeneration of the Tooth-Pulp," Eugene S. Talbot, Chicago, Ill.

8. "The Pulp," Jos. Arkövy, Budapest, Hungary.

9. "A System for Surgical Treatment of Harelip, Cleft Palate, and Facial Deformities and Post-Operative Speech Education," George V. I. Brown, Milwaukee, Wis.

10. "Multiple Fracture of Lower Jaw complicated by Simultaneous Fracture of the Upper Jaw," Thomas L. Gilmer, Chicago, Ill.

11. "Impacted Teeth: Their Diagnosis, Liberation, and Extraction," Matthew H. Cryer, Philadelphia, Pa.

12. "Ankylosis of the Jaw," G. Lenox Curtis, New York City, N. Y.

13. "Necrosis of the Bones of the Face," Stewart L. McCurdy, Pittsburg, Pa.

14. "Treatment of Pathological Irregularities of the Teeth," M. H. Fletcher, Cincinnati, Ohio.

15. "Report of a Case of Vincent's Angina and Stomatitis, with Photographs," George C. Crandall, St. Louis, Mo.

16. "Oral Infection and Sterilization," M. L. Rhein, New York City, N. Y.

17. "Concerning Changes in the Salivary Secretions as affected by Systemic Disease," Heinrich Stern, New York City, N. Y.; William Lederer, New York City, N. Y.

18. "Prophylaxis in Relation to Tooth Environment and to the Prophylactic Value of Materials employed," Chas. F. Allan, Newburgh, N. Y.

19. "The Physician's Duty to the Child from a Dental Standpoint," Alice M. Steeves, Boston, Mass.

20. "Ethics," Adelbert H. Peck, Chicago, Ill.

DR. GEORGE F. EAMES, *Chairman.*
EUGENE S. TALBOT, *Secretary.*

NORTHERN INDIANA DENTAL SOCIETY.

THE sixteenth annual meeting of the Northern Indiana Dental Society will be held in Huntington, Ind., on October 4 and 5, 1904.

Arrangements are being made to make this the greatest convention ever held in Northern Indiana. Already some of the best talent in the country has been secured.

OTTO U. KING,
Secretary.

DENTAL COMMISSIONERS OF CONNECTICUT.

THE Dental Commissioners of Connecticut hereby give notice that they will meet at Hartford on May 14, as prescribed by law, and will adjourn to July for the summer examinations, so as to enable those students who do not finish their college or other educational course until June an opportunity to secure a license to practise without the long delay now made necessary because of being required to wait until November.

Hereafter the November examinations will be dispensed with until further notice.

Examinations to secure a license to practise dentistry in Connecticut will be held July 14, 15, and 16, 1904, at Hartford, Conn.

Full particulars will be published in the dental journals, or may be secured of the Recorder.

By direction of the Dental Commissioners.

J. TENNEY BARKER,
Recorder.

WALLINGFORD, CONN.

CALIFORNIA STATE DENTAL ASSOCIATION.

THE Joint Clinic of the California State Dental Association and the Alumni Association, Dental Department, University of California, will be held May 16 to 19, 1904, in San Francisco.

Dr. Hart J. Goslee, of Chicago, will give a series of clinics on Porcelain, Dr. Henry A. Baker, of Boston, will give a series of clinics on Orthodontia and the Baker Anchorage, and a large local clinical programme is being arranged.

All the leading manufacturers have signified their intention of making an exhibit of their products, and the local dealers will also be represented.

The session is expected to surpass any previously held in this State.

GUY S. MILLBERRY,
Secretary.

MINNESOTA STATE BOARD OF DENTAL EXAMINERS.

THE Minnesota State Board of Dental Examiners will hold a special meeting for the purpose of examining applicants for license, June 13, 14, and 15, 1904.

No applications received after 12 M. June 13. Meeting held at the Dental Department of the State University at Minneapolis.

C. H. ROBINSON,
Secretary.

WABASHA, MINN.

THE

International Dental Journal.

| VOL. XXV. | JUNE, 1904. | NO. 6. |

Original Communications.[1]

DEVICE FOR EXTENSION CROWN.[2]

BY HENRY W. GILLETT, D.M.D., NEW YORK.

MR. PRESIDENT AND GENTLEMEN,—I am moved to make these few remarks, which can scarcely be dignified by the name of a paper, by the following train of circumstances.

I received recently, from Chicago, a circular describing the conditions to which a so-called extension crown is applicable as an aid in securely anchoring lower partial plates, and offering a license for the use of the patented process for the sum of fifty dollars.

The documents, which very carefully avoided any description of the device, I mailed to Dr. J. N. Crouse for his information, but the point of particular interest in them for me was the name extension crown, because for some years I have been using a device to which the name might apply. Asking one of our leading Chicago dentists about the device offered in the circular led to

---

[1] The editor and publishers are not responsible for the views of authors of papers published in this department, nor for any claim to novelty, or otherwise, that may be made by them. No papers will be received for this department that have appeared in any other journal published in the country.

[2] Read before the American Academy of Dental Sciences, Boston, February 3, 1904.

my also asking if the device I use is generally known and used, and if it had ever been described so as to safeguard it from patents. His verdict that it ought to be so described and your committee's request for a paper were coincident in time.

The kernel of the matter I want to put before you is the principle involved in the providing of a fixed point of support for certain classes of partial plates. I think most of us are quite ready to admit that fixed bridge-work is less cleanly than removable pieces, but oftentimes the superior firmness it offers is so essential as to more than offset that defect, and lead to its use, where we would prefer to advise partial plates. Removable bridges, strictly so classed, often call for so much destructive cutting as to rule them out. I think you will bear me out in the statement that many times these two points lead to the use of a plate, which the operator recognizes as less effective as a masticator than the bridge that might be used.

Dr. Bonwill showed us years ago one way of overcoming this difficulty when dealing with spaces having molars and bicuspids on each side. You remember, and without doubt practise, his valuable method of supplying a hook or lug to bear on the occlusal ends of adjoining teeth, and so provide rigid support for small pieces, and you are also familiar with Dr. Head's use of it in connection with porcelain work. I recently saw a most successful application of the principle from Dr. Rhein's hands, the large rectangular lug in this case being let into the surface of a large gold filling in a molar, so as to stand flush with the occlusal surface, and its generous proportions and parallel sides serving to steady the piece against torsional strain.

Modifications of the Bonwill lug are to me invaluable, in a certain type of fixed bridge—but that is another story, and one which Dr. S. S. Stowell has told in detail. Minor objections to Dr. Bonwill's way of applying the lug sometimes present in cases of close bite, where convenient space for it cannot be arranged, or where the shape of occlusal surfaces and the angle at which the teeth stand is unsatisfactory.

The place where we need its help most, however, and where it entirely fails us, is in the cases where we want and often must have rigid support if we are to attain even mediocre success in restoring the masticatory apparatus to real usefulness,—namely, those cases where we have only the six front teeth for our anterior support, or often in the lower jaw for the sole support, and where the occlusion is such as to readily allow these teeth to yield and move forward if pressure is made against them. Even in the cases where the Bonwill lug is readily feasible, it seems to me a better application of the principle to place the point of support nearer the neck of the tooth—not that I discard entirely the Bonwill device, for it is often very useful. Placing the point of support at the neck of the tooth often results in a cleaner piece, because it presents less crevices and corners for débris lodgement. It renders possible the balancing of the strains thrown on the supporting tooth, and when the tooth utilized is one of the six anterior teeth it seems the only practicable point for such attachment.

My first use of the device grew out of my need for solving the problem presented by a case in which an upper partial rubber plate carrying molars, bicuspids, and one cuspid, and bearing heavy stress, kept presenting for repairs. It was observed that the plate was constantly driving up and the upper front teeth, by a process familiar to all of you, were being forced forward quite rapidly. A molar on each side at the back gave opportunity for using Bonwill lugs, but until the left lateral (and later the right cuspid) broke off and needed crowning, no stable support could be found at the front. When the lateral crown was made, a modified Richmond provided the needed help, and later, with the same device on the cuspid, stability was gained which revolutionized the conditions in the mouth.

You have, of course, already grasped the point that this support was provided by a projection and strengthening of the top of the gold cap on the palatal side of the crowns, and the insertion in the rubber plate of a bit of gold plate to rest on this projection. Since that I do not remember to have used the principle in connection with rubber plates, but repeatedly I have found it so indispensable in partial gold plate work, that I have extended its application to all cases where it is feasible to provide the support.

The advent of the so-called staple or Marshall crown has been very helpful in providing means for this support, and I do not hesitate to utilize a half-jacket of the staple class on the palatal surface of cuspids, or even centrals if it is needed.

These half-crowns or jackets provide attachment for simple projections, hooks, or hooked arms as needed, upon which the gold plate may rest. The stress is applied in the line in which the tooth is best able to bear stress, and without torsional or wrenching strain, as when a fixed bridge is used. What lateral strain there is can be easily balanced by contact with the artificial appliance near the occlusal surfaces. The teeth utilized for such support are still left in the best condition to withstand the extra strain put upon them.

In Fig. 1 I present at *a* the simple projection from the side of a molar gold crown; at *b*, a hook sometimes useful when there

FIG. 1.

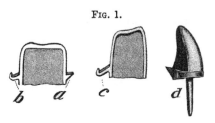

is a possible spreading tendency of the appliance as it rests between the teeth on each side; at *c*, a more extended hook which I have had occasion to use but once; and at *d*, a projection from the band of a gold-banded porcelain crown.

FIG. 2.

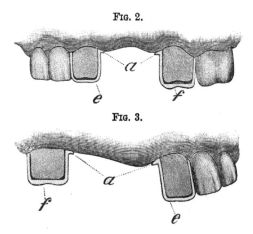

FIG. 3.

In Fig. 2 we have the left side, and in Fig. 3 the right side, of the upper jaw of a heavy strong man, for whom it was necessary to shoe with 18-carat gold the upper six front teeth and open the bite. This, of course, called for rigid support against stress tending to drive the appliances towards the gum, and on the right side I did not dare put so long a span on a fixed bridge, and so expose the only remaining molar on that side to such severe stress. Simple lugs like *a*, of Fig. 1, on the molar gold crowns (*f*) and on staple half-crowns (*e*) on the cuspids provided the desired rigid support for the small plates used. On the lower jaw the same principle of support was supplied, using the first bicuspids to support half-jackets, carrying the necessary projections. Lower bicuspids lend themselves readily to such a device, and in patients of the usual age needing them the pulps have generally become small enough to permit of the comparatively small amount of grinding needed on the lingual, mesial, distal, and occlusal surfaces for the proper fitting of staple crowns. In these teeth I often prefer to get my grip on the tooth, with two 21-guage iridio-platinum pins extending into dowel-holes in the occlusal end, rather than to cut the grooves in the sides for the so-called staple.

FIG. 4.

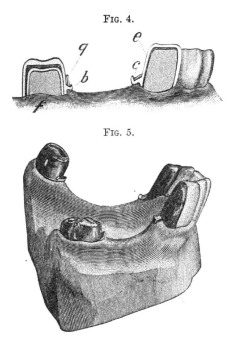

FIG. 5.

Figs. 4 and 5 show a case over which I have had one of the hardest struggles of my professional life, and in which I have gained what I consider a conspicuous degree of success. Previous plates before my first attempt had been worn mostly in the bureau drawer. The first one I made, with elaborate attention to perfection of detail, shared a similar fate. It had Bonwill lugs on the molars, and rested with broad contact against the slanting lingual surfaces of the six unusually thick rooted lower front teeth. The first day, or sometimes two days, in the mouth it would work perfectly, and then it would have to go on furlough till the bruised gum got well. Repeated relieving of the bearing at the sore points did no good. The ridge is large and firm, and because of its firmness bruised easily. Note the square effect of the cutting edges,[1] and you will realize that I had an edge-to-edge incisor bite to deal with, and the result of a day's mastication on the plate was to force the front teeth outward just a little, and that little allowed impingement of the plate upon the gum sufficient to cause trouble.

The problem was solved in this way. A gold crown was made for the left molar, and it and the gold crown already on the right one were provided with hooks like *b* of Fig. 1. The lower edge of the clasps (*g*) engaged these hooks so that they helped to resist any tendency of the plate to move forward. The lingual and approximal sides of the cuspids were provided with gold jackets of " staple" crowns, anchored by grooves cut into the sides of the teeth. The gold was cut away till it did not show at all on the labial aspect and at the lower edge a hooked arm like *c* of Fig. 1 was soldered. This form was necessary because of the sharp upward slant of the gum at that point, so that a plain lug on that angle would probably result in permitting the same forward movement of the teeth, and because the position of the teeth was such that it was found that a lug set at any other feasible angle interfered with the insertion of the plate. A suitable recess was made in the plate to engage the hooked arm. These devices have solved the problem to the entire satisfaction of the patient and operator, and while the much remodelled plate is not as pretty to look at as at first, it does its whole duty three times a day.

In making these devices, I usually find it best to make all crowns and lugs first and take impressions with the crowns in place. If some settling of the plate is desired, the cast may be run without the crowns and the resulting plaster duplicate of the

---

[1] Not sufficiently pronounced in the cut.

crown may be built up at the point of support as much as is desired, and the plate struck over it.

In such a case as the lower plate just described, it is better to work directly to the crowns themselves, striking up the plate free from contact with the crowns and taking impression with it and the crowns in place, and make the needed additions when you have cast with all parts in place on it. To do this calls for the same absolute accuracy of detail as the highest grade of bridge-work.

A REVIEW OF SOME METHODS OF CROWNING TEETH.

BY GEORGE F. GRANT, D.M.D., BOSTON, MASS.

It is not intended by this article to lay down any special system of making crowns, but rather to consider and compare results of some systems which have come under my observation, in a practical way, at a considerable period of time after their insertion. In this connection we will consider porcelain crowns only. There was a time when they were called pivot teeth; later they were called dowel teeth; then crowns. When they took on this new title our troubles multiplied tenfold, because we tried to do so many needless things.

First, the root must be banded to insure greater strength, so that, with the band and pin together, a crown was supposed to be secured for all time. You then had a combination five times the strength of its weakest part,—to wit, the tooth. To prevent fracture of the porcelain all sorts of expedients were resorted to, until many so-called porcelain crowns could be better described as gold teeth with porcelain inlay.

The Logan has been quite extensively used, but has to my mind one great defect,—viz., the fixed position of the pin in the crown is often fatal to the proper adaptation in many cases, unless the root is so greatly weakened by enlarging the canal to accommodate the pin that, when all is completed, there remains the danger of a split root.

It would be interesting to know just the percentage of success of the Logan crowns. It is only just to say that my remarks upon

them are based entirely upon observation of such as have come
under my care for replacement, as I could never feel sufficient
confidence in them to justify their use. This feeling of doubt has
been greatly strengthened by the large percentage of cases in which
the roots have been found in almost hopeless condition, either
through fracture or greatly impaired strength, caused by too much
reaming of the canal in the original setting of the crown.

At this time it is well to say that if you wish to lay up comfort for the future, and would avoid one of the pitfalls of the
whole science, discard every material for posts except platinized
gold or platino-iridium. All others will in time cause you to
regret that you are still alive, for you may be sure that they will
stretch or bend or corrode, or do anything that they should not do,
and for that sin of small economy you will pay dearly.

The porcelain and platinum banded crown, in which the tooth
and band are fused to the pin with high-fusing body, is very strong
at all points; in fact, is least liable to fracture of any crown
made, one point only being likely to give trouble or impair its
appearance,—that is, that the enamel is very likely to flake from
the band, probably caused by vibration in use. This is likely to
happen after a year or two of wear. You know that the proper
time to judge a crown is about the fifth year of wear.

It is by no means certain that with a good healthy root the
band is not rather a doubtful factor. I believe that, when there
are conditions even fairly good, it is better to do without the
band and depend upon a perfect joint at or near the gum margin.
This can always be assured by placing a piece of pure gold about
No. 60, or ribbon gold if preferred, upon the prepared root, per-
forating and passing the post through it into the root. If the
perforation in the plate or foil is slightly smaller than the post
before it is pushed through, you may withdraw plate and post
together in their proper relation, and, holding the post by the
end, a little solder and a Bunsen flame unite them in a moment.
Replace upon the root and mallet the gold as you would condense
a filling, holding the post firmly meanwhile, and you may be
certain that your cast made from an impression taken with this
base and pin in position will give you all that is needed as a base
upon which a perfect fitting crown can be adjusted.

This is not new, but only brought in as an illustration of one
of the most successful and durable forms of crown,—one which

I left for a time to try banded crowns, and the one to which I return with confidence and a feeling of security.

About fifteen years ago I designed a form of removable crown which has proved a great success. It was suggested to my mind by the difficulty of replacing the porcelain facing, which *would* break. The plan was a square tube or socket into which the post (square also) was accurately fitted. The socket with the post inserted was first set in cement in the root, the post withdrawn after the socket was secure and levelled to the surface of the root. The post was then passed through the perforated gold base as described above, and all completed as by the first process.

A square or triangular post is always best, as there can be no danger of loosening by rotation, which I find is a greater factor in displacing of crowns than is generally considered.

A crown so constructed can be removed at any time by means of a strong, straight pull, usually by a ligature of strong silk, which will injure nothing. I have made such crowns in duplicate for patients who were likely to need a repair in places where attention could not be readily obtained, or in any case a simple direction would simplify the situation.

Though the crown was held simply by perfect contact of the sides of the post with the tube, I have never heard of one becoming loose; in fact, it requires quite a considerable force for its removal.

It is in order to say that this was before the day of the detachable facing. I find that even now it is easier to put a new facing on the old base than to find a sufficient number of detachable facings from which to make a suitable selection.

The best thing about the band crown is that it can be so efficiently applied to cases in which the post cannot be used. Many times it is imperative that crowns be supplied where the natural crown has been lost through fracture or so reduced in length by abrasion as to require it.

As it often happens that such teeth are " full of life," the process of devitalizing before crowning is undesirable, in fact, sometimes next to impossible. The way out of this difficulty seems to lie through the band crown. To illustrate, I will describe an operation which helped me out of a difficulty and made a patient happy for years. The case was one so commonly met with when the only teeth remaining in the mouth were the six anterior teeth of the lower maxilla. An artificial upper set, also lower bicuspids and molars, had been worn for some years. The difficult feature was that the six natural teeth, though healthy and firm, were so short that it was impossible to restore the face to its normal appearance unless the teeth could be lengthened. So I decided that a little experiment could do no harm. With this end in view six crowns were fitted, retained entirely by the band of each accurately fitted after slightly bevelling the anterior face of each tooth to give a good gum line. These crowns had rather a shallow seat, still the band of each was so fitted that each would stand up without cement, though of course they were finally cemented. The prosthetic work was completed to conform to the new condition established by the lengthened lower teeth. This was done in 1895. This autumn (1903) the patient desired some new plates, so that I had the opportunity of examining the six crowns. They were perfectly firm after the eight years of service, some part of which time they must have received the whole burden of mastication, as the bicuspids and molars of the lower plate had settled far below the possibility of occlusion with the upper teeth (a good argument for the use of the banded crown) ; for, supposing those teeth to have been devitalized in order to use posts, it is probable that they would have all loosened before this time, as the patient was at least fifty years of age at the time of the operation.

It has been my practice for many years to use a crown with band and without a post in anterior teeth, whenever devitalization has not been effected, for the reason that in all cases where it can be done upon the live stump the danger of the band coming into sight after a year or two does not exist. It is only the devitalized root that lengthens in that way, and it is especially true in the mouths of patients of mature age, say thirty-five or beyond.

Such crowns are easily repaired without injury to the stump, for if the porcelain breaks while the band holds, you have only to open the band on the palatal side to remove it. You also have the evidence of an accomplished fact that no chain can be stronger than the weakest link.

Along the lines of experience in retaining crowns by the narrow band has perhaps been built up the new system of jacket crowns, the basic principle of which is good, the conservation of the tooth-pulp.

SOME METHODS OF TEACHING ELEMENTARY OPERA-
TIVE DENTISTRY.[1]

BY WILLIAM H. POTTER, D.M.D., BOSTON, MASS.[2]

AT the present day much is said as to the most approved
methods of imparting information. It is generally conceded that
the highest degree of success cannot be attained by the average individual unless the method employed is of the most approved sort.
The methods of dental education have advanced coincidentally with
those of other branches of education. If we go back twenty years
we will find that the way by which a man was taught the elements
of operative dentistry was to allow him to operate upon a patient.
The mouth of the patient was his work-bench and his subject for
operation. He sat down or stood up to it and began to learn the
nature of his instruments. He tried them in the mouth to see
how they fitted different situations there to be found. He thus
became acquainted with his instruments. He found that certain
of them would not cut tooth-substance, and that certain of them
would. He discovered the necessity for curves and angles. He
found out the methods of applying force in the mouth, and so
controlling it that it would go no farther than desired. This last
piece of information was usually obtained through great hardship
to the patient, as was evidenced by the laceration of parts surrounding the teeth due to the slipping of instruments. To be
sure, these elementary things about operative dentistry were not
learned from the patient with absolutely no preliminary training.
It was the custom to set up teeth in plaster and work upon them
before going into the mouth. But the operations upon teeth so set
up were rather unsatisfactory, owing to the difficulty of mounting
them in such a way as to imitate the conditions found in the
mouth. Hence it was that students were very quickly put upon
actual cases and allowed to acquire by the aid and forbearance
of the patient the elements of operative work. This method was a
decided injustice to the patient, and was undesirable for the

---

[1] Read before the American Academy of Dental Science, Boston, Mass.,
April 6, 1904.
[2] Assistant Professor of Operative Dentistry, Harvard Dental School.

student, inasmuch as it surrounded him with too many difficulties all at one time.

Modern methods of teaching operative dentistry insist, first of all, upon a knowledge of dental anatomy. This anatomy implies more than is likely to be learned from the course in general anatomy. It has to do with the external contour of the teeth, the peculiarities which distinguish one tooth from another, the number and location of cusps and fissures, the size and shape of the pulp-cavity, the proper occlusion of the teeth. Without the knowledge gained by such study it is inevitable that the beginner will make many false steps; as, for instance, the forming of undercuts in such a manner as to expose the pulp; the failure to find and properly treat all the root-canals; the improper use of drills in root-canals whereby false passages are made from the root-canal to the socket of the tooth. As a general surgeon who proposes to cut into the tissues of the arm should know in advance what muscles and vessels he will encounter, so the dental operator should first be sure of his anatomy before venturing to do the simplest work in the mouth. This seems a self-evident proposition, and yet only in comparatively recent time have we given sufficient importance to it. After the student has acquired dental anatomy, the modern method puts him at work upon teeth that are so arranged as to simulate the conditions found in the mouth. Great improvements have been made since the time when two or three teeth were set up in plaster on which the student began his work in operative dentistry.

I wish here to describe an apparatus which I came across in Vienna four years ago and which is now used at the Harvard Dental School. This apparatus is called in Vienna a " Phantom," and it came into existence in this way: It had been the custom in the Dental Department of the University of Vienna to use a human skull provided with full dentures for the demonstration of operations upon the teeth and for the first work of students in operative dentistry. This skull was mounted upon a standard and brought into such a position that it could be readily operated upon. In Vienna it is a comparatively easy matter to obtain a skull with a good set of teeth, and the expense of a skull is not great. Such a skull offered an excellent means for teaching students the methods of operating upon the teeth, and also gave them useful practice. If skulls were plenty enough, no better method could be devised than to use them in the teaching of the rudiments of operative dentistry. But even in Vienna, so bountiful in its supply of anatomical material, suitable skulls and teeth might not always be available, and it occurred to Messrs. Weiss & Schwartz, of Vienna, to make the apparatus which I have alluded to as a " Phantom," and which takes the place of the skull. The " Phantom" consists of two iron jaws bolted together so as to imitate the positions of the superior and inferior maxillæ. The two jaws are also attached to a post which can be clamped to a dental chair in place of the usual head rest. Thus fixed, it occupies the same relative position which a human head would occupy when undergoing a dental operation. The iron jaws are so arranged that extracted teeth can be inserted and fixed by means of plaster of Paris. Here, then, we have a simple apparatus which when filled with teeth simulates in the most important particulars the conditions found in the human mouth. On it the student can begin his operative experiences; he can get used to his instruments and learn how to apply force in the mouth. While the " Phantom" imitates the conditions of the mouth, it is undoubtedly easier to operate upon it than upon the mouth. The saliva is absent, the resisting lips and cheeks are absent, and, of no small importance, the nerves of the patient are absent. Thus for the beginning student some of the difficulties are removed and he is able to master the elementary things and be prepared for the more difficult. It is the custom at the Harvard Dental School to require each student to perform the more common operations upon the " Phantom" before they are performed in the mouth.

I am aware that there are sundry devices now made which are calculated to perform the same service as the " Phantom." There are rubber jaws in which teeth can be inserted and operated upon, and which are useful as far as they go. And then there are very complicated and expensive manikin heads, in which teeth can be placed. They are very useful, but are so expensive that they cannot well be furnished for each student. Composition teeth of celluloid and rubber have been made for operative purposes, but there is always the objection to artificial teeth that the student is cutting a substance which is essentially different from dentine or enamel.

A final point which I wish to touch upon is the method of teaching cavity preparations by means of plaster teeth of a size of perhaps ten times that of natural teeth. Such teeth, so far as I know, cannot be bought and must be manufactured at one's own laboratory. Here is a bicuspid form which I have used during the past year. I carved the original one myself, and then reproduced it by means of the fusible metal moulds which I show. It is rather a rough affair, but it serves accurately to express the teacher's idea as to how a cavity should be prepared. It is my custom to ask students to prepare cavities in these models and bring them to the class for criticism. It is thus possible to know with certainty whether a student has understood what has been said to him.

THE SUPERIORITY OF HIGH-FUSING PORCELAIN FOR DENTAL PURPOSES.[1]

BY DR. HERBERT L. WHEELER, NEW YORK.

THE terms used in the title of this paper are somewhat arbitrary, and express the meaning which I desire to convey to you only in a general way. The manufacturers of low-fusing materials have been pleased to call their product enamels, etc., and to consider any material which baked below the melting point of gold as low-fusing; and any material with which gold could not be used as a matrix, because the heat required to bake it was greater than the fusing-point of gold, as high-fusing material. It is probably impossible to state just where the line should be drawn which separates a high- from a low-fusing porcelain, except so far as I am acquainted with the low-fusing product at present obtainable for dental purposes.

There seems to be two methods of obtaining a powder that will fuse at a temperature so far below the melting-point of gold that there is no danger in using this metal as a matrix. One of these methods seems to produce a real porcelain in that it contains ingredients which are not changed or fused in the baking process. This quality is secured by the use of artificial flux, either in the mix with the color frit, or by adding quantities of pulverized glass of a variety that contains lead oxide, to lower the degree of temperature required to cause the fusible parts of this material to melt. This

---

[1] Read before the Academy of Stomatology, Philadelphia.

particular quality increases the liability of the color to flee and the probability of gassing or bubbling. Experience has demonstrated that this substance is sooner or later effected unfavorably by the fluids of the mouth, a discoloration or a disintegration of the surface of an inlay made from this substance taking place in many instances. The other process is somewhat different and is, I think, made in the following manner: Felspar, which will fuse at a low temperature, is procured by either an admixture of different varieties or by recalcining and rebaking a felspathic rock several times; or perhaps both methods are used to secure the desired results. For it is well known that the baking of porcelain and repulverizing lowers the fusing-point without correspondingly producing loss of color in overbaking; and the porcelain enamel on the market in some of its qualities seems to indicate that this process may have been used in its manufacture. Except that the color flees so quickly after the glazing-point has been reached, I doubt if the recalcining process is used to any extent in the making of this material. While there may or may not be oxide of lead used in this latter class, I still consider it as a glass rather than a true porcelain; because, as near as I can judge by careful observation, all the component parts are fused in the baking process.

The most representative product now on the market of the first class above mentioned is the Ash & Sons low-fusing mineral bodies. The only representative of the second class, so far as I know, is the Jenkins enamel. If one is to use a low-fusing material, it seems to me the Ash & Sons product is quite superior in many respects. Its color is less apt to flee in the baking process, it can be shaped to any desired form with much greater certainty of retaining that form when baked, and the color frits are so well mixed and the substance of such a quality that it forms a much more translucent inlay than does the Jenkins enamel. On the other hand, in negative qualities the Jenkins enamel seems to be less desirable, because of the general opaque appearance, its tendency to spheroid or ball up in the baking process, its great shrinking tendency, and the temperature at which the color will flee and the number of degrees between which glazing takes place and loss of color occurs, being less than any ceramic material used for dental purposes to-day. However, my belief is, after several years observation, that no low-fusing material for porcelain inlays has ever fulfilled the hopes of those that have been induced to use it, when subjected to the test of time. The Ash & Sons material has been with us a long time; and who has not seen cases where a roughening or disintegration of the glazed surface has occurred, resulting in a changed and blackened appearance of the filling, which has entirely ruined it from an æsthetic point of view. Take also the Jenkins enamel, the formula for which has been constantly changed, if one can judge by the oft-published statements of the manufacturer who produces it. Even with this constant change, who has not seen instances of roughened surfaces, more or less disintegrated and blackened, of inlays made of this material, which is always perfect and yet is ever being perfected.

Now, I do not wish to say that low-fusing porcelain or enamels are useless. But what I do wish to impress upon you is this: that in a general way, to lower the fusing-point of an enamel means to increase the ingredients that contain alkaline salts, and that in a general way, in proportion as the alkaline parts are increased, the strength of the enamel and its ability to withstand the solvent action of the fluids of the mouth is decreased. Probably many of you know that the clay kaolin, which is one of the materials used in making porcelain, is nothing more nor less than disintegrated felspar, in which the most of the alkaline constituents, such as potassium, sodium, magnesium, etc., have been washed out by being exposed to the elements during the ravages of time. If, then, felspathic rocks are utterly destroyed or disintegrated by the action of the wind and rain, are there not great possibilities for disintegration in the fluids of the mouth, when you come to consider that in all low-fusing bodies the alkaline, or soluble, proportions are greatly increased by artificial means? And I do think that those of us, who have the best interests of our patients at heart, will be very cautious about the use of these enamels, until their permanency, under all reasonable conditions, are much better established, than they are at present.

Another very disappointing place in which I have had the misfortune to use the Jenkins enamel several times is this: it is my habit to rearrange porcelain crowns, facings, etc., by grinding in some places, adding contour in others, by means of baking on new porcelain, in order to reproduce the individual peculiarities of the teeth in different patients. Now, it has been my experience in using the Jenkins enamel for this purpose that it invariably crackled badly. The reason for this is, I think, the difference in contraction between this body and all the different bodies used in making porcelain teeth or crowns. In a good high-fusing porcelain the amount of alkaline proportions is reduced to the minimum quantity required to obtain a homogeneous mass; also at the present stage of electric ovens it is necessary to have a material that does not fuse much above 2400° F., for the reason that both the clay and the platinum will not stand a higher heat than this for any length of time without causing disaster to the oven.

There are, as you probably know, certain chemical changes that take place during the baking process of porcelain, and these processes can be varied somewhat by changing certain qualities of the ingredients without changing the proportions; that is to say, it would be quite possible to have the formula of two bodies apparently identical, but the silica in one might be much more finely powdered than in the other. The result would be that the one with the finely powdered silica would fuse at a lower temperature, the color would more readily disappear, and the strength would, I think, not be as great. On the other hand, it might be possible to leave the silica so coarse and put in such a small proportion of felspar that the glazed surface would not be perfectly smooth. It is my opinion that a material of this latter quality might have greater strength than the more homogeneous and more artistic product with the finely pulverized silicon. The silica in high-fusing bodies prevents shrinkage or retards it, and overcomes the tendency to warp or change shape noticeable in the more easily baked lower-fusing bodies. A fair amount of this ingredient gives that quality, so necessary in some cases, that admits of building out corners to a sharp edge, or of producing those concavo-convex inlays sometimes so necessary for the proper reproduction of the natural shape of a tooth at the cervical margin of the crown. This material also seems to increase the strength of porcelain. It is this ingredient that breaks up the rays of light in a porcelain body and still permits of translucency. Those low-fusing enamels which do not contain silica would be transparent like glass were it not for coloring-matter or the quality of clay used, which seems to prevent translucency to some extent and to produce a slight opacity. Then, too, the greater stability of the high-fusing material permits the work being done with much less time spent in close observation of the baking process; but the most valuable quality of a high-fusing porcelain lies in its greater resistance to chemical action by the fluids of the mouth and its less probability to disintegration and roughening of its surface.

That a translucent substance is necessary for a resemblance to the natural appearance of a tooth seems to be generally agreed upon. If it were not for this, manufacturers would doubtless be producing and selling teeth made of a material quite similar to the Jenkins enamel, especially as this low-fusing material, so far as the cost of ingredients goes, would be much less expensive than the high-fusing compounds already in use. It seems rather astonishing when one considers that inlays have been made now and then since 1857 of high-fusing material, and so far as I know there has never been a complaint of destructive action of the fluids of the mouth upon this material. On the contrary, I do not know and never have heard of a low-fusing enamel of which there were not reports from various sources of its disintegration and destruction from the action of the fluids of the mouth.

The first porcelain inlays I have seen a record of were described by Dr. A. J. Volck in the *American Journal of Dental Science* for July, 1857. These were set by packing gold around the inlay between it and the cavity margins. Down to the present time this method has remained somewhat in vogue, and I have, within two years, seen the tip of a central incisor restored by Dr. J. Morgan Howe twenty or more years ago, and the porcelain and fastenings were still apparently perfect. In spite of its great disadvantages, this method of grinding already baked porcelain to fit a cavity has some things to commend it, especially to the beginner and the man who has time. The material itself is usually of superior texture to the average inlay made in a dentist's office, because it is made of higher-fusing material and is more skilfully baked and annealed than most inlays, in consequence of having been made by the skilled hands employed by the manufacturer.

The present method of making porcelain inlays by baking in a matrix which has previously been accurately fitted to the cavity was, I think, originated by William Rollins, of Boston, and first described by him in a paper read before the Society of Oral Science, in June, 1880. Dr. Rollins also originated the gas furnace for porcelain work. His ideas seem to have been seized upon by Dr. Land and exploited as his own; he also had them patented.[1]

---

[1] Independent Practitioner, June, 1888.

In speaking upon the history of porcelain, in a paper read by me before The New York Institute of Stomatology, last year, and published in the May, 1903, INTERNATIONAL DENTAL JOURNAL, I relied somewhat upon an article of Dr. Bruck's, which was translated by Dr. Jenkins, for my data, and I find, upon a more careful examination of the facts, that the statements of Dr. Bruck are quite inaccurate or lack any published record to support them.

About the strength of the various porcelains and enamels upon the market, the reckless assertions of the superior strength of low-fusing enamel stimulated me to make a few experiments for myself, and while I have only made a beginning, they serve to show that the low-fusing products are decidedly inferior in the matter of strength. I secured these results by baking two platinum pins in a block of porcelain, each piece being made in the same mould, and subjecting them to a tensile strain until the block of enamel broke. The power required to break them was averaged up as I repeated the experiment from four to eight times, the results in pounds being as follows: Jenkins enamel, $32\frac{1}{2}$; Ash & Sons low-fusing, $30\frac{1}{2}$; Ash & Sons high-fusing, 45; this latter result was so high because of one remarkable block which was mixed with water instead of the fluid furnished by Ash & Sons, which stood a strain of $60\frac{1}{2}$ pounds. The consolidated inlay material which was originally made by Mr. Whiteley averaged 39; the material now made by Mr. Whiteley, 41; the Brewster enamel, 19; S. S. W. material, $33\frac{1}{2}$. A block of the very high-fusing body made by Dr. Parker, of Boston, would not break, the pins breaking first, leaving the body intact.

I was so firmly impressed, by watching the fusing in these cases, that the fusing-points given by Mr. Hammond in my original paper were erroneous, that I decided to try them for myself. In order to more closely observe the fusing process in high-fusing material I am accustomed to using colored glasses to protect my eyes. I obtained the following results, though I may say the Jenkins enamel was over-baked, lost color, and was stronger as a result. The degrees are Farenheit. Jenkins enamel, 1552°; Ash & Sons low-fusing, 1580°; high-fusing, 2084°; Consolidated, 2084°; Whiteley's, 2228°; Brewster's, 2084°; S. S. W., 2228°; Parker's, 2588°. A special lot sent me by Mr. Whiteley fused at 2264° and held its color in the baking process remarkably well. This also stood a strain of forty-eight pounds in the tensile tests.

In the matter of shrinkage the Parker body showed the least and stood up well at the corners. S. S. White's and the Whiteley bodies came next in these qualities. The Consolidated, Ash & Sons high-fusing, and Brewster's were next, then Ash & Sons low-fusing, and the greatest shrinker of all was the Jenkins enamel; this also showed the least tendency to retain its form when baked.

It is to be borne in mind that in the matter of strength much depends upon a proper cooling or annealing. *You can not bake a porcelain in a Bunsen flame, leaving it unprotected from the atmosphere of the room, and get good results where any resistance or strain is to be borne.* The very ease and carelessness with which low-fusing material is baked is against it because the weaknesses of structure thus produced are not immediately visible. There is no good reason why the manufacturers should not furnish an inlay material as good and as high-fusing as their teeth, except the one previously mentioned,—viz., that most furnaces will not stand the strain, though I have reason to believe the Hammond will for a time, at least. Some few members of our calling have been securing this material by breaking up teeth, reducing them to a powder, and rebaking, and I am informed from an authoritative source that the S. S. White Company are now making teeth of their enamel and without pins to sell for this very purpose. I really think that thus far this provides the very best method I know of for securing desired color and a superior quality and strength in the inlay.

Reviews of Dental Literature.

SOME NOTES ON THE ENAMEL. By Douglas E. Caush, L.D.S.I.

MR. PRESIDENT AND GENTLEMEN,—In the paper I have the honor of readng before you to-night it is not my intention to deal with the question of the development of the enamel to any extent, but to bring before your notice a series of experiments I have carried out, and, as a result of these, to draw your attention to what appears to be some variations from the accepted theories of the microscopic structure of this tissue.

These experiments were commenced in the year 1888 for the

purpose of finding, if possible, a reason for the staining of the enamel of human teeth by copper and other amalgams, the object being to stain the enamel, either from the outside or through the pulp; and at the same time to find out what portion of the tissue would take the stain, if any of it stained at all.

After a large number of experiments had been carried out, I found the following methods of staining were by far the most successful of all that were tried:

1. A number of teeth were placed in a five per cent. solution of chloride of gold for various times extending from two to ten days, after which the teeth were taken out of the stain, washed, and ground down until they were quite thin; these sections were then placed in distilled water, and exposed to the sunshine until they were almost black; they were then rubbed down between ground glass to get rid of the surface stain, and at the same time to make the sections thin enough for examination when they were mounted in balsam.

2. Teeth were placed in alcohol for some days, after which they were placed in an alcoholic stain of fuchsin for several weeks, in some cases even months; on taking them out of the stain the teeth were ground down in the usual manner and mounted for examination.

3. The teeth were placed in alcohol for a few days, then placed in a quantity of hot fuchsin stain and kept in a hot chamber for twenty-four hours, after which they were allowed to cool; when the teeth were ground down in the usual manner and mounted for examination. This method produced very good results, but the heat made the enamel much more brittle than the previous methods of staining.

After years of apparent failure I had almost given up hope of ever staining the enamel, when, a few months since, on examining one of the earlier prepared slides with a more powerful eye-piece, to my astonishment, and, I may say, delight, I found the enamel in the slides thus prepared had been much more thoroughly stained than at first appeared. This led to further experiments with eye-pieces of various powers. As a result of these experiments, I now use a compensating ocular × 18, with a comparatively low power objective (either eight or sixteen millimetres apochromatic), and find that I can see much more of the structure of the enamel, owing to the larger field, greater depth of focus, and the more perfect correction of color of the apochromatic lens, than when I use the microscope in the ordinary manner.

During the past six months a large number of sections (both longitudinal and transverse) have been prepared.

I have not confined myself to human teeth, but from *Primates* have made slides of the teeth of man and gorilla; *Carnivora,* fox and dog; *Ungulata,* cow, pig, and horse; *Rodents,* rats; all of which have been successfully stained by one of these processes.

In all cases the staining has been accomplished prior to the cutting of the sections of the teeth; and in no case have acids of any kind been used, either before or during the preparation of the teeth for the microscope. I have avoided the use of acids to prevent the possibility of any alteration of the tissues by decalcification.

Although for years I could see no staining of the enamel, at the same time I learnt much from the examination of these slides. Among other things, my attention was drawn to the fact that in every case those peculiar and constantly occurring portions of this tissue, known as the enamel spindles of Von Ebner, were always stained in the same manner as the tubuli of the dentine, whatever stain was used.

This led me to suppose, and I think proves, that there is a connection, or at least a means of communication, between the tubuli of the dentine and these spaces in the enamel. It also proves that the contents of these spaces are of an organic nature, uncalcified, probably protoplasmic in character, and possibly similar to the contents of the tubuli of dentine.

The staining also proves that there is direct communication between the pulp and these spindles. (Fig. 1.)

The constant and regular occurrence of these cavities shows that they are not pathological, as has been suggested by Mr. Charles Tomes, but normal, and probably play an important part in the life of the enamel. They vary very much in size, shape, and number, but in every case I think their existence is due to a check, or checks, in the calcification of the cells forming the enamel, during the process of development.

Besides the regular, uncalcified contents of these spaces, there are at times to be seen certain small glistening bodies, known as Römer's corpuscles. When they exist they are, I believe, composed of minute particles of calcified enamel. In all the experi-

FIG 1.

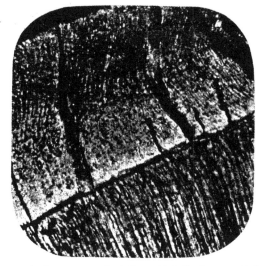

Showing connection between enamel spindles and tubuli ; also enamel-tubes × 200.

FIG. 2.

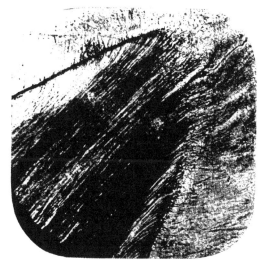

Bundles of enamel-tubes and connection with tubuli of dentine. × 100.

ments made I have not been successful in staining them, and it is easy to understand how readily small, isolated, and calcified enamel cells may become surrounded by the non-calcified tissue in the early stages of development.

I do not think Von Ebner was correct when he suggested that these spindles contained air, and I am certain these cavities are not produced by the shrivelling up of the cement substance, as he suggests.

In those cases where air has been enclosed, if such a condition exists, it may be the result of having allowed the teeth to dry for some time prior to the sections being made from the teeth, for examination; even in these cases I have found that the action of the alcohol is to displace any air and to allow the stain to easily penetrate into the tissues; this is well demonstrated by the hot method of staining.

As far as my examination of the teeth of animals has gone, it is very unusual to find any pronounced cavities corresponding to the enamel spindles of man, though in some animals I have found what appears to be a modification of these spindles.

At the same time, in the teeth of all the animals from which sections have been made I have found that there is a means of communication between the pulp and the enamel, in the form of certain tubes or tube-like processes distributed through this tissue. So constant were they, that they could not be considered as other than normal.

As there appears to be no record of their existence, I shall, for the purpose of describing them, call them "enamel-tubes." There is apparently no sheath to these tubes, their position is between the enamel prisms; the calcified prisms forming their walls. They are, I think, produced by the non-calcification of the tissue (cement substance or otherwise) between the enamel prisms.

These tubes vary somewhat in size, according to their position in the tissue. Near the neck of the teeth they usually appear as short, separate, and distant tubes, but as we approach the cutting edge of the incisors and canines they are frequently to be found grouped together in bunches or bundles, as well as in separate tubes. These tubes also take this form very pronouncedly in the crowns of the bicuspids and molars. (Fig. 2.)

The arrangement of the tubes in these bundles is frequently that of a spiral, with the upper portion branching into two or more divisions. They sometimes radiate from their base like a fan, and as a consequence it is impossible to get the whole of the bundles into focus at once.

The connection between the pulp and these enamel-tubes is proved by the fact that they take the stain readily. For these tubes to be thus stained, the stain must pass through the pulp or pass in from the outside. Experiments show that it is easier to stain through the pulp than to stain direct through the enamel.

That these enamel-tubes are distinct canals or tubes containing uncalcified tissue may also be assumed from this staining, as well as from the fact that wherever there are cut ends they are always stained in the same manner as the cut ends of the tubuli of the dentine.

That they are not pathological is clear from the fact that they occur in the teeth of the gorilla, fox, dog, cow, pig, horse, rat, and alligator, as well as in human teeth. (All the animals I have at present examined.)

It is interesting at this point to trace the connection between the tubuli of the dentine and both the spindles and the enamel-tubes. Immediately under the enamel the tubuli of the dentine branch very much and frequently anastomose, thus forming a complete net-work of small tubes under the enamel margin.

In the pig the branching is more pronounced, and a rudimentary granular layer is seen. In the fox the granular layer is more pronounced, whilst in the cow there is a perfect granular layer, corresponding to, and continuous with the granular layer between the dentine and the cementum.

The tubuli of the dentine terminate in this layer on the one side, and the enamel-tubes often pass into it from the other side; thus making the ends of the tubuli and the granular layer the means of communication between the two tissues.

Besides the enamel spindles and tubes there appears to be a more or less complete net-work of uncalcified tissue passing between the prisms and capable of being stained. This continues until the outer portion of the enamel is reached, when we find a series of larger tubes passing from the outside towards the central portion of this tissue.

This method of staining enables us to follow the curvature of the prisms both in man and animals. In the incisors and canines this curvature is not very pronounced, except at or near the cutting edges, but in the bicuspids and molars the reverse is the case, for in both the curvature of the prisms are very pronounced; and I believe there is a very good reason for their existence.

We all know the ease with which the enamel can be cut along the line of fracture, where the prisms are straight and comparatively parallel, but try to do the same on the crown of a molar, and you will find the resistance is very great. The cause of the resistance is the curvature, and the crossing of the prisms: the reason for this curvature of the prisms is that they may overcome the strain put upon these organs during the process of mastication.

The enamel-tubes that appear on the outer portion of this tissue and pass inward are usually very regular, and generally run parallel to each other in human teeth, whilst in the cow, with these tubes are frequently to be found bundles of tubes similar to the bundles found on the inner surface of the tissue.

I said in the earlier portion of my paper that these tubes and spindles played a very important part in the life of the enamel. The following, I believe, are some of the functions of both enamel spindles and tubes: (1) To convey sensation from the outside of the enamel to the pulp, especially in cases of erosion, and sensitive enamel; (2) to allow for any expansion, or contraction that may take place in the enamel; (3) as a means of conveying nourishment to the enamel during the life of the pulp, as, unless there is some way of conveying nourishment to this tissue it must of necessity be a dead tissue from the time of its development.

I think it is the existence of these tubes that has misled Dr. Bödecker in the theory propounded by him in his work on the enamel. Trying to harmonize the theories expressed by him, with the views of the writers on this side of the water, I carefully prepared a number of sections according to his method, and certainly there was apparently much, at first sight, to substantiate the views expressed by him, but for this fact, he evidently had not taken into consideration the action of the acids used in his method of preparing the slides of enamel, and as a consequence drew wrong conclusions from the sections thus prepared.

That which Dr. Bödecker designated the enamel-fibre is probably that portion of the enamel which has taken the stain in the slides I have prepared, whilst the other portion (the reticulum) described by him I do not think exists in the enamel under ordinary conditions; it has been artificially produced, as the result of the partial decalcification of the enamel prisms by the acid used in preparing the sections.

There are two other portions of this tissue to which I wish to call your attention: (1) the brown striæ of Retzius; (2) Schreger's lines.

(1) The brown striæ are, I believe, produced as a result of a difference between the refractive index of the enamel prisms and the tubes between the prisms.

Mr. Leon Williams, when referring to the brown striæ, says, " These markings are due to pigmentation." This, I think, is not quite correct, for in those sections where the enamel is very thin the prism between the tubes is as free from color or pigment as it is in any other portion of the tissue; whilst the tubes themselves are well colored and very pronounced. In thicker sections there is the appearance of pigmentation. This is due to the fact that where there is more than one layer of cells the tubes are not directly under each other, and the difference between the refractive index of the tubes and prisms produces the results seen.

In transverse sections stained in this manner the striæ are well shown, and it is not at all unusual to find a small portion of more perfectly calcified tissue on either or both sides of these markings, which by contrast makes the striæ appear more pronounced. May not these more perfectly calcified portions indicate that there were times of rest as well as times of activity in the development preceding, or following, the formation of the striæ?

In some sections, owing to the angle at which they are cut, the ends of these tubes form a continuous line of colored dots along the line of the striæ.

These brown striæ are not confined to human teeth, as I have found them in the teeth of some of the animals examined.

(2) Lines of Shreger. In these lines, though the cause is the same as in the brown striæ of Retzius, the appearance is quite different, and this is accounted for by the fact that in the brown striæ the stained tubes run parallel to each other, and those forming one of the sections of the brown striæ are very much in the same plane. This is not so in those markings known as the lines of Schreger. The tubes and prisms in Shreger's lines are very much curved, and the optical effect of this curvature is to produce the peculiar cloud-like markings characteristic of these lines. But if,

whilst examining these lines under the microscope, the focussing is altered, it is possible to follow the course of these lines, and the the cloud-like effect is the result of the softening produced by the curvature of both prisms and the tubes.

As I said at the beginning of my paper, it is not my intention to deal to any extent with the development of this tissue. That subject is so vast, that were I desirous of doing so, the time at my disposal would be far too short. At the same time, as far as my study of this fascinating subject has gone, I think the theory expressed by Mr. Charles Tomes is more correct than that of Mr. Leon Williams.

If we accept Mr. Tomes's theory, that the enamel is produced as the result of the direct calcification of the enamel-cells, all the modifications I have shown to-night are easily explained, and their development can be readily understood. If, on the other hand, we accept the theories propounded by Mr. Leon Williams on the development of this tissue, so clearly and ably expressed in that splendid monograph of his on " The Enamel," these variations cannot exist, or, if they do exist, then there is much Mr. Williams has left unaccounted for.

To illustrate one point. Mr. Williams says, whilst discussing the theories of Von Ebner on the formation of the brown striæ, " that the idea is a mistaken one, first, because these supposed canals have no existence; and, secondly, because the ground-off ends of the enamel prisms do not appear except when the section of the enamel is ground at a certain angle."

In the face of such pronounced differences, pronounced with regard to the development of this tissue, what a splendid work our Society would accomplish if it were possible for them to appoint a committee to investigate this important matter. Should our Council see their way clear to carry out such a scheme, I shall be delighted to lend my slides to them for the purpose of examination and comparison with other slides to try and find out what is true in this matter.

In bringing this, my imperfect, and I am afraid somewhat rambling, paper to a conclusion, I believe your attention has been directed to the portion of the enamel that is stained by copper and other amalgams.—*Transactions of the Odontological Society of Great Britain.*

ON ELECTRIC STERILIZATION OF ROOT-CANALS. By Dr. W. D.
Miller, Berlin, Germany.

MR. PRESIDENT AND GENTLEMEN,—About two hours ago I was
absolutely innocent of any design of occupying your attention this
evening, but I happened to ask Mr. Mummery, when dining with
him, whether he had ever made use of electric sterilization in the
treatment of pulp-canals. He said he had not, and immediately
pounced upon me for remarks on the question this evening. The
subject of electro-sterilization of pulp-canals and diseased condition of teeth and the surroundings is by no means new. You are
no doubt acquainted with the work done some four or five years
ago by Zieler, a Russian dentist, residing in Würzburg. He made
a number of experiments, using an apparatus very similar to that
which we use for cataphoresis, conducting a current of about three
milliampères through the root-canals for ten minutes; he reported
most favorable results.

Slightly previous to this a dentist in Vienna, Dr. Brauer, also
published results which tallied with those of Zieler. The matter,
however, rested as it was until about six months ago, when one of
my colleagues at the Dental Institute of the University of Berlin,
Dr. Hoffendahl, came to me and reported enthusiastically about the
results he had obtained by the use of an electric current in the
treatment of root-canals. He cited a number of cases of chronic
abscesses and fistulæ which had been treated in the ordinary way
without any result being obtained, and other cases in which the
teeth remained comfortable as long as no filling was inserted, but
the moment the filling was inserted the teeth began to hurt. By
treating those canals with the electric current he was able to reduce the inflammation, and repeatedly he noticed that the suppuration stopped entirely after two or three treatments, and that the
teeth could be filled without any discomfort. That brought the matter again to my attention, and I decided to look into it a little closer,
and make some bacteriological experiments. I repeated the experiments, I think, in all some twelve or fifteen times, taking
freshly extracted putrid teeth, conducting an electric current of
one and one-half to two milliampères through the canals for ten
minutes, and, in order to bring about conditions as similar as possible to those of the mouth, I took the head of a calf, spread the
jaws open, and implanted a tooth containing a putrid pulp in the
anterior part of the upper jaw. The positive pole of the battery

was inserted in the root-canal and the negative applied to the anterior part of the lower jaw. That gave a current passing through the whole head of the calf. In dealing with a patient we put the positive pole in the canal of the tooth we wish to treat, and the patient takes the negative pole in his hand, so that the current passes through two or three feet of tissue. We were able to determine, in nearly all cases, that the bacteria were completely destroyed by the current of one and one-half to two milliampères passing through the root-canal for a space of ten minutes. Experiments were made by testing the contents of the canal before beginning the experiment for the presence of bacteria, and also again after five minutes and after ten minutes, and in the majority of cases, after ten minutes, there were no living bacteria to be found, and usually after five minutes the number was very materially reduced. I also made experiments with *Staphylococcus pyogenes aureus* by infecting the canal with this bacterium, and found the same results. In order to determine whether the electric current would have the effect of sterilizing the contents of abscesses, I constructed a little apparatus consisting of a glass tube broadened at one end and drawn out at the other to a fine point, somewhat like a funnel. The positive pole was placed at the narrow end of the glass, representing the root of the tooth, and the broad end was supposed to represent the abscess. This was fixed into a plate of thick cardboard, and filled with a solution of bouillon that had been infected with Prodigiosus. The current was conducted through this solution, the negative pole being on the opposite end of the cardboard, after the whole had been impregnated with chloride of sodium, so as to make a conductor and get about the same conductivity as we have in the tissues of the human body. After ten minutes no diminution in the number of bacteria had taken place; but after twenty minutes the number had been reduced about half, and in thirty minutes, with a current of one and one-half to two milliampères, the number had been reduced to about one-fifth of the original number on starting. So that we see there is a certain action upon bacteria even in larger cavities. In this case I used a tube about ten to twelve millimetres in diameter, which represents perhaps something larger than the abscesses with which we usually have to deal.

The canal is kept moist with a physiological solution of common salt during the operation, and the sterilizing action is not due to the direct action of the electric current, but to that of the products of electrolysis, in particular to that of chlorine.

The bacteriological results I obtained were, on the whole, very favorable, confirming those obtained by Brauer and Zieler, and showing beyond a doubt that we are in a position to diminish, if not completely destroy, the bacteria by the use of the electric current. If that should turn out to be applicable in practice, it would be of immense value to us. We all know how difficult it is to treat the buccal roots of upper molars, or the mesial roots of the lower molars, and how impossible it is sometimes to penetrate them with the finest broaches. And if we are able to put an electric current, something as subtle, if not more subtle than the bacteria themselves, on their track and to penetrate the finest canals, exerting a destructive effect on the bacteria, it would be a most beneficial and wonderful advancement in dental surgery. The results which I have obtained in the application of this method in the dental clinic have been, on the whole, very favorable. In one case in particular we had to treat an upper central incisor, which for five weeks had been under the direction of one of the assistants, who had never been able to close it up without producing pain on the following day. Dr. Hoffendahl gave it one treatment, and sealed the tooth up, and the patient came next day and had not had the slightest trace of pain.

Nearly all the cases we have treated have turned out very favorably. In one case, however, the day following the treatment a large swelling on the cheek occurred. In this case we had used the electric current without cleaning out the root-canal at all, and it occurred to me afterwards that possibly the electric current had had the effect of conducting the ptomaines in the root-canal through into the tissue and brought about infection. I wrote to Zieler, who is now in Hamburg, and asked him whether he had given up the method. He said he had not given it up, but owing to his being continually moving about he had been unable to continue his work, but he was thoroughly convinced of the great utility of the method. I asked him if he had ever had a case of swelling occur after application of the current, and he said that he had not. I advise any one using the method to first clean out the root-canal as far as possible, or at least the easily accessible portions, before applying the electric current, because it seems to me there is a possibility of ptomaines present in the pulp being conducted into the tissue.

We are, as I say, at present at work on this method, and I have not given any particular attention to the battery. I am using a chromic acid battery of thirty to forty cells with rheostat, provided me by Dr. Hoffendahl. We begin with a very low current, a fraction of a milliampère, and gradually increase the current to one and one-half or two milliampères, and let it pass through for ten minutes. The patient, in the majority of cases, experiences no inconvenience whatever. Sometimes they say they have a slight sensation, not amounting to pain. After ten minutes the current is removed, and the tooth may be filled. The experiments, however, are only in progress at present, and I would prefer that you should not make use of it until you receive the result of our further experiments, because methods of this kind cannot be tested too thoroughly. New methods are often introduced, and give wonderful results at the beginning; but later on we find the results were only fictitious, and that the method has to be given up. I will take the liberty of keeping you informed of what further results we may obtain, and, if they continue to be as favorable as they have been heretofore, I shall be able to advise you to make experiments in the same line.

The President, while he could not help admiring Dr. Miller's persistence in his careful experimentation, felt still more admiration for the interesting and frank way in which he had stated the unsuccessful experiment, and for the warning he extended to dental surgeons not to play with the method until a little more information had been received from head-quarters. The most interesting point was that of the uncleaned canal. At first sight it seemed that the method would afford a delightful way out of the difficulties of dealing with those irregular canals which refused to be treated by ordinary methods of bristles, and so forth. He had felt that perhaps the current might be able to go where the bristles would not, and at least as far as the bacteria could permeate. But apparently it was necessary to be very careful, and await a further communication from Dr. Miller at some later date.—*Transactions of the Odontological Society of Great Britain.*

STARTING-PITS: THEIR USE AND ABUSE. By S. H. Guilford, D.D.S., Ph.D.

The advisability or inadvisability of the use of starting-pits in the placing of gold fillings has long since ceased to be a subject for discussion either in the journals or the societies. The line of

division between those who believe in their value or those who do
not has been pretty sharply drawn, and each side seems satisfied
with its respective method.

The subject would not now be revived in this journal were it not
for the fact that a few examining boards have recently taken occasion to express strong disapproval of their employment when recent
graduates were doing their practical work before them.

That small pits or depressions as aids in the starting of gold
fillings were in very general use a quarter of a century ago, and
that their employment has very greatly decreased since then, is
certainly true; but that quite a number of practitioners still find
them serviceable in certain cases is also true.

The decline in the use is most probably due to two causes,—
first, their too general and often improper employment; and
second, the advancement made in the methods of shaping cavities
and inserting fillings.

They were called " retaining pits" originally, and this misnomer
probably caused much of the prejudice which grew up against them.
In many cases they were employed for purposes of retention, because the practitioner had a wholesome dread of his fillings dropping
out and desired to take every precaution against such an unfortunate mishap.

The shaping of cavities to give them a proper retentive form
was not so well understood in those days as it is now, but even
when improvement came in this direction the " starting-pit," as it
came to be called, continued to be used for the more secure anchorage of the first pieces of gold placed in a cavity.

Through ignorance and lack of experience their use often led to
abuse, and so they fell more and more into disfavor. As used by
Webb and other renowned operators, the starting-pit was made
with a very small drill, and besides being very shallow, it was
formed in the dentine very near to the enamel.

Others, less skilful or less prudent, made them large and deep,
and often located them very near to the pulp.

There could be but one result in such cases,—namely, the death
of the pulp with its unfortunate consequences. That a reaction
should follow such practice was not only natural but inevitable.

In the more recent methods of shaping cavities, as advocated
by Black and others, the cavity, if a compound one, is largely flattened at its cervical aspect, thus forming angles with the lateral
walls. These angles in the dentine are intensified for the double

purpose of more readily starting the filling and for its more secure retention.

In cavities of this class very few operators, if any, make use of a starting-pit, because the newer method does away with its necessity. In simple cavities on the approximal surfaces of teeth, however, especially the incisors and cuspids, a small, shallow starting-pit, properly located so as to avoid all danger to the pulp through thermal changes, has certain advantages, as many believe.

Each practitioner is naturally governed by his experience in the use or non-use of this aid to filling, but with the student who has had little opportunity to gain experience, and whose skill in overcoming difficulties has not had time to develop, the case is different.

Probably nothing proves so discouraging to the student in his efforts to acquire the art of properly introducing a filling as to have it shift its position when once started, or possibly come out entirely after it is completed, because its position has changed without his knowledge.

Teachers often find it necessary to advise and encourage their students to take advantage of certain aids which will assist them in their work and inspire confidence, knowing full well that as they advance in knowledge and experience many of these aids will be laid aside.

Thus we find students adjusting the rubber dam in all or nearly all cases where a gold filling is to be inserted and encircling each included tooth with a ligature.

Later, experience teaches them that in many simple cases both dam and ligatures may be discarded in favor of the napkin, to the advantage of the patient and themselves.

Excessive undercutting of cavities and the over-annealing of gold are excesses often practised by students in their overanxiety to secure a successful result.

Nearly all good points of any operative procedure are likely to be carried beyond the bounds of advisability by the inexperienced, but all these matters right themselves in time.

Students are usually taught correctly, and while the advantages of certain methods are pointed out, it is also made plain to them that the same methods carried to excess may result in injury instead of good.

We cannot expect a recent graduate to be as proficient as he is likely to become after years of practice.—*The Stomatologist.*

17

Reports of Society Meetings.

THE NEW YORK INSTITUTE OF STOMATOLOGY.

A MEETING of the Institute was held at the "Chelsea," No. 222 West Twenty-third Street, New York, on Tuesday evening, February 2, 1904, the President, Dr. Brockway, in the chair.

Owing to the amount of material in the regular transactions, the communications on theory and practice were omitted.

The regular subject of the evening, Oral Hygiene and Prophylaxis, was discussed.

Dr. Sinclair Tousey stated that Dr. Leo Green and he had been working for some time on a method for the treatment of pyorrhœa alveolaris by means of the X-ray apparatus. They had quite a number of successful results to report later, but as yet they were not quite ready. Any members of the society who were interested he would like to invite to a demonstration of the apparatus, either at the St. Bartholomew's clinic or at his office. He also had a specimen of radium. He would also demonstrate a method he had perfected of the immediate development of the picture taken by means of the X-ray machine and without any dark room, only a comparatively dark space being necessary. The print could be ready for exhibition in five minutes after the exposure.

Upon motion, the thanks of the Institute were extended to Dr. Tousey for his kind offer.

Dr. E. S. Gaylord, of New Haven, stated that the subject for this evening, oral prophylaxis, was a most important and interesting one, yet he had not prepared a paper, and the little he had to say would be more in description of the work of another than anything he had been able to accomplish himself. In July last it was his good fortune to receive an invitation from Dr. D. D. Smith, of Philadelphia, to attend a clinical examination of a number of his patients' mouths who had been under his care for several years. There were eleven other dentists from different parts of the country in attendance. Dr. Smith had made appointments with his patients, to avoid confusion, and upon arrival, they were introduced, and a brief description given of the prior condition of the mouth by Dr. Smith, supplemented by the patient. Each gentleman was given the opportunity to thoroughly examine the mouth, Dr. Smith requesting not only a thorough examination, but to criticise whatever they might find. The first patient arrived soon after nine in the morning, the list of patients was completed a little after four, and they had examined twenty-nine mouths. Until about a dozen patients had been examined, it was his impression (and, he afterwards learned, that of others) that they were examining selected cases, and certainly those that required no dental operations, being in condition of perfect health. Their verdict was unanimous: positively there was no room for criticism, either of the fillings, crowns, or bridges, or general condition of the mouths; they seemed as nearly perfect as possible. In November last he again received an invitation from Dr. Smith, and with seventeen other dentists, representing nearly as many States, they spent nearly the entire day in examination of the mouths of thirty patients. Thus he has seen over fifty of Dr. Smith's patients, ranging from the ages of six to sixty-five. In many there were evidences that they had not been in a normal condition, and by the testimony of the patient, they learned there had been much suffering, both physical and mental, prior to Dr. Smith taking them in charge. Pyorrhœa in its worst form had been perfectly eliminated, and around the teeth was to be seen the beautiful restorations of the gingivæ, teeth firm in their sockets, entire surfaces beautifully polished, striations of the gums, giving evidence of a condition with which, in their own practice, they thought themselves unfamiliar; indeed, there was such sameness and perfect condition, that, as some one remarked, it seemed monotonous. In children's mouths they saw no evidence of caries having occurred, and he believes he is safe in affirmation that no caries occur in any of these mouths when well under treatment, and here it seems to him is where Dr. Smith is deserving of so much praise, in conceiving and executing the necessity of frequent treatments, which consist in systematically polishing the entire surfaces of the teeth every month with pumice and orange-wood stick, at the same time massaging the gum margins, thus not only preserving a condition of health, but seemingly a restoration or preservation of their natural colors; certain it is there was little variation in the shade of the teeth, even in different mouths. Dr. Smith asserts, and it seems reasonable, this rubbing with stick and pumice stimulates circulation within the tooth, thereby preserving natural hues and normal conditions. Dr. Smith has designed a set of scalers, both unique and unusual in form (made by J. W. Ivory), in that they are to be used in the manner of a file, with draw cut, which after removal of the calculus, leaves the surface of the teeth smoother than the ordinary scaler, and able to follow into pockets farther with greater ease and less pain than with any other form with which he was familiar. After thorough scaling, the teeth are thoroughly polished with the orange-wood and pumice, held in a very neat form of porte-polisher of his own device, and each tooth is polished, not only on its crown, but, where pyorrhœa exists, to the bottom of each pocket; the pockets are then washed with a strong solution of phenol sodique, after which, in severe cases, a deliquesced solution of zinc chloride is carried in with the point of a small stick, the ordinary wood tooth-pick shaved thin serving a good purpose. Dr. Gaylord regards the opportunity of seeing this method of treatment of more value than he can well express, and he has carried it into his own practice with results that are so pleasing to his patients and himself that he will never abandon it. He would urge all to investigate, particularly the young men, as he believes it possible to conduct a practice, beginning with children, carrying them along through life with no fillings (except in imperfections in fissures), without the loss of a single tooth, and pyorrhœa absolutely unknown to them.

Dr. C. W. Strang was reminded of what Dr. Dio Lewis had said many years ago, that a clean tooth never would decay. If Dr. Lewis had stated that a perfectly formed tooth, properly kept clean, would never decay, Dr. Strang would feel more like agreeing with him. For that thing to be accomplished, the patient must polish his teeth almost every minute of the day. Dr. Strang mentioned the case of an old patient of thirty years' standing in his practice who from year to year had had very little to be done with the exception of the removal of a little soft tartar and the polishing of the teeth. Occasionally there had been a little filling to be inserted. About two years ago that gentleman's health had failed, and six months ago Dr. Strang had seen the patient and noted evidences of a change in the condition of his mouth. At that time he had been entered upon his books to be seen again in six months. At the end of this six months he was surprised to see the ravages of disease in that mouth. Dr. Strang believed that such progress of dental caries as this was due principally to the vitiated condition of the secretions of the mouth, more than to deleteriorations of tooth-structure. Dr. Black has told us that there is very little difference in the various specimens of dentine that he had examined. In the enamel there is a great difference. About five years ago Dr. Strang had ·made the statement before a local society in Providence that if we took patients in early life and were systematic and careful in cleansing and polishing their teeth we would have very little trouble from the development of pyorrhœa alveolaris in these cases. Dr. Strang had been fortunate enough when in college to be under the tuition of Dr. James Truman. Dr. Truman had always tried to impress upon the minds of the students the importance of keeping the teeth of every patient clean; that the younger men could not hope to compete with the older practitioners in many things, but they could compete in cleanliness. Dr. Strang had always endeavored to follow this teaching to his very best ability. At first the instruments obtainable for this purpose were very crude, but with time these had improved. He had been conscientiously trying for the past thirty-five years as far as possible to remove the deposits of tartar from his patients' teeth, but he did not believe he was any better able to do it to-day than he was five years ago, except that now he was equipped with a little better instruments. If anybody had told him two years ago that he was not doing as well by his patients as he ought, he would not have believed them; indeed, he would have been willing to compare any twenty-five or thirty of his patients with those of any other practitioner. He was glad that Dr. D. D. Smith had not had an opportunity to accept such a challenge. If any one had told him two years ago that teeth could not be properly cleansed with the dental engine, Dr. Strang would have said that he knew better. When he had seen the results of the work in Dr. D. D. Smith's office, it did not take him long to be convinced that he had been doing the work improperly. He had been so thoroughly convinced that since last July he had used the dental engine but three times in cleansing teeth, and then only to remove some stains.

Dr. Alfred C. Fones stated that he claimed little or no originality regarding the thoughts he wished to express on this subject. Our chief object should be the prevention of dental diseases, rather than being content with the repairing of the damages wrought. He said that micro-organisms, with their action upon food débris, were the cause of most of the pathological conditions found in the mouth. As it was seemingly impossible to entirely rid the mouth of these organisms, we should adopt some plan or system whereby our patients could keep their mouths clean and free from the accumulations of food products. The teeth presented about twenty-five square inches of surface. Now, if we compared the relative difficulties of cleansing a piece of smooth and then of ground glass of about this surface, the importance of keeping the teeth smooth and polished could readily be seen. The method used to produce this mirror surface was that advocated by Dr. D. D. Smith, using pumice and orange-wood sticks carried in holders, such as furnished by J. W. Ivory of Philadelphia. All surfaces of the teeth are thoroughly rubbed, considerable pressure being used, the edge of the stick kept sharp, in order to reach under the margin of the gums. Particular attention is paid to the necks of the teeth. Polishing strips are used on the proximal surfaces. It takes, generally, a number of thorough treatments to produce this high polish, but when once secured it may easily be maintained by monthly treatments of about a half-hour.

He said it was absolutely impossible to get the desired results unless we had the thorough co-operation of our patients and were arbitrary with them in insisting upon their systematically cleansing their teeth with tooth-brush and dentifrice. We should also pre-scribe the kind of brush and kind of dentifrice, and when and for how long they should cleanse their teeth. If we would be arbi-trary in these matters it would be done as we directed and we would soon begin to get results. The average person spends, per-haps, twenty to thirty seconds brushing the teeth, in spite of what we all have heard them affirm,—that they spent fully five minutes at it,—evidently never having timed themselves. It was impossible to get proper results in less than ninety seconds for thoroughly cleansing the teeth and imparting a vascular stimulus to the gums.

Dr. Fones stated that he had some forty patients under prac-tical treatment in this manner, and was much pleased with the results obtained. Through Dr. Smith he had become somewhat in-terested in the system some five years ago, but had not then realized its full value. He believed it was along the line of prophy-laxis that future progress in the profession of dentistry would be made. He believed that the art of restoring lost tooth-structure had about reached its zenith, unless perhaps the ideal filling, a porcelain cement, might be discovered. The work of the future in preventing dental caries and the development of pyorrhœa would be found in extreme cleanliness. He said it was an ideal treatment for children's teeth and for adults who were susceptible to dental decay. After a thorough instrumentation in cases of pyorrhœa, he believed it to be the most effective treatment known.

Regarding the theoretical side of pyorrhœa alveolaris, Dr. Fones considered the disease divided into (1) interstitial, (2) phagadenic pericementitis, and (3) gouty pericementitis, the third being rare, the first and second being conditions we were constantly meeting. It had been estimated that sixty-five per cent. of the teeth lost were lost from results of this disease. Although caries was more prevalent, it was not so fatal. He thought that the development of the disease might be placed under two general heads, one due to susceptibility and the other to a local exciting cause.

Every person, after passing the age of thirty-five, was susceptible to this disease; it was simply a question of degree. After this age the peridental membrane gradually became thinner, the alveolar process more dense, and there was a lessened vascularity and resistant power. Susceptibility of the patient was increased by nervous disorders, lowering the vitality, faulty metabolism, etc. The exciting cause was almost entirely produced by the irritation of the toxins and ptomaines generated by the action of micro-organisms on food débris around the necks of the teeth. Its quick response to extreme cleanliness and antiseptic treatment seemed to prove it. The stimulus imparted to the gums by the thorough and systematic brushing was imparted in turn to the underlying tissues, which lessened their susceptibility by increasing their vascularity.

To what degree these nervous disorders and faulty metabolic conditions were caused by systematic infection due to unsanitary mouths, it was difficult, at present, to predict. Chronic indigestion, neurasthenia, malarial symptoms, periodic headaches, throat troubles, and bad breath were cured or showed marked improvement in a comparatively short time. He believed there was a condition here producing systemic disturbances that the great majority of the medical profession had not dreamed of. The time was coming when the first law of hygiene would be recognized as a clean and sanitary mouth, and the assistance of the dental practitioner would prove indispensable to his medical brother in restoring many of his patients to health without the use of drugs.

Dr. Fones believed that the dental profession will owe Dr. D. D. Smith a debt of gratitude for demonstrating and calling our attention to this field of prophylaxis which is now opening up before us.

Dr. L. C. Taylor merely wished to reinforce the statements made. He thought the subject of Oral Hygiene and Prophylaxis a very important one. A vast number of people are to-day suffering directly or indirectly from mouth infection, and many cases of so-called stomach trouble can be cured by proper attention to oral cleanliness. It requires great skill to treat a set of teeth properly where pyorrhœa alveolaris is present. He mentioned a friend who thought a higher grade of skill is necessary than in an operation for appendicitis.

Several cases were mentioned of invalids being entirely cured by a careful attention to the septic condition of the mouth and polishing off the bacterial plague on the teeth. They had been suffering from mouth infection and nothing more. We have had ample description and abundance of literature upon the different kinds of bacteria found in the oral cavity. Dr. Andrews, Dr. Williams, Dr. Black, and may others have given us the result of their researches, but none have told us how to get rid of this infection. It is time that we get to the business side of it. We know these bacteria existed, we have seen them repeatedly, but have we seen the beautiful healthy mouth and the resulting tone of the whole system? This is what we want. It is a high ideal, but it is one worth attaining.

Regarding the much talked of connection between uræmia and pyorrhœa, and the consequent desirability of a systemic treatment for pyorrhœa, Dr. Taylor did not know of a single instance where a systemic treatment had cured a case of pyorrhœa, but he could mention numbers of cases where, the pyorrhœa alveolaris being cured, the uræmia had disappeared. It was another case of intestinal derangement due to mouth infection.

Dr. Taylor does not believe any living man can properly treat pyorrhœa of the mouth with the dental engine. He mentioned in this connection that the first practical teaching of oral hygiene and prophylaxis in any dental college was established in a dental school in New York City. He said he thought New York would see the time when she would be proud of this pre-eminence.

Dr. Taylor spoke with praise of the work done by Dr. D. D. Smith, of Philadelphia. He thoroughly approves his methods. He does not believe that in many cases it is possible at one sitting to get perfect health of the mouth. It will require from twelve to twenty consecutive months before that mouth will be satisfactory to the practitioner. The first two or three sittings will be sufficient to render the teeth mechanically clean, and thereafter each month the teeth may bé gone over in thirty or forty minutes, but it will take months for the mouth to reach what might be called a perfect state of health.

Dr. Tousey stated that in the work at the St. Bartholomew's Parish, it was noticed that an unhygienic condition of the patient's mouths existed almost without exception, and in order to stimulate the children to be more cleanly they were taught to play what was known as the " tooth-brush game." The game had become very popular, and it was seen that some of the elders and parents were playing the game also.

Dr. Green stated that Dr. Fones's remarks about the care of children's mouths had led him to call attention to other features in this connection. He believed that prophylaxis should be extended to include proper nourishment even before the eruption of the teeth. He had noticed, especially among the children of wealth, that the modified forms of milk so commonly given to children had a very deleterious effect upon their teeth. These foods seemed to lack the essential properties required in tooth building. Furthermore, Dr. Green thought, where children are given over to a wet-nurse, too much attention could not be given to the condition of the mouth of the nurse. Dr. Green had been preparing statistics upon this subject, but as yet was not prepared to place them in the hands of the society.

Dr. Locherty stated that he would like to hear more concerning the medicines used in connection with this mechanical cleansing. He had himself, in the case of very persistent green stain, applied the rubber dam and first used iodine, following this with hydrogen peroxide in connection with a heated instrument, thus bleaching the surface and afterwards polishing. The results in these instances had been very satisfactory.

Dr. F. Milton Smith stated that in regard to this subject and the claim of Dr. D. D. Smith, of Philadelphia, it seemed to him that this perfect cleanliness of the teeth and mouth was the goal after which every man here was striving. That Dr. Smith succeeded better than any other man he knew he was willing to admit. He had seen a dozen or fifteen of these cases, and he hoped the time would come when he would be able to do as well by his own patients. However, he did not believe Dr. Smith was the first man to preach that cleanliness was the best thing we could accomplish for our patients. If he had understood Dr. Gaylord, Dr. D. D. Smith claimed nothing new except persistence. He was very glad to hear this. He had made a statement himself to the effect that he believed the chief point in Dr. Smith's method was thoroughness, which is another word for persistence. However, according to his own understanding of the case, this was not all that Dr. D. D. Smith had claimed for his method. He had claimed something entirely new and something that he alone had advanced. There seemed to be some mystery about this point. He himself believed and it was generally conceded that a thorough polishing of the teeth, even as often as once in two weeks or once a month was a very beneficial thing, and he had several cases where he had proved the efficacy of this. Dr. Gaylord had stated that he formerly believed the teeth could be thoroughly cleansed with the engine. Dr. Smith had never believed that. However, he believed that with the dental engine, with scalers, files, and scrapers, with the polishing sticks and pumice, with the floss-silk, and with every other means available, it would be possible to pretty nearly remove all the foreign substances from the teeth, and when this was done as thoroughly and as frequently as it was done by Dr. D. D. Smith the results would be marvellous.

The President stated that he was most favorably impressed with the prophylactic method under consideration, and had read all the papers describing it, published by Dr. D. D. Smith, with great interest and profit. As he had remarked on a former occasion, he was an easy convert to the idea, for the first operation at which he was set by his preceptor at the beginning of his study of dentistry was the cleansing and polishing of teeth in the mouths of his patients. His preceptor had been a strong believer in the value of such service, and Dr. Brockway had always retained and practised what he was then taught.

He thought, however, that few if any of us had carried the cleansing process to the extent and thoroughness of Dr. Smith, which is its most important and distinguishing feature, and for this Dr. Smith has rendered our profession and the public which we serve what Dr. Brockway considers the greatest service of our time.

At first he was inclined, as were others, to take issue with Dr. Smith on his emphatic declaration that this work could not be accomplished by the engine, and while Dr. Brockway still holds that much of it can more easily be done thereby, it is perhaps necessary to supplement its use by hand-work with the porte-polisher and similar adjuncts for the purpose of obtaining the stimulating effect aimed at.

In this connection he wished to call attention to the value of tecum fibre as a most efficient article for the purpose of polishing the approximal surfaces of the teeth where the floss-silk and tape are generally used, this being fine, strong, and charged with native grit, silex, like the cortex of a reed, making it most admirable for the purpose required. It can be drawn between the most closely set teeth with the aid of a little vaseline, in extreme cases, which does not seem to impair its efficiency. Dr. Brockway thought that probably this article was not new to most of the men present, but, never having seen any mention of it in the discussions of this subject, he could not refrain from calling attention to its merits.

A vote of thanks was extended to the gentlemen who had so kindly presented this subject to the Institute.

Adjourned.

FRED. L. BOGUE, M.D., D.D.S.,
Editor The New York Institute of Stomatology.

ACADEMY OF STOMATOLOGY.

THE regular meeting of the Academy of Stomatology of Philadelphia was held on the evening of Tuesday, December 22, 1903, at the rooms of the Academy, 1731 Chestnut Street, the President, Dr. L. Foster Jack, in the chair.

A paper was read by Dr. M. H. Cryer, entitled " Impacted Teeth: Their Diagnosis, Liberation, and Extraction," and illustrated by the use of lantern slides.

(For Dr. Cryer's paper, see page 321.)

DISCUSSION.

Dr. E. T. Darby.—If we were to study carefully, in this relation, every mouth we look into, we would probably find few people who have thirty-two teeth fully erupted. Out of the six or eight patients I saw to-day, but one had the full complement. One woman thirty years of age had never had any third molars.

It has been said that the size of the human jaw has been deteriorating for hundreds of years. I remember hearing, some twenty-five or thirty years ago, in our State Society, a paper by Dr. Welcher, in which he took the ground that the wisdom-tooth was unnecessary, and that in time there would be no wisdom-teeth in the mouth. When in Egypt, over thirty years ago, I examined hundreds of ancient skulls, but did not find a single jaw which was not large enough for thirty-two teeth. I do not remember seeing any with the wisdom-teeth missing where the subject had been old enough to have them. If it be true that the jaw is deteriorating in size, that may account for the present frequency of impaction of wisdom-teeth.

In the case of a young woman of twenty-six or thirty, seen in my practice, who never had had a lateral incisor, there was a bulging just under the lip near the nose. Suspecting an impacted tooth, I made an incision, which revealed the central incisor twisted around the lateral in a perfect hook. The question arises as to what was the cause of this.

The fact that so many inferior wisdom-teeth are tipped forward, with the occlusal surface abutting against the distal surface of the second molar, raises the question as to whether the tooth can be extracted without injury and a great deal of trouble. I have for years been in the habit of sending such cases to Dr. Thomas. He has often advised the removal of the second molar, hoping that the third molar might right itself and take a normal position; but, experience proves that this tooth rarely becomes useful. In such a case a perfectly sound second molar has been lost and a tooth that is of little value has been saved. When I find a molar tipping forward in that way, with its occlusal surface against the distal surface of a second molar, I prefer not to risk the possibility of fracture at the ramus; on the contrary, I much prefer to cut down with a large bur, exposing the anterior portion of the ramus, and take out the tooth through the opening thus made.

Dr. F. C. Van Woert, Brooklyn.—I am here mainly in the interests of the X-ray, being thoroughly convinced that when these obscure cases are presented to us, as general practitioners we should refer them to specialists in that particular line. I cannot quite agree with Dr. Cryer in some of his deductions regarding the X-ray, and yet I fully realize how difficult it is to diagnose some of these skiagraphs.

I have brought over some slides and shall be pleased to show them and tell you some of the difficulties of making a diagnosis from them. The skiagraph does not always present a clear definition owing to the superimposition of one shadow upon another. One requires at times some clinical knowledge of the case itself, otherwise the readings from the skiagraph may possibly be misleading. In such a case as this, which was referred to me by Dr. S. G. Perry, you can plainly see that there are two permanent laterals. The crowns were equally good, and upon the possible condition of the roots depended the extraction of one of the teeth for orthodontic purposes, as you see the root of the lateral next the one to be moved, and which would naturally be extracted, is better than that of the other lateral. Upon the valuable evidence of the skiagraph the distal lateral was removed.

In some of these other cases the evidence is not so clear. An interesting discussion was precipitated during the exhibit between Drs. Van Woert and Cryer, the latter claiming that the location of an impacted lower molar could not be determined by a skiagraph, whereas Dr. Van Woert held that the intensity of the shadows of the alveolar process would give a fairly approximate idea as to whether a tooth lay to the buccal or the lingual side of the lower jaw, while the outline of the tooth would give its other position.

Dr. M. K. Kassabian.—Dentistry and medicine have derived equal benefits from the introduction and use of the X-rays. I will confine my remarks to one class of dental anomalies for the treatment of which this discovery can be utilized,—*i.e.,* unerupted teeth. Many difficult cases have been brought to my attention by the dental profession at large, and especially those which have been kindly referred to by Dr. Cryer. Most of Dr. Cryer's cases were those of an obscure nature, and with great difficulty and skilful use of the explorer he diagnosed the conditions which I confirmed by using the Röntgen rays, thus showing and proving the existing conditions by skiagraphs. The ordinary method of probing with an explorer did not always locate the absent tooth, especially in some cases of bicuspids and third molars. These had insinuated themselves deeply beneath other teeth, and the alveolar process was so dense that nothing but the X-ray would locate and determine their position.

An invaluable return from using the X-ray in these dental cases is the exact and precise results obtained. It not only locates the unerupted tooth, but also determines the position in which it is resting. For the benefit of those who are not conversant with X-ray work, I will describe how the location and position of a tooth can be best gotten.

Two skiagraphs are taken from two angles or directions, to determine whether we have a buccal, lingual, distal, or mesial presentment, and I might mention here that Dr. Cryer suggested that I make stereoscopic skiagrams, which permit viewing by a reflecting stereoscope, and as a result, instead of observing flat pictures, we obtain a relief or stereoscopic perspective effect. I have received very good results with my stereoscopic skiagrams at the Philadelphia Hospital, where I use a special table which I had built for that purpose. I employ two methods for skiagraphing dental conditions, —A, the intra-oral method; B, the extra-oral or buccal method.

A. The intra-oral method is proceeded with by inserting a small piece of film (which is light and moisture-proof) over the gum tissue at a point where trouble is suspected, placing the tube in such a position that perpendicular rays will be cast upon the teeth and film. This method covers a smaller area, but produces a picture with very sharp detail, and is especially recommended for anterior teeth.

B. The extra-oral or buccal method requires that a plate 5 x 7 be brought in contact with the jaw at the region of suspected trouble. The patient is directed to incline the neck and head to an angle measuring about forty-five degrees. The tube is now placed over the shoulder on the opposite side at a distance of twenty inches from the face, to avoid superimposition of the jaws. This process produces a picture of great area, and is intended for bicuspids and molars.

During exposure of this plate it is wise to insert a block of wood about two inches square between the teeth, which prevents the patient from closing the mouth. These methods produce pictures which to the novice appear difficult to intelligently read, but, as in other lines of our professional work, only time and experience teach and give masterly results.

The slides exhibited here this evening show the great progress that has been made in this line of work and how much assistance is rendered in diagnosing unerupted teeth by the aid of the X-ray.

Dr. Pfahler.—As Dr. Cryer has told you, I am not a dentist, but as a doctor of medicine I have done some X-ray work. Just as Dr. Cryer has learned to use his probe most skilfully, so in X-ray work we must learn to use the X-ray skilfully; and in order to obtain results we must do two things,—make good negatives, and know how to read them. The mistakes which seemed to be so prominent to-night were, I think, no fault of the X-ray, but rather of the man who read them. This subject is still in its infancy. Some one asked why the shadow of the loose piece of bone lying in a pus-cavity was darker than the surrounding bone. If you will look at that carefully you will find that the shadow was not darker than the surrounding bone, but it stood out more prominently, because of the light area surrounding it. The difficulty Dr. Cryer has mentioned in the case of an impacted tooth is not one that cannot be overcome. Their exact location can be determined by the method which Dr. Van Woert has shown you, and again brought out by Dr. Kassabian. You can determine the proximity of a foreign body to the plate by the sharpness of the shadows and by their overlapping. Another method is by fluoroscopic study. This is not yet thoroughly worked out, but will be in a short time. By these various methods we locate foreign bodies, and can probably come within a millimetre of the exact location of one of these teeth. All these difficulties can be overcome as our experience increases.

Dr. Cryer (closing).—Dr. Darby asked about the cause of impaction. I tried to make that plain in my paper. If we study the anatomical structure of normal bone of the jaw, the lower for instance, we find that the cancellated portion slides within the cortical portion from the back forward. This sliding is accomplished as the teeth are developed. It has been demonstrated that the development of the teeth changes their relation to the mental foramen until the latter, instead of being at the base of the cuspid tooth, comes to be between the two bicuspids, and in some cases under the first molar. This sliding motion allows the teeth to move into their proper position. If this motion is interfered with we have impaction. The occurrence of an inflammatory condition in the cancellated bone near the cortical will cause the osteoblasts to build bone at that point, which will lock them together. The teeth being developed in little bony capsules, these will be cemented to the cortical portion of the bone, which does not move. It appears to me, that this is the reason of impaction. To avoid this condition, we must constantly keep the mouths of our children in perfect health, and allow nothing to exist which will cause a productive inflammation.

In answer to Dr. Van Woert, I do not consider the X-ray of little use to us. It is bound to be of great use to us, but, as Dr. Pfahler has said, we must learn to read the pictures. The pictures which Dr. Van Woert has shown prove conclusively to my mind that he cannot tell what he sees in these pictures. In one case he said he could not tell whether it was bone until it was removed. The most important use of the X-ray in this connection will be in the region of the canine, lateral, and central teeth.

OTTO E. INGLIS,
Editor Academy of Stomatology.

Editorial.

THE NATIONAL ASSOCIATION OF DENTAL FACULTIES.

IT is possible that by the time this reaches our readers the National Association of Dental Faculties will have met at Washington, D. C., and may have concluded its deliberations.

This body has ceased to be a mere instrument to meet annually and to voice the aims and aspirations of the dental colleges. It has become more than this, and it stands to-day as the exponent of the advanced thought of the dental profession of America, and by America is meant not merely the limited boundaries of the United States, but the entire continent. This is written advisedly, for dentistry, as taught since the organization first met has sent its young graduates everywhere, and these represent the thoughts and highest aims of this organization.

If, then, the " Faculties" has become, as represented, the mouth-piece of the profession, it has, as its most important duty, to guard its portals that nothing may enter to mar the confidence heretofore reposed in its decisions.

This body will meet at Washington, D. C., June 9. The writer in a previous number discussed this plan, as at that time proposed, and endeavored to show that no provision was made in the laws governing the organization to warrant any meeting except that provided by the laws heretofore adopted. This, apparently, had no deterring influence, for, upon a vote taken by mail, the majority, it is presumed, decided it was wise to hold this meeting five months after an equally irregular one held at Buffalo in January last, thus making three meetings within ten months for this Association,—those of Asheville, Buffalo, and Washington.

No attempt has been made to disguise the purpose of the two called meetings. It is well known that a certain number of dental colleges are in direct opposition to the course of four years, that went into operation the present session of 1903–04. At the time of the original passage of this act there was but feeble opposition to this measure. It was demanded by the National Association of Dental Examiners and by some of the State boards. Hence opposition, if felt at that time, was silenced.

The meeting at Asheville, N. C., was held preceding the period fixed for beginning this course. The colleges had had no experience as to the results of this advanced time. Harvard refused to comply with the decision of the Faculties, and resigned.

The National Association of Dental Examiners offered a loophole for the weaker dental colleges to escape this, to them, oppressive statute, and then began the efforts to bring about a return to a three years' course. It was attempted at Buffalo and failed, but, not discouraged, the opposition set to work to secure a meeting before the regular period, which would be the last of August at St. Louis. Under the specious pretence that time would not permit careful consideration of other matters at this time, with the National Organization and the Congress to care, for, a note was sent round demanding a vote for certain places and for a meeting in June. The result was, it seems, fixed as before stated, at Washington. Who ordered this vote is unknown to the writer, but it is presumed it originated at Buffalo. As this meeting was irregularly called, no authority existed there or elsewhere to call another meeting save and except that provided for under the rules.

The meeting has, therefore, been convened for a special purpose.

What that may be cannot positively be decided at this writing, but presumably it will give an opportunity for those colleges interested in a retrograde movement to push the matter to a finality. The motive which underlies this effort is not difficult to determine. As the course stands at present, it is not to the financial interests of many of the independent dental colleges to continue the extended period. The meeting must be held to meet the time at which announcements are usually issued, and if this retrograde action were adopted it must be entered therein, or a delay of one year would follow. No attempt has been made to disguise this motive by those working in the interest of a three years' course.

The arguments used to sustain this retrograde movement have been previously alluded to and answered, but one used at Buffalo was so intrinsically weak that surprise must generally be felt that men of intelligence could have entertained it as a process of reasoning. This was that three years of nine months would be practically equal to four years of seven months, the first making a college course of twenty-seven months and the latter one of twenty-eight. It seems to have been forgotten that the most strenuous advocates of the four years have been the departments of universities, and these have had, for a number of years, courses of nine months each. The results have not been satisfactory, and they have insisted on an extension of time. That the schools not equally as well fitted for training undergraduates should be able to accomplish what these have found beyond their power must impress itself upon every logical mind.

At this writing, a month in advance of the meeting, it is impossible to foretell with any accuracy what may result from this meeting, but it is earnestly desired that wise counsels may prevail and that the standard will be left as it is at present.

Most of the dental colleges of this country are organized upon a weak financial foundation. The majority are comparatively new and are dependent upon the income from students, and it is natural that the faculties view the prospect with serious misgivings. It means, from their view, a dissolution of the faculties and serious financial loss. They will therefore, be unable to regard the ethical side of the question at Washington, and if able to force their opinions it may be that their retrograde ideas may prevail and a three years' course be ordered.

The object of this article is not to influence legislation on this subject, for it will be too late even to be read by those most interested. Its motive is to give the world at large an insight into the influences that have led up to this effort. If this be successful, those interested in advanced dental education should understand the influences leading to such a disastrous ending of twenty years of earnest work.

It is a mistake to suppose that this first year of the four years' course represents the future. It will, of course, require some years to accustom the minds of parents and guardians to the new order of things, but experience has demonstrated that financially the schools are, in the end, equally as well off with the higher standard as they were with the lower. Every advance in dental teaching has been followed by a period of depression, to be again followed by an enlarged matriculation list, and this means more than mere financial benefit, for it brings with it a higher class of men and an equally higher standard of character.

The writer has, however, very little interest in the commercial side of dental education. The aim of the active workers has been, from the time of Harris and Hayden, to carry dental training to its utmost limits, and if this means the destruction of means and methods that may have become antiquated or insufficient, the earlier this is accomplished the better it will be not only for our profession, but for the world at large.

CORRECTION NOTICE.

In Dr. H. A. Baker's paper on "Treatment of Protruding and Receding Jaws," published in the May number, there occurred a very regrettable transposition of two cuts,—Fig. 13 should have occupied the place filled by Fig. 9, and the latter in the former, showing the completion of the work and the correction of the irregularity.

No doubt all our readers made the correction for themselves, as the transposition was clearly made evident in the character of the illustrations.

Bibliography.

Irregularities of the Teeth and their Treatment. By
Eugene S. Talbot, M.S., D.D.S., M.D., LL.D., Professor of
Stomatology, Illinois Medical College; Honorary President
of the Dental Section of the Tenth International Medical
Congress, Berlin, 1890, etc., etc. Fifth Edition. Five hun-
dred and eighty-one Illustrations. The S. S. White Dental
Manufacturing Company, Philadelphia, 1903. ·

This work of Dr. Talbot was very thoroughly reviewed in a
former edition, and it is, therefore, not possible and perhaps unnecessary to enlarge upon the previous judgment. It comes to us
in this edition without any change from that of the fourth; the
text, paging, and binding are in this followed with scrupulous
exactness. The author gives the reason for this in the fact that
" Since the fourth edition of this work appeared, practically no
modifications of the general principles therein outlined have been
made. The laws by which deformities of the jaws and irregularities of the teeth are governed had been worked out on broad
scientific lines." The author, however, adds an " Introduction,"
not in former editions, in order to " outline . . . the working of
the developmental principles governing heredity and environment
as to facilitate their application to the topics discussed in the
different divisions of the subject."

The author in this assumes that the human face is gradually
deteriorating, for he states: " The human face, with all its beauty,
considered from the stand-point of food-getting, chewing, and combat is, as Minot has shown, assuming an embryonic type. The
jaws are needed less and less for the purpose mentioned, hence,
under the law of economy of growth, the resultant disuse sacrifices
them for the benefit of the growing brain and nervous system and
the dermal elements of the skull." This assertion is made, it seems
to the writer, without sufficient proof to give it support. It is a
recognized fact that at no period in the history of the human race
has there been more evidence given of brain activity and conse-

Bibliography.
453

quently brain development, than during the nineteenth century, and, judging the race *en masse,* there certainly is no marked evidence of jaw deterioration for "the benefit of the growing brain and nervous system and the dermal elements of the skull." It is thought, therefore, that the Introduction, while it may briefly cover the thoughts of the author, does not strengthen the edition. This may be a matter for regret, for the author, more than any other writer, has bróadened the scientific view of irregularities. of the jaws and surrounding parts. He has taught the professional mind to probe deeper into the mysteries of development and has shown that if we expect to comprehend irregular presentations we must understand the changes that have gradually, through generations, led up to this. Hence this work has forced its way through four editions, necessitating a fifth to meet the demand.

To perform a practical piece of work in the regulation of teeth may seem to the average dental mind simply as a mechanical problem. If success follows this superficial idea it must be regarded as accidental. All treatment of abnormal conditions must be based on a thorough understanding of the processes that have led up to the deterioration. If this be not done then treatment becomes wholly empirical.

It is to the credit of leading writers on orthodontia that this important foundational idea has not been lost in the effort to appeal to the practical man. Dr. Talbot has, in all probability, aecomplished more than others in this direction, in that he has worked out his problems upon lines of development and carried these logically to the given result.

It is thought the author has been wise in not making any change in this edition. The, so-called, practical man will object to the limited space devoted to appliances and methods of use. This remains the same as in the fourth edition. The value of this work cannot be based on this, but upon the research given and preceding this, to make orthodontia something more than a series of screws, springs, and bands, but problems that require for their solution a knowledge of changes produced by heredity, evolution, and environment, and when these are understood the difficulties may be scientifically conquered. To this end our author has marked a path for all to follow. The book should be in the library of every practitioner of this very difficult branch of dental practice.

IRREGULARITIES OF THE TEETH AND THEIR CORRECTION. By J. N. Farrar, M.D., D.D.S.

Dr. Farrar has for a long time been considering the advisability of publishing an edition of his work, " Irregularities of the Teeth and their Correction," in smaller volumes, to be sold at two dollars and fifty cents per volume, so that the younger members of the dental profession may obtain a volume treating upon any particular case desired, at a less price than the larger volumes. But by dividing each of the large volumes (published) into three small volumes, and the third large volume (which is in process to be published) is added, they all would make nine volumes, which, at two dollars and fifty cents per volume, would amount to twenty-two dollars and fifty cents for the full set, in cloth binding, which would be four dollars and fifty cents more than his former price.

As there would be an extra expense in making so many small volumes, Dr. Farrar has finally decided that instead of issuing his work in smaller volumes, it would be better for the dental profession, as well as all other parties interested, to lessen the usual prices by curtailing some of the sale expenses, and making some personal reductions, thereby permitting a material reduction. For illustration, a volume in cloth would be only four dollars instead of six dollars, the usual price, and for the higher grade of binding the same reduction of two dollars per volume would be made. At this rate per volume, in cloth binding, " Irregularities of the Teeth and their Correction," when all are published, will be obtainable at the remarkably low price of twelve dollars for the complete work of three volumes, of which two volumes are now published and the third is being prepared for the publisher; being pushed as fast as the author's leisure time will permit of the proof-reading. Dr. Farrar's manifold professional labors do not permit him to progress as rapidly as we would like.

SUNSHINE THOUGHTS FOR GLOOMY HOURS: PROSE AND VERSE. By Geo. H. Chance, D.D.S., M.D., J. K. Gill Company, Publishers, Portland, Ore.

It seems not a very long time in the history of this country when all that the East knew of Oregon was from the travels and descriptions of intrepid explorers who braved exposures, Indian raids, and months of travel overland that curious readers might be made familiar with this far away western border of our Continent.

The writer's boyish imagination revelled in the thought of the time when he possibly might investigate personally this new life as it was then pictured; but that time never came, and now cities and towns have made the Pacific Coast so populous that no longer is there any wild country there or between the great oceans, and at the base of Mount Tacoma and Ranier we find the same æsthetic tastes as in the older settled regions.

Now comes ´our old friend Chance, of Portland, Ore., with the sunshine of his thoughts,—and who that has ever been an hour in his society has not felt their warming and enlivening influence. Dr. D. Solis Cohen, in his "Introduction," says that "the optimist is one of the world's treasures," and this he applies very truly to the author of this book of "Sunshine Thoughts."

The latter divides the book into articles of prose and verse. Treating themes "Patriotic," and again he discourses on "Fads, Facts, and Fancies;" then becomes "Fraternal," and enters into the domain of Freemasonry. Here the author seems much at home, as he writes himself as a 33°; also, as an "Odd Fellow," he grows enthusiastic over the good deeds of that Order; and finally he descends from Parnassian heights to measure his muse with his prosaic profession.

The near approach of the Fourth International Dental Congress at St. Louis seems to make appropriate the following extract from the address the author delivered at the opening of the Pacific Coast Dental Congress in 1897.

> "And when this congress stands adjourned,
> May those from near and far
> Reach each his home in blissful mood,
> Without a pain or jar.
> But, when adjourned, be not in haste
> To reach your Eastern homes,
> Till you have seen the Cascade Range,
> Its snow-capped peaks and domes."

The altruistic thought permeating these effusions of our author will be apparent in every line, but especially so in the last "International Anthem" to "England and America," which seems to the writer to be the best in the collection. The author has evidently lived to carry sunshine everywhere, and those who have known him best can well understand that these poems simply typify the soul of the man enshrined in words.

Obituary.

RESOLUTIONS OF RESPECT TO DR. OTIS AVERY.

THE Lackawanna-Luzerne Dental Society, at a regular meeting, held March 15, 1904, adopted the following resolutions upon the death of Dr. Otis Avery, an honored member of the Dental profession for more than seventy years, and who passed away in his ninety-sixth year.

WHEREAS, It has pleased the Divine Ruler to remove from this life Dr. Otis Avery, who passed to the great beyond February 22, 1904; and
WHEREAS, The dental profession recognizes the benefits received through his having lived, and by his life given us an example of a true, courteous, professional gentleman; therefore be it
Resolved, That in the death of Dr. Avery our profession has lost a man of sterling worth, whose progress in the profession was a source of pride to his colleagues. And for whose example we return thanks to the Divine Ruler; also,
Resolved, That we condole with his bereaved family, and a copy of the resolutions be sent to his widow and to the dental journals, and also be inscribed on our official records.

C. L. BECK,
W. A. SPENCER,
E. J. DONNEGAN,
Committee.

Current News.

PENNSYLVANIA STATE DENTAL SOCIETY.

THE Pennsylvania State Dental Society will hold its thirty-sixth annual meeting at Wilkes-Barre, Pa., on the 12th, 13th, and 14th of July, 1904.

GEORGE W. CUPIT,
Secretary.

UNIVERSAL EXPOSITION.

DAVID R. FRANCIS,   HOWARD J. ROGERS,
President.   *Director of Congresses.*

FOURTH INTERNATIONAL DENTAL CONGRESS.

(*St. Louis, August 29 to September 3, 1904.*)

Committee of Organization.   *Local Committee of Arrangement.*
H. J. BURKHART, *Chairman.*   WILLIAM CONRAD, *Chairman.*
E. C. KIRK, *Secretary,*   SAM. T. BASSETT, *Secretary,*
Lock Box 1615, Philadelphia.   457 Century Bldg., St. Louis.

WE, the Committee on Local Information, submit the following facts, important for the success of the Fourth International Dental Congress:

Every member of the profession who has at heart the welfare of dentistry should give it support financially and by action.

We, as American members of the dental profession, would well keep in mind that the Congress will be held in our great country, and pride should prompt us to action to make the meeting one of great magnitude and far excel its predecessors.

Let every dentist take hold with a will and push it to a successful issue.

This Congress should be of great interest to all of the profession. There is planned a monster clinic from the best clinicians of the world, scientific papers from the pens of the most noted and scholarly men of the profession, and an exhibit to excel all others.

The section meetings, the clinics, and the exhibits will be held in the great Coliseum, where ample accommodations are secured.

Hotel Jefferson, the general head-quarters of the Dental Congress, one of the most fashionable and complete hotels in the West, if not in America, is located on Twelfth Street, one block from the Coliseum. Hotels of St. Louis will be sufficient to meet all requirements.

The Information Bureau of the Exposition has a list of ninety-seven well-established hotels now doing business in St. Louis, with a capacity for twenty-one thousand guests, at prices ranging from fifty cents a day up on the European plan, and from one dollar a day up on the American plan. These established hotels have been supplemented during the year 1903 by thirty-five new permanent hotels now opening or about to open, increasing the permanent hotel capacity to forty-seven thousand guests, at prices ranging from one dollar a day up. The Exposition management holds the signed agreement of the leading hotels that " rates shall not be increased during the World's Fair period." Prices are now lower in St. Louis than in any other city for similar hotel accommodation and service.

The Exposition Information Bureau list of one hundred and thirty-two permanent hotels includes only the better class. There are now one hundred and seventy-three hotels, large and small, in operation in the city, and the new hotel enterprises being inaugurated justify the belief that the number will reach two hundred and fifty before the opening day of the World's Fair.

Besides hotels with accommodations for more than two hundred thousand guests, the Exposition Information Bureau has a list of boarding-houses and rooming-houses of respectable character on the street-car lines with lodgings for fifteen thousand guests, and a list of private houses that will let rooms for twenty thousand persons.

All over the city, apartment-houses and rooming-houses are available for those who prefer rooms away from crowds, with meals at the restaurants.

There are four hundred and eighty-five restaurants in St. Louis that have a reputation for good fare, good service, cleanliness, and moderate prices. Twenty of these four hundred and eighty-five restaurants can take care of forty thousand patrons.

The climate of St. Louis is temperate in summer and most delightful in the spring and fall. It is the most central and accessible of the four large cities of the United States, twenty-seven more railways entering it, and passenger steamers on the Mississippi reaching it from north and south.

World's Fair cheap rates on railways and steamboats will be offered during the whole Exposition season. The New England Passenger Association, Trunk Line Association, Central Passenger Association, and Southeastern Passenger Association have adopted the following rates, which will be on sale from April 15:

Season tickets for eighty per cent. of double one fare, good to return until December 15.

For sixty days, one and one-third fare, not good to return after December 15.

For ten days, one fare plus two dollars, from points within two hundred and fifty miles of St. Louis.

For fifteen days, one fare plus two dollars, from points over two hundred and fifty miles from St. Louis.

St. Louis is the fourth city of the United States in point of population, having seven hundred and fifty thousand people. Certainly, no city is more attractive with interest for the student of nature, science, history, etc. There are twenty-four public parks containing over two thousand one hundred acres, all well improved.

The World's Fair Grounds lie five miles from the river on the western edge of the city, and are reached quickly and comfortably by steam railway and fast trolley lines.

The visitors reach the city through the largest and most beautiful railway station in the world.

Thirty-two tracks run into the station side by side, and the midway or glass-roofed hall in front of the gates to the trains will hold thirty thousand people.

Most of the hotels, except the temporary ones near the World's Fair Grounds, are within ten minutes' ride of the station in the heart of the business district. Street cars, reaching all of the hotels for one fare, run by the station, and the cab, carriage, and baggage system is excellent.

The great Music Hall and Coliseum Building that is secured for the meetings of the International Dental Congress is down town, on Olive Street, between Thirteenth and Fourteenth Streets, within easy walking distance of Union Station, the hotels, and the business district. It has a seating capacity for eight thousand people, with section rooms that will be arranged for the various committees and exhibitors.

Naturally, every member attending the Fourth International Dental Congress will wish to see the World's Fair. This will be the most magnificent the world has ever seen, and it will probably be the last great exposition to be held in this country for many years, because of the enormous expenditure of labor and money attending it.

Congressman Bartholdt, in a recent speech made before Congress, said, " The Universal Exposition at St. Louis is the apotheosis of centuries of civilization. It is the culminating perfection of those wonderful international spectacles which have served to impress on our minds that it is good to be a living participant in the glories of this world.

" A decade of human achievement has elapsed since the Columbian pageantry of progress at Chicago. Every American who saw the ' White City' thrilled with the thought that the nations of the earth had assembled in the greatest republic to do homage to the genius of enlightenment.

" Triumphs of the emperors of imperial Rome were but the mock pomp of childish fancies compared to the triumphs of peace as celebrated by such a labor of love at St. Louis. On the May day of this year the gates of welcome will be flung wide open, and the vision of the century will then unfold its prophetic beauty for the uplifting of humanity.

" All in all, the Universal Exposition of 1904 will be the sensational climax of the twentieth century, the grandest victory of peace and civilization, the greatest triumph human genius has yet achieved. To millions of its visitors it will be an academy of learning, an inspiration, and an inexhaustible source of genuine delight, and the memories of the Ivory City will live and bear fruit in ages yet to come."

We appeal to all reputable, legally qualified practitioners of dentistry to interest themselves in the success of this great international meeting.

Let every dentist in America put forth his greatest effort to advance the cause. Make application at once through your State chairman for a membership certificate. See that your fellow-practitioner is enrolled, and then, and not till then, will you have done your full duty.

The membership fee to the Congress will be ten dollars. It will entitle the holder to the official badge and all the rights and privileges of the Congress. He will also receive one copy of the transactions. Without a membership certificate, it will be impossible to get into the general meeting, sections, or clinics, or attend any of the various entertainments given during the Congress.

This great Congress presents to the American dentist an opportunity to see and hear the brightest and most learned men of the profession from all parts of the world,—men of international reputation that shine as clinicians and men of great renown of the inventive turn of mind. This international meeting will be the Mecca of the profession of the world. We will all receive new light and be stimulated to a higher appreciation of our noble profession.

The Local Committee of Arrangements and Reception, with its various minor committees, are working with increasing energy, and will be ready to meet you and extend you a most hearty welcome. Any further information can be obtained from the committee.

D. O. M. LeCron, *Chairman*, Missouri Trust Building,

Max Fendler, *Secretary*, Missouri Trust Building,

George H. Gibson,

H. F. D'Oench,

G. L. Kitchen,

S. H. Voyles,

Orem H. Manhard,

Permanent Local Committee and Bureau of Information.

NATIONAL ASSOCIATION OF DENTAL EXAMINERS.

The National Association of Dental Examiners will hold their annual meeting in the Coliseum Building, corner of Thirteenth and Olive Streets, St. Louis, Mo., on the 25th, 26th, and 27th of August, beginning promptly at 10 A.M. Telephone and telegraph offices in the building. Hotel accommodations will be secured for the members. Special railroad rates will be secured for those in the East desiring to attend, trains leaving on the 23d from New York.

The Committee on Railroad Accommodations for the East have made arrangements for fast through Pullman service to St. Louis from New York with the Delaware and Lackawanna Railroad. Two special Pullman cars will leave New York Tuesday, August 23, at 10 A.M. The cost of our excursion including berth each way will be $35.50. A proportionate reduction is made for those going from Buffalo, Toledo, Fort Wayne, and cities on the line connecting with the Wabash Railroad. To those desiring to go in the special cars, send notice to Charles A. Meeker, D.D.S., Secretary of the National Association Dental Examiners, or to Guy Adams, General Passenger Agent of the Delaware and Lackawana Railroad. Accommodations have been secured for the National Association of Dental Ex-

aminers at the Franklin Hotel, northwest corner of Sarah and
Westminster Place, with rates from $1.50 to $6.00 per day, Euro-
pean plan. Hotel first-class. Secure rooms by writing to E. C.
Dunnavant, St. Louis Service Company, Seventh and Olive Streets,
St. Louis, Mo.

CHARLES A. MEEKER, D.D.S.,

Secretary.

FOURTH INTERNATIONAL DENTAL CONGRESS, ST.
LOUIS, MO., AUGUST 29 TO SEPTEMBER 3, 1904.

Committee of Organization.—H. J. Burkhart, Chairman, Ba-
tavia, N. Y.; E. C. Kirk, Secretary, Lock Box 1615, Philadelphia,
Pa.; R. H. Hofheinz, Wm. Carr, W. E. Boardman, V. E. Turner,
J. Y. Crawford, M. F. Finley, J. W. David, Wm. Crenshaw, Don
M. Gallie, G. V. I. Brown, A. H. Peck, J. D. Patterson, B. L.
Thorpe.

The Department of Congresses of the Universal Exposition, St.
Louis, 1904, has nominated the Committee of Organization of the
Fourth International Dental Congress which was appointed by the
National Dental Association, and has instructed the committee thus
appointed to proceed with the work of organization of said Congress.

Pursuant to the instructions of the Director of Congresses of the
Universal Exposition, 1904, the Committee of Organization pre-
sents the subjoined outline of the plan of organization of the Dental
Congress.

The Congress will be divided into two departments: Department A—SCIENCE (divided into four sections). Department B—
APPLIED SCIENCE (divided into six sections).

DEPARTMENT A—SCIENCE.

I. Anatomy, Physiology, Histology, and Microscopy. Chairman, M. H. Cryer, 1420 Chestnut Street, Philadelphia, Pa.

II. Etiology, Pathology, and Bacteriology. Chairman, R. H.
Hofheinz, Chamber of Commerce, Rochester, N. Y.

III. Chemistry and Metallurgy. Chairman, J. D. Hodgen, 1005
Sutter Street, San Francisco, Cal.

IV. Oral Hygiene, Prophylaxis, Materia Medica and Therapeutics, and Electro-therapeutics. Chairman, A. H. Peck, 92 State
Street, Chicago, Ill.

DEPARTMENT B—APPLIED SCIENCE.

V. Oral Surgery. Chairman, G. V. I. Brown, 445 Milwaukee Avenue, Milwaukee, Wis.

VI. Orthodontia. Chairman, E. H. Angle, 1023 North Grand Avenue, St. Louis, Mo.

VII. Operative Dentistry. Chairman, C. N. Johnson, Marshall Field Building, Chicago, Ill.

VIII. Prosthesis. Chairman, C. R. Turner, Thirty-third and Locust Streets, Philadelphia, Pa.

IX. Education, Nomenclature, Literature, and History. Chairnian, Truman W. Brophy, Marshall Field Building, Chicago, Ill.

X. Legislation. Chairman, Wm. Carr, 35 West Forty-sixth Street, New York, N. Y.

COMMITTEES.

Following are the committees appointed:

Finance.—Chairman, C. S. Butler, 680 Main Street, Buffalo, N. Y.

Programme.—Chairman, A. H. Peck, 92 State Street, Chicago, Ill.

Exhibits.—Chairman, D. M. Gallie, 100 State Street, Chicago, Ill.

Transportation.—(To be appointed.)

Reception.—Chairman, B. Holly Smith, 1007 Madison Avenue, Baltimore, Md.

Registration.—Chairman, B. L. Thorpe, 3666 Olive Street, St. Louis, Mo.

Printing and Publication.—Chairman, W. E. Boardman, 184 Boylston Street, Boston, Mass.

Conference with State and Local Dental Societies.—Chairman, J. A. Libbey, 524 Penn Avenue, Pittsburg, Pa.

Dental Legislation.—Chairman, Wm. Carr, 35 West Forty-sixth Street, New York, New York.

Auditing.—(Committee of Organization.)

Invitation.—Chairman, L. G. Noel, 527½ Church Street, Nashville, Tenn.

Membership.—Chairman, J. D. Patterson, Keith and Perry Building, Kansas City, Mo.

Educational Methods.—Chairman, T. W. Brophy, Marshall Field Building, Chicago, Ill.

Oral Surgery.—Chairman, G. V. I. Brown, 445 Milwaukee Avenue, Milwaukee, Wis.

Prosthetic Dentistry.—Chairman, C. R. Turner, Thirty-third and Locust Streets, Philadelphia, Pa.

Local Committee of Arrangements and Reception.—Chairman, Wm. Conrad, 3666 Olive Street, St. Louis, Mo.

Essays.—Chairman, Wilbur F. Litch, 1500 Locust Street, Philadelphia, Pa.

History of Dentistry.—Chairman, Wm. H. Trueman, 900 Spruce Street, Philadelphia, Pa.

Nomenclature.—Chairman, A. H. Thompson, 720 Kansas Avenue, Topeka, Kan.

Promotion of Appointment of Dental Surgeons in the Armies and Navies of the World.—Chairman, Williams Donnally, 1018 Fourteenth Street N. W., Washington, D. C.

Care of the Teeth of the Poor.—Chairman, Thomas Fillebrown, 175 Newbury Street, Boston, Mass.

Etiology, Pathology, and Bacteriology.—Chairman, R. H. Hofheinz, Chamber of Commerce, Rochester, N. Y.

Prize Essays.—Chairman, James Truman, 4505 Chester Avenue, Philadelphia, Pa.

Oral Hygiene, Prophylaxis, Materia Medica and Therapeutics, and Electro-therapeutics.—Chairman, A. H. Peck, 92 State Street, Chicago, Ill.

Operative Dentistry.—Chairman, C. N. Johnson, Marshall Field Building, Chicago, Ill.

Resolutions.—Chairman, J. Y. Crawford, Jackson Building, Nashville, Tenn.

Clinics.—Chairman, J. P. Gray, 212 North Spruce Street, Nashville, Tenn.

Nominations.—Chairman, A. H. Peck, 92 State Street, Chicago, Ill.; W. E. Boardman, 184 Boylston Street, Boston, Mass.; M. R. Windhorst, 3518 Morgan Street, St. Louis, Mo.; Wm. Conrad, 3666 Olive Street, St. Louis, Mo.

Ad Interim.—Chairman, G. V. I. Brown, 445 Milwaukee Avenue, Milwaukee, Wis.

The officers of the Congress, president, vice-presidents, secretary, and treasurer, will be elected by the Congress at large at the time of the meeting, and will be nominated by the Nominating Committee.

The Fourth International Dental Congress, which will be held August 29 to September 3, inclusive, 1904, will be representative of the existing status of dentistry throughout the world. It is intended further that the Congress shall set forth the history and material progress of dentistry from its crude beginnings through its developmental stages, up to its present condition as a scientific profession.

The International Dental Congress is but one of the large number of congresses to be held during the period of the Louisiana Purchase Exposition, and these in their entirety are intended to exhibit the intellectual progress of the world, as the Exposition will set forth the material progress which has taken place since the Columbian Exposition in 1893.

It is important that each member of the dental profession in America regard this effort to hold an International Dental Congress as a matter in which he has an individual interest, and one which he is under obligation to personally help towards a successful issue. The dental profession of America has not only its own professional record to maintain with a just pride, but, as it is called upon to act the part of host in a gathering of our colleagues from all parts of the world, it has to sustain the reputation of American hospitality as well.

The Committee of Organization appeals earnestly to each member of the profession to do his part in making the Congress a success. Later bulletins will be issued setting forth the personnel of the organization and other particulars, when the details have been more fully arranged.

H. J. BURKHART, *Chairman.*
E. C. KIRK, *Secretary.*

Approved:
HOWARD J. ROGERS,
Director of Congresses.
DAVID R. FRANCIS,
President of Exposition.

COMMITTEE ON STATE AND LOCAL ORGANIZATIONS.

(J. A. Libbey, Chairman, 524 Penn Avenue, Pittsburg, Pa.)

The Committee on State and Local Organizations is a committee appointed by the Committee of Organization of the Fourth International Congress with the object of promoting the interests of the

18

Congress in the several States of the Union. Each member of the committee is charged with the duty of receiving applications for membership in the Congress under the rules governing membership as prescribed by the Committee on Membership and approved by the Committee of Organization. These rules provide that *membership in the Congress shall be open to all reputable legally qualified practitioners of dentistry.* Membership in a State or local society is not a necessary qualification for membership in the Congress.

Each State chairman, as named below, is furnished with official application blanks and is authorized to accept the membership fee of ten dollars from all eligible applicants within his State. The State chairman will at once forward the fee and official application with his indorsement to the chairman of the Finance Committee, who will issue the official certificate conferring membership in the Congress. No application from any of the States will be accepted by the chairman of the Finance Committee unless approved by the State chairman, whose indorsement is a certification of eligibility under the membership rules.

A certificate of membership in the Congress will entitle the holder thereof to all the rights and privileges of the Congress, the right of debate, and of voting on all questions which the Congress will be called upon to decide. It will also entitle the member to one copy of the official transactions when published and to participation in all the events for social entertainment which will be officially provided at the time of the Congress.

The attention of all reputable legally qualified practitioners of dentistry is called to the foregoing plan authorized by the Committee of Organization for securing membership in the Congress, and the committee earnestly appeals to each eligible practitioner in the United States who is interested in the success of this great international meeting to make application at once through his State chairman for a membership certificate. By acting promptly in this matter the purpose of the committee to make the Fourth International Dental Congress the largest and most successful meeting of dentists ever held will be realized, and the Congress will thus be placed upon a sound financial basis.

Let every one make it his individual business to help at least to the extent of enrolling himself as a member and the success of the undertaking will be quickly assured. Apply at once to your State chairman. The State chairmen-already appointed are:

General Chairman.—J. A. Libbey, 524 Penn Avenue, Pittsburg, Pa.

Alabama.—H. Clay Hassell, Tuscaloosa.

Arkansas.—W. H. Buckley, 510½ Main Street, Little Rock.

California.—J. L. Pease, 1016 Clay Street, Oakland.

Colorado.—H. A. Fynn, 500 California Building, Denver.

Connecticut.—Henry McManus, 80 Pratt Street, Hartford.

Delaware.—C. R. Jeffries, New Century Building, Wilmington.

District of Columbia.—W. N. Cogan, The Sherman, Washington.

Florida.—W. G. Mason, Tampa.

Georgia.—H. H. Johnson, Macon.

Hawaii.—M. E. Grossman, Box 744, Honolulu.

Idaho.—J. B. Burns, Payette.

Illinois.—J. E. Hinkins, 131 East Fifty-third Street, Chicago.

Indiana.—H. C. Kahlo, 115 East New York Street, Indianapolis.

Iowa.—W. R. Clark, Clear Lake.

Kansas.—G. A. Esterly, Lawrence.

Kentucky.—H. B. Tileston, 314 Equitable Building, Louisville.

Louisiana.—Jules J. Sarrazin, 108 Bourbon Street, New Orleans.

Maine.—H. A. Kelley, 609 Congress Street, Portland.

Maryland.—W. G. Foster, 813 Eutaw Street, Baltimore.

Massachusetts.—M. C. Smith, 3 Lee Hall, Lynn.

Michigan.—G. S. Shattuck, 539 Fourth Avenue, Detroit.

Minnesota.—C. A. Van Duzee, 51 Germania Bank Building, St. Paul.

Mississippi.—W. R. Wright, Jackson.

Missouri.—J. W. Hull, Altman Building, Kansas City.

Montana.—G. E. Longeway, Great Falls.

Nebraska.—H. A. Shannon, 1136 " O" Street, Lincoln.

New Hampshire.—E. C. Blaisdell, Portsmouth.

New Jersey.—Alphonso Irwin, 425 Cooper Street, Camden.

New York.—B. C. Nash, 142 West Seventy-eighth Street, New York City.

North Carolina.—C. L. Alexander, Charlotte.

Ohio.—Henry Barnes, 1415 New England Building, Cleveland.

Oklahoma.—T. P. Bringhurst, Shawnee.

Oregon.—S. J. Barber, Macleay Building, Portland.

Pennsylvania.—H. E. Roberts, 1516 Locust Street, Philadelphia.

Rhode Island.—D. F. Keefe, 315 Butler Exchange, Providence.

South Carolina.—J. T. Calvert, Spartanburg.

South Dakota.—E. S. O'Neil, Canton.

Tennessee.—W. P. Sims, Jackson Building, Nashville.

Texas.—J. G. Fife, Dallas.

Utah.—W. L. Ellerbeck, 21 Hooper Building Salt Lake City.

Vermont.—S. D. Hodge, Burlington.

Virginia.—F. W. Stiff, 2101 Churchill Avenue, Richmond.

Washington.—G. W. Stryker, Everett.

West Virginia.—H. H. Harrison, 1141 Main Street, Wheeling.

Wisconsin.—A. D. Gropper, 401 East Water Street, Milwaukee.

For the Committee of Organization,

EDWARD C. KIRK,

Secretary.

MEETING OF THE COMMITTEE OF ORGANIZATION.

At a meeting of the Committee of Organization of the Fourth International Dental Congress held in St. Louis, Mo., April 9, 1904, the following action was taken:

In accordance with the understanding at the last meeting of the committee, held at Washington, D. C., February 23, 1904, that a Nominating Committee for the purpose of nominating officers for the Fourth International Dental Congress be elected at the next meeting of the committee, Dr. M. F. Finley made the following motion:

" That a Committee on Nominations be elected at this time for the purpose of proposing names for the officers of this Congress, and that Drs. A. H. Peck and W. E. Boardman, representing the Committee of the National Dental Association, and Drs. M. R. Windhorst and Wm. Conrad, representing the Committee of the Fédération Dentaire Internationale, be constituted the Committee on Nominations, to present nominations for the officers of the Fourth International Dental Congress, and that said nominations be presented at the present meeting of the Committee of Organization."

The motion was unanimously carried, and Drs. A. H. Peck,

W. E. Boardman, M. R. Windhorst, and William Conrad were elected as the members of the Nominating Committee.

At a subsequent session the Nominating Committee presented the following report:

" Your committee begs to report the following nominations for officers of the Fourth International Dental Congress:

"*President.*—H. J. Burkhart, Batavia, N. Y.

"*Honorary Presidents.*—James Truman, Philadelphia, Pa.; A. H. Fuller, St. Louis, Mo.; G. V. Black, Chicago, Ill.; Thomas Fillebrown, Boston, Mass.; S. G. Perry, New York, N. Y.; Gordon White, Nashville, Tenn.; E. T. Darby, Philadelphia, Pa.; A. W. Harlan, Chicago, Ill.; James McManus, Hartford, Conn.; W. W. Walker, New York, N. Y.; J. N. Crouse, Chicago, Ill.; G. A. Bowman, St. Louis, Mo.; H. A. Smith, Cincinnati, Ohio; T. W. Brophy, Chicago, Ill.; Wm. Jarvie, Brooklyn, N. Y.; Wm. Conrad, St. Louis, Mo.; M. R. Windhorst, St. Louis, Mo.; S. H. Guilford, Philadelphia, Pa.; J. D. Patterson, Kansas City, Mo.; C. C. Chittenden, Madison, Wis.; Wm. Carr, New York, N. Y.; E. H. Smith, Boston, Mass.; M. H. Cryer, Philadelphia, Pa.; E. A. Bogue, New York, N. Y.; V. E. Turner, Raleigh, N. C.; A. L. Northrop, New York, N. Y.; J. H. Moore, Richmond, Va.; C. Newlin Peirce, Philadelphia, Pa.

"*Vice-Presidents.*—A. H. Thompson, Topeka, Kan.; J. G. Reid, Chicago, Ill.; George Fields, Detroit, Mich.; D. O. M. Le-Cron, St. Louis, Mo.; Garrett Newkirk, Los Angeles, Cal.; R. Ottolengui, New York, N. Y.; R. M. Sanger, East Orange, N. J.; D. N. Rust, Washington, D. C.; N. S. Hoff, Ann Arbor, Mich.; L. P. Bethel, Columbus, Ohio; Jules J. Sarrazin, New Orleans, La.; C. L. Alexander, Charlotte, N. C.; C. H. Darby, St. Joseph, Mo.; B. C. Nash, New York, N. Y.; G. S. Vann, Gadsden, Ala.; B. F. Luckey, Paterson, N. J.; E. R. Warner, Denver, Col.; Williams Donnally, Washington, D. C.; Frank Holland, Atlanta, Ga.; C. A. Meeker, Newark, N. J.; W. P. Dickinson, Minneapolis, Minn.; E. K. Wedelstaedt, St. Paul, Minn.; Adam Flickinger, St. Louis, Mo.; V. H. Jackson, New York, N. Y.; J. M. Whitney, Honolulu, Hawaii; B. Holly Smith, Baltimore, Md.; Louis Ottofy, Manila, P. I.; C. M. Gingrich, Baltimore, Md.; H. B. Tileston, Louisville, Ky.; Wm. Crenshaw, Atlanta, Ga,; J. F. Dowsley, Boston, Mass.; J. W. David, Corsicana, Tex.; Geo. E. Hunt, Indianapolis, Ind.

"*Secretary-General.*—Edward C. Kirk, Philadelphia, Pa.
"*Treasurer.*—M. F. Finley, Washington, D. C.
"*Committee to Nominate Honorary Presidents and Vice-Presidents for Foreign Countries.*—Edward C. Kirk, Philadelphia, Pa.; Edward H. Angle, St. Louis, Mo.; Wilbur F. Litch, Philadelphia, Pa.

(Signed)   "A. H. PECK,
"WALDO E. BOARDMAN,
"WM. CONRAD,
"M. R. WINDHORST,
"*Committee on Nominations.*"

The above report was adopted by the Committee of Organization subject to ratification by the Congress in general session.

It should be understood that the foregoing list of nominations is necessarily incomplete and subject to future correction and amendment, depending upon individual acceptances and the addition of new names.

EDWARD C. KIRK,
Secretary Committee of Organization.

NEW JERSEY STATE DENTAL SOCIETY.

THE thirty-fourth annual session of the New Jersey State Dental Society will convene in the Auditorium, Asbury Park, N. J., at 10 A.M., Wednesday, July 21, 1904, and continue in session Thursday and Friday. Asbury Park is one of the great Atlantic coast watering-places contiguous to New York and Philadelphia. The Auditorium will hold three thousand people, and is open on every side.

Fifty clinics will be given by men from North, South, East, and West most eminent in their profession, and will include the newest advances in all that pertains to operative and mechanical dentistry. In the exhibits the society feels that the latest and largest number of adjuncts to the successful practice of modern dentistry will repay a visit and inspection. The essays will consist of five already accepted and the best obtainable.

The social to members and visiting friends will be, as usual, provided for, and on Thursday evening at 10.30 a smoker will be provided.

The Columbia Hotel will be the head-quarters, with rates of $2.50 to $3.00 per day. Those desiring rooms must send in notices by July 1. The programme, as usual, will be replete with information.

CHARLES A. MEEKER, D.D.S.,

Secretary.

29 FULTON STREET, NEWARK, N. J.

FOURTH INTERNATIONAL DENTAL CONGRESS—
GENERAL INFORMATION.

THE Fourth International Dental Congress, to be held in St. Louis, August 29 to September 3, inclusive, 1904, will convene in the Coliseum, a building most favorably adapted to the holding of such a gathering and possessing accommodations so ample that all of the features of the Congress will be held under one roof and without interference one with another. This great structure occupies two blocks between Olive and St. Charles, and Thirteenth and Fourteenth Streets; it covers an area of nearly four acres, with a floor space for exposition purposes of three hundred thousand square feet.

The Coliseum is one of the largest and most commodious convention halls ever built, and is practically fireproof. It contains a large theatre capable of seating two thousand five hundred people, which will be used for the general sessions of the Congress, and ten additional meeting-rooms, furnishing ample accommodations for the simultaneous meeting of the ten sectional divisions of the Congress; a large hall for exhibits, covering nine thousand square feet of floor space, practically all of which has been taken by intending exhibitors; and a well-lighted gallery for clinics, capable of accommodating the one hundred chairs which have been provided for that purpose. In addition to the foregoing, numerous committee-rooms and telegraph, telephone, and postal facilities will be provided in the building, and it is expected also that a well-ordered café will be in operation during the time of the Congress.

In connection with the building, and under the same roof, is the Coliseum proper, where nineteen thousand persons may be comfortably seated, exclusive of the stage, and it is anticipated that this

audience-room will be used for one of the social features of the
Congress, constituting an entertainment unique of its kind.

Besides the advantages of its ample accommodations for the
Dental Congress, the Coliseum building has the advantage of being
located in the heart of the business section of St. Louis, and at considerable distance from the Exposition, so that the meetings will be
less disturbed by the diverting attractions of the great Exposition
than if the Congress were held within the Exposition grounds.

ACCOMMODATIONS.

The Local Committee of Arrangements has selected the Hotel
Jefferson as the general head-quarters of the Dental Congress. This
is one of the most fashionable and complete hotels in the United
States, and is located on Twelfth Street, one block from the
Coliseum. In addition to the Hotel Jefferson as head-quarters, the
hotel accommodations of St. Louis will be sufficient to meet all
requirements. The Information Bureau of the Exposition has a
list of ninety-seven well-established hotels in St. Louis, with a
capacity of forty-one thousand guests, at prices ranging from fifty
cents a day upward on the European plan, and from one dollar a
day upward on the American plan. These established hotels have
been supplemented during the year 1903 by thirty-five new permanent hotels, increasing the permanent hotel capacity to sixty-
seven thousand guests, at prices ranging from one dollar a day upward. The Exposition management holds the signed agreement of
the leading hotels that " rates shall not be increased during the
World's Fair period." Prices are now lower in St. Louis than in
any other city for similar hotel accommodations and service.

The Exposition Information Bureau's list of one hundred and
thirty-two permanent hotels includes only those of the better class.
There are now one hundred and seventy-three hotels, large and
small, in operation in the city, and the new hotel enterprises being
inaugurated justify the belief that the number will reach two hundred and fifty.

Besides hotels with accommodations for more than two hundred
thousand guests, the Exposition Information Bureau has a list of
boarding-houses and rooming-houses of a respectable character on
the street-car lines with lodgings for sixty-five thousand guests, and
a list of private houses that will let rooms for twenty thousand
persons. All over the city permanent houses and rooming-houses

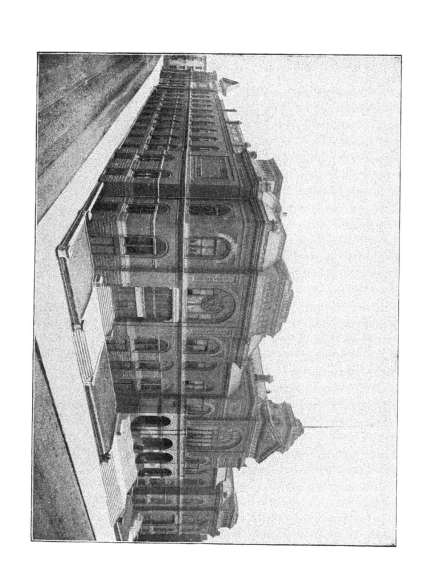

are available to those who prefer rooms away from the crowds, with meals at the restaurants. There are four hundred and eighty-five restaurants in St. Louis that have a national reputation for good fare, good service, cleanliness, and moderate prices; twenty of these four hundred and eighty-five restaurants can take care of forty thousand patrons.

ST. LOUIS AND ITS SURROUNDINGS.

The climate of St. Louis is temperate in summer and most delightful in the spring and autumn. The weather which visitors to the Louisiana Purchase Exposition may expect is shown by the " normals" at St. Louis, taken from the records of the United States Weather Bureau. These " normals" are the averages of the temperatures at St. Louis during the thirty-three years that the Weather Bureau has had a station in St. Louis. The " normals" are as follows: May, 66.1; June, 75.4; July, 79.4; August, 77.6; September, 70.2; October, 58.7; November, 44.3. How closely the actual temperature for any one year follows the normal is well shown by the mean temperature for the month taken by the Weather Bureau at St. Louis during the past year. These temperatures are: May, 71.8; June, 74.2; July, 80.3; August, 76.4; September, 66.4; October, 62.2; November, 63.3. The weather at St. Louis during October and November is particularly pleasant. It is the " Indian summer" of the Middle States.

St. Louis is the most central and most accessible of the four large cities of the United States. Twenty-seven railways enter it, besides passenger steamers on the Mississippi reaching it from the north and south.

World's Fair cheap rates on railways and steamboats will be offered during the whole Exposition season as follows: Season tickets for eighty per cent. of double one fare, good to return until December 15. For sixty days, one and one-third fares, not good to return after December 15. For ten days, one fare plus two dollars, from points within two hundred and fifty miles of St. Louis. For fifteen days, one fare plus two dollars, from points over two hundred and fifty miles from St. Louis.

St. Louis is the fourth city of the United States in point of population, having seven hundred and fifty thousand people. It presents peculiar attractions for the student of nature, science, history, etc. There are twenty-four public parks, containing over

two thousand one hundred acres of well-improved property. The
World's Fair grounds lie five miles from the Mississippi River
on the western border of the State, and are reached quickly and
comfortably by steam railways and electric lines. Visitors reach
the city through one of the largest railway stations in the world;
thirty-two tracks enter the station side by side. Most of the hotels,
except those in the World's Fair grounds, are within ten minutes'
ride of the station, which is in the heart of the business district.
Street-cars reaching all of the hotels for a single five-cent fare
pass the station, and the cab, carriage, and baggage system is
excellent.

Nearly every member of the Fourth International Dental Con-
gress will wish to see the World's Fair. The Local Committee of
Arrangements has already planned a special " Congress day" at the
Exposition, and ample opportunity will be provided for members
to enjoy visiting this greatest of all expositions. Congressman
Bartholdt in a recent speech made before the Congress of the
United States, among other things, said, " All in all, the Universal
Exposition of 1904 will be the sensational climax of the twentieth
century, the grandest victory of peace and civilization, the greatest
triumph human genius has yet achieved. To millions of its visitors
it will be an academy of learning, an inspiration and an inexhaustible source of genuine delight, and the memories of the ' Ivory
City' will live and bear fruit in the ages yet to come."

VISITORS FROM ABROAD.

Extensive preparation is being made for the hospitable care and
entertainment of all members attending the Dental Congress. The
General Committee of Reception, aided by the local committees,
is making every effort to provide for the comfort and care of all
visitors. Dr. D. O. M. LeCron, Missouri Trust Building, St.
Louis, chairman of the Permanent Local Committee and Bureau
of Information, will be pleased to answer all inquiries regarding
the accommodations for those who desire to secure them in advance
of the Congress. A subcommittee of the General Reception Committee has been appointed to meet and give information and dirce-
tion to those arriving from Europe and elsewhere at the principal
ports of entry of the United States, and to arrange the details of
transportation from the sea-board to St. Louis. These committeemen will answer inquiries as to hotels, railways, etc. The subcom-

mittees of the General Reception Committee for the principal ports of entry are:

New York.—Drs. W. C. Deane, 114 East Sixtieth Street, and Gladstone Goode, 35 West Forty-sixth Street.

Philadelphia.—Drs. J. D. Thomas, 1122 Walnut Street, Joseph Head, 1500 Locust Street, and Julio Endelman, Southeast corner Twelfth and Chestnut Streets.

San Francisco.—Drs. H. P. Carlton, 62 Crocker Building, and P. D. Gaskill, Crocker Building.

New Orleans.—Drs. J. J. Sarrazin, Godchaux Building, and R. H. Welch, Godchaux Building.

Baltimore.—Drs. Cyrus M. Gingrich, 608 St. Paul Street, W. G. Foster, 813 North Eutaw Street, and B. Holly Smith, 1007 Madison Avenue.

In other cities not ports of entry, but which may be visited by members from abroad, the following committeemen will furnish all desired information

Buffalo.—Drs. F. E. Howard, 331 Franklin Street, C. W. Stainton, 47 North Pearl Street, S. Eschelman, 421 Franklin Street.

Chicago.—Drs. T. L. Gilmer, 31 Washington Street, J. W. Wassall, 92 State Street, W. V-B. Ames, 31 Washington Street.

St. Louis.—Dr. Wm. Conrad, 3666 Olive Street (chairman Local Committee of Reception and Arrangements).

Washington.—Drs. H. C. Thompson, 1113 Pennsylvania Avenue, N. W., W. E. Dieffenderfer, 616 Twelfth Street, Williams Donnally, 1118 Fourteenth Street, N. W., and W. N. Cogan, " The Sherman."

The rate for the round trip from New York, exclusive of sleeping-car charge and subsistence, is $32.35. Arrangements have been made for any who may desire to return from St. Louis *via* the Big Four, Lake Shore, and Michigan Southern and the New York Central railways to New York.

MEMBERSHIP IN THE CONGRESS.

The following are the rules governing membership in the Fourth International Dental Congress, submitted by the Committee on Membership and approved by the Committee of Organization:

1. All reputable practitioners of dental and oral surgery who are entitled to membership in representative State, district, or local dental associations where they reside are eligible for membership in the Congress.

2. The State conference committees in America, and the national chairman of each foreign country have authority to receipt for the membership fee, which, with the application for membership, shall be forwarded to the chairman of the Finance Committee, Dr. C. S. Butler, 680 Main Street, Buffalo, N. Y., who will thereupon forward the official credentials conferring membership in the Congress.

3. If any difference of opinion arises in State committees or national committees as to the eligibility of an applicant for membership, the question shall be referred to the Committee on Membership of the Congress.

4. The wives and children of the members of the Congress may be admitted upon special request and by consent of the Committee on Membership.

5. A uniform fee of ten dollars shall be paid for each membership, and each person whose name appears on the programme either as essayist or clinician must be a paid member of the Congress.

J. D. PATTERSON,
Chairman Committee on Membership.

KANSAS CITY, MO., U. S. A.

Membership in the Congress will entitle the holder to all the privileges of debate and discussion of papers, and the right to vote upon all questions which the Congress will be called upon to decide. It will also entitle the members to participate in all the social functions of the Congress under the same conditions as enjoyed by others; to the official badges and insignia of the Congress; to one copy of the complete volumes of the Transactions, which it is anticipated will comprise not less than four volumes of about five hundred pages each. Judging from the material already offered, it is believed that the Transactions of the Congress will be the most complete exposition of modern dentistry yet published. This work will be sent to every member, whether he is able to be present at the Congress or not.

In order to avoid confusion and crowding of work at the last minute, those intending to apply for membership in the Congress are urged to send in their applications at once, which will give time to correct any error should one by chance occur.

All communications of a scientific nature must be submitted to the Committee on Essays for approval before final acceptance for a place upon the programme. All communications to the literary programme of the Congress from foreign countries must receive the approval of the national committee of the respective countries from which they are sent before they can be accepted by the Committee on Essays of the Congress. Each essay must be accompanied by a *résumé* giving the substance of the communication in an epitomized form, which must be in the hands of the Essay Committee thirty days before the opening of the Congress, in order to give opportunity for translation and printing in advance of the Congress, and in order to secure a position upon the official programme. All essays, titles of essays, and *résumés* thereof should be forwarded to Dr. Wilbur F. Litch, 1500 Locust Street, Philadelphia, Pa., U. S. A., or to the secretary of the Committee of Organization.

CLINICS.

All who intend to give clinical demonstrations should communicate with Dr. J. P. Gray, 214 North Spruce Street, Nashville, Tenn., U. S. A., chairman of the Committee on Clinics, who will make the necessary arrangements and supply suitable patients as far as may be possible. The rules governing the approval of literary communications by the several national committees will govern also the clinical demonstrations, and all arrangements for clinical demonstrations must be completed by August 1 in order to secure space and a place upon the programme.

EXHIBITS.

All exhibits of a technical character relating to dentistry will be arranged for by the chairman of the Committee on Exhibits, Dr. D. M. Gallie, 100 State Street, Chicago, Ill., U. S. A., to whom all applications should be made for space. All exhibits relating to dental education will be provided for upon application to Dr. Truman W. Brophy, Marshall Field Building, Chicago, Ill., U. S. A., chairman of Section IX.,—Education, Nomenclature, Literature, and History.

PRIZES.

The Committee of Organization offers two prizes,—viz., a handsome gold medal for the best essay on any subject pertaining to dentistry, and a similar medal for the best exhibit of an archæological character illustrating the development of dental art. All essays in competition for the gold-medal prize are to be forwarded to Dr. James Truman, 4505 Chester Avenue, Philadelphia, Pa., U. S. A., chairman of the Committee on Prize Essays, without the name of the author attached, and designated by a motto, accompanied by a sealed envelope containing the name of the author and bearing upon its outside a duplicate of the motto upon the essay. The committee after having decided upon the respective merits of the essays, and after having selected that one deemed worthy of the medal, will open the envelope bearing the duplicate motto and announce the name of the successful author. The other communications will be destroyed *incognito* six months after the Congress closes unless return of the unsuccessful essays be requested by the authors thereof within that period; or, at the option of the writers, the competing essays which fail to secure the medal may be referred to the Essay Committee for presentation before the Congress. The successful prize essay will be published as a part of the proceedings of the Congress.

The awarding of the prize for the archæological exhibit will be made by a committee to be appointed specially for that purpose. All exhibits competing for this medal will be cared for by the chairman of the Committee on Exhibits, Dr. D. M. Gallie, 100 State Street, Chicago, Ill., U. S. A.

PRESENT STATE OF ORGANIZATION.

The chairman of the Committee of Organization through Senator Depew has secured from Secretary of State the Hon. John Hay a promise to send through our foreign ambassadors and representatives an invitation, on behalf of our government, to all governments with which the United States is in diplomatic relation to send an official delegate to the Congress, and the Secretary has received notification that these invitations have been issued.

Upward of twenty nations have signified their intention to take part in this great Congress. No fewer than fifteen hundred committeemen are now actively at work promoting the success of the meeting. Every State and Territory in the United States is in charge of a State committee actively at work in developing the details of the Congress in a local way. So that the prospect of an unusually large attendance is practically assured, and it is confidently expected that the membership in the Fourth International Dental Congress will be much in excess of any other dental meeting ever held. The number and character of essays already prepared, the number and character of the clinical demonstrations, the magnitude of the exhibits already arranged for, will surpass in these features all previous dental meetings. The work which has been accomplished by the Committee on Education, Legislation, and Dental History will constitute the most extensive contributions to these departments yet made.

The social features of the Congress are being provided for upon an elaborate plan. Receptions, lunches, and various forms of entertainment are being arranged on a scale commensurate with the magnitude and importance of the meeting, and as much time will be given to the amenities of social intercourse as may be consistent with the more serious features of the programme.

The Fourth International Dental Congress is now an assured success, and, judged from any stand-point, it will be a meeting which will not only adequately set forth the most recent developments of dental science and art, but it will constitute a liberal education in dentistry which no progressive practitioner can afford to miss.

An efficient corps of interpreters has been provided to assist those visiting members who are unfamiliar with the English language.

EDWARD C. KIRK,
Secretary Committee of Organization.

DENTAL COMMISSIONERS OF CONNECTICUT.

THE Dental Commissioners of the State of Connecticut hereby give notice that they will meet at Hartford, on Thursday, Friday, and Saturday, July 14, 15, 16, 1904, respectively, to examine applicants for license to practise dentistry, and for the transaction of any other proper business.

The practical examination in operative and prosthetic dentistry will be held Thursday, July 14, at 9 A.M., in Putnam Phalanx Armory, corner Haynes and Pearl Streets.

The written theoretic examination will be held Friday and Saturday, July 15 and 16, at the Capitol.

All applicants should apply to the Recorder for proper blanks, and for the revised rules for conducting the examinations.

Application blanks must be carefully filled in and sworn to, and with fee, twenty-five dollars, filed with the Recorder on or before July 7, 1904. Examination Fee must be forwarded by Money Order or Certified Check.

By direction of the Dental Commissioners.

J. TENNY BARKER,
Recorder.

COLORADO STATE BOARD OF DENTAL EXAMINERS.

THE regular semi-annual meeting of the Colorado State Board of Dental Examiners will be held in Denver, June 7, 8, and 9, 1904. The examination will be both theoretical and practical, and applicants for the examination must be prepared to do such prae-tical work as is required. All applications must be filed before June 7. For particulars address,

M. S. FRASER, *Secretary,*
407 Mack Building, Denver, Col.

GEORGIA STATE DENTAL SOCIETY.

THE thirty-sixth annual meeting of the Georgia State Dental Society will be held in Athens, Ga., June 28, 29, and 30, 1904. Arrangements are being made to make this the greatest convention ever held in Georgia. All ethical practitioners are cordially in-vited.

A. M. JACKSON,
President.
D. H. McNEILL,
Corresponding Secretary.

NORTHERN OHIO DENTAL ASSOCIATION.

THE forty-fifth annual meeting of the Northern Ohio Dental Association will be held in Cleveland, Tuesday, Wednesday, and Thursday, June 7, 8, and 9, 1904. The programme is a strong one, and will be of exceptional interest to the general profession. The motto for the year is " Annihilation of Pain in Dentistry." Essay-ists and clinicians have been selected with this thought ever fore-most. The best authorities and the most successful men in this line of work will be at this meeting. The members of the profession are cordially invited to attend. It is expected that we will have the largest attendance of any meeting ever held in this section of the country. You cannot afford to miss it. Come!

W. G. EBERSOLE,
Corresponding Secretary.

THE

International Dental Journal.

VOL. XXV.   JULY, 1904.   No. 7.

Original Communications.[1]

SOME THOUGHTS REGARDING METHODS, AND A NEW
APPLIANCE FOR MOVING DISLOCATED TEETH
INTO POSITION.[2]

BY GEORGE C. AINSWORTH, D.D.S., BOSTON, MASS.

IT has been suggested to assume that my audience is totally
unfamiliar with everything connected with this subject except that
they are dentists.

I wish to say that the time at my command since accepting the
invitation to appear before you this evening has not been sufficient
to accomplish all that I desired, more especially since some of the
pictures which will be shown have necessarily been made from old
models that were made with no thought of the importance of perfection, and simply for study models. Some of the appliances, too,
in their application to the models are not perfect in their adaptation,
but simply gotten up to demonstrate the theory of their application.

It is my purpose, this evening, to place before you *three* appliances, all of which I have been using for some time with much
satisfaction, and while the principles involved are not new, the

---

[1] The editor and publishers are not responsible for the views of authors
of papers published in this department, nor for any claim to novelty, or
otherwise, that may be made by them. No papers will be received for this
department that have appeared in any other journal published in the
country.

[2] Read before The New York Institute of Stomatology, March 1, 1904.

manner of applying them *is,* so far as I have been able to learn.
The first is a self-acting spreading appliance, the second is an
inclined plane for jumping the bite and adjusting the occlusion,
while the third is a simple retaining appliance.

To appreciate the increasing need of orthodontic services, one
has but to observe the faces of the rising generation we meet every
day. The causes are many and the conditions alarming. Indeed,
the patient whose teeth cannot be improved by the orthodontist
seems the exception rather than the rule.

It also seems to be the opinion of those best able to judge, that
this work should be largely done by the specialist. Certain it is
that the successful orthodontist must be a man of large resource,
—in art, in mechanics, and in patience,—for there is no hard and
fast rule for the solution of all cases, and while we may classify
them in general terms, there still remains an individuality which
necessitates an independent solution of the case in hand according
to its merits.

Nevertheless, while conditions remain as they are the average
dental practitioner, especially in the smaller districts, will be called
upon to do more or less of this work. It then becomes a duty
for us to be keenly alive to any methods which may promise the
greatest good with the least amount of suffering to the patient, as
well as the least draft upon the time of the operator.

We should study to simplify methods and appliances, to minimize pain, and to economize time. Along these lines I have expended much time and thought to produce something that should
be self-acting, requiring little attention, and which should interfere
as little as possible with the ordinary functions of the teeth and
mouth, not forgetting cleanliness, which presupposes simplicity
and a due regard for one's appearance.

Teeth are made irregular by pressure, of one sort or another,
and without pain. Why, then, should we not expect to make them
regular by pressure without pain? In the first instance, the pressure
is against nature, while in the second it is in accordance with her
design. It seems, then, to be a question of applying the necessary
force to move them in a proper way.

We have two kinds of force at our command,—the intermittent,
as applied by the screw, and the constant, as applied by the spring,
the lever, the ligature, and the elastic.

The claim has been made in favor of the screw pressure, that force thus applied was attended with less soreness and consequent discomfort; that there should be periods of rest between the periods of movement such as might be obtained by turning the screw each day; that the force having spent itself, the tooth rested until the next turn of the screw. That claim, it seems to me, is not borne out by facts; and while it undoubtedly is true that force applied by an elastic band or rubber wedge is attended with more soreness and consequent pain, it seems to be owing to that peculiar quality of elastic force as applied by rubber, and which differs from force as applied by a spring. What seems to be tolerated most kindly is a firm, gentle pressure, be it intermittent or otherwise. When a tooth first starts it is usually attended with slight tenderness, which, as a rule, quickly subsides without a letting up of that force; then, if the force is continued in a reasonable way, all goes well.

It is idle, perhaps, to talk about pleasure to the patient in having teeth regulated. Nevertheless, there are different degrees of comfort, and it is to obtain the maximum that we are striving. To do this the work had best go on slowly. The effort to accomplish an extensive piece of work in orthodontia in a remarkably short time seems to me to be ill advised, and not likely to be attended with as satisfactory results as it would have been had the change been conducted more gradually. All these changes are accomplished by force, which, if applied too suddenly, or too severely, renders nature antagonistic and rebellious, as evidenced by pain, heat, redness, and swelling,—she recognizes an enemy; whereas, if the force is applied gradually and gently, she looks upon you as a friend trying to help her, and takes kindly to your efforts, falling into line with all the assistance of which she is capable.

Again, where teeth are moved slowly they are less liable to be drawn out of, or away from, their tissue environment,—a matter of much importance, particularly when elongating teeth.

We come now to a consideration of the self-acting spreading appliance, which may have a double action,—*i.e.,* it can be so adjusted as to spread the arch and, when desirable, retract the incisors at the same time, or, by the addition of ligatures, the front teeth may be moved forward or elongated. In accomplishing the first two, it is entirely self-acting and requires very little attention, allowing the absence of the patient two, four, or even eight weeks at a time, yet its action is under the control of the patient at all times.

In the second instance, where ligatures are employed it requires closer attention, but where wire ligatures are used, even those allow the absence of the patient for some days. Yet I find many occasions to use silk ligatures, even though they require more constant attention, for the sake of cleanliness.

This appliance, in its simplest form, is composed of three members (Fig. 1, A),—two anchors and a wire spring, while the compound form has two springs. Each anchor is made up of three pieces,—a piece of seamless tubing, with 30-gauge walls, of suitable size and length to be fitted to the tooth chosen for anchorage, after the manner of forming a band for a gold crown. To this is soldered, on the palatal side and at right angles with the band, a piece of 16-gauge wire running along the border of the arch, with a bearing on and of sufficient length to engage all of the teeth to be moved on that side; while on the buccal side of the anchor band is soldered a short piece of 16-gauge seamless tubing running parallel with the band, to receive the end of the spring-wire,—the active principle of the appliance. These anchors, when completed, are adjusted to the teeth selected, and cemented firmly into place (Fig. 1, B)—one on either side of the arch, after which the two ends of the spring wire, bent at right angles to itself, are sprung into the tubes provided for them (Fig. 1, C). The inside bar is designed to move the bicuspids and molars as a unit without the aid of ligatures.

This case seems to be an unusually favorable one for this appliance, which in its operation has a double action. The sides of the arch are to be equally expanded and the incisors moved in (Fig. 1, D). The teeth to be moved out include the cuspids, the bicuspids, and the first molars. The spring, being adjusted to bear firmly on the labial surface of the incisors, presses those teeth in as the side teeth move out. The teeth chosen for attaching the anchor bands should be midway between the two points of resistance, and this perhaps more often fails on the first bicuspid than otherwise, though sometimes it may be the second bicuspid, or even the first molar.

My estimate of the central point of resistance in this case is the first bicuspid, the cuspid and first molar being the extreme points. You will readily see that if the pressure be applied in the molar region it would not expand the arch at the cuspid, which tooth offers marked resistance. If, however, during the operation you

FIG. 1.

A B

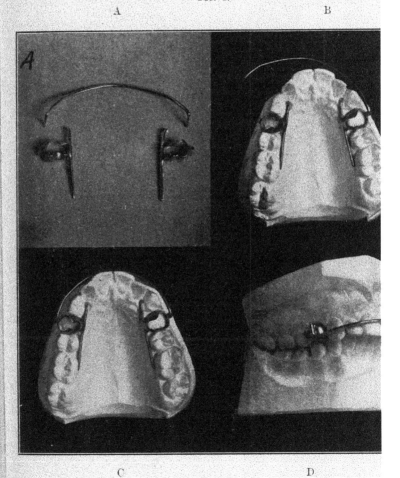

C D

FIG. 2.

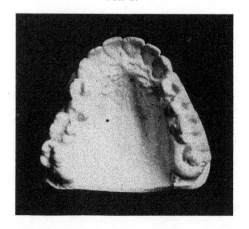

FIG. 3.

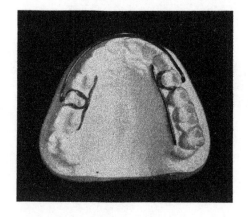

FIG. 4.

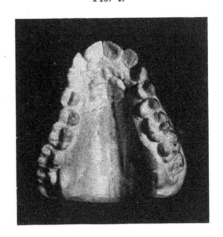

FIG. 5.

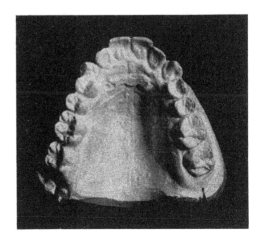

FIG. 6.

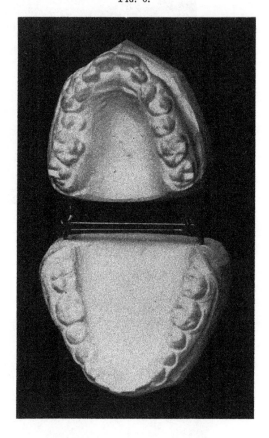

find your judgment has been in error for any reason, it is not a difficult matter to change the attachment to a more favorable location.

The time required to accomplish the desired change depends upon the age of the patient and the adjustment of the spring. I should not hesitate to dismiss this patient for two months after adjusting the appliance, but where convenient I would look at it about once in two weeks, always directing that if anything seems wrong, or soreness develops, to report at once. The spring, as you see, can be readily removed and readjusted by the patient.

Fig. 2 shows another case for the simple appliance. All the teeth seem in satisfactory relation excepting the second upper bicuspid on the right side, which occludes inside the arch.

The appliance was adjusted here to pit the resistance of the five teeth on the left—all the teeth from the cuspid to the second molar—against the resistance of the one displaced tooth on the right.

In eight weeks the tooth had moved to the position as you now see it (Fig. 3), with practically no attention or change, and, if I may believe the patient, without any pain or inconvenience whatever. Undoubtedly, had the tooth not been locked in by the approximating teeth, it would have moved to position in half the time. The small wire on the inside was put on as a precaution, lest the tooth should start suddenly, when it had progressed far enough to throw off the lateral resistance, and come out too far. On its completion the appliance was removed and a retainer, consisting of a simple band, cemented to the tooth, to the buccal side of which was soldered a piece of gold wire, similar to the one shown on the palatal side, the ends of which rested against the buccal surfaces of the approximating teeth.

Fig. 4 shows a case where the simple appliance would be appropriate, but where I should choose the second bicuspid for anchorage of the bands and place the spring-wire tubes at the antero-buccal surface.

Fig. 5 shows a case now under treatment where the slight contraction of the arch has forced the centrals and cuspids to assume a position outside of the arch, or perhaps, more correctly speaking, the bicuspids are inside of the arch. The simple appliance has been adjusted, anchored to the first bicuspids, and the arch is gradually spreading. I see the patient once a week, just to keep an eye on it, but as yet have made no change. In eight weeks, I should judge, the expansion will be sufficient to allow the turning of the cuspid teeth into position.

I have been asked to explain why I commenced work on the upper teeth instead of the lower. It is not always easy to give a lucid explanation of the reason for doing a certain thing, although one follows the dictates of his judgment—*instinct,* perhaps. It is true, nature begins her work in the adjustment of her masticatory apparatus by the development of the lower teeth first, but the conditions under which she does it are different from those presented to us for correction. She moves the teeth upward and downward on a line with the axes of the tooth, while we are called upon to move them sidewise. Again, the lower teeth are inferior in size and stability to the upper, which, when fully developed, have a larger controlling influence, and it seems to me as a rule easier to expand the larger arch first after which the smaller is more easily adjusted to it, especially as the upper jaw is stationary, while the lower is not. In other words, there are limitations to the possibilities of movement or adjustment in the upper jaw that do not obtain in the lower.

It is, however, perfectly practicable with this appliance to carry both upper and lower along simultaneously, sometimes a matter of much importance, since it lessens the number of visits and expedites the work. Indeed, there are many cases where inconvenience and discomfort are lessened by having the upper and lower carried on together.

Fig. 6 shows another case,—that of a nervous, excitable, young lady thirteen years of age. The parents dreaded the commencement of the operation, lest it upset her entirely. The simple appliance has been on now four weeks, with perfect comfort and happiness; in fact, I think she rather enjoys it. Her visits are made once a week in company with a young lady friend undergoing the same sort of an operation, and there is invariably a controversy between them as to which shall occupy the chair first. My attendant usually settles it by having them draw lots. I speak of this merely to show that the work is not always dreaded.

You will notice (Fig. 7) that the molars on one side occlude inside the arch, while the bicuspids are not yet far enough advanced to determine exactly where they would come. The appliance is anchored to the first molars, while the inside bar is so arranged

FIG. 7.

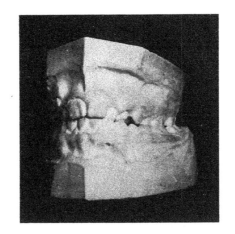

FIG. 8.

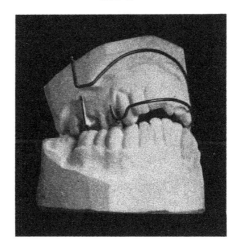

Fig. 9.

B

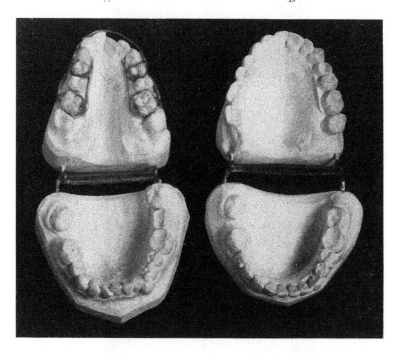

as to guide the bicuspids out into a proper position. During the four weeks the arch has expanded three-sixteenths of an inch.

Of course, there is nothing remarkable in what is being accomplished in most of these cases, excepting the satisfaction of seeing them progress so favorably without laborious and painful attention. The gums are clean, healthy, and comparatively free from irritation.

Fig. 8 represents the teeth of a lady from forty-five to fifty years of age, and introduces the addition of another spring-wire and its attachment to the simple appliance, making a compound, self-acting appliance which is applicable to those cases where *much* pressure is required at both the cuspid and molar region. The longer spring, acting on the molars, may be adjusted high up under the lip entirely out of sight, while the shorter one, acting on the cuspids, may be adjusted lower down at the pleasure of the operator.

All the teeth are present excepting the lower second molar on the right and the four wisdom-teeth (Fig. 9, A). The upper bicuspids and molars occlude inside the arch on both sides, the front teeth badly bunched, giving to the mouth a decidedly unpleasant expression, the lips closing over them with difficulty. The lower arch is of normal width, but the teeth are somewhat out of position in the left cuspid region, that tooth being, perhaps, one-sixteenth of an inch short.

The simple, one-spring appliance was put on this case in June, with the longer wire, as here shown, adjusted to the molar bands, while the appliance here shown represents what I would use were I to conduct the case again. If I remember correctly, I saw the patient three times before I went on my usual August vacation, but made no change in the appliance. On my return, early in September, I found the arch widened at the molar region fully one-half inch (Fig. 9, B), with the assurance from the patient that she had suffered no inconvenience whatever; in fact, she said she could not believe for a long time that it was accomplishing anything, it was so comfortable. The arch was spread at the cuspid region by a jack-screw running from cuspid to cuspid on the palatal side, after which the alignment was accomplished by the well-known arch band anchored to the molars. Fig. 10 shows the case completed.

You will observe that the tubes on the molars (Fig. 8) run

high up opposite the ends of the roots. This was for the purpose of applying the expanding pressure in such a way as to move the roots and process at that point, the long ends of the spring-wire being bent out at such an angle as to apply force *there* when inserted in the tubes. It is also perfectly practicable to insert the wire the other way,—*i.e.,* at the top of the tubes,—and .thus apply the force high up, overcoming the tipping tendency sometimes met with in other appliances.

Thus you will see that this appliance offers the possibility of many variations through additions and modifications, which unfold every day in our experience, to solve the problems as they are presented.

Figs. 11 and 12 show a case where the inside bar is used in connection with the ordinary arch band. The cuspids and bicuspids are to be moved out a little, while the front teeth are to be elongated and brought in.

The objection to the self-acting appliance here is the limited downward pressure obtainable with the spring-wire attached to the first bicuspids, besides the possibility of moving those teeth forward while in the act of pressing the front teeth in. If we anchor to the molars we shall not spread the arch at the cuspids and bicuspids without the addition of several ligatures, around those teeth. The same objection applies to the ordinary arch band, anchored to the molars with nuts at the distal ends of the tubes, but by combining the inside bar with this appliance we do away with all such ligatures, substituting one between the cuspid and first bicuspid on either side connecting the inside bar with the spring of the outside band. This will move those teeth out and not materially interfere with the downward spring of the arch band.

The inside bar soldered to the anchor band around the molar counteracts the tendency to the tipping of that tooth, which might be experienced by raising the arch band up and ligating to the front teeth.

The following case is shown, not because of its connection with any appliance presented, but for the reason that it is in some respects quite remarkable.

The gentleman presented at the age of forty-nine. The only contact between the upper and lower teeth was on the right side, between the second molars, which, instead of meeting each other squarely, passed by each other, wearing an inclined plane on either

FIG. 10.

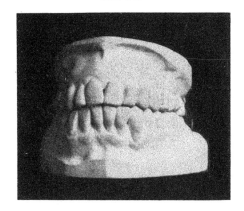

FIG. 11.

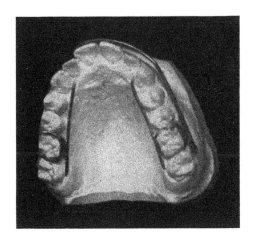

FIG. 12.

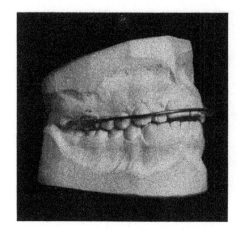

FIG. 13.

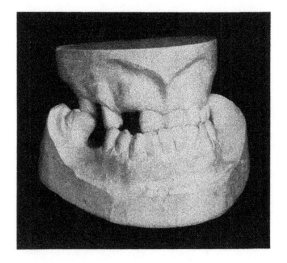

FIG. 14.

A   B

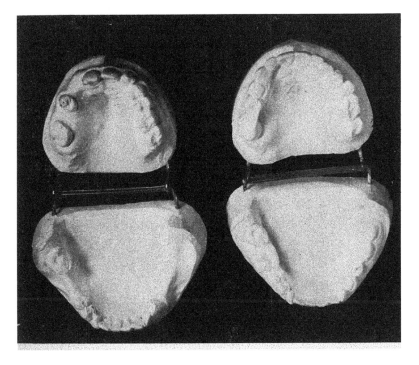

FIG. 15.

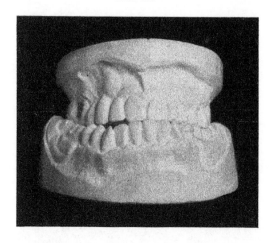

FIG. 16.

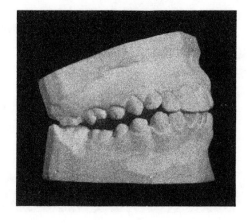

tooth (Fig. 13). The jaws closed much beyond the normal point, giving a most unpleasant expression to the face.

One molar and lateral are missing on the upper left side, and on the right side two molars, one bicuspid, the cuspid, and the lateral, seven teeth in all (Fig. 14, A). In consequence, the contraction of the jaw has been such that all the upper teeth strike well inside the lower arch, the incisors fully one-half inch.

On the lower jaw every tooth back of the first bicuspid on the left side had been extracted, and the right first and second molars were also missing. The question asked by the patient was, " Can you do anything for me, or must I be turned out to pasture to die like an old horse? I cannot chew as I am."

Three months' study of the case and models was necessary before a possible solution of an apparently hopeless case was determined upon. Artificial plates alone were out of the question, because of the great discrepancy in size of the two arches.

It was decided to attempt to widen the upper arch in order to bring the molars and bicuspids as nearly as possible over the lower, since every particle of movement in that direction would be a distinct gain; and to move the incisors as far forward as might be to improve the appearance, though it seemed absolutely out of the question to obtain an occlusion of the incisors.

In four months the result was beyond the most sanguine expectations entertained at the start, and a temporary retainer was inserted for the summer (Fig. 14, B).

In the fall a combined bridge and retainer in one continuous piece was made for the upper, using as abutments the molar and first bicuspid on the left side and the molar and second bicuspid on the right, swinging the missing intervening teeth on as dummies. The missing teeth on the lower jaw were supplied on a partial gold clasp-plate.

The result is a good masticating contact on either side back of the cuspid teeth and a reduction of the antero-posterior distance between the incisors to one-eighth of an inch (Fig. 15).

MAKING THESE APPLIANCES.

In making these appliances ordinary German silver is used for all except the spring-wire, which is eighteen per cent. nickel especially drawn for the purpose, with the maximum amount of spring obtainable consistent with toughness. If too hard, it is apt to break and cause annoyance. This I have obtained of the Holmes, Booth & Haydens Company, of Waterbury, Conn. The tubing, of various sizes, is seamless drawn, and especially made for me by J. Briggs & Sons' Company, 65 Clifford Street, Providence, R. I.

Ordinary plate, of German silver or gold, may be used, with platinized gold wire for the spring, if one prefers, but I have found the German silver to answer every purpose, and in some respects it is superior. Seamless drawn tubing possesses a marked advantage, particularly when soldering the small tubes to the anchor bands. The appliance when completed is gold-plated.

In making the appliance the method of procedure is as follows: After cutting off a piece of seamless tubing of the proper size, anneal it, and with a pair of contouring pliers form it into a sort of barrel-shaped cylinder; next, with a small pair of scissors cut away a part of one end to approximately correspond to the gum line around the tooth; then gradually work it up into position, perhaps a little under the gum, take an instrument and mark around at the gum line; also at the top, so that there shall be a small projection left after trimming to turn over the edge of the tooth into the sulci, giving the band a firm seat when finally cemented to place. After trimming, the two bands are placed in position and a *plaster* impression taken; *this,* in my judgment, is important, as accuracy counts for much when one comes to set the appliance.

As a rule, it is reasonably possible to force a band of 30-gauge walls between the teeth, but sometimes, as an aid, I draw in some sort of a wedge for fifteen minutes or an hour, as the case may be. A rubber wedge works well for that length of time. Then, again, the edges of the band may be thinned a little and smeared with vaseline; one band may be crowded in a trifle and left while proceeding with the other. In short, a variety of expedients may be resorted to, that will be suggested to the mind of the resourceful man.

After the impression has been removed from the mouth the bands are carefully taken off and replaced in the impression, and the usual detail of making the model gone through with, the bands appearing on it exactly as they will stand in the mouth. Proceed then to adjust the palatal wires to fit the model as desired, being *particularly* careful, if intending to move the cuspids out, to turn that end of the wire well up under the gum in such a way as to engage that tooth above the bulge of enamel; otherwise, when the spring pressure is applied that end of the wire will slide down the incline plane surface of the cuspid instead of moving the tooth, resulting in a troublesome elongation of the tooth banded.

When these wires have been properly fitted, hold them in position by pieces of binding wire passed around them and through the model, twisting the ends till taut.

Next, to adjust the small tubes for receiving the ends of the spring-wire, pass an ordinary pin through them into the model in such a way as to hold them in position while being soldered.

Next, bur out a little of the plaster from within the anchor band opposite the points where the solder is to flow, and proceed to the soldering, which is done on the model.

The next step is to remove, finish, polish, and gold plate.

The labial spring-wire is usually fitted into position after the anchors are placed in the mouth, sometimes before cementing, sometimes after. If the front teeth are to be moved in and spaces closed up, the wire is adjusted to bear as firmly as possible on those teeth; if the front teeth are to be moved out, the wire is adjusted to stand out a bit to admit of the ligatures doing their work. Under favorable conditions, the fitting of the anchor bands and taking the impression can be accomplished in an hour.

PLATING PLANT.

Some sort of a gold-plating plant seems an important auxiliary to the dental equipment of to-day. A simple one is made up of a glass jar of convenient size with a cover to prevent evaporation and exclude dust, containing a fluid composed of thirty grains of chloride of gold, sixty grains of cyanide of potassium, and one-half pint of distilled water, operated by a single-cell Sampson battery. A piece of pure gold is attached to the carbon wire and suspended in the fluid, while the article to be plated is attached to the zinc wire and likewise suspended, care being taken that the gold and the article to be plated do not come in contact while in the solution.

In place of the Sampson cell, the wires may be connected with the ordinary electric lighting supply, in which case the current is run through a series of lamps to reduce it.

In the latter case the piece to be plated is left in the solution perhaps three minutes, when it is taken out and polished; this process is repeated several times according to the amount of plate desired.

In summing up the advantages of this appliance, its *simplicity* seems to stand out as a key-note far and above everything heretofore in use. Being simple, it is *cleanly,* doing away largely with ligatures, *always painful to apply and uncomfortable to wear.*

It is *effective,* because it is worn twenty-four hours every day, and the power is applied directly to the teeth to be moved. It interferes as little as possible with the ordinary functions of the teeth and mouth, besides minimizing the deleterious effect sometimes noticed from wearing a more complicated appliance.

It is automatic in its work, and may be adjusted so as to have a double or, by the addition of ligatures, a triple action,—*i.e.,* it will spread the arch, move the front teeth in, and elongate at the same time.

As it is automatic in its action, it requires less attention, and consequently produces less inconvenience and pain, which should lend value to our services.

It is equally applicable to the upper or lower teeth and may be used on both simultaneously.

It is conveniently adjusted to bring pressure to bear on the roots and alveolus, and thus has a tendency to overcome the outward tipping of the anchor teeth sometimes encountered in spreading the arch.

And lastly, it is not unsightly, since it admits of greater cleanliness.

INCLINED PLANE.

The next appliance shown is an inclined plane fixed to the teeth, for "jumping the bite" and adjusting the occlusion.

It sometimes happens in regulating teeth that the lower jaw is all at sea as regards an occlusion of the teeth. It is equally bad in two or three different positions. It becomes then a question of compelling one, and only one, closure in order to give the teeth a chance to adjust themselves to each other after nature's design.

It is particularly applicable where there is excessive overbite of the front teeth, such as usually accompanies a case of thumb-sucking.

Fig. 16 shows such a case, after the upper teeth had been brought into an approximately correct arch relation. An attempt was made to establish a correct occlusion by constructing gold

19

FIG. 17.

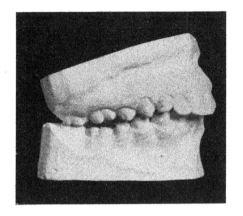

FIG. 18.

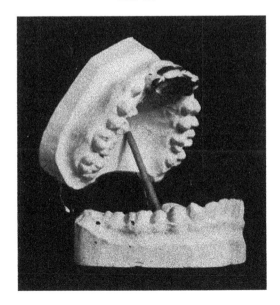

Fig. 19.

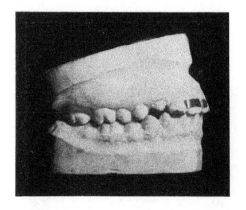

Fig. 20.

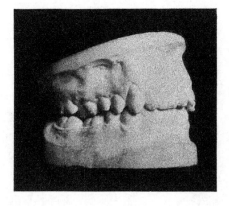

. crowns for the upper sixth-year molars with grinding surfaces corresponding to those on the lower teeth when in correct relation, thus allowing the twelfth-year molars, which were just beginning to show through the gum, to erupt into their proper relation. Thus far everything seemed satisfactory, but the gold crowns being removed, observe what happened. The patient instead of adopting the correct occlusion, just shown in the last picture, found the one now on the screen more agreeable and effective, thus defeating the attempt to correct the overbite (Fig. 17).

The obvious objections to an inclined plane in connection with a plate led to the application of the same principle involved in a plane soldered to bands encircling the upper centrals and to lugs engaging the cutting edges of the laterals (Fig. 18), to prevent undue depression of the centrals. This resulted in establishing the correct occlusion shown in Fig. 19.

This appliance may seem at first an uncomfortable one to wear, but this young man affirms that after the first day or two he paid no attention to it, and like reports come from similar cases.

This was the first appliance of the kind I made. I now have them made with a round wire lug to rest over the end of the lateral, as more cleanly and less likely to injure the tooth, and for the same reason have the gold dressed away from the palatal side of the laterals as much as possible to avoid contact. The bands on the centrals cover nearly the whole palatal surface and are firmly cemented on. The inclined plane surface is made from a fairly heavy piece of platinized gold plate.

Fig. 20 shows a case of a young man, twenty-one years of age, where the overbite completely covers the lower front teeth; the lower incisors badly bunched; one central having been extracted. Notice the discrepancy in the length between the front and back teeth on the lower jaw (Fig. 21, A). Both arches were spread, the lower front teeth were somewhat improved and an inclined plane adjusted, as in the previous case. This not only held the teeth apart and facilitated the regulation of the lower front teeth, but it depressed the upper and lower front teeth in their sockets, while the back teeth were free to elongate and meet each other under natural conditions. The final result is seen in Fig. 22.

The time required to produce the desired change varies from perhaps four to twelve months, according to the age of the patient and the amount of elongation to be accomplished.

Some of the teeth to be lengthened in the first case were banded with thin gold, pin-heads being soldered to the bands in such a way that an intermaxillary elastic band could be attached at night and produce an elongating pull, but this was soon abandoned as unnecessary.

The inclined plane need not, as a rule, be as wide as the one shown, and may be reduced as the work progresses. This appliance sometimes facilitates the work of the automatic spreading appliance, and may be worn in conjunction with one of those appliances on the lower teeth. It may also be incorporated with a retainer for the upper teeth such as shown in Fig. 23.

The advantages of this appliance are, first, its simplicity—no ligatures or rubbers required. It is cleanly and effective, automatic in its action, and requires no attention from either patient or operator after it is adjusted. It is not painful, and the patient makes less complaint than the parent.

RETAINING APPLIANCE.

The next, and last, appliance to be shown is a simple retaining appliance, designed to securely hold the teeth after regulating until they have become fixed in their new position.

The requirements in such an appliance are *security, cleanliness, comfort, appearance.*

The appliance here shown (Fig. 24) combines all these to a marked degree. Like the self-acting expanding appliance (which is an outgrowth from the retaining appliance), it is composed of anchor bands with small tubes attached to the buccal sides, into which are inserted the ends of a labial wire, bent at right angles to itself. The inside wire differs from that of the self-acting appliance in that it is continuous around the arch, thus holding all the teeth that may have been moved out, while the labial wire holds the front teeth in.

This appliance is securely cemented into place and worn without discomfort.

An important and pleasing feature is the removability of the labial wire, as it sometimes happens that a young lady wishes to avoid its appearance for an evening. The wire is readily taken out and readjusted by the patient. In cases where the front teeth have not been moved in, it can be dispensed with altogether, otherwise the appliance is not particularly conspicuous.

FIG. 21.

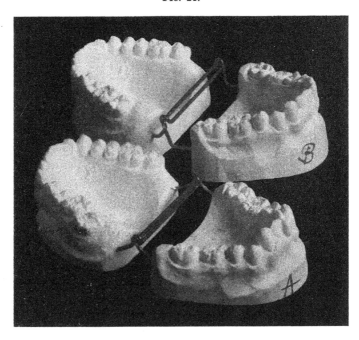

FIG. 22.

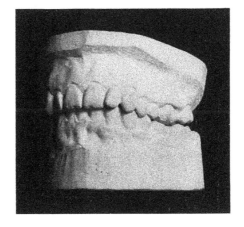

Fig. 23.

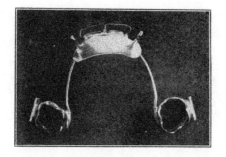

Fig. 24.

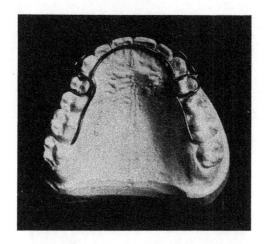

Fig. 25.

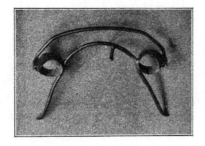

The labial wire is usually smaller than in the self-acting appliance.

Additions may be made to this appliance, as, for instance,
when a tooth has been rotated, it may be banded and the band
soldered to the inside wire, thus becoming a part of the retaining
appliance.

And again, when it is desired to tip a front tooth or teeth
inward, moving the apex of the root outward, spurs may be soldered
to the inside wire at right angles to it in such a way as to rest on the
palatal or lingual surface of the root high up under the gum, exerting, when adjusted, an outward pressure, while the labial spring-
wire is adjusted to bear hard on those teeth well down towards the
cutting edge (Fig. 25). The result is obvious.

This completes what I have to show this evening, and while
it may not all be new to you, I hope some of it is. It has been
my desire to make the subject clear. If I have not, I shall be
glad to do so later. And if any of you can derive the satisfaction
from the use of these appliances that I have, it will be an added
source of pleasure to me.

RADIOTHERAPY IN PYORRHŒA ALVEOLARIS, AND DENTAL RADIOGRAPHY.[1]

A DEMONSTRATION OF THE X-RAY, THE ULTRA-VIOLET RAY,
HIGH-FREQUENCY CURRENTS, AND RADIUM, THE AUTHOR'S
X-RAY TUBE FOR THE TREATMENT OF THE TEETH, AND
HIS METHOD OF RADIOGRAPHY.

BY SINCLAIR TOUSEY, A.M., M.D.[2]

DURING the past two years a very great deal has been done
with the X-ray and kindred applications as an adjunct to the
mechanical and chemical treatment of the fatal disease of the
teeth known as pyorrhœa alveolaris, or Riggs's Disease. During
this time reports upon the subject of pyorrhœa have been published
by Finsen, Custer, Parker, Hickey, Guy, Schwartz, Robin, Römer,
Achorn, Suye, Talbot, Logan, Stewart, Newell, Goadby, Burchard,

[1] Read before The New York Institute of Stomatology, March 1, 1904.
[2] Attending Surgeon St. Bartholomew's Clinic. Assisted by Leo Green,
D.D.S., of the Dental Department of St. Bartholomew's Clinic.

Ames, Grieves, Cook, Bödecker, Choteau, Rhein, Peacock, Bester, V. Wolrozynickie, and in *Dental Annals,* 1903, *Odontologie,* 1903, *Pathologie der Zähne,* 1903.

From the reports we gather that the probability is that the ordinary pus organisms, such as the staphylococcus, the bacillus pyocyaneus, bacillus coli communis, etc., have no direct share in the production of pyorrhœa alveolaris, and that the pneumococcus is also absent. Probably a member of the yeast family is the pathogenic germ. The constitutional conditions are often due to poisoning by toxins, and a filtered broth culture from these teeth kills guinea-pigs (Goadby). The constitutional cause is frequently rheumatism or gout (Newell). The teeth themselves are generally free from caries and the dental tissues hard and highly organized. Some cases (1) arise from a primary gingivitis, with the formation of hard, scaly, dark calculi beneath the gum margin. In other cases (2) the gingivitis is not marked, early deposits may be absent, and there is phagedenic pericementitis. In still other cases (3) degeneration and necrosis of the pericementum and deposits of calculi occur upon the lateral aspects of the tooth root, the gum margin being normal (Burchard).

The clinical appearance is described by Guy in an article in the *Dental Record,* reviewed in the *Dental Digest* for September, 1903. In his patient there was chronic enlargement of the submaxillary glands; the lower incisors, cuspids, and premolars were all very loose; the gum festoons hung patulous away from them; the gums were unhealthy, spongy, livid, and almost purpuric; pus exuded freely from about the roots of the teeth; the two upper incisors and a number of roots required extraction. The teeth were hypersensitive to heat and cold, and the patient had to warm his beer and cool his tea, and was quite unable to use his teeth.

In one of my own patients, the radiograph of whose lower front teeth, taken by the process described later, is shown herewith (Fig. 1), there was such great pain all along the right half of the lower alveolar margin as to make her sick in bed for several weeks, during which time the dentist had to visit her twice a day. She came to me six months later for constitutional treatment for indefinite digestive distress, with rheumatic or neuralgic pains, and with an excess of uric acid and a large amount of sugar in the urine. This is a condition which yields to the application of high-frequency currents and vibratory massage, and these were

FIG. 1.

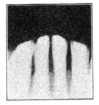

FIG. 2.

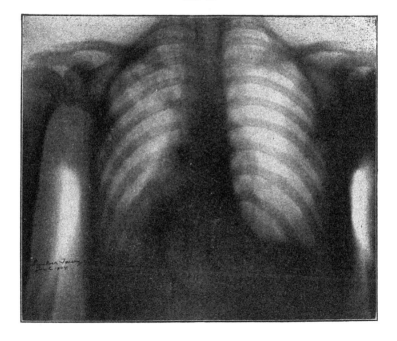

FIG. 3.

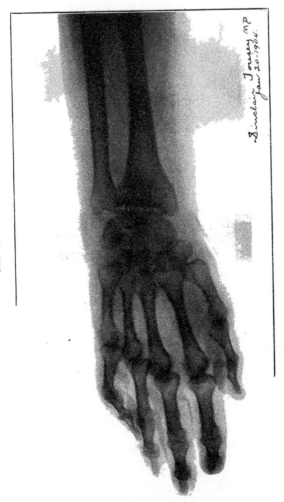

Sinclair Tousey M.D.
Jan 20. 1904.

applied over the abdomen and spine, and over the affected joints. A few applications of the X-Ray by my special tube were made to the teeth. The result is apparently a perfect cure, but could not have been accomplished without the local applications by the dentist.

Turning now to a demonstration of X-ray and phototherapeutic methods and apparatus, I call your attention to some X-ray pictures.

Fig. 2 is a radiograph of the chest and shoulders of a patient whom I am treating for tuberculosis of the larynx and lungs. The picture shows the right shoulder-joint and the shoulder-blade completely, with the ribs showing through the shoulder-blade, the picture being taken from behind. It also shows both clavicles. Shining through the entire thickness of the chest, it shows the heart area, and the area of the stomach, liver, and spleen. In three weeks' treatment the expectoration, which had been so profuse as to choke her, and had been full of the tubercle bacilli, entirely ceased; and at the end of a month's treatment the larynx was examined by a throat specialist, who found that the area of ulceration and redness below the vocal cords had decidedly diminished in size and that the hoarseness of the voice had much improved. She had also gained in weight and strength.

Fig. 3 is a picture of the hand and forearm which was taken at the patient's home, she being an old lady who had sustained an injury to the wrist which was feared might be a fracture. The picture was taken to make sure that the bones were in the correct position. It was taken right through the splints and bandages. It shows no fracture, but is interesting as a beautiful picture, and also because it shows rheumatic enlargement of the finger-joints.

Fig. 4 is the elbow-joint of a patient whom I was treating for chronic rheumatism by use of the X-ray and high-frequency currents, and who has spent a quarter of his time for the last twenty-seven years in hospitals being treated for rheumatism,—being filled with medicine, having his joints baked with a temperature of three to four hundred degrees, and being treated by different forms of electricity. A few months of treatment by means of the X-ray and high-frequency currents have made a new man of him. The picture shows the lower end of the humerus with the two condyles and the olecranon fossa, at which point the bone is transparent and must be very thin. It shows the radius with its head taking part in the formation of the elbow-joint and also articulating with the ulna, and shows the ulna overlapping the radius, the entire outline of both bones being visible. The olecranon process is clearly shown.

Fig. 5 is a picture of the teeth of a young lady in whom there is such a wide separation between the upper central and incisors as to present a disagreeable appearance and cause a certain degree of hissing in the voice, and the occasional flying out of a little drop of saliva in the face of any one to whom she might be talking. This is a patient of Dr. Leo Green, at whose request I took this picture in order to make sure that there was no supernumerary tooth or other reason why these teeth should not be brought together. The picture shows that there was nothing between the roots, and he accordingly regulated the teeth.

For the X-ray light we get the power by means of the street current which comes into the office as a continuous direct current of one hundred and ten volts. It has to pass through an interrupter, which consists of an outer jar in which one of the lead connections drops into dilute sulphuric acid, and an inner jar in which there is another lead connection also in dilute sulphuric acid. This inner jar has a certain number of perforations which permits of the passage of an electric current from the outer to the inner plate. As soon as the current is turned on hydrogen and oxygen gas are produced by the decomposition of this liquid by the current, and bubbles of this gas block up the small perforations in the inner jar, and in that way interrupt the current. No sooner is the current interrupted than the bubbles escape to the surface of the liquid and the current begins to flow again. This interruption takes place in some of my interrupters at the rate of ten thousand times a minute, and in others still more rapidly, and thus we have a series of ten thousand currents a minute and an intensity of one hundred and ten volts through the primary coil, each one producing a current of very much greater intensity in the secondary coil; the intensity in the second coil being dependent upon the very large number of turns of wire. In that coil there are about one hundred thousand feet of wire, so that when the current is turned on full we have about one million volts in the secondary coil.

This current is allowed to pass through the X-ray tube, which contains a partial vacuum through which the current is carried,

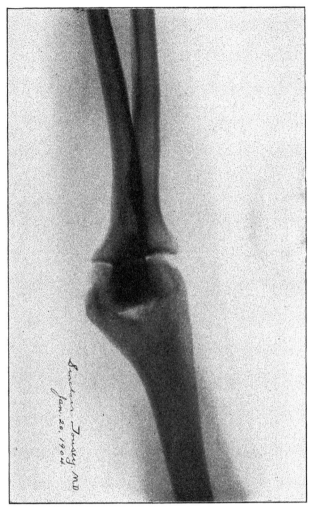

FIG. 4.

FIG. 5.

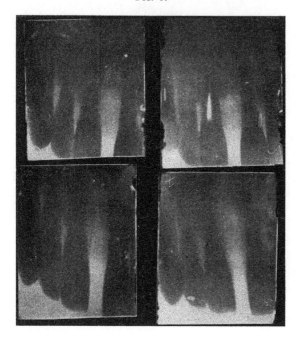

not as a tremendous spark or flame, as would be the case if the two points were in the open air, but as a very fierce bombardment of molecules which strike on the platinum disk in the centre of the tube and there break up into the form of motion which we know as the X-ray.

To see the bones of the hand, etc., by means of the X-ray, we have to employ a fluoroscope, which consists of a box into which we look, the bottom of it being coated with a chemical substance which becomes fluorescent under the influence of the X-ray. Very often people looking through the fluoroscope will be surprised when they discover later that the bottom of the box is an opaque piece of cardboard, the fluorescence being so brilliant that it seems as if they were looking through a piece of glass. Every substance is more or less transparent to the X-ray, but the more solid substances—metals and bones—cast deeper shadows than those less solid, like the flesh, etc. A piece of glass is relatively quite opaque to the X-ray, while wood is very transparent. Aluminum is very transparent, but lead is very much less so, and very often when treating a patient with the X-ray and in taking an X-ray picture we use a piece of lead to protect the portions which we do not want exposed to the rays.

The degree of penetration and the brilliancy of the light can be regulated by means of raising or lowering the degree of the vacuum in the tube, and all of the best tubes are provided with arrangements for this purpose. Of course, the strength of the current also has to be adjusted to the purpose in hand.

The ordinary X-ray tube, which I here show (Fig. 6), has its main portion spherical and the entire half of the tube in front of the plane of the platinum disk is brilliantly lighted up by a green light. The special X-ray tube which I have devised for the application of the X-ray to the treatment of Riggs's disease is made of lead glass, opaque to the X-ray except a cylindrical prolongation, from the end of which the rays go in a straight line, and none of the X-ray goes in any other direction, the light being absolutely localized to an area about an inch and a half in diameter, and the end of the tube is so shaped as to be convenient for application to the gums. If a great many treatments are necessary, of course the X-ray, if allowed to shine through the lips, would eventually cause a loss of the hair upon the lip, so that in such cases this special tube of mine ought to be applied with the lips separated.

For a few applications, or for the purpose of taking a picture, the X-ray can be allowed to shine right through the lips without any disturbance of any kind being produced.

The process by which I take pictures of the teeth, the roots of the teeth, supernumerary teeth, fractures of the jaw, etc., employs a piece of sensitized paper which is wrapped in opaque black paper and protected by thin rubber tissue; it is placed inside the mouth and pressed against the jaw, the light being allowed to shine from the outside of the face, and it is not necessary to use a special X-ray tube, the large spherical X-ray tube being perfectly adapted to the purpose. The distance is about ten inches, and the time of exposure required is from twenty seconds to a minute.

After making this exposure, we will take the piece of sensitized paper out of this envelope and drop it into a developing solution, and then later drop it into a fixing solution, and in five minutes we have a complete picture which may very probably show not only the roots of the teeth but also the entire pulp-cavity of the teeth extending down to the tips of the roots. In one picture, which I show you here (Fig. 7), we can see a gold crown upon the second molar, with a root filling from the same extending down about one-thirty-second of an inch into each root, instead of all the way; as it was supposed to be. The adjacent tooth, which appears to be sound, shows very perfectly the entire pulp-cavity of the root-canals. Pictures of this sort are, of course, necessary in making the diagnosis of supernumerary teeth, fractures of the jaw, impacted and displaced teeth, etc.

I now demonstrate to you the fluoroscope which I have devised for the immediate examination of the teeth and jaws with the X-ray. It is shaped like a dental mirror, but instead of a reflecting surface has a barium platino-cyanide surface protected from moisture by a sheet of transparent celluloid, and when in use instead of a reflection of the teeth we see a complete X-ray picture covering the whole surface of the fluoroscope. For satisfactory examinations the room ought to be darkened and the X-ray tube itself wrapped in a black cloth, these precautions being taken to exclude ordinary visible light and to cause the image upon the fluoroscope to become more brilliant by contrast. Figs. 8 and 9 show the appearance of this fluoroscope.

Another patient to whom I would like to refer is a lady whom

FIG. 6.

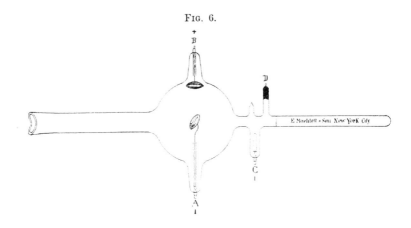

FIG. 7.

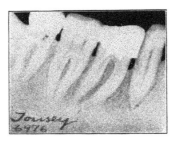

FIG. 8.

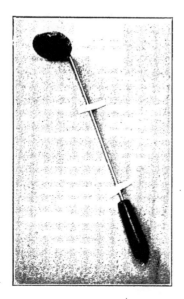

Dr. Tousey's fluoroscope for X-ray examination of the teeth and jaws.

I have treated for Riggs's disease by means of the X-ray and high-frequency currents. These high-frequency currents are produced by the same X-ray coil, with the addition of a D'Arsonal transformer and vacuum electrodes. These vacuum electrodes are simple glass tubes which contain a partial vacuum. They are of various shapes and are applied directly to the surface of the body, and when the current is turned on ten thousand waves of the violet-colored light pass down through the vacuum and disappear in the body every minute. The test by means of Willemite, which is also used for testing radium, shows the presence of ultra-violet rays in very rich abundance in this light. From these tubes there is produced a large amount of ozone right on the surface of the body, and this is carried in by the current. The electric current itself passes into a metallic handle which is held by the patient, and when the vacuum electrode is applied to the seat of disease the current passing through the patient has greater efficiency than can be applied in any other way.

The whole application is devoid of any uncomfortable sensation. In fact, there is practically no sensation except that of the actual contact of the glass with the surface. It is used by me with very great success in the treatment of rheumatism, gout, sciatica, paralysis, neuralgia, and as an adjunct in the treatment of tuberculosis.

One case of Riggs's disease which I have treated had been treated for a couple of months by Dr. Jones, a dentist in Birmingham, Ala. The treatment had been very successful, indeed, and consisted of almost daily applications of some caustic substance which destroyed the inflamed and necrotic tissue about the roots of the teeth. This subsequently gave place to a new and firm tissue, with the loss of only two teeth. She had been suffering from the disease for some six years before this course of treatment was undertaken, and when she came to New York there was very little of the original condition to be seen, and that little had disappeared entirely under the use of the vacuum electrodes and high-frequency currents applied through the lips. At the same time this patient has been cured of an epithelioma of the face by the X-ray.

The next part of the apparatus to be shown is the lamp which produces the ultra-violet ray. This is Dr. Piffard's modification of the Görl lamp, and is actuated by the X-ray coil with the addition of the Leyden jar, serving as a condenser. The lens in front of the lamp is made of quartz crystal, and, as you see by the experiment that I show you, the light produces a brilliant green fluorescence in a piece of Willemite; but this invisible ultra-violet ray will not pass through the thinnest piece of tissue-paper, and as I interpose such a piece of paper between the lamp and the Willemite you will see that the fluorescence is entirely prevented. The same takes place when a piece of glass is interposed between the lamp and the Willemite, although light appears the same when looking at it through a piece of glass.

The treatment of these conditions about the mouth, and also for lupus, consists in holding the lamp as close as possible to the affected surface. It seems to be something more than a merely antiseptic action which produces the benefit in these cases.

The next part of the apparatus to be seen is the Cooper-Hewitt light, a large cylinder of glass containing vapor of mercury, through which a current of very high intensity passes. The light appears white and is of four hundred candle-power, but the spectrum seems to be almost a pure violet, and anything red, like the beautiful bunch of roses which I have here, appears to be dark purple, from the absence of the red rays and the abundance of the violet element in the light. This light contains practically the chemical and life-giving properties of sunlight, about one hundred times intensified, and is applied directly over the bare chest at a distance of about four inches, and without danger of burning or discomfort. It is one of the parts of my treatment for tuberculosis.

The next part of the apparatus which I show you is the static machine, and its principal use for dental cases is for neuralgia; and I would very strongly advise any dentist, in treating a case of neuralgia apparently due to teeth, to do whatever is necessary in the way of treatment of the teeth, but not to consider extraction until the case has been treated by the static form of electricity. My own nurse suffered very much from neuralgia for two years, and two apparently healthy teeth were opened and the pulp-cavity disinfected and filled, but the neuralgia still persisted. The teeth were finally extracted, but the neuralgia continued worse than before, so that now for about a year she has suffered very much, indeed, in cold and wet weather, and has been unable to take solid food at such times. Finally, I gave her one or two treatments with high-frequency currents, which did not seem to agree with her; then about a month ago I gave her a single treatment with the static machine, which has resulted in the complete and entire

FIG. 9.

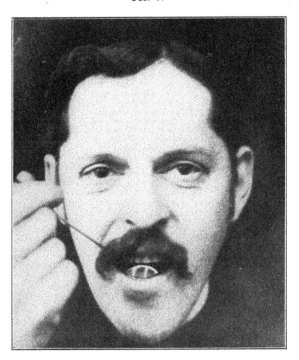

Illustrating the use of Dr. Tousey's fluoroscope in X-ray examination of the teeth.

disappearance of the neuralgia, although, as you know, there have been a great many cold and wet days since that time.

Now examine the specimen of radium, which, as you see, I keep in a small safe purchased for the purpose—the idea being not that I am so much afraid of losing it, as to prevent the radiation from this substance saturating everything in the room and interfering with the X-ray photography, which is so essential a part of my work. The radium, as you see, is a white powder about one-tenth gramme in amount, and its radial activity is twenty thousand times that of uranium. Now, if we turn out the light entirely, we see a faint glow, and holding a piece of Willemite near this tube, the Willemite is lighted up quite distinctly. A diamond, which I borrow from one of the gentlemen, is also lighted up. The other day a Spanish doctor from Porto Rico was here, and we exposed his diamond to these rays for such a long time that it became quite radio-active itself, and for the balance of the afternoon, instead of looking at the bones in his hand through the fluoroscope, I caught him every once in a while looking down at this sparkler on his finger, which was glowing in the darkness.

This electric vibrator which I show you now is a very essential part of the treatment for the uric acid condition upon which so many of these cases depend. It is applied over the abdomen and up and down the spine, and acts in a certain way like massage; but the vibrations are very, very rapid, and stimulate the action of the liver, intestines, stomach, and all spinal centres. I find it of the greatest service as an adjunct to high-frequency currents in the treatment of rheumatism, sciatica, and neuralgia, and in the treatment of obesity and of sluggish portal circulation, which come to so many people after middle life if they are prosperous and have heavy dinners and comparatively little exercise. Such ladies have the pleasurable experience of going to the expense of buying new corsets after taking in the old ones about two inches; and even gentlemen often take this treatment for the improvement in their figures and the very marked improvement in their condition of physical health.

Now we will take this X-ray picture, the patient being a young lady about twenty-three years old, with two temporary teeth (bicuspids) in the upper jaw and no evidence of permanent teeth, the question naturally being whether the permanent teeth are present and ready to make their appearance if these temporary teeth were to be extracted. The X-ray picture which we take is developed right here before you without requiring the use of a dark room, and shows no sign of permanent teeth. It shows that the roots of these permanent teeth are comparatively short, absorption having taken place very much as if the permanent teeth were present to take their place. Naturally, our advice to our friend, Dr. Green, is to preserve these primary teeth as long as possible.

Another patient shown now by Dr. Green is a woman about thirty-five, with pyorrhœa of the lower incisors, who shows marked improvement since the X-ray was begun at St. Bartholomew's clinic a few days ago. We will now treat this case with my special X-ray tube, applying the light directly to the affected gums for about three minutes, and this will be used twice a week.

BIBLIOGRAPHY.

Harlan, A. W. Dental Hints, January, 1904 (reviewed from Items of Interest).

Parker, C. H. Dental Cosmos, December, 1903.

Ames, W. V. B. Dental Cosmos, May, 1903.

Grieves, C. J. Dental Cosmos, January, 1904.

Cook, Geo. W. Dental Digest, December, 1903.

Newell, E. B. Dental Digest, May, 1903.

Hickey, P. M. Dental Digest, May, 1903.

Guy, Wm. Dental Record (London), 1903, p. 162.

Bödecker, C. W. Dental Review, 1903, p. 110.

Schwartz. Montpel. Méd., 1903, p. 494.

Choteau. Dictionaire Dentaire.

Ames. Dental Cosmos, 1903, p. 355.

Rhein. Dental Cosmos, 1903, p. 369.

Robin. Journ. dè Méd. de Paris, 1903, p. 135.

Custer. INTERNATIONAL DENTAL JOURNAL, 1903, p. 247.

Römer. Schweizer Vierteljahrschr. für Zahnheilk.

Achorn. Dental Cosmos, 1903, p. 189.

Peacock. Dental Record, 1903, p. 123.

Besten. Deutsche Monatschr. für Zahnheilk., 1902, p. 581.

Weil, C. Pathologie d. Zähne, 1903.

Odontologie, Paris, 1903, p. 365.

Schwartz. Archiv. d'Elec. Méd., 1903, p. 611.

Suye. Odontologie, Paris, 1903, p. 201.

V. Wolrozynickie. Wiener med. Wochenschr., 1903, p. 1245.

Talbot. Dental Summary, 1903, p. 538.

Logan. Brit. Dental Soc. Tr., 1903, p. 546.

Stewart. Memphis Med. Monthly, 1903, p. 345.

Dental Annual, 1903.

A REPLY TO DR. RHEIN'S ANSWER.

BY E. K. WEDELSTAEDT, ST. PAUL, MINN.

I HAVE read the "Answer" of Dr. Rhein, which appeared in the March number of this journal, also his remarks, which appear in the *Dental Cosmos* for April.

As was stated in my discussion, when a man of the doctor's standing will make changes in his methods, there is hope for others. After comparing the terms which he uses in his essay with those he is quoted as using in the *Dental Cosmos,* I feel, if nothing is gained otherwise, that the educational value of the discussion of his ideas is productive of great good. Dr. Rhein is to be congratulated for placing to one side the use of ambiguous terms and using in their place definite terms. With this example before us, there is a chance that the use of such terms as "floor of the cavity," "putting in fillings in the mouth," "cavities between the teeth," "anterior," "posterior," "canine," etc., etc., will soon disappear from print and exact terms be used.

There is so much to be discussed, and so little time mine in which to formulate ideas, that I am compelled to write most hastily. Let the reader understand what is meant by the use of the two terms, cohesive or annealed gold, and soft or unannealed gold. By cohesive gold is meant gold which is annealed just prior to being placed in the cavity. By soft gold is meant gold which is not annealed prior to being placed in the cavity. What is printed on the book in which the gold comes from the dental depot makes no difference. In using these terms in this way, there cannot be any "soft cohesive" gold.

An examination of a section of a tooth which has had a cavity in the proximo-occlusal surface filled with gold, anchoring the gold in cement, which has been "plastered over the floor of the gingival seat" prior to placing the gold, will show a layer of cement between the tooth and the gold. Has not the doctor become somewhat mixed in the use of terms? It is a very difficult matter for me to believe the statement as it appears before me in print. If Dr. Rhein means what he says, then I have no time at my disposal to spend in discussing any such unscientific method.

It is alleged in the "Answer" that a certain gold filling condensed with the electric mallet had a specific gravity of 19.87.

The usual specific gravity which is accredited cast gold is 19.3. Higher specific gravities, such as 19.42 for hammered gold, have been obtained. A specific gravity of 19.3 for pure gold has, however, been accepted by all scientists. When, therefore, it is alleged that a specific gravity of 19.87 has been obtained, and that by using an electric mallet for the purpose of condensing the gold to a certain filling, all thinking men are compelled to ask, first, will the doctor please send the filling to another chemist and obtain a certificate from him regarding the specific gravity? Secondly, if he is unwilling to do this, will he not ask his chemist to make another specific gravity after first balancing his scales? It is an easy matter to obtain a specific gravity, but very often errors creep in.

Some time ago a man, who for twenty years had used the electric mallet, made some fillings for me in the steel cavity block, using a No. 3 Webb plugger in his mallet for condensing the gold. The gold used was Williams's No. 4 cohesive foil. A sheet of foil was divided into thirty-two equal pieces, and each piece rolled into a loose pellet. Each piece of gold was annealed just prior to being placed into the cavity. Not less than thirty-five seconds of malleting was given any of the pieces of gold, and so many pieces received seventy-five seconds that I was first inclined to adopt the last-named figure as the average. A number of specific gravities were made by two different persons, and but ten specific gravities could be obtained.

Some reference has been made to the exhibit of fillings which can be found on pages 749 and 750 of the *Dental Cosmos* for 1895. The operator who made fillings Nos. 41, 42, and 43 has used the electric mallet for twenty-two years, and he informs me that he knows how to use it also. I am conversant with the manner as well as the method used in making these fillings. Anybody who is interested in this subject can make a comparison of the different specific gravities in the exhibit and draw his own conclusions. It is not necessary for me to say anything regarding the differences existing between the different specific gravities. They tell their own story. I am, however, very sorry to say that there seems to be a very great difference between 10.7 and 19.87, or even between 13.2 and 19.87.

Others are now beginning to discuss our expressed views. They have said something about the use of cohesive and soft gold, as well as polished enamel margins. This is about the place that calls for some plain English. I do not care to give expression to thoughts which but few will believe, notwithstanding the fact that they may be but too true. But if the issue is forced upon me, it is an easy matter to say what is necessary. Altogether too many men become possessed with ideas, and too often it is imagined that these ideas are facts. Too often when we come to simmer down many of these ideas, we find that they are based upon the veriest suppositions. We have made many contentions regarding them, and when we find that they are worthless, how many men have the moral courage to go into print and acknowledge the error? Well, not very many. There are many men in our profession who imagine that they are making water-tight margins with cohesive gold against polished or even planed enamel margins. I do not care to enter into a lengthy discussion regarding any man's ability to do this, and I wish to say right here that unless I had been perfectly aware of what I was writing about I should not have said what I did about polished enamel margins and the use of adhesive gold. For the past thirteen years I have been making a careful study of this subject, and I have also spent much time in observing the methods employed by other operators while packing cohesive gold. This is neither the time nor the place to discuss the value of cohesive or soft gold, for every man of any knowledge in our profession knows how valuable both these materials are in their proper place. The quickest way for the reader to satisfy himself regarding the relative value of using cohesive and soft foils is to obtain two glass tubes, three millimetres in diameter. These glass tubes can be cemented into a block of wood in such a manner that the cavity in the glass tube will be about two and one-half or three millimetres deep. These two glass tubes can be filled, one with cohesive and the other with soft gold. After the fillings have been made, they can be removed from the wood, examined, and thereafter tested in aniline. An examination of the fillings prior to their being placed in aniline will tell a far better story of the relative value of the different golds used than any words of mine. In the aniline test it will be found that both fillings leak. If there is a desire on the part of the experimenter to test his ability for making water-tight margins with cohesive gold, let him grind the inside of one of the glass tubes with a coarse stone, fill it with cohesive gold, remove it from the block,

and test it in aniline. A number of the members of the Black Club
have made this experiment, and have made non-leakable fillings.
No man has, however, ever succeeded in adapting cohesive gold
against the polished surfaces of glass tubes and made a non-leakable filling. (See page 955, *Dental Cosmos,* 1891.) But cohesive
gold has been packed against the roughened surfaces of glass tubes,
and water-tight fillings have been made. I merely give the results
of my own experiments, and leave it for the reader to draw his
own conclusions regarding the ability of any man to pack cohesive
gold against differently prepared enamel margins.

After making about so many experiments with gold, a man
begins to have a certain respect for cohesive gold which he did
not imagine it was possible for mortal to have. It may be an easy
matter to handle cohesive gold, but I am free to confess that the
more of it I use, the greater is my respect for it and the more
dissatisfied I become with myself, my operations, and the gold.
And in conversation with others who have also made laboratory
experiments, studied filled extracted teeth, and who know much
more than I shall ever know, I find that they give expression to
similar opinions, which are based upon the results of experimental research, observation, and a study of the gold itself. Where
a man says that it is an easy matter to make tight margins with
cohesive gold, I am quickly made aware that that man has much
more to learn than he knows of, for had he any knowledge of the
action of cohesive gold under the plugger-point he would be more
careful in his statements. Where men say that they can do this,
that, and the other thing with cohesive gold, I merely wish to
observe their methods while operating. Let me illustrate what I
mean. Recently, while at a public clinic, a man came to me and
said, " Come across the room with me, for I wish you to see the
best operator in this country pack gold." I accompanied the young
man as was requested. When we reached the operator's chair he
had his back turned to us and was just placing a mat of gold to
his partly completed operation. It was only necessary to observe
the methods which he employed in condensing the piece of gold
which he had just placed to his filling to prove that the man did
not have the remotest idea of handling his gold. He displayed a
total lack of knowledge regarding the important part of employing lines of force and principles of instrumentation. He was in
total ignorance of any knowledge pertaining to these subjects. I

observed the man place his second mat of gold, and thought, here is a chance to do some real charity work. Before, however, I had a chance to say anything to him, he turned and said to me, " How do you like it? Is it not fine? There is no man in this country my equal when it comes to 'putting in' gold." I wisely held my peace; silence is often golden. Perhaps such might have been the case in this discussion, and yet the individual *per se* is of little importance, but the advance and progress of the men in the dental profession is all important. Whether it is possible for Dr. Rhein to have me look at his methods from his stand-point, or whether I be able to have him look at things from my point of view, makes little difference; but it is of greatest value to us all if some of the readers of these words become sufficiently interested to make the experiments to which attention has been called.

It makes very little difference to the seeker of truth what either Dr. Rhein or I say. Two men with such widely diverse views can never convince each other, so it remains then for the reader to take the best out of what has been written, make the experiments, and judge for himself. Discussions of any subject should be the means of assisting others to get a better hold on the truth, which should enable them to be of greater use to humanity by placing the truth in use. Personalities, ridiculing the expressed views of others, etc., are displays of weakness, and have no place in a discussion of scientific subjects. Readers of dental periodicals wish the salient features brought out, and in any discussion all that is necessary is an expression of opinion which should be the means of assisting others towards having a better understanding of the essentials. If the reader of these words will but make the experiments to which attention has been called, he can ascertain for himself all that is necessary.

There has been a discussion in the " Answer" of the electric mallet. If we believe in the theory that it is necessary to use certain lines of force in packing gold, then the electric mallet has but a limited use. (As cavities in the proximo-occlusal surfaces of molars and bicuspids have been dealt with, my discussion will be confined to dealing with the cavities spoken of.) The electric mallet can only be used for packing gold in cavities in the mesial surfaces, with here and there a cavity in the distal surface. The cavities are opened from the occlusal surface, and direct access can thus be obtained and correct lines of force used in packing the gold. Where the cavity is situated in the distal surface of molars, and more especially lower bicuspids, the electric mallet is absolutely useless, provided correct lines of force are to be used. Reverse instruments are, however, absolutely necessary if the operator desires to use correct lines of force, which must be used, provided watertight fillings are to be made. Nor is this all. The condensing power of the electric mallet is so slight that it can readily be called a mere surface condenser. It has no value as a condensing instrument *per se.* To prove this assertion take a piece of smooth lead or a piece of smooth wood. With a No. 3 Webb plugger in the electric mallet, make a row of indentations across one end of the lead or board. Remove the plugger from the mallet and make a row of indentations by using the hand-mallet on the end of the plugger. Another row of indentations can be made by using hand-pressure. If a comparison with the power of an automatic mallet is desired, place the same sized plugger in it and make a row of indentations. Anybody making this experiment will be in a position to know whether or not there is any truth in my allegation that the electric mallet is merely fit for surface condensation. (See remarks made by Dr. Perry, on page 221, *Dental Cosmos,* 1878.) Those interested should make this experiment, for to comprehend we must first apprehend, and this apprehension leads to our having an understanding of the subject. After the experiment has been made, we can better comprehend the experiments of Dr. Black (see pages 741–746, *Dental Cosmos,* 1895), and are capable of better understanding the efforts which he displayed in obtaining a specific gravity of 19.42. If it was necessary for him to use the methods which he employed for this purpose to obtain any such result, how is it possible to condense gold with an electric mallet, that condenses the surface only, to obtain a specific gravity of 19.87? I could with equal truth say, I took four ounces of gold and refined it four times. Thereafter I took it to Dr. Lehnen, a well-known chemist of this city, who assured me that it was 27-carat fine. Should such a thing happen to me, I should at once question the sanity of Dr. Lehnen and in future consult with a different chemist. I should not publish Dr. Lehnen's statement and ask the men in the dental profession, " Am I too presumptuous in claiming that gold" of greater purity than 24-carat can be obtained?

Here are four facts with which all thinking dentists are conversant:

1. Where cohesive gold fillings have a specific gravity of 17 or 18 we all know what a difficult matter it is to cut into them for the purpose of anchoring a proximating filling. A bur will slip and slide and will not " bite." A drill must be used to enter the filling.

2. Every man with any experience knows that gold fillings condensed with the electric mallet are as easily entered with a bur as cutting so much putty. In his essay and in the answer to my discussion, Dr. Rhein speaks of using a bur on that portion of the filling previously placed and recommencing the packing of the gold on this freshened surface.

3. Since this " Answer" has been published every man I have asked has informed me that where he attempted to anchor one filling into another, he having made the original filling, he was compelled to start in a definite retention pit in the filling. I do not believe a union of the kind Dr. Rhein speaks of can be made if the gold is cohesive gold and of 18 specific gravity. Even if it could be made, the gold would be held together by interserration, and not molecule adhering to molecule.

4. It is a fact that gold fillings condensed with the electric mallet are always so odoriferous. Remove one of these fillings from the teeth, roll it between the thumb and the finger for an instant, and then smell your finger. This will tell its own story. In drilling into one of the fillings condensed with the electric mallet more than one patient has exclaimed, " My! Excuse me, but there is something rotten in Denmark." If such fillings had a specific gravity of 17 or 18, the different layers of gold would not be filled with the products of fermentation. This process goes on between the different layers of gold which have not been properly condensed. Later on it will be discovered that these ill-smelling fillings are filled with micro-organisms which materially interfere with the health of the individual in whose teeth such corruption exists.

It is not necessary to enlarge upon these four facts. There remains, then, but one thing to discuss, and that is the doctor's expressed views regarding the uselessness of definite knowledge. I am very sorry that Dr. Rhein said what he did about my statement of the size of the cavity in the lower left first bicuspid. The size of the cavity in two directions, the size of the gingival seat, as well as the size of the first three pieces of gold used, were all given. This was done for the reason that anybody who was interested and who had a Boley gauge, could make a similar operation and thus ascertain for himself whether or not the contention which I had made was correct. I try to be definite and to so place matters before the members of the profession that others can prove my results, provided there is any question regarding them. I must leave for others to judge whether or not this is the right way of doing things. In all kindness, however, I feel that it is preferable to go into detail and be exact, than to place into print under my name, " A cavity, a distal approximating occlusal cavity, in a molar." Over two-thirds of the discussions which take place on all topics are on account of men not being exact in their statements. If I am to judge from the contents of seven different dental journals which come to me each month, I can readily say that there is a constant increase in the ranks of those who are using more exact terms and who are following more definite methods. It is to be deplored that any man should be willing to go into print and acknowledge that he was opposed to definite knowledge. The use of the Boley gauge and a dentometer will increase as the value of definite knowledge is more greatly appreciated, Dr. Rhein's unfortunate remarks to the contrary notwithstanding.

I have a certain kind of respect for a man who will discuss scientific subjects from a scientific basis. I have too little time at my disposal to waste it in being personal and in ridiculing what I know nothing about. If I could not be foremost in assisting others to obtain definite knowledge, I should at least do the best that I could for them. And if I could not help others to raise the standard to a higher plane, I should not allow my name to stand at the head of an answer of the kind Dr. Rhein has sent to my discussion of his ideas.

(On account of the limited time at my disposal, I have been compelled to dictate this answer in greatest haste and at different times, therefore every apology is offered for the same.)

TEETH DURING PREGNANCY.[1]

BY THOMAS J. GIBLIN, D.M.D., BOSTON, MASS.

You are to have an opportunity later in the evening to learn more about the very interesting subject of Orthodontia from one who is not always with you. That you may not be held too long in suspense I shall make my paper brief and touch upon only a few of the topics that my subject suggests.

Some eighteen years ago a woman, accompanied by her husband, visited my office. She was suffering intensely from periodontitis about an upper bicuspid. The husband told me his wife was pregnant about seven months, which was obvious. It was her intention, as soon as she was able, to have her upper teeth removed for the purpose of inserting an artificial denture, but just at that time she desired to have the troublesome tooth extracted. Her physician had told her to have it done if her dentist considered it would be right. As had been my practice for a few years previously, I administered gas and removed the tooth. Some time after the husband called at my office and in a disagreeable manner said, "Well, what are you going to do about my wife's illness?" For the first time I learned that his wife had had a miscarriage, was attended by several physicians and two nurses, and had passed through a very severe and critical experience. I was a young man, about to be married, and with much at stake, and the picture I conjured of law-suits, damages, and deterrent advertising was horrible. I insisted that I had used due care and had followed the usual practice in what I had done; that I was not responsible for his wife's illness, and consequently would not be responsible for the expense attending it.

I maintained that the remedies she had used and the long suffering she had endured previous to my attendance would account for the result. However, rather than at that time face the disagreeable alternative of the law-court, through my attorney I compromised with him and settled the case.

About two months ago I filled with gold a labial cavity in a lower cuspid for a young woman. The excavation was difficult, the tooth very sensitive, and the patient extremely nervous. She

---

[1] Read before the Harvard Odontological Society, May 26, 1904.

started at the appearance of the excavator or the bur. However, the filling was finally inserted, another appointment was made for further work, and the patient was dismissed. The subsequent appointment was not kept. After a few weeks she called and informed me that she had been ill; that she had had a miscarriage, and had been critically ill. Her physician ascribed as the cause the dental operation of a few days previous. As I had no knowledge of her condition, which was only about ten weeks' pregnancy, I was not held responsible.

These reminiscences have prompted me to offer this caution to young men for pregnant women,—defer all but absolutely necessary operation until the patient is in a more favorable condition. Use soothing, palliative measures, temporary fillings, etc. I have asked several students from different colleges how they were instructed, and found that it was taught that pregnancy is not a valid objection to extraction when extraction is advisable.

I do not believe that specific rules are possible, either in medicine or dentistry, to deal with the intricate and varying problems, and I respectfully dissent from the inference that it makes no difference whether or not a woman is pregnant in performing dental operations. The intimate relation between mother and child should be borne in mind. Whatever of physical or mental character affecting the mother may also affect the child. Causes of miscarriage may be violence, idiosyncrasy, disease of general or local character, reflex influence, mental, moral, or nervous, whether upon the uterine contractions or indirectly through the circulation upon the fœtus. That dental operations upon pregnant women may be the exciting cause of miscarriage I am fully convinced, and I have made it my practice, when I am aware of such condition, to do only such work as will prevent or relieve pain, and to carefully avoid nervous shock.

Passing from this topic, let us for a few minutes consider another.

It is a generally accepted fact that the teeth during pregnancy are very often attacked by rapidly developing caries. It has often been my experience to have been startled by destruction that has gone on during a comparatively short time upon the teeth of some woman whom I had seen previous to and subsequent to pregnancy. I have no doubt that you have each one had similar experience.

How can it be accounted for, and what preventive measures may be suggested?

Not so very long ago it was taught that during the growth of the fœtus the mother was called on to supply through the circulation of the blood the necessary lime salts; if the ingesta failed in supply, the bones of the mother, through the process of absorption, were called on to supply the deficiency. Thus it was supposed that even the teeth were rendered soft and readily susceptible to decay. This theory has been shown to be erroneous, because the teeth are not supplied with any system of absorbents, whereby the lime salts can be abstracted.

Even the bones, which are supplied with lymphatics, give no evidence that absorption goes on during this period.

As a matter of fact, the teeth once formed are least liable, of all the tissues of the body, to undergo changes dependent upon nutrition. While the theory was in vogue we frequently recommended an increased phosphate diet, in the form of certain kinds of food which contained an abundance of lime and magnesium salts, and even in the administration of the hypophosphites. The result was that we so overfed the mother that many cases of parturition were made difficult by the advanced calcification of the fœtus.

The conclusion of empiricism—and most of the conclusions of medicine are empiric—is that the mother normally ingests sufficient phosphates for the necessary work of gestation.

It is much more rational to explain the ravages upon the teeth during pregnancy by directing our search and examination of the environment of the teeth during gestation. We are all convinced of the theory of caries as advanced by Miller,—lactic acid and bacteria, the lactic acid acting upon the tooth and, later, furnishing soil for the culture of bacteria.

I made a request of the house physician of one of our lying-in hospitals here in Boston to make certain tests for me. He reported to me yesterday that he examined the mouths of twenty pregnant women, of from five to nine months, and in every case found the saliva strongly acid, in both the morning and evening tests.

Here we have ready complete and sufficient explanation of the cause of rapid caries during pregnancy. If we add to this cause the action of the acid of the stomach following the "morning sickness" and the frequent neglect of the usual care of teeth by

women in this condition, we no longer wonder at the destruction
we are so often called upon to repair.

If you agree with me in the conclusion at which I have arrived,
—that during pregnancy the environment of the teeth is dangerous
to the integrity of that organ,—how shall we best prevent the
harm?

By instructing those patients where possible that exceptional
care must be exercised during that period, and in particular calling the attention of a physician, friend, or patient to the facts I
have laid before you, and urge him to prescribe to every pregnant
woman an alkaline mouth-wash as a *sine qua non.*

DR. MEYER L. RHEIN'S TECHNIQUE.

BY DR. CHARLES SOUTHWELL, MILWAUKEE, WIS.

Dickens, in speaking of Daniel Doyce, said, " Showed the whole thing
as if the Divine artificer had made it and he happened to find it. So
modest was he about it, such a pleasant touch of respect mingled with
his quiet admiration of it and so calmly convinced that it was established
on irrefragible laws."

DR. MEYER L. RHEIN, of New York City, read a paper entitled
" The Technique of Approximal Restorations with Gold in Posterior Teeth," before the Academy of Stomatology, in Philadelphia, in February, 1903. The paper appears in the INTERNA-
TIONAL DENTAL JOURNAL, September, 1903, in which number may
also be found an extended discussion at page 711. A *résumé* by
Dr. Wedelstaedt may be found on page 25 in the January, 1904,
number of the same journal. Dr. Rhein's reply to Dr. Wedelstaedt may be found in the March, 1904, number.

When an essayist appears before the Academy of Stomatology
of Philadelphia, a body of gentlemen composed of professors, clinical teachers, and accredited experts, it is to be presumed that his
effort will approach the scientific, and that any new data or expedient offered the subject under consideration will have sufficient
dignity to warrant an introduction, and furthermore that the dic-
tion be clear in construction and chosen with a distinct desire to
be instructive and deferential in view of the attainments of his
audience.

To one critically inclined a close examination of Dr. Rhein's paper reveals marked ability in the construction of a very presentable garment out of old material and a distinct effort of the writer to interject inconsequent somethings, all of which when published in dental journals pictures Dr. Rhein as a sizar of operative dentistry, and places before the inexperienced teachings that are unavailing if not mischievous. Much if not all of the commendable matter in his paper may be safely said to have been covered by others in the past.

Taking up the components of his paper *seriatim,* attention is directed to the title, The Technique, etc. He might have said "a history of," or "some suggestions in," or "a later-day consideration of," and one may be excused in noting the modesty.

On page 654 he directs that the cervical wall (meaning foundation or floor) be "made perfectly flat, in order to form a stable foundation for the filling." Dr. Rhein's plethora of the theoretical compelled him to say perfectly flat when he meant reasonably flat. He immediately follows this with the statement that any deviation from such an ideal lessens the ability of the filling to withstand the strain of usage. Viewed from a practical standpoint this is theoretical rot, in the estimation of the writer, for the suggested change from a "natural rounded outline of the cervical margin, especially at the angles," is obviously for extension only. Certainly not for stability, for it should be obvious that a V-shaped filling, broad or wide, and with bevelled margins at the masticating surface, may end in an edge at the cervical margin at the centre of the interspace, and be as enduring, so far as stress is concerned, as any other filling, if usual undercuts and good condensation be had. If it fails, it will be from a recurrence of decay on one or both sides of the cervical end of the V. This clearly points to extension for prevention only. Should a filling of the character referred to by Dr. Rhein need a flat floor for stability (and it is not admitted), that requirement may in part be better provided by bevelling the coronal or masticating ends of the walls, a procedure (mentioned by Dr. Rhein) that has been audited for many years.

He argues against undercuts, and, referring to Fig. 1, states that "the real anchorage seat of all fillings of this nature depends on the dovetailed occlusal step cut at right angles into the occlusal surface," following this with directions for the cutting of a non-carious occlusal surface. Can any exigency in the preparation of approximal cavities justify the mutilation of a non-carious fissure in a bicuspid to the degree necessary to form " the real anchorage"? And yet he clearly directs this to be done. If the fissure be not involved, the walls will accept a liberal undercut. If the fissures be involved, the step may be relied on for anchorage, but as no such distinction is made in his paper, it is reasonable to assume that he dispenses with required undercuts in the cavity proper, and, depending largely on the step, mutilates all innocent fissures. In a bicuspid this is malpractice, and in a molar inexcusable.

He decries undercuts, but advises dovetailing. All very pretty on paper or in pine, but so far as the weakening of the walls is concerned, wherein lies the difference? As to the forming of undercuts and dovetailing, the former may be undulating, following the lines outlined by caries, and are quickly made with a bur, while the latter dictates a straight wall in which the dovetail is laboriously and painfully made with edge tools.

It should be obvious to any one of extended experience that undercuts need not be deep enough to weaken the walls. Moderate undercuts, but little more than sufficient to keep the filling from rocking during the packing of the foil, will retain a perfectly packed filling of foil if mainly cohesive.

Passing some commendable matter, in which he directs the packing of the gold, we arrive at the injunction to wash the cavity " with a few drops of ten per cent. solution of formalin and then thoroughly dry." How profound! Does he imagine that any one in his audience or elsewhere, deciding that formalin be advisable, would use a teaspoonful or a hose? Dry it thoroughly, he says, quite as a kindergartner might say, after the tots are ready to be sent home, " Now, children, do not get your feet wet."

It is next directed that a small piece of one of the plastic forms of gold be placed on the electric annealer.

A small amount of oxyphosphate is now mixed to the consistency of thick cream, and an amount equal to the head of a pin is placed carefully *along* the inner half of the floor, being careful not to allow any of this small amount to remain on the margins. This caution to that audience!

The " very small piece" of plastic gold which has flocked all alone on the electric annealer, at Dr. Rhein's direction, is now to be remembered and " carefully laid in position over the cement."

A small round burnisher, which these gentlemen are directed to "keep thoroughly polished" (is there no limit?—no constitutional nerve paste?), is used to work the gold into the film of cement. Why not interject a direction about the oiling of the hand-piece? This cement suggestion as a starting base for the foil is so extremely puttering and unnecessary that it might better be omitted from a paper aiming to be scientific. It is this that I would characterize as an inconsequent something, for in years of practice equal to those of Dr. Rhein the necessity of its adoption has not even occurred to the writer. Its adoption by skilled operators is so improbable that one need be concerned only about its influence on the inexperienced, to whom the writer would say that it is far more expeditious, to put it mildly, having discreet undercuts in the floor and walls, to gather a mass of slightly annealed cylinders sufficient to cover the floor undercut liberally, and after locking the mass securely with hand-pressure to begin with the elected dynamic method.

In the time required for the hardening of the bit of cement to be of the conjectured aid every operator of ordinary ability with ordinary methods would have the filling well started, and many would have it one-third completed.

He sweetly, confidently, aye, benignly, next says, as if to some of second years, the cavity is now ready for the "strip of freshly annealed gold-foil" (tells these gentlemen how wide to cut it), which is malleted against the gold starting-point "cemented to the dental floor." If he has ever tried this on a flat cervical foundation devoid of undercut he has omitted to say how often it was found in the lap of the patient or on the floor.

At another point, in speaking of "a few moments for the small amount of cement to harden," he has the charming effrontery again, as if to a class of students, to direct his hearers to employ the time in cutting gold, yet fails to direct what the capable assistant, referred to in the next paragraph, is to do while the operator is cutting the gold.

He next says, "The filling is now brought in an even manner from the bottom upward, advancing no part of the gold beyond another part. This requisite evenness of surface is best accomplished by wiping the gold with a plugger, hammering away from *side to side,*" "ironing" (my italics). How scientifically clear. "Hammering away [like a nailer] from side to side," and yet "advancing no part of the gold beyond another part."

This " requisite evenness" of the upbuilding is denied, for the reason that it is unavailing, inconsequent, and unnecessarily laborious to the operator and taxing to the patient.

While positive solidity throughout may be permissible, it is not a requisite for good service, and I would go so far as to aver distinctly that in many instances homogeneous impacting of gold is ill-advised and excessive, and furthermore that the even building up of a filling is inexpedient.

A broad foot-plugger is absolutely necessary to expeditiously create a hard regular surface to an increasing contour, and advance work with round pluggers by hand or otherwise in the undercuts, filling them liberally, will enable an operator to pack three-fourths of the approximal gold with the foot-plugger suggested, thereby accomplishing a saving of half the time required by the procedure outlined by Dr. Rhein. (Fig. 1.)

A homogeneous packing of the foil as a requisite is denied. Having the undercuts well packed by hand, the body or interior of the filling may be condensed but little better than could be well accomplished by hand if followed by perfectly condensed margins and surfaces, and such a filling will endure just as well as though perfectly condensed throughout.

On page 661 he offers another choice remark, where he states, " In fact, the best results are generally attained where the lower third or half of the filling is inserted at one sitting and the operation completed at a later time." In the language of the lurid litterateur, words fail me in attempting to characterize this puerility.

In the succeeding paragraph it is directed that the " matrices be removed occasionally," to see if the filling is loose. He gives his procedure a deserving negative in that very direction, and I truly believe with him that, with no undercut whatever in the foundation and none in the walls, the filling should be under suspicion at all times. Why conceive, much less exploit, a procedure so unassuring when positive methods have been in practice so long that many operators cannot remember when they last tested a filling for insecurity during its upbuilding.

He next says, " Care must be taken that all overhanging bits of gold should be removed and the polishing done without *in any way* [my italics] defacing or marring the enamel margins." This is an injunction impossible to adopt. Any means for the reduction

FIG. 1.

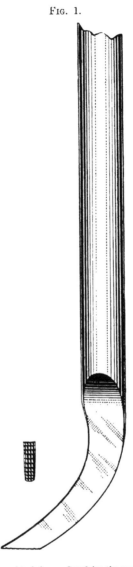

A cut of the plugger referred to is here offered for the reason that it is not to be found in catalogues or on sale. It is after one of a set received from Dr. Bonwill many years ago, and with four sizes of this one shape I pack *more* than half of the gold I use. Attention is directed to the serrated surface being at right angles to the shank, making the blow as direct and forceful as if the plugger was straight. Enlarged ten times the size.

of a rough surface of gold to a smoothness "resembling polished enamel" would affect the contiguous enamel, and it is impossible to reduce a filling to the directed degree of smoothness without "in any way defacing the enamel margins," no matter how much care is exercised. Care of the cervical enamel margins has been obligatory for so long that pointed cautionary reference to it in a paper to-day to an audience of past masters is not excessively deferential.

A strip or disk or file has some unavoidable effect on the contiguous cervical enamel, and may only be met by including these surfaces in the polishing process. The contiguous cervical enamel usually more or less disintegrated should be jealously conserved, and it is to be regretted that the essayist did not direct how it may be done without it "in any way defacing or marring the enamel margins."

Speaking of "best results," especially in distal cavities, it is not only very frequently humane, effective, and considerate to adopt a limited base of standard alloy (voicing my preference), and, as it may be made quite smooth by almost any wiping means, it offers practical immunity in the polishing to the glaze overlying the more or less disintegrated contiguous cervical enamel.

On page 662, in speaking of the finishing of this portion of the filling, he suggests that the day's work "stop at that point." Were this to be taken literally, one might inquire where the next "day's work" ceased. In the same paragraph he suggests (or audits) that the insertion of the filling be divided into several short sittings. The next bit of choice teaching is the frequent changing of the matrices to thinner ones, "until the very thinnest is used at the place mapped out for the marble-like contact points." These and the cement suggestion are of the same order. We are told that cement "sets in a few moments," that "best results are generally attained" by packing a part of the filling one day and completing it another, or *others* (dentistry as a pastime); that the matrix is to be removed occasionally (what joy!), to see if the filling is loose (what confidence!), and replaced with thinner ones, as if this were the only way or even an acceptable way of restoring contour. And yet, Dr. Rhein, in his reply to Dr. Wedelstaedt, says "that it becomes a difficult matter to reply to the same and preserve the temperate demeanor, which is only becoming to scientific discussion," implying thereby that he, Dr. Rhein, was and continues to be scientific.

The amount of time required to follow the technique urged by Dr. Rhein demands a clientele composed exclusively of the wealthy, enduring, and appreciative. I am free to urge that many patients have not these requisites sufficient to warrant, or the discrimination to appreciate, severely correct methods. Yielding to a maudlinity of theory, essayists so often seem unable to remember the realities of every-day practice, urging procedures that are decidedly inconsiderate of the consideration due the average patient.

By coupling vain theories with want of an ardor, a combination is created that is decidedly negative in many instances, and who can say how many teeth are lost or curtailed in usefulness because the discouraged patient, going to the other extreme, employs " Doctor Pusil," or neglects the dentist altogether. The suggestions by Dr. Rhein of two or more sittings offers no remedy in lessening the stress unless the patient possesses means; and. furthermore, the adjustment of the dam, clamps, etc., two or more times would indicate an amount of patience and endurance sufficient unto the stress of a restoration of any size at one sitting, except possibly in very rare instances. Perfect indication for two or more sittings for a single restoration are too rare to warrant the teaching that, " In fact, the best results are generally attained where the lower third or half is inserted at one sitting and the operation completed at a later time."

Ideal restorations are indicated perfectly only when the patient offers the usual combination of means, endurance, and discriminative appreciation, and in the degree that these favoring conditions are absent, a discreet operator lessens the amount of theory. With rare exceptions the capable operators throughout our profession do not and should not advise restorations that are taxing in every respect at all times, and what they do perform under the circumstances is in no wise culpable. The operator is not called upon, nor can he afford an extra hour of unremunerated finesse, any more than many patients are in a position to audit it financially or otherwise. Absolute homogeneity of impact in the average case is as unwise as unnecessary. Pursuing the subject to a greater attenuation, is it not reasonable to inquire what becomes of those cavities in which it is impossible to use a dynamic method throughout, wherein, as a result of the necessity of hand-pressure, a portion of the filling is not homogeneous to the degree pictured by Dr. Rhein? All operators of experience know that such a filling with condensed margins and surfaces is destined to last as long as one perfectly condensed throughout. In fact, we all audit imperfect condensation in many of the gold fillings we insert in daily practice, and if very fair condensation be audited at this point and at that because perfect condensation is denied, why not audit it for the major portion of the heart of the filling. Who can say but that it was this almost fanatical adherence to an ideal that contributed largely to the lamentable and untimely death of Dr. Marshall H. Webb, whose operations cannot be too highly extolled. I am personally indebted to him, and at the time of his death there were those in a memorial session of the Wisconsin State Dental Society who were moved to tears.

There can be no objection to ideally perfect condensation throughout, other than the unnecessary tax on the patient and operator, but as a matter of daily practice, if the comfort and well-being of the patient and operator are of any moment, I raise my voice against perfervid zeal as being ill-advised and intemperate.

To sum up Dr. Rhein's paper frankly, I am willing to believe that it is not his habit nor the habit of any good operator to mutilate a non-carious fissure, especially in a bicuspid, and, if that be the case, why mention a teaching so mischievous. Again I am willing to believe that he very rarely adopts the cement suggestion, and, if that be the case, why parade a teaching so puttering and unavailing?

As to his paper being lacking in deference, I hardly think that what I have said and implied needs modification.

THE COLLECTION OF BILLS.[1]

BY LESLIE BARNES BOUTWELL, D.M.D.

MR. PRESIDENT AND FELLOW-MEMBERS OF THE HARVARD ODONTOLOGICAL SOCIETY,—Many years ago, at a district school which I attended as a small boy, there was an occasional morning set apart for declamation, or " speaking pieces," as we used to term it,

---

[1] Read before the Harvard Odontological Society, April 28, 1904.

and the favorite effort of the average badly scared youngster used
to be a choice excerpt which began thus :

> "You'd scarce expect one of my age
> To speak in public on the stage."

I will spare you the description of how the knees would knock
together, the cold sweat stand out upon the body, and the tongue
and brain refuse their co-ordinate labor as the declaimer faced
the combined stare of schoolmates, friends, relatives, and the occasional committeeman, and merely call your attention to the paral-
lelism of the present case and that of the youngster alluded to.
You will probably discover the analogy for yourselves as this effort
continues.

It is useless to attempt to give you gentlemen any information from a dental point of view, and the choice of a subject is
a most serious one to the poor unfortunate drawn as an essayist ;
and any essay in that direction would hardly instruct, though it
probably would amuse you. When you go back mentally to that
time in your early practice that you faced your first problem, in,
for instance, trying to combat some carefully cherished fallacy in
a patient, real or prospective, and endeavoring to make him believe that a perfect-fitting artistic denture cannot be made for
five dollars, or a large contour gold filling inserted at the advertised price of one dollar, even though you carefully explain that
the aforesaid attractive advertisement was not fathered by you,—
in such cases they have a sincere belief in the old adage, "What
man has done, man can do,"—such problems fade into insignifi-
cance beside the momentous one of what to talk to you about.

I have therefore chosen for a subject one that will at least interest you, and one on which from many years of business experience
I can speak with some authority, and that is, the collection of bills,
and in combining enough of business principles with our profession to render that collection easier and more systematic, the latter
being, in my opinion, the great desideratum ; and I might preface
my few remarks with a text from the "good book" as follows:
"And he took him by the throat, saying, Pay me that thou owest."
Do not be alarmed because I have begun with a text. This
sermon will hardly go beyond "Firstly, my brethren." Probably
the creditor in the foregoing was a dentist who had been unfortunate enough to do two hundred pence worth of work for one

hundred, and after much unsuccessful dunning was endeavoring
to forcibly collect his little bill, and although in the present civilized age we can scarcely go to the extent of bodily punishment
for delinquent debtors, yet there is so little change in human nature
in 1900 years, that we sympathize with the man of old who resorted
to extreme measures in collecting from a particularly exasperating
case. You who have threshed out your wheat, and have gathered the
kernels of experience from years of practice, have also, to a greater
or less extent, so sifted that practice that you have comparatively
little trouble in collecting; but to us who are starting—particularly those of us who have a fairly large transient practice—it
is a serious question when, and when not, to give credit, and when
credit is given and abused more or less, how far are we justified
in pushing our claims?

From a twenty years' experience as credit man in commercial
life, I incline to the radical course of "taking them by the throat"
and collecting anyway—peaceably if possible, forcibly if necessary; and as to the various methods, steps, and gradations of
appeal to the debtor before invoking the aid of the law, each professional man has his choice, but it is all a means to an end, as
the debtor who requires urging to settle is truly an "absent-
minded beggar," and, therefore, the burden of our song to him
should be insistently, "pay—pay—pay." I believe that in ninety-
nine cases out of a hundred the patient is honest and means to
pay. The one-hundredth one must be dealt with rigorously, and
usually a mild pacific course, such as intimating ever so slightly
that the account will be placed in a lawyer's hands for collection
if not paid before a certain time, is vastly insufficient. I find
that a statement to the effect that the poor debtors' court will be
the ultimate result if payment is not forthcoming at once usually
makes an impression and brings about a state of mental dis-
quietude, which ceases only when the bill is paid. You have given
of your best, time, material, and, greatest of all, nervous energy,
and your charge should be paid gratefully, but if after repeated
duns payment is not made, then make up your mind that you would
lose the patient anyway, and take such action as will secure the
bill, lest eventually you lose both.

Of course, such cases are rare, happily, but they are like the
poor, "always with us," and unfortunately there is more joy over
collecting one such bill than over those of "ninety and nine just

men." It is a problem you are constantly called upon to decide, and while we are urged to err if necessary upon the side of mercy, yet why should we be incessantly asked to extend mercy to those who have no mercy upon us,—the very ones, usually, who have taxed our nervous energy the most. I believe that there is a lack of simple business principle in most professional men, particularly in sending out bills and statements, regularly and impartially, to all patients, and which lack results in much monetary loss.

The condition of mind which enables a debtor to disregard the receipt of two or more bills will usually enable him to sleep peacefully, even though he eventually does not pay the bill at all, and for such cases the cure is a sharp, harsh remedy analogous to the surgeon's knife, rather than the bloodless method; and then again, if financial care is not possible, excision is the most conducive to your future comfort, as well as a lesson to the delinquent not to assume financial obligations too easily. It might be laid down as a cardinal principle, that a man who is offended at receiving a bill is not a desirable addition to one's list of patients.

You and I receive bills the first of the month (not often, we will hope), and esttle them as promptly. Why, then, should we give more credit than we ask? Understand me—it is the debtor who makes no response at all to bills, statements, and letters that I refer to; patients that eventually pay in full, even though but a little at a time, are desirable ones to most of us. It is the conscienceless one who remains silent to all appeals, after he has got his work finished with you, at whom these strictures are directed. To such I personally show not a particle of consideration, and have collected my bill in all cases of the kind (where the debtor has not defaulted) by carrying them to court, even though it cost me nearly the whole amount of the bill, as there are few who care to have the stigma of such a conclusion fixed upon them.

Among all the problems outside the actual practice of dentistry, but within its province, I regard collection of bills as the one requiring the most tact, persistency, and knowledge of human nature. It also necessitates the most delicate " touch" known to mankind,— that which touches the pocket-book.

Several members of our profession have said, apropos to following up deliquent debtors closely, that they did not care to go too far, for fear of incurring the ill-will of the debtor, and the consequent loss of not only his patronage, but the loss of the persons who might be influenced by his recommendation as future patients.

I argue that a man who is so lacking in common honesty that he will not pay his bills, is also dead to any generous feeling that he will hardly go out of his way to influence new patients to come to us, and the chances are that those he did recommend would be of the same stamp as himself.

There is no question but that we all wish to collect our bills promptly, but I find many dentists who, after sending a few statements and meeting no response, cease to urge payment, and my effort here to-night is to suggest the same persistency applied to such cases as would be given to a difficult case in office practice. Each instance may require a different method of procedure,—one case may be necessary to be dealt with severely, and the next merely necessitate a call, to bring about a settlement.

In a few cases I have found that frequent visits by a youthful collector armed with the bill, and sent to the man's place of business with instructions to present it and ask for payment audibly enough so that by-standers may hear, is wonderfully effective as a last resort. I do not advocate extreme measures. I do, however, advise frequent calls, as I find that method successful when all sorts of written appeals fail. At least, that is my experience. The proportion of beats is small, I am glad to say, for out of the first five hundred names in my own practice I find only ten uncollectible bills, and of those the largest was under twenty dollars. The number, however, would have been larger but for a general adherence to the importance of persistent dunning.

Reviews of Dental Literature.

OXYGENATED DENTIFRICES. NEW CALCIUM AND OXYGEN COMPOUND INTRODUCED INTO DENTISTRY.—At a meeting of the New York Odontological Society, held at the Academy of Medicine, 17 West Forty-third Street, New York, on Tuesday evening, April 19, Eustace H. Gane, of New York, the secretary of the Scientific Section of the American Pharmaceutical Association, gave a demonstration of the properties and dental applications of some new oxygen compounds.

Mr. Gane pointed out that considerable attention was being devoted, by chemists and physicians, to the problem of manufacturing substances which would readily part with oxygen, on account of the value of this element in its nascent state as a harmless germicide and antiseptic. The only compound hitherto available was hydrogen dioxide, which could be prepared only in the form of dilute solutions. Quite recently the ingenuity of American chemists had resulted in the discovery of several new compounds, which were available both for the dentist's and the physician's use. Thanks, too, to the development of the electric industries at Niagara, it was now possible to prepare these on a commercial scale at a reasonable cost. There were two of these oxygen compounds in particular which promised to be of great value to the dentist. These were the sodium and oxygen compound, which had been called "natrozone," and the calcium and oxygen compound, which was called "calox."

Mr. Gane showed a number of interesting experiments to illustrate the ease with which these compounds gave up oxygen. The most luminous one was the gentle heating in a glass tube of some iron filings with the calcium compound, when the oxygen united so rapidly with the iron as to raise the latter to a white heat.

The sodium and oxygen compound would bleach teeth discolored by age, decay, or even smoking, restoring them to their pristine whiteness without destroying the pulp, for, while oxygen was death to germs and destroyed dead organic matter, it was without action on healthy cells or tissues.

The calcium and oxygen compound would make an excellent tooth-powder, and, the speaker said, if the public could be induced to use such a preparation, which would not only clean the teeth, but sterilize the mouth, it was not too much to say that most of them would be saved from the terrors of the dental chair.

The paper was discussed by Dr. D. W. Ward, Professor of Chemistry at the New York Dental School, and by T. J. Keenan, associate editor of the *American Druggist*.

Mr. Keenan said that, in his long experience as a pharmacist, he had seen the rise and fall of many a much-vaunted dentifrice compound. Pharmacists had dentists to thank for many a new and wonderful mixture, each succeeding one of which was to be the acme of perfection, as regards antiseptic and detergent power. A simple compound of camphor and chalk, in the proportion of one part of the former to three of the latter, long held sway, but the use of some detergent, such as soap or alkali, later came to be considered indispensable, and some awful messes resulted in consequence. Charcoal was popular for a time on account of its supposed deodorant property, but it is not much used nowadays, as much because it caused discoloration by getting between the gums and the teeth as from a growing scepticism regarding its antiseptic value.

The speaker said that pharmacists were indebted to the dental profession for many useful suggestions regarding the nature of desirable additions to tooth-powders, as well as regarding what should be left out. For example, it was not so long since pharmacists had learned that the use of gritty and abrasive substances, like pumice-stone and cuttlefish-bone, was highly objectionable, because of the abrading action which such substances exerted on the delicate enamel of the teeth.

Of late years the main effort in the formulation of dentifrice recipes had been directed to the bringing together of ingredients which would, upon application to the teeth and gums, produce a refreshing sense of coolness, combined, of course, with real antiseptic power. The acid dentifrice of the French Codex was, he said, a good example of this class of compounds, consisting, as it did, of a mixture of cream of tartar and sugar of milk highly flavored with oil of peppermint. One ingenious investigator had hit upon potassium chlorate as a valuable addition to tooth-powders, being doubtless impelled to its use by a knowledge of its well-known antiseptic properties, and possibly having a vague idea that it would part with its oxygen readily. The antiseptic action of potassium chlorate, when applied as a tooth-powder, was more or less chimerical, and powders of this kind never became really popular, for what the laity wanted in a tooth-powder was a combination of substances and flavors that would leave a pungent and slightly sweetish taste in the mouth.

Referring to Mr. Gane's application of the medicinal peroxides as dentifrice compounds, Mr. Keenan said that this clearly marked a new era in the history of dentistry. The discovery was more important, as a matter of fact, than the discovery of radium, for it was more practical. When calcium dioxide, applied as a dentifrice to the teeth and gums, was brought into contact with the fluids of the mouth, it was split up into milk of lime and hydrogen dioxide, so that an antacid as well as a germicidal action was attained, the hydrogen dioxide being, of course, decomposed into water and liberating oxygen, which was supposed to combine with any organic matter that might be present in the teeth. He congratulated the New York Odontological Society in being selected as the medium through which the first announcement of the discovery was to be made public.—*American Druggist.*

THE MECHANISM OF THE ERUPTION OF THE TEETH.[1] By J. Thornton Carter, L.D.S. (Eng.), F.Z.S.

Whilst studying the teeth and jaws of fishes I was much struck by the fact that in all the skulls I had the opportunity of observing and examining, if the successional teeth were formed in crypts, a foramen always existed leading to the reserve tooth and transmitting a band of fibrous tissue to the capsule of the tooth. In tooth-bearing reptilia I have observed the same condition, and in mammalia it is a common feature. That these are not merely nutrient foramina seems evident, for the bundles of fibrous tissue which they transmit do not appear to be very vascular.

It would seem strange if a rudiment, absolutely functionless, were to be found so widely distributed throughout the animal kingdom, and I am of the opinion expressed by the " older anatomists" that the gubernaculum is concerned in some way in directing or effecting the eruption of the teeth.

The manner in which this takes place I shall endeavor to state briefly in the remainder of this paper, and though there may be auxiliary forces operating, such as blood-pressure, as Mr. Constant has so ingeniously brought forth, I believe the most important factor, and the only one which provides a satisfactory working hypothesis for the practitioner in dealing with cases of irregularity of the teeth, to be the force exercised on the tooth through the gubernaculum. This motive force I believe to be derived from absorption and deposition of bone (not merely of the free edges of the alveolus) operating on the muco-periosteum of the mouth, and to make clear how this takes place it is necessary for me to trespass on your time and patience by briefly outlining the mode of growth of the jaws.

Owing to the facilities afforded by the mandible for the investi-

---

[1] Abstract taken from the British Dental Journal of February, 1904.

gation of this subject, it has been mainly on this bone that the inquiry has been carried out, but the method of growth in the maxilla has been found to be of a similar nature.

The invaluable researches of the late Sir John Tomes, whom we revere as the founder of our profession as a scientific body, and whose work should never be out of reach of the earnest practitioner, show that the arch occupied by the deciduous teeth corresponds very closely with that occupied by their immediate successors, and that any alteration is referable " to deposition on the exterior surface and not to any fundamental alteration or interstitial growth."

Moreover, he found that the distance between the lingual surfaces of the second deciduous molars is almost the same as that between their successors, the second bicuspids or premolars; and drawing a line forward to the spina mentalis from the centre of a line connecting these latter teeth, he found the length to be about the same in the child where the deciduous molars were standing as in the case of the adult. But if the line were produced to the external alveolar plate a great difference would be apparent; " in point of fact, contemporaneously with the development of the crypts of the permanent teeth inside them, the temporary teeth and their outer alveolar plate are slowly pushed outward, a process the results of which we see in the separation which comes about between each one of the temporary teeth prior to their being shed, when the process of dentition is carried on in a perfectly normal manner."

His researches have shown that the growth of the mandible takes place mainly by deposition on the posterior border of the ascending ramus with coincident absorption over its anterior border, and by additions to the outer surface of the horizontal ramus.

Also, that the portion of the mandible lying below the level of the inferior dental canal practically reaches its full development, excepting the angle, by the age of seven years, but that the portion above the canal undergoes great change between this time and adult age.

During these years the vertical growth of the horizontal ramus takes place almost entirely in the alveolar portion,—*i.e.*, that portion which depends for its existence on the presence of teeth; for when these are lost this part of the bone is almost completely absorbed. There is also a considerable increase in the depth of the ascending ramus by deposition under the interarticular fibrocartilage, which in this position partakes somewhat of the nature of an epiphyseal cartilage.

This constant and rapid growth of the anterior surface of the horizontal ramus and more rapid but intermittent growth of the alveolar portion of the bone causes the muco-periosteum covering the jaw to be at times in a state of considerable tension. That this is so is apparent on looking into the mouth of a child between the years of two and seven, and that this tension exercises a force leading to change of position of teeth is plainly seen. To take a single example in the case of the first permanent molar: at the age of two years the follicles of the deciduous molars lie immediately over the tooth-sacs of the first permanent molars. As the jaw lengthens backward these tooth-sacs are borne backward by the tension and consequent extension of the muco-periosteum to which they are attached.

As before mentioned, the deciduous teeth are never completely roofed in by their crypts, but lie in incomplete alveoli; as the growth of the jaw goes on, the tension on the anterior fibres causes absorption to start at the anterior border of the crypt, this being the part where pressure first pulls. This absorption continues until the tension is relaxed and the tooth free to emerge from its crypt, when it is gradually raised to the surface by the constant thickening of the outer alveolar plate operating on the membrane covering the jaw, the posterior alveolar plate acting as a more or less fixed *point d'appui.*

The edges of the crypt, relieved from the pressure which caused their absorption, immediately assume a period of great activity (contrary to the steady continuous growth of the outer plate), growing up around the neck of the tooth to afford it support, prevent its displacement, and to protect the remainder of the tooth-germ during its completion.

Meanwhile, the calcification of the permanent teeth and the steady growth of the jaw continue, until the mucous membrane of the mouth is again in a condition of tension. This causes the peridental membrane ensheathing the root of the deciduous tooth to change its function, and, since steady pressure causes absorption, either to become or to give origin to an absorbent organ, the absorption starting at the point where the pressure is greatest.

Coincidentally with the process of absorption there is a deposition of bone immediately beneath, so that ultimately the crown alone remains attached to the gum and separated from the bone roofing over the crypt of its successor by the absorbent organ only.

As before stated, the follicle of the permanent tooth retains its connection with the mucous membrane of the mouth by means of the gubernaculum, the fibres of which pass upward through the iter dentis, and diverging radially blend with the fibrous elements of the gum.

The tension produced by the unequal growth of the jaw acts first on the anterior fibres of the gubernaculum, causing the labial margin of the iter dentis to be absorbed, and the crypt is open sufficiently to permit the egress of the partially formed tooth which is gradually raised to its place in the dental arch in the same manner as were the deciduous teeth.

We have another instance of a somewhat similar process taking place. In Heisler's "Text-book of Embryology" it is stated that in the case of the descent of the testis, the inguinal ligament or gubernaculum testis does not grow, whilst the surrounding tissues do grow, and that by this means it is displaced downward from its original position, attributing little or no part to the unstriped muscle fibres which it contains.

Comparative anatomy appears to lend support to the views enunciated above. In plagiostomous fishes (standing as they do at the very base of the vertebrate phyllum) the simplest conditions are found, and since the parts have not undergone great specialization, investigation of the process of development and eruption in this sub-order is comparatively simple when contrasted with the conditions obtaining in the more specialized groups, where a more highly specialized organ is needed leading to a corresponding complexity of the formative process.

THE USES OF SWISS BROACHES. By Otto E. Inglis, D.D.S., Philadelphia, Pa.

The Swiss broach is an invention from the watchmaker's art which has become almost a necessity in root-canal treatment. These broaches, as sold by the jeweller's finders, consist of a handle, or thumb-shank, like that on the ordinary barbel broach, and a foil-like polygonal blade, tapering to a fine point.

The broaches vary in size, from extremely fine to comparatively thick. They may be purchased of very hard temper and of very soft temper. The latter renders the broach useless except for barbing, and the former makes it so exceedingly brittle as to render it useless as purchased. The high temper may be very readily reduced, however, by placing a few broaches in a test-tube, and holding the latter over a flame, allowing the flame to impinge upon that part of the tube over which the shanks of the broaches lie. As the correct heat is approached, the blade of the instrument will change to a straw color, then to a bright blue. This change will appear first near the shank, and, if the tube be moved slowly, the color will creep along the blade until the extreme tip is tempered. The broach may then be thrown out to cool on anything that will not burn. The operation may be done with a single broach over a tiny flame, or near the flame of a match, but the results are much inferior, as a rule.

This tempering changes the broach from a useless article to one which may be tied in a knot without breaking, but may be used to penetrate a canal, offering some resistance, without the maddening result of bending upon itself into a crumpled mass of useless steel.

In the selection of the broaches, only those having a distinct taper to the blade should be bought, as those with blades of even diameter throughout are very liable to bend.

The uses of these little instruments are varied.

As explorers for fine points of exposure, they are admirable, entering the small orifice readily, and, while producing the sensation desired as a diagnostic, they do not make painful compression of the pulp.

As explorers of canal apertures for the determination of the size and direction of the canal, they are very useful, and may be filed to an extreme thinness to enable them to enter the finer canals.

As reamers of canals, they also do admirable work. Successive sizes, beginning with the finest, are passed into the canal and rotated with the fingers. Acids tend to injure these instruments, so that they may break, but this does not occur, as a rule, unless undue force be used.

As carriers of cotton for the swabbing out of canals for any object, they are indispensable, though of course an analogous instrument may be constructed by filing the fine truncated end of a Donaldson bristle to a polygonal form. Their value, in this connection, lies in their smooth taper and unround form, which permits the cotton to be quickly rolled upon them, and, when charged with the canal contents, to be removed; the cotton is readily removed without soiling the fingers by grasping the broach with the finger and thumb of the left hand at a point near the shank, and back of the loose fibres of cotton; the shank is held with the thumb and finger of the right hand, and with a quick pull the cotton is slipped off the broach as a neat cone.

The same instrument may be used to place cottons in canals as temporary dressings. This may be done by using the broach, mounted in a chuck handle, as a canal plugger, but the dressing is more easily done by another method, especially in the finer canals.

The cotton is wound on the broach, as previously described, with as few fibres about its end as possible, as all bulk interferes with canal penetration. If the canal be very fine, the broach which explored it may be filed down, and again smoothed by drawing it through a folded cuttle-fish disk. In dressing the canal, the broach, with the cotton upon it, is passed in with a twist to the right to engage the fibres with the canal walls; when solidly placed, a couple of twists to the left are made to loosen the broach from the centre of the cone. It is then withdrawn about a sixteenth of an inch, and then pressed in again, an act which crimps the cotton cone upon itself.

This may be done, even if the broach be bent so as to enter mesial canals of lower molars. If desired, the broaches may be many times bent and again straightened without injury, but it is well to avoid too much of this without annealing, as all steel is finally injured by the disarrangement of its molecules.

The rolling of the cotton upon the broach is done by first laying a few loose fibres upon the forefinger of the left hand. The broach is placed upon it, allowing a few fibres to lie beyond its end. Next, the thumb is lightly pressed upon the broach. The shank is then quickly rotated with the right thumb and forefinger, and, as the cotton is rolled up, the left thumb and forefinger are used to stroke it into a symmetrical cone. If the pointed broach be used, it will be noted that there is a tendency on its part to penetrate the end of the cone of cotton. This may be obviated by slightly truncating the end of the broach with scissors. This penetration of the cotton is annoying from the fact that apical tissues are liable to be irritated, and that the broach is liable to be stripped of the cotton which crowds back upon it as it comes into friction with the canal walls. In use as a swab-carrier, the broach is constantly twisted to the right, if twisted at all. To remove cotton, it may be twisted in this manner into the loose fibres until these are tightly engaged; but, as a rule, an old, barbed broach, or Donaldson cleanser, is preferable for this purpose.

Any one who has used as a cotton-carrier a broach which requires a wire brush, or burning off, to free it, will be much relieved by the adoption of this method.—*Stomatologist* for November.

Reports of Society Meetings.

THE NEW YORK INSTITUTE OF STOMATOLOGY.

A MEETING of the Institute was held on Tuesday evening, March 1, 1904, at the " Chelsea," No. 222 West Twenty-third Street, New York, Dr. Brockway, the President, in the chair.

The minutes of the last meeting were read and approved.

Dr. G. C. Ainsworth, of Boston, read a paper entitled " Some Thoughts regarding Methods and a New Appliance for moving Dislocated Teeth into Position."

(For Dr. Ainsworth's paper, see page 481.)

Dr. Sinclair Tousey, A.M., M.D., read a paper at a meeting held at his residence, March 1, 1904, on the " Radiotherapy in Pyorrhœa Alveolaris, and Dental Radiography."

(For Dr. Tousey's paper, see page 495.)

Dr. E. A. Bogue stated that he had found Dr. Ainsworth's methods such a revelation to him that, so far as he had understood them, he had adopted them in several cases. Regarding the inclined plane shown by Dr. Ainsworth, Dr. Bogue thought if it would work as well for the rest of us as it did for Dr. Ainsworth it would assist very materially in obtaining a proper occlusion in certain cases. Dr. Bogue would also like to call particular attention to these little tubes that Dr. Ainsworth solders to the bands. These tubes accurately fit the spring-wire they are made to hold, so that there is no lost motion and the tooth is moved exactly as desired by properly bending the wire.

In considering the three appliances of Dr. Ainsworth, it seemed proper to call attention to a few collateral facts. The first was the contraction of the upper arch. He had noticed this in examining his own models, and his attention had also been called to it by other orthodontists. Dr. Stanley had confirmed these observations recently, asserting that seventy per cent. of the cases that needed regulating had contracted upper arches. If this were anything like the proportion, and Dr. Bogue believed it to be within the limits, there was a broad field for the use of Dr. Ainsworth's appliance among persons who could not give a great deal of time to having their teeth regulated. It was also a great saving of time and attention to those who were going to do the regulating. Without claiming that Dr. Ainsworth's method was applicable in all cases, it seemed to Dr. Bogue that it was a decided advance for a great many. Dr. Bogue would give an example or two. Among the lantern slides that he exhibited before this Institute a year ago was one of a little girl whom he had sent to a friend in Paris for treatment. This friend had applied to her teeth the Angle arches, above and below, making an admirable attachment and ligating the teeth so well that the fixtures, when Dr. Bogue first saw them, had been on about ten months. He had taken careful impressions and made models of the teeth as they then were. The gain in expansion of the entire arches had been very little. He could judge of this accurately, as he had the original models, and he measured them as they were originally and as they came to him about two years later. The little girl was impatient of pressure and intolerant of pain. He found that with a single nut at the end of each screw of the expansion arch those nuts could never be kept tight twenty-four hours. The moment the teeth responded to the immediate pressure the nuts became loose and turned backward. He sent this child to Dr. Ainsworth, who put on to the upper teeth such a fixture as he had described this evening. Dr. Bogue had replaced the Angle appliance on the lower teeth, but had taken the precaution to put two nuts on the screw at each end. By actual measurement, more progress was made in three weeks than had been made in the previous ten months, and this without pain. The patient was about thirteen years of age. Dr. Bogue had noticed recently that a new regulating appliance had been under discussion in the American Dental Club of Paris since this child had gone back.

Another case was that of a little girl seven years of age upon whom he had placed this fixture. He had seen her again after two days and again after two weeks. The gentleman into whose hands he had sent her reported that aside from drawing a developing central incisor slightly forward, he had had nothing to do but to keep the fixtures in place. He said the case might be regarded as practically completed; for, having moved the temporary molars and cuspids and the permanent central incisor out of the way of the lower teeth, the child had voluntarily assumed the proper occlusion; and the principal upper molars, which when he began had occluded one full cusp in advance of their proper position, now occluded with the anterior buccal cusp in the buccal depression of the lower molars, leaving plenty of room for the comfortable cruption of all the remaining teeth.

It was well to notice, as Dr. Ainsworth said, that the tooth may sometimes start suddenly and come out too far. Dr. Bogue had seen three cases where the expansion arch had pushed or pulled the teeth in a direction exactly opposite from that which was intended, because the gentleman into whose hands the cases were sent had failed to take cognizance of the fact that the arch is at work the entire twenty-four hours of the day, although the patient might not be aware that it was doing anything.

Dr. Bogue would take issue with Dr. Ainsworth when he stated that the lower teeth were inferior in stability to the upper ones. It seemed to him that the teeth in the lower jaw were far more stable than those in the upper jaw, and more difficult to move.

Dr. Ainsworth made an admirable use of his expansion arch in correcting deformities in the middle-aged. If we were not discussing his three regulating appliances only, he would feel like making his compliments to Dr. Ainsworth for the case of restoration shown, the patient being forty-nine years of age.

He would like to ask Dr. Ainsworth what solder he used in making these regulating appliances.

Dr. Bogue's attention had been attracted to this method, especially for use with little children, in which cases it had shown itself to be particularly well adapted to do the work required quickly and with little if any pain.

Dr. Bogue had been frequently asked why the permanent teeth should be so much larger than the temporary teeth they replace, and why these teeth should seem so out of proportion to the mouths in which we found them. He would like to ask a question,—Why are the feet of a pup so out of proportion to the size of the animal? Do we remove some of the toes lest the dog should seem to be all feet?

The retaining appliance shown commended itself, particularly for its cleanliness, acuracy, and comfort.

Dr. Rolof B. Stanley stated that the spirit which prompted him to take part in the discussion was born of a desire to learn rather than criticise. He had tried to analyze with an unbiassed mind Dr. Ainsworth's method of treatment of malocclusion and the application of the mechanical principle of his appliance. Dr. Stanley trusted he might be pardoned if for a moment he dwelt upon the A, B, C, of orthodontia, so familiar to all. It might serve to bring out more clearly the points he wished to make. Problems of orthodontia were problems of malocclusion, and restoration to the normal was the essential object. The first and most important step in any case was a correct diagnosis. The ability to make a correct diagnosis implied a knowledge of normal occlusion, of the fundamental types of malocclusion, and an appreciation of the harmony of facial lines. We must classify these cases and establish hard and fast rules, else the work savored of the experimental, or the operator must be guided by instinct alone. The only part individuality played in any case was in the degree of deviation from the normal. We could never bring order out of chaos if the individuality of the patient, as well as that of the operator, was allowed to play so important a part to the exclusion of fixed rules. With the knowledge of the normal occlusion and of the fundamental types of malocclusion, the deviation from the normal could be seen at a glance. It was the position of the teeth collectively that we must first consider, then the teeth separately, and an appliance should be chosen that would embody, in the order named, efficiency, simplicity, and inconspicuousness. Under the head of efficiency, the ideal appliance was one of standard pattern, no matter what the pattern might be, which would meet all the requirements from start to finish of all forms of malocclusion, and exclude the necessity of mechanical skill and ingenuity on the part of the operator. By simplicity was meant not only simplicity of mechanical construction, but freedom from an array of modifications or additions necessary to effect all changes in a given case, for the farther we wandered from the straight and narrow path of one fixed appliance the greater would be the confusion in the mind of the operator.

To consider the appliances shown, Dr. Stanley failed to see where they covered all the requirements, or how they were capable of accomplishing restoration to the normal in all cases. That they

would bring about results in certain cases was proved by some of
the photographs shown, but he doubted if they were available for
all forms of malocclusion. For instance, where it was necessary
to lengthen one or both lateral halves; where it was necessary to
expand but one lateral half; where it was necessary to contract the
lateral halves. Or, in the use of the inclined plane, how could
the mesio-distal relation of the molars and bicuspids on one side
only be restored; or in a case where the lower molars and bicuspids
on one side are mesial or anterior and on the other distal or posterior to normal; how could the normal occlusion be restored
by the use of the inclined plane or by any appliance or combination
of appliances shown to-night? Dr. Stanley could cite many other
cases that had come to his mind while listening to the paper, but
thought these sufficient to emphasize the points he wished to make.
They were all possible cases and cases that he had had in his practice during the present winter.

The question of discomfort to the patient and the length of
time of treatment was of some moment. He believed in making
orthodontic treatment as easy for both patient and operator as
possible, both in application of the appliance to the teeth, the force
used, and the time consumed, but he did not believe it to be of
advantage to allow the patient to operate the appliance at will, since
he did not appreciate the normal conditions. In conclusion, efficiency had been sacrificed in applying the principle of the expansion
arch in the manner shown. While in some cases the ligature had
been done away with to simplify the manipulation of the expansion
arch, in as high as seventy per cent. of cases its use was required,
either for carrying the incisors forward or for rotating them.
Again this appliance presupposed that each tooth in the lateral
halves was to be removed equally, which was far from the case
generally. So with the inclined plane, the device might restore
normal mesio-distal relation where both of the lateral halves required it, but could not where but one of the lateral halves required
it. Cases of this type were as frequent as the bilateral. To meet
all conditions, no matter how extreme, with one form of appliance
certainly simplified treatment and promoted proficiency in its use.

Dr. J. Bond Littig was gratified to hear such a paper, and was
going away with something new. He would especially commend
the movable character of the appliance for retention. He thought
there was great danger in an appliance impossible of removal. He

had had two cases at least where, although thorough instructions had been given as to the proper cleansing of the immovable appliance, there had been a certain amount of disintegration of the enamel.

As to the inclined plane illustrated, Dr. Littig thought one principle was applied here that he had never seen before. We had all used the rubber plate, thickened in front to reduce the lower teeth or lengthen the molars, but he had never seen an appliance whereby the upper and lower teeth could at the same time be shortened.

Dr. C. F. Allan said that the paper had been most interesting to him. That effectiveness, simplicity, and cleanliness were salient points called for in all regulating and retaining appliances, and Dr. Ainsworth possibly more than anybody had attained these conditions. His only criticism would be the name of the paper. It seemed to him that the terms occlusion and malocclusion are much more properly descriptive of the conditions under consideration.

The inclined plane attached to the teeth of the upper jaw was the most individual of all the valuable appliances Dr. Ainsworth had shown, and Dr. Allan expected to put it in use immediately. Dr. Allan expressed his thanks to Dr. Ainsworth for the many good points he had given.

Dr. J. Morgan Howe, in expressing his gratification at the instructive paper, thought Dr. Ainsworth had presented an entirely new method of the application of springs. His own experience was that the movement of teeth by means of metal springs was the least painful of any of the various methods except the screw. The screw, however, requires more attention. Dr. Ainsworth's method certainly accomplished results in an easier and quicker way than those in general use. Whether or not it was universally applicable, it had added a new means of applying force and accomplishing results in certain cases at least. All of the presentations Dr. Ainsworth had made had been most interesting and instructive.

Dr. C. F. Allan stated that he wished to call attention to the necessity for always cementing on any appliance to be worn in the mouth and which cannot be removed for cleansing.

In putting on bands the teeth should be smeared with cement as well as the bands, and that this was imperatively necessary to prevent the possible rapid disintegration of the teeth over which appliances were placed, and in this matter one could not be too particular.

Dr. Bogue agreed with Dr. Allan regarding the cement under the bands of regulating and retaining appliances. He recalled one case at least from an exceedingly eminent orthodontist where, had the teeth been in his own mouth, he would rather have had them in any condition of dislocation than in the condition in which he found them. Dr. Bogue was not impressed with the fact that this appliance of Dr. Ainsworth could be removed to permit of a good appearance when the young lady went to a party. It was liable to form a habit that might be indulged in at other times.

Dr. Ainsworth, in closing the discussion, stated that he wished to disclaim all intention of developing a system of appliances to take the place of those now in use, or supplying them commercially; that he believed, as a rule, the appliance should be especially made for the case in hand. He had come here in response to the solicitations of members who were acquainted with what he was doing, to show what experience had dictated to him as improvements in the conduct of some cases. It had been claimed that seventy per cent. of all regulating cases required expansion of the arch. He thought this a sufficient apology for his demonstration of a self-acting appliance to do this work. Dr. Ainsworth had stated that this appliance was under the control of the patient by removing the front wire, but practically it was a control seldom exercised, as the appliance was so comfortable. It was very different from a rubber plate or an appliance that interfered with the functions of the mouth. It had been his experience that with such appliances the patient left them out much of the time.

These appliances were not perfect. The ideas were offered with the hope and belief that if intelligently applied they would be found to possess much merit. The principles might be applied in connection with other devices.

Dr. Charles O. Kimball, in proposing a vote of thanks to Dr. Ainsworth for coming on from Boston to give us this demonstration of his method, wished to call attention to two or three points; in the first place, to the simplicity, efficiency, and cleanliness of his apparatus, and no less so to the clear and simple and remarkably terse way in which he had demonstrated it by means of his photo-

· graphs and his paper. Dr. Kimball would move a vote of thanks from the society to Dr. Ainsworth.

Motion seconded and carried.

Adjourned.

FRED. L. BOGUE, M.D., D.D.S.,
Editor The New York Institute of Stomatology.

Editorial.

ANTISEPTIC SCIENCE IN CHICAGO.

IN January last a paper was read before the Chicago Dental Society, by Hermann Prinz, M.D., D.D.S., of St. Louis, on "A Few Facts concerning the Action of Antiseptics." This paper was given to readers of dental subjects in the *Dental Review,* of Chicago, May 15, 1904. The essay was an able *résumé* of the subject, largely made up, outside of the author's own opinions, with the history of the subject and the theories and investigations of other minds. Very little original work by the writer appears in the article. This, however, did not militate against its interest, but rather enhanced its value as a contribution to the knowledge of the subject. It brought forth an interesting discussion in which the author of the paper naturally took an active part.

In the course of his remarks he went out of his way to scarify the present writer, because in a recent review he had the audacity to express certain convictions regarding the action of silver nitrate on tissue.

The remarks of Dr. Prinz, as reported, were as follows: "As to metal salts, I have looked into them very thoroughly. It is almost incredible to believe that a man like Dr. Truman, of Philadelphia, stands by a statement to-day that he made six years ago. In one of the latest numbers of the INTERNATIONAL DENTAL JOURNAL, in reviewing a book on modern therapeutics by Stevens, he attacks the statement made by Stevens as to the limitation of silver nitrate in tissue, saying that it does not exist; that he has demonstrated this in test-tubes, etc. I have worked in the mouths of poor patients; I have taken the lower second molar, in which there was deep caries; placed in there pure nitrate of silver, sealed it in for

months, and after a while extracted the tooth, and it has shown
distinctly the limitation of nitrate of silver. My observations have
convinced me that nitrate of silver is self-limiting in its action.
It precipitates albumin and silver albumin will not allow the
smallest particle of silver to penetrate any farther. It will not do
so, no matter what the test-tube shows. Living subjects are the
ones in which to make these experiments, and experiments show
that there is a resisting force in the tissue. There it stops. There
is no force behind it."

The personal part of this quotation is not regarded as of any
importance by this writer. The editor of this journal has long
since ceased to reply to mere personalities, and would have allowed
this to sink into forgetfulness were it not for the fact that this
paragraph contains either important truths, or serious errors, of
grave concern to all practising dentists. Is the dental profession
prepared to accept the dictum that silver nitrate can be applied
to a tooth *ad libitum,* and that without producing discoloration?
If they are willing to accept Dr. Prinz's dogmatic assertion as the
truth, then they can apply this metal salt without fear to any and
all teeth with which we have to deal; but if they doubt his conclusions, they will agree with the writer and wait further investigations
before risking their reputations on the mere statement that silver
nitrate is self-limiting.

Dr. Prinz has poor patients. That is commendable. He takes
a " lower second molar and applies silver nitrate and seals it there
for months." He speaks of " deep caries," but does not state
whether the pulp was exposed, gangrenous, or whether he applied
the silver salt to a clean, dry canal, or whether the application
was in crystal form or solution. It is taken for granted that the
pulp was not exposed, and that he placed the silver nitrate in the
cavity in crystals upon the open ends of the tubuli of the dentine.
After months he extracted the tooth. It was certainly kind in this
poor patient to submit to this mutilation in the cause of science.
It is another item for the Antivivisection Society to record, and
might be of value to the Society for Prevention of Cruelty to
Children, providing St. Louis supports such an organization. This
question can best be settled by those most interested. The writer
would suggest to Dr. Prinz that when he makes further experiments
in this direction, he take a number of vital teeth, and not confine
his work to one. Place the silver nitrate in the cavity in solution

and not in crystals. Saturate cotton with it so that it will remain for a definite period in contact with the living protoplasm of the tubes. If after several months he finds, upon extraction and sectionizing these teeth, that the silver salt has not coagulated the organic material, he will be able to assert, with some degree of positiveness, that silver nitrate " precipitates albumin and silver albumin will not allow the smallest particle of silver to penetrate any farther." Silver nitrate is not deliquescent. It will remain as he placed it, unchanged indefinitely, and it is doubtful whether the salt thus placed will penetrate deeply. It has also to be proved to what extent vitality resists the progress of a coagulant. It has been fully and completely demonstrated that dead protoplasm offers no obstruction to its progress in the tabulated structure of dentine. This the writer demonstrated years ago, and Dr. Prinz can read the results as published at the time, if not already familiar with them.

The evidence furnished by Dr. Prinz, in his one tooth, that vitality is a resisting force is not sufficient. The evidence offered by Dr. Stebbins is probably the only test of much value in this direction, and this is not conclusive, for while working on poor children he failed to extract the teeth. Dr. Stebbins, then unknown to fame, called the writer's attention to a group of children with him, while the latter was in attendance at the American Dental Association at Saratoga. His statement that he had been using silver nitrate in some of the cavities for a period of six years was received by the writer with marked evidence of incredulity. The facts, however, were too positive to be set aside without further and more careful examination. Some of these deciduous teeth were vital, and, as far as the observer could determine from external examination, they were not seriously discolored. This was, then and now, attributed to the fact that Dr. Stebbins had *carefully removed all excess* of the silver nitrate, to avoid, if possible, any deep penetration and, at the same time, secure the antiseptic property of the agent. In this he succeeded, and in teeth exposed to the destructive action of the fluids of the mouth there was no evidence of deterioration from caries. Dr. Stebbins had, however, no thought of determining the resisting power of living tissues. That this is a factor to be considered requires no argument, but the extent of the resisting force has, as yet, not been formulated, and the writer may be pardoned if he is sceptical as

21

to Dr. Prinz's success in proving it to be an assured fact. It seems
to the writer that the essayist's descent from the sublimity of scientific statements, in his paper, to the paragraph quoted from the
discussion, is a remarkably good illustration of a descent from the
elevated in writing to the bathos of speech.

Some years since, when the question of the penetration of coagulants was a warm subject for dispute in our national conventions,
the action of silver nitrate came up for consideration in the American Dental Association. Those who advocated its use in pulp-canals
took practically the same position as Dr. Prinz,—that it would not
penetrate the tubules, that its penetration would be prevented by
its own coagulant, etc. Specimens were handed around to prove
this; human teeth in microscopic sections. The result had its
amusing side for those who had contended that silver nitrate was
not self-limiting, for all of these sections clearly demonstrated that
it had entered the tubes to a considerable extent; in fact, was only
self-limiting up to the quantity used. So far as it went, it ef-
fectually discolored the protoplasm in the tubes.

The writer is aware that mere opinions are not worthy of much
consideration upon a matter of this character, but there must
have been some clinical evidence that led to the universal teaching,
for a half-century and longer, that silver nitrate would discolor
tooth-substance if brought in contact with organic matter. This
was the universal opinion; it was universally taught and as universally accepted. When one as prominent in professional circles
as the writer of the paper mentioned takes great pains to assure
the rising professional generation that it will not discolor, that it
will not penetrate beneath the surface, that it can be used with
safety, and that " silver is one metal of all others, no matter what
statements are made to the contrary, which is best tolerated by the
tissues," he is bound to prove it beyond all fear of successful criticism.

The writer's experiments, alluded to by the essayist, were not
made especially to prove the penetrating power of silver nitrate,
but they were conducted through months and in a variety of ways
to demonstrate the action of coagulants in the presence of albumin. Silver nitrate was one of many. In regard to this the writer
entertained the opinions universally held by writers, including the
author of the paper, that the action of this metal salt was superficial. To his great surprise he found that in sealed capillary tubes

filled with egg albumin the penetration was continuous until the entire mass was coagulated. The experiments were then transferred to human teeth. The same results followed, many sections showing deep discoloration throughout the tubulated structure. If these experiments are not satisfactory to Dr. Prinz, it belongs to him to originate more positive methods. It seems to the writer that the older theories that have attempted to describe its action in the presence of albumin need revision, and it might be instructive to the coming generation of dentists if Dr. Prinz would extend his laboratory experiments from one tooth to many.

This sort of teaching has given dentists the courage to use silver nitrate indiscriminately; indeed, we find one prominent writer recommending it as an occasional mouth-wash in solution. A conservative estimate of its value is, therefore, greatly needed.

The writer still remains of the opinion that silver nitrate is *not self-limiting,* and that the reason why it does not always penetrate deeply is simply that the agent was used in too limited a quantity to permit active coagulation upon the deeper layers of albumin. The question is, therefore, one of quantity in solution and continuance of action.

MEETING OF THE "FACULTIES" AT WASHINGTON, D. C.

THE meeting of this organization at Washington, D. C., June 9 to 11, 1904, must be regarded as the most important held in recent years by that body. While the one which decided to advance the dental course to four years marked an epoch in dental education, it did not compare, in point of interest, to the one that has just closed its sessions.

It was generally understood that a determined effort would be made to return to three years and six or seven months, and those who attended the meeting were not disappointed. The subject was the main topic that occupied the thoughts of the members; in fact, but little else was considered of moment in comparison. The members discussed it in meetings and in the hotel corridors. The result was at all times in doubt, for it was plainly evident that a very large number of the dental colleges of the country were earnestly in opposition to a further continuance of the four years' course.

It was the general opinion that the question, in all its length and breadth, had been discussed as no other question had been in the past at meetings of this organization. Upon both sides there had been exhibited an earnest effort to meet the problems connected with the question with the dignity due to its importance and to the interests involved. It was very evident that the motive for a retrograde action was mainly one of finance. The large majority of the schools desiring a change were being seriously affected by the four years' course; indeed, with some it had become a matter of life and death. This was fully appreciated by those in opposition to any change, and there was felt, and openly expressed, much sympathy for those who had tried the lengthened course and had severely suffered by the experiment. Especially was· this felt for the Southern schools. Notwithstanding this sympathy, the determination to maintain the higher standard was not in the least lessened.

The anxiety to know how the Association stood on the question resulted in the adoption of a motion to take an informal vote upon it, but this was to be considered simply in the light of a test. The result was a surprise to both sides, as it demonstrated that the section in the Association advocating a return to three years must increase the vote if there was to be any change. This informal vote stood 19 to 27. The hope that this margin might be lessened if not entirely obliterated, by earnest efforts caused a caucus to be held and every effort made to influence those in doubt. The majority was not very hopeful of final success, and hence the interest and anxiety on both sides were intense, and were not removed until the final vote was announced and the question decided by 24 in opposition to change, to 21 in favor, and 2 not voting. This was not a very reliable majority, but it was sufficient, and the tension was greatly relieved.

Before the final adjournment, upon motion of Dr. Black, it was decided, by a vote of colleges, to give the weaker schools some relief, and the final vote was cast for four years with a six months' course. This was not altogether satisfactory to several of the colleges, for these desired three years with a nine months' course, and one or two openly stated that their schools would probably be forced out of the Association.

The final vote does not influence those departments of universities that have persistently held to four years with a nine months' course. These will continue to uphold the higher standard.

It is thought, by those best qualified to judge, that the cutting down of the matriculating list in the Freshman year will be but temporary, and that in a year or two an equilibrium will be established and the classes will resume the normal number. If this should prove not to be the case, the question may again, in the near future, cause a repetition of the effort to reduce the time, but for the present it must remain practically without alteration.

The Association made another important move in the direction of more liberal treatment of those applying for advanced standing. The " Count System" was adopted, which will permit dental colleges to place a certain valuation upon studies taken in other than strictly dental colleges. This will greatly simplify the question of entrance and do away with many unjust decisions, forced upon colleges in deciding applications for advanced standing. This decision does not apply to, nor does it affect, the preliminary entrance standards already in force.

The vote in detail upon the question will be found upon another page, and it will bear careful inspection and will doubtless be of interest to all dental educational circles in this country.

Bibliography.

INDEX DER DEUTSCHEN ZAHNÄRZTLICHEN LITERATUR UND ZAHN-ÄRZTLICHE BIBLIOGRAPHIE. Bearbeitet von Prof. Dr. Port in Heidelberg. Hörning und Berkenbusch, Heidelberg, 1904.

This very important work which, as the title implies, covers the German dental literature and the bibliography of dentistry, the latter in part only, as the author has confined the notices of the work of foreign writers to the brief abstract translations into German found in the periodical literature of those speaking and writing that language. This makes the book imperfect so far as the dental literature of the world is concerned.

This " Index" had its origin at the annual meeting of the Central Association of German Dentists, held at Munich, 1902, at which a commission was appointed to prepare an index of dental literature. The following were named to serve in that capacity: Julius Parreidt, Leipzig; Schäffer-Stuckert, Frankfort a/M.; Sternfeld, Munich; Professor Witzel, Essen; and the author, Professor Port.

The Index covers one hundred and eighty pages, the subject-matter being divided into the various branches practised in dentistry. This includes not only elaborate works, but papers as they have appeared in various periodicals. This has involved an enormous amount of labor upon the part of the author. The patient research made necessary to perfect this deserves the special thanks of the author's co-workers among German-speaking peoples.

The book has, of course, but a limited value for those who confine their reading to English. The intention of the author not to enter thoroughly into foreign work has necessarily reduced his notices of English and American writings. This seems unfortunate, as the author's ability and industry applied to all countries would have made this the most valuable book of reference for the literature of dentistry ever published. As it is, the English reader must wait, it is feared, a long period for some industrious compiler to prepare this much-needed work.

On carefully scanning the pages of this book one is struck with the fact that much of minor importance finds a place there, and much of real value, in the world's work, is omitted. It is rather surprising that Black's labors have not found any notice in German periodical literature; at least, our author makes no mention of his name. Nothing has been said of Farrar, Angle, and Talbot in Orthodontia, or of the latter in his elaborate work on "Interstitial Gingivitis." This means that not only these books, but many others of equal value, are unknown to German readers. Upon the other hand, the long list of valuable works printed in German are absolutely unknown to American readers, beyond, in some instances, a mere abstract of contents. Until all readers become linguists, or the world has a universal language for scientific publications, this ignorance must continue to produce a narrow conception of the work of each branch of science in foreign tongues. Many books have been published in German in recent years, of very great value, but so far these have not found translators, consequently those who might materially benefit by the reading are shut out entirely from large stores of knowledge. All this may be changed in the not far distant future, through greater attention paid in the schools to the study of modern languages. This has become imperative through the constant intermingling of nationalities. In the mean time the writer would express the hope that in the near future some American would follow the good example of Professor Port and prepare an index of American writings and American authors, such as we find in this volume devoted to German dentistry.

To those who can read German this Index will prove of great value as a work of reference, and it can be recommended to fill worthily a place in all libraries.

Obituary.

JAMES SMITH TURNER.

DENTISTRY knows no country, nor is it possible for it to lose interest in those not immediately connected with its local work. American dentists to-day mourn with our English brethren the loss of one of the most faithful exemplars of the best in our profession. For this, J. Smith Turner's name has become a household word among English-speaking dentists the world over. His death, therefore, at threescore years and ten, must be regarded as something more than a national loss. His activity up to the period of his last illness was seemingly equal to that of any former period of his life.

James Smith Turner belonged to a race of men who, having formed a standard of character, endeavor to live up to it, and no exertion was too great to have other men realize that the standard of ethics he had formulated for himself was the one to meet the highest needs of his profession. As the *British Dental Journal* says of him, " He was a strong man, raised up to fight a long and stubborn battle; he was always fighting, always winning in the end. . . . He always thought of the cause, and never of himself, and how he wore himself out to win not recognition, honors, wealth, or even professional success, but a solid, honorable, legalized status for the profession to which he belonged."

Such was the man, unselfish, devoted, sacrificing the good things

of life that dentistry in Great Britain might occupy worthily a
place among the honored professions.

James Smith Turner passed away from his earthly activities on
Monday, February 22, 1904, and the interment took place at St.
George's Cemetery, Ealing.

He was born at Edinburgh in 1832, and received his education
in that city. He was apprenticed to an Edinburgh dentist by the
name of Mien, and when he reached his twenty-first year he removed
to London. This was in 1853. In 1857 he became a member of
the College of Dentists. In 1863 he passed the necessary examinations and became an M.R.C.S. and an L.D.S. He was for forty-
five years connected with the Middlesex Hospital. He delivered
lectures there on dental surgery and acted as Dental Surgeon, and
for many years was Consulting Surgeon to the Hospital.

He was subsequently elected to fill the position of Lecturer on
Dental Mechanics in the London School of Dental Surgery. This
position he held until 1879.

On July 26, 1880, the dental profession presented Mr. Tomes
a portrait of himself and to Mr. Turner an inscribed clock and a
purse of money.

In 1888 Mr. Turner was actively engaged in the management of
the Dental Hospital of London.

He was a member of the " Odontological Society." The British
Dental Association, in which he was an ever active member and
later its President, presented Mr. Turner, in 1890, with his portrait,
and a replica was also presented to Mrs. J. Smith Turner.

These facts, culled from the *British Dental Journal,* simply
show the high appreciation in which J. Smith Turner was held by
his colleagues, but they do not show the great work performed
by this man. His labor was unceasing to advance dentistry in
Great Britain. This was markedly in evidence in the labor he gave
to the passing of the " Dentists' Act." " For weeks, months, years,
night and day, the business was in hand. Parliamentary committees had to be attended and the House of Commons frequented
night after night."

This was the man that the dentistry of Great Britain honors
in memory to-day, and the dentists of the United States join with
their brethren there in mourning the fact that one of the few
laborers in the ranks who have unselfishly worked that the profession might live has passed away to be known no more among

men. The writer of this never knew J. Smith Turner personally. That fact is of no material consequence. The spirit that actuated this man has no need of personal recognition. It permeates space and becomes part of the moral force of the universe, recognized everywhere by those energized by the same power. It will live, and J. Smith Turner, though dead, will rouse up others in all lands to go forward in a crusade against the commercial, selfish spirit that has gradually attempted the destruction of the very heart of professional life. It is such as he that has made the dentistry of Great Britain a model for the best in the United States to copy. May the dentists of this land take seriously to heart the life of this man. It is the one great lesson needed here. The golden age is measured by many, not from the results following a high ethical standard, but by that which glitters for a season. That which is born to live must be that which the J. Smith Turners of all lands and of all ages have lain down their lives to bring to perfection.

Miscellany.

A More Simple Way of Making a Crown.—A more simple way of making the crown described in the October issue, page 796, is as follows:

After the tooth is prepared, swage a gold cap to fit the case, reinforce the cusps with solder, cut out the buccal surface, and prepare as described. Then fuse the Jenkins body to this surface, and there you have it. This body can be baked before 18-carat, or even 14-carat, solder will flow.—N. A. Stanley.

New Application of Soft or Velum Rubber (Joaquin Plet, *La Odontologia,* Madrid, October, 1903).—In the class of cases where the two cuspids may be the only remaining teeth, with large crowns and narrow necks, the close adaptation of hard rubber in a denture around these teeth becomes impossible. The case is then flasked and the wax removed in the ordinary way. The plaster teeth may have been previously trimmed slightly, then completely encircled by packing liberally the soft rubber.

Around this is then packed the rubber ordinarily used, when the case is vulcanized as usual. Care should be observed in finishing not to use scrapers or files, but a sharp knife, with both the knife and rubber wet. Some little force will be required to press the plate to place, when a snug adaptation will be attained, offering support to the plate superior to clasps and less harmful to tooth-structure.—P. B. McC.

Current News.

FOURTH INTERNATIONAL DENTAL CONGRESS, ST. LOUIS, MO., AUGUST 29 TO SEPTEMBER 3, 1904.

Committee of Organization.—H. J. Burkhart, Chairman, Batavia, N. Y.; E. C. Kirk, Secretary, Lock Box 1615, Philadelphia, Pa.; R. H. Hofheinz, Wm. Carr, W. E. Boardman, V. E. Turner, J. Y. Crawford, M. F. Finley, J. W. David, Wm. Crenshaw, Don M. Gallie, G. V. I. Brown, A. H. Peck, J. D. Patterson, B. L. Thorpe.

The Department of Congresses of the Universal Exposition, St. Louis, 1904, has nominated the Committee of Organization of the Fourth International Dental Congress which was appointed by the National Dental Association, and has instructed the committee thus appointed to proceed with the work of organization of said Congress.

Pursuant to the instructions of the Director of Congresses of the Universal Exposition, 1904, the Committee of Organization presents the subjoined outline of the plan of organization of the Dental Congress.

The Congress will be divided into two departments: Department A—SCIENCE (divided into four sections). Department B—APPLIED SCIENCE (divided into six sections).

DEPARTMENT A—SCIENCE.

I. Anatomy, Physiology, Histology, and Microscopy. Chairman, M. H. Cryer, 1420 Chestnut Street, Philadelphia, Pa.

II. Etiology, Pathology, and Bacteriology. Chairman, R. H. Hofheinz, Chamber of Commerce, Rochester, N. Y.

III. Chemistry and Metallurgy. Chairman, J. D. Hodgen, 1005 Sutter Street, San Francisco, Cal.

IV. Oral Hygiene, Prophylaxis, Materia Medica and Therapeutics, and Electro-therapeutics. Chairman, A. H. Peck, 92 State Street, Chicago, Ill.

DEPARTMENT B—APPLIED SCIENCE.

V. Oral Surgery. Chairman, G. V. I. Brown, 445 Milwaukee Avenue, Milwaukee, Wis.

VI. Orthodontia. Chairman, E. H. Angle, 1023 North Grand Avenue, St. Louis, Mo.

VII. Operative Dentistry. Chairman, C. N. Johnson, Marshall Field Building, Chicago, Ill.

VIII. Prosthesis. Chairman, C. R. Turner, Thirty-third and Locust Streets, Philadelphia, Pa.

IX. Education, Nomenclature, Literature, and History. Chairman, Truman W. Brophy, Marshall Field Building, Chicago, Ill.

X. Legislation. Chairman, Wm. Carr, 35 West Forty-sixth Street, New York, N. Y.

COMMITTEES.

Following are the committees appointed:

Finance.—Chairman, C. S. Butler, 680 Main Street, Buffalo, N. Y.

Programme.—Chairman, A. H. Peck, 92 State Street, Chicago, Ill.

Exhibits.—Chairman, D. M. Gallie, 100 State Street, Chicago, Ill.

Transportation.—(To be appointed.)

Reception.—Chairman, B. Holly Smith, 1007 Madison Avenue, Baltimore, Md.

Registration.—Chairman, B. L. Thorpe, 3666 Olive Street, St. Louis, Mo.

Printing and Publication.—Chairman, W. E. Boardman, 184 Boylston Street, Boston, Mass.

Conference with State and Local Dental Societies.—Chairman, J. A. Libbey, 524 Penn Avenue, Pittsburg, Pa.

Dental Legislation.—Chairman, Wm. Carr, 35 West Forty-sixth Street, New York, New York.

Auditing.—(Committee of Organization.)

Invitation.—Chairman, L. G. Noel, 527½ Church Street, Nashville, Tenn.

Membership.—Chairman, J. D. Patterson, Keith and Perry Building, Kansas City, Mo.

Educational Methods.—Chairman, T. W. Brophy, Marshall Field Building, Chicago, Ill.

Oral Surgery.—Chairman, G. V. I. Brown, 445 Milwaukee Avenue, Milwaukee, Wis.

Prosthetic Dentistry.—Chairman, C. R. Turner, Thirty-third and Locust Streets, Philadelphia, Pa.

Local Committee of Arrangements and Reception.—Chairman, Wm. Conrad, 3666 Olive Street, St. Louis, Mo.

Essays.—Chairman, Wilbur F. Litch, 1500 Locust Street, Philadelphia, Pa.

History of Dentistry.—Chairman, Wm. H. Trueman, 900 Spruce Street, Philadelphia, Pa.

Nomenclature.—Chairman, A. H. Thompson, 720 Kansas Avenue, Topeka, Kan.

Promotion of Appointment of Dental Surgeons in the Armies and Navies of the World.—Chairman, Williams Donnally, 1018 Fourteenth Street N. W., Washington, D. C.

Care of the Teeth of the Poor.—Chairman, Thomas Fillebrown, 175 Newbury Street, Boston, Mass.

Etiology, Pathology, and Bacteriology.—Chairman, R. H. Hofheinz, Chamber of Commerce, Rochester, N. Y.

Prize Essays.—Chairman, James Truman, 4505 Chester Avenue, Philadelphia, Pa.

Oral Hygiene, Prophylaxis, Materia Medica and Therapeutics, and Electro-therapeutics.—Chairman, A. H. Peck, 92 State Street, Chicago, Ill.

Operative Dentistry.—Chairman, C. N. Johnson, Marshall Field Building, Chicago, Ill.

Resolutions.—Chairman, J. Y. Crawford, Jackson Building, Nashville, Tenn.

Clinics.—Chairman, J. P. Gray, 212 North Spruce Street, Nashville, Tenn.

Nominations.—Chairman, A. H. Peck, 92 State Street, Chicago, Ill.; W. E. Boardman, 184 Boylston Street, Boston, Mass.; M. R. Windhorst, 3518 Morgan Street, St. Louis, Mo.; Wm. Conrad, 3666 Olive Street, St. Louis, Mo.

Ad Interim.—Chairman, G. V. I. Brown, 445 Milwaukee Avenue, Milwaukee, Wis.

The officers of the Congress, president, vice-presidents, secretary, and treasurer, will be elected by the Congress at large at the time of the meeting, and will be nominated by the Nominating Committee.

The Fourth International Dental Congress, which will be held August 29 to September 3, inclusive, 1904, will be representative of the existing status of dentistry throughout the world. It is intended further that the Congress shall set forth the history and material progress of dentistry from its crude beginnings through its developmental stages, up to its present condition as a scientific profession.

The International Dental Congress is but one of the large number of congresses to be held during the period of the Louisiana Purchase Exposition, and these in their entirety are intended to exhibit the intellectual progress of the world, as the Exposition will set forth the material progress which has taken place since the Columbian Exposition in 1893.

It is important that each member of the dental profession in America regard this effort to hold an International Dental Congress as a matter in which he has an individual interest, and one which he is under obligation to personally help towards a successful issue. The dental profession of America has not only its own professional record to maintain with a just pride, but, as it is called upon to act the part of host in a gathering of our colleagues from all parts of the world, it has to sustain the reputation of American hospitality as well.

The Committee of Organization appeals earnestly to each member of the profession to do his part in making the Congress a success. Later bulletins will be issued setting forth the personnel of the organization and other particulars, when the details have been more fully arranged.

H. J. BURKHART, *Chairman.*
E. C. KIRK, *Secretary.*

Approved:
HOWARD J. ROGERS,
    Director of Congresses.
DAVID R. FRANCIS,
    President of Exposition.

COMMITTEE ON STATE AND LOCAL ORGANIZATIONS.

(J. A. Libbey, Chairman, 524 Penn Avenue, Pittsburg, Pa.)

The Committee on State and Local Organizations is a committee appointed by the Committee of Organization of the Fourth International Congress with the object of promoting the interests of the Congress in the several States of the Union. Each member of the committee is charged with the duty of receiving applications for membership in the Congress under the rules governing membership as prescribed by the Committee on Membership and approved by the Committee of Organization. These rules provide that *membership in the Congress shall be open to all reputable legally qualified practitioners of dentistry.* Membership in a State or local society is not a necessary qualification for membership in the Congress.

Each State chairman, as named below, is furnished with official application blanks and is authorized to accept the membership fee of ten dollars from all eligible applicants within his State. The State chairman will at once forward the fee and official application with his indorsement to the chairman of the Finance Committee, who will issue the official certificate conferring membership in the Congress. No application from any of the States will be accepted by the chairman of the Finance Committee unless approved by the State chairman, whose indorsement is a certification of eligibility under the membership rules.

A certificate of membership in the Congress will entitle the holder thereof to all the rights and privileges of the Congress, the right of debate, and of voting on all questions which the Congress will be called upon to decide. It will also entitle the member to one copy of the official transactions when published and to participation in all the events for social entertainment which will be officially provided at the time of the Congress.

The attention of all reputable legally qualified practitioners of dentistry is called to the foregoing plan authorized by the Committee of Organization for securing membership in the Congress, and the committee earnestly appeals to each eligible practitioner in the United States who is interested in the success of this great international meeting to make application at once through his State chairman for a membership certificate. By acting promptly in this matter the purpose of the committee to make the Fourth

International Dental Congress the largest and most successful meeting of dentists ever held will be realized, and the Congress will thus be placed upon a sound financial basis.

Let every one make it his individual business to help at least to the extent of enrolling himself as a member and the success of the undertaking will be quickly assured. Apply at once to your State chairman. The State chairmen already appointed are:

General Chairman.—J. A. Libbey, 524 Penn Avenue, Pittsburg, Pa.

Alabama.—H. Clay Hassell, Tuscaloosa.

Arkansas.—W. H. Buckley, 510½ Main Street, Little Rock.

California.—J. L. Pease, 1016 Clay Street, Oakland.

Colorado.—H. A. Fynn, 500 California Building, Denver.

Connecticut.—Henry McManus, 80 Pratt Street, Hartford.

Delaware.—C. R. Jeffries, New Century Building, Wilmington.

District of Columbia.—W. N. Cogan, The Sherman, Washington.

Florida.—W. G. Mason, Tampa.

Georgia.—H. H. Johnson, Macon.

Hawaii.—M. E. Grossman, Box 744, Honolulu.

Idaho.—J. B. Burns, Payette.

Illinois.—J. E. Hinkins, 131 East Fifty-third Street, Chicago.

Indiana.—H. C. Kahlo, 115 East New York Street, Indianapolis.

Iowa.—W. R. Clark, Clear Lake.

Kansas.—G. A. Esterly, Lawrence.

Kentucky.—H. B. Tileston, 314 Equitable Building, Louisville.

Louisiana.—Jules J. Sarrazin, 108 Bourbon Street, New Orleans.

Maine.—H. A. Kelley, 609 Congress Street, Portland.

Maryland.—W. G. Foster, 813 Eutaw Street, Baltimore.

Massachusetts.—M. C. Smith, 3 Lee Hall, Lynn.

Michigan.—G. S. Shattuck, 539 Fourth Avenue, Detroit.

Minnesota.—C. A. Van Duzce, 51 Germania Bank Building, St. Paul.

Mississippi.—W. R. Wright, Jackson.

Missouri.—J. W. Hull, Altman Building, Kansas City.

Montana.—G. E. Longeway, Great Falls.

Nebraska.—H. A. Shannon, 1136 " O" Street, Lincoln.

New Hampshire.—E. C. Blaisdell, Portsmouth.

New Jersey.—Alphonso Irwin, 425 Cooper Street, Camden.

New York.—B. C. Nash, 142 West Seventy-eighth Street, New York City.

North Carolina.—C. L. Alexander, Charlotte.

Ohio.—Henry Barnes, 1415 New England Building, Cleveland.

Oklahoma.—T. P. Bringhurst, Shawnee.

Oregon.—S. J. Barber, Macleay Building, Portland.

Pennsylvania.—H. E. Roberts, 1516 Locust Street, Philadelphia.

Rhode Island.—D. F. Keefe, 315 Butler Exchange, Providence.

South Carolina.—J. T. Calvert, Spartanburg.

South Dakota.—E. S. O'Neil, Canton.

Tennessee.—W. P. Sims, Jackson Building, Nashville.

Texas.—J. G. Fife, Dallas.

Utah.—W. L. Ellerbeck, 21 Hooper Building Salt Lake City.

Vermont.—S. D. Hodge, Burlington.

Virginia.—F. W. Stiff, 2101 Churchill Avenue, Richmond.

Washington.—G. W. Stryker, Everett.

West Virginia.—H. H. Harrison, 1141 Main Street, Wheeling.

Wisconsin.—A. D. Gropper, 401 East Water Street, Milwaukee.

For the Committee of Organization,

EDWARD C. KIRK,
Secretary.

DENTAL COMMISSIONERS OF CONNECTICUT.

THE Dental Commissioners of the State of Connecticut hereby give notice that they will meet at Hartford, on Thursday, Friday, and Saturday, July 14, 15, 16, 1904, respectively, to examine applicants for license to practise dentistry, and for the transaction of any other proper business.

The practical examination in operative and prosthetic dentistry will be held Thursday, July 14, at 9 A.M., in Putnam Phalanx Armory, corner Haynes and Pearl Streets.

The written theoretic examination will be held Friday and Saturday, July 15 and 16, at the Capitol.

All applicants should apply to the Recorder for proper blanks, and for the revised rules for conducting the examinations.

Application blanks must be carefully filled in and sworn to, and with fee, twenty-five dollars, filed with the Recorder on or before July 7, 1904. Examination Fee must be forwarded by Money Order or Certified Check.

By direction of the Dental Commissioners.

J. TENNY BARKER,
Recorder.

FOURTH INTERNATIONAL DENTAL CONGRESS BANQUET.

THE Fourth International Dental Congress Banquet will be held on September 1, 1904, at 8 P.M., in the Coliseum Building adjoining the Congress Hall. The price per plate is three dollars. It is requested that all who expect to attend will send their names and money to Dr. A. H. Fuller, P. O. Lock-Box 604, St. Louis, Mo., at once, and not later than August 20. Arrangements to pay can be made with Dr. A. H. Fuller at the time of registration, provided notice is given before August 20.

G. A. BOWMAN,
A. H. FULLER,
ADAM FLICKINGER,
Banquet Committee.

NATIONAL ASSOCIATION OF DENTAL EXAMINERS.

THE National Association of Dental Examiners will hold their annual meeting in the Coliseum Building, corner of Thirteenth and Olive Streets, St. Louis, Mo., on the 25th, 26th, and 27th of August, beginning promptly at 10 A.M. Telephone and telegraph offices in the building. Hotel accommodations will be secured for the members. Special railroad rates will be secured for those in the East desiring to attend, trains leaving on the 23d from New York.

The Committee on Railroad Accommodations for the East have made arrangements for fast through Pullman service to St. Louis from New York with the Delaware and Lackawanna Railroad. Two special Pullman cars will leave New York Tuesday, August 23, at 10 A.M. The cost of our excursion including berth each way will be $35.50. A proportionate reduction is made for those going from

Buffalo, Toledo, Fort Wayne, and cities on the line connecting with the Wabash Railroad. To those desiring to go in the special cars, send notice to Charles A. Meeker, D.D.S., Secretary of the National Association Dental Examiners, or to Guy Adams, General Passenger Agent of the Delaware and Lackawana Railroad. Accommodations have been secured for the National Association of Dental Examiners at the Franklin Hotel, northwest corner of Sarah and Westminster Place, with rates from $1.50 to $6.00 per day, European plan. Hotel first-class. Secure rooms by writing to E. C. Dunnavant, St. Louis Service Company, Seventh and Olive Streets, St. Louis, Mo.

CHARLES A. MEEKER, D.D.S.,
Secretary.

AMERICAN SOCIETY OF ORTHODONTISTS.

A SPECIAL meeting of the American Society of Orthodontists will be held in the rooms of the Orthodontia Section of the Fourth International Dental Congress, in the Coliseum, St. Louis, at 10 A.M., August 29, 1904.

ANNA HOPKINS,
Secretary.

" F. D. I." FÉDÉRATION DENTAIRE INTERNATIONALE.

THE next (fourth annual) meeting will be held in the Coliseum Building, St. Louis, Mo., August 26 and 27, 1904. The first session will convene under the presidency of Dr. Charles Godon, at 11 A.M. There will be a meeting of the Executive Council on Thursday, the 25th, at the Hotel Jefferson, at 10 A.M.

The Section on Education will meet at 3 P.M. Friday; the Section on Hygiene and Public Dental Service, at 3 P.M. Friday; the Section on International Dental Press, at 4.30 P.M. Friday.

The officers of the Sections are:

Education.—President, Dr. T. W. Brophy; Vice-Presidents, Dr. E. C. Kirk, Dr. W. B. Paterson, and Dr. O. Zsigmondy; Secretaries, Dr. M. Roy and Dr. R. B. Weiser.

Hygiene and Public Dental Service.—President, Dr. W. D. Miller; Vice-Presidents, Dr. Cunningham, Dr. Forberg, Dr. Jenkins, and Dr. Rose; Secretaries, Dr. R. Heide, Dr. Sauvez, and Dr. R. B. Weiser.

Commission of the International Dental Press.—President, Dr. E. Forberg; Dr. A. W. Harlan; Secretary, Dr. E. Papot.

Executive Council.—President, Dr. Charles Godon; Vice-Presidents, Dr. A. W. Harlan, Dr. W. D. Miller; Secretary, Dr. E. Sauvez; Treasurer, Dr. F. Aguilar.

Members.—Dr. George Cunningham, Dr. E. Forberg, Dr. R. B. Weiser, Dr. J. E. Grevers, Dr. F. Heisse, Dr. Klingelhofer.

On behalf of the Federation,

A. W. HARLAN,
Vice-President.

1122 BROADWAY, NEW YORK CITY, June 16, 1904.

NATIONAL ASSOCIATION OF DENTAL FACULTIES.

THE vote upon the motion to change the present order of four years with a seven months' course to three years and a seven months' course, was as follows: Those marked ✕ voted yes; those marked O no. The result will be seen to have been 21 yes, 24 no, and 2 not voting.

O 1. Baltimore College of Dental Surgery, Baltimore, Md. Dr. M. W. Foster, Dean, No. 9 West Franklin Street.

✕ 2. Pennsylvania College of Dental Surgery, Philadelphia, Pa. Dr. Wilbur F. Litch, Dean, 1507 Walnut Street.

✕ 3. Philadelphia Dental College, Philadelphia, Pa. Dr. S. H. Guilford, Dean, 1728 Chestnut Street.

✕ 4. New York College of Dentistry, New York City. Dr. Faneuil D. Weisse, Dean, 205 East Twenty-third Street.

O 5. Tufts College Dental School, Boston, Mass. Dr. Harold Williams, Dean.

O 6. Dental College of the University of Michigan, Ann Arbor, Mich.

O 7. University of Iowa College of Dentistry, Iowa City, Iowa. Dr. W. S. Hosford, Dean.

N.V. 8. Chicago College of Dental Surgery, Chicago, Ill. Dr. Truman W. Brophy, Dean, 126 State Street.

O 9. Dental Department University of Pennsylvania, Philadelphia, Pa.   Dr. E. C. Kirk, Dean, corner Thirty-third and Locust Streets.

X   10. Ohio College of Dental Surgery, Cincinnati, Ohio.   Dr. H. A. Smith, Dean, 116 Garfield Place.

X   11. University of California College of Dentistry, San Francisco, Cal.   Dr. H. P. Carleton, Dean, Crocker Building.

O   12. Kansas City Dental College, Kansas City, Mo.   Dr. Charles C. Allen, Secretary.

N.Y.   13. Dental Department of Washington University (Missouri Dental College), St. Louis, Mo.   Dr. J. H. Kennerly, Dean, 2639 Locust Street.

X   14. Department of Dentistry of Vanderbilt University, Nashville, Tenn.   Dr. D. R. Stubblefield, Dean.

X   15. Indiana Dental College, Indianapolis, Ind.   Dr. George E. Hunt, Dean, Ohio and Delaware Streets.

O   16. Northwestern University Dental School, Chicago, Ill. Dr. G. V. Black, Dean, corner Lake and Dearborn Streets.

O   17. University of Tennessee, Department of Dentistry, Nashville, Tenn.   Dr. J. P. Gray, Dean, Spruce and Church Streets.

18. School of Dentistry Meharry Medical College, Nashville, Tenn.   Dr. George E. Hubbard, Dean.   (Not represented.)

X   19. Southern Dental College, Atlanta, Ga.   Dr. S. W. Foster, Dean, 63 Inman Building.

X   20. Louisville College of Dentistry, Louisville, Ky.   Dr. W. E. Grant, Dean.

21. Dental Department of the National University, Washington, D. C.   Dr. J. Roland Walton, Dean, 700 Tenth Street, N. W. (Not represented.)

X   22. Dental Department University of Maryland, Baltimore, Md.   Dr. F. J. S. Gorgas, Dean, 845 North Eutaw Street.

23. Dental Department of Columbia University, Washington, D. C.   Dr. J. Hall Lewis, Dean, 1023 Vermont Avenue, N. W. (Not represented.)

O   24. Royal College of Dental Surgeons of Ontario, Toronto, Canada.   Dr. J. B. Willmott, Dean.

O   25. College of Dentistry University of Minnesota, Minneapolis, Minn.   Dr. W. P. Dickinson, Dean, Andrews Building.

O   26. Dental Department of Detroit Medical College, Detroit, Mich.   Dr. H. O. Walker, Secretary, 27 Adams Avenue, East.

2?. Western Reserve University, Cleveland, Ohio. Dr. W. H. Whitslar, Secretary, 29 Euclid Avenue. (Not represented.)

X 28. Western Dental College, Kansas City, Mo. Dr. D. J. McMillan, Dean, Eleventh and Locust Streets.

X 29. University of Buffalo, Dental Department, Buffalo, N. Y. Dr. W. C. Barrett, Dean, 208 Franklin Street.

O 30. University College of Medicine and Surgery, Dental Department, Richmond, Va. Dr. L. M. Cowardin, Dean.

31. Birmingham Dental College, Birmingham, Ala. Dr. Chas. A. Merrill, Dean, Cholifoux Building. (Not represented.)

X 3?. Atlanta Dental College, Atlanta, Ga. Dr. H. R. Jewett, Dean, 515 The Grand.

33. Cincinnati College of Dental Surgery, Cincinnati, Ohio. Dr. G. S. Juukerman, Dean, 231 West Court Street. (Not represented.)

O 34. Dental Department of Howard University, Washington, D. C. Dr. F. J. Shadd, Secretary, 901 R Street, N. W.

X 35. Marion-Sims Dental College, St. Louis, Mo. Dr. M. C. Marshall, Dean, 610 Chemical Building.

X 36. New York Dental School, New York City. Dr. C. Milton Ford, Dean, 21S West One-Hundred-and-Thirty-fifth Street.

X 37. College of Dentistry Ohio Medical University, Columbus, Ohio. Dr. L. P. Bethel, Dean, Columbus, Ohio.

O 38. Baltimore Medical College Dental Department, Baltimore, Md. Dr. W. A. Montell, Dean, 833 North Eutaw Street.

O 39. Milwaukee Medical College Dental Department, Milwaukee, Wis. Dr. H. J. Banzhaf, Dean, Ninth and Wells Avenue.

O 40. North Pacific Dental College, Portland, Ore. Dr. H. C. Miller, Dean, Oregonian Building.

O 41. Dental Department University of Omaha, Omaha, Neb. Dr. A. O. Hunt, Dean, Bee Building.

O 4?. Colorado College of Dental Surgery, Denver, Col. Dr. W. T. Chambers, Dean California Building.

O 43. Pittsburg Dental college, Department of Western University of Pennsylania, Pittsburg, Pa. Dr. W. H. Fundenburg, Dean.

X 44. Dental Department College of Physicians and Surgeons, San Francisco, Cal. Dr. Charles Boxton, Dean.

X 45. Medico-Chirurgical College of Philadelphia, Department of Dentistry, Philadelphia, Pa. Dr. R. H. Nones, Dean, Cherry Street above Seventeenth.

X   46. College of Dentistry University of Southern California, Los Angeles, Cal.   Dr. Garrett Newkirk, Dean, 203 South Broadway.

O   47. School of Dentistry University of Illinois, Chicago, Ill. Dr. B. J. Cigrand, Dean.

X   48. Central College of Dentistry, Indianapolis, Ind.   Dr. M. F. Ault, Dean.

O   49. Georgetown University Dental Department, Washington, D. C.   Dr. W. N. Cogan, Dean, The Sherman.

O   50. New Orleans College of Dentistry, New Orleans, La. Dr. A. G. Frederichs, Dean.

X   51. Keokuk Dental College, Keokuk, Iowa.   Dr. B. C. Hinkley, Dean.

O   P. and S. of Wisconsin.

O   Lincoln Dental College.

BANQUET TO DR. SCHOLL.

In honor of Dr. W. H. Scholl, who is next to the oldest practising dentist in this section of the State, the members of the Lebanon Valley Dental Association, which met in Reading, gave a complimentary banquet at the Mansion House to Dr. and Mrs. Scholl.

The banquet was a handsome compliment to the guests of the evening, who occupied posts of honor at the head of the tables.   The latter sparkled with silver and cut glass.   The carnations used in the decorations were presented by Dr. and Mrs. Charles R. Scholl, the former being a son of the couple.   Covers were laid for more than sixty guests.   Quite a number of the members were accompanied by their wives.

In responding, Dr. Scholl thanked the members for the handsome compliment to Mrs. Scholl and himself, and said it was appreciated at its true value.   He reviewed at length his forty-five years' experience as a practising dentist, and gave many interesting reminiscences.   He said he was the first graduate in dentistry to practise in this county, and that many changes had occurred in methods since that time.   When he first entered the profession everything was done by hand, as no machinery had been introduced.

" The modern appliances do not only make the work easier and quicker, but the comfortable chair affords the patient a good resting-place, in comparison with the chair used forty years ago. Creosote and chloroform were our alleviators.

" It is well to remember, however, especially the younger members of the profession, that our advanced position is due to the unselfishness of the pioneers and their successors who made known their discoveries through teaching, through the dental journals, and, best of all, through the dental associations. There were men who did as fine work in operative dentistry as any that is done to-day—without the rubber dam."

The guests wore badges which bore excellent portraits of Dr. and Mrs. Scholl.

LEBANON VALLEY DENTAL ASSOCIATION.

THE annual meeting of the Lebanon Valley Dental Association, held at the Mansion House, Reading, Pa., was one of the most interesting gatherings of the profession held for several years. The turnout was larger than usual.

The greater part of the session to-day was devoted to clinics and demonstrations. Dr. P. K. Filbert, of Pottsville, had a clinic on " Gold Filling," while Dr. C. R. Scholl, of Reading, followed and spoke on " Porcelain and Gutta-Percha Fillings." Dr. H. W. Bohn, of Reading, had a clinic on " Porcelain Fillings."

These were followed by demonstrations by the exhibitors who are attending the convention: Demonstration of Hammond electric furnace by S. S. White Dental Manufacturing Company, Philadelphia; demonstration of Jenkins low-fusing porcelain by L. D. Caulk, Philadelphia; demonstration of Sharp's seamless crown machine by Gideon Sibley, Philadelphia; demonstration of Price furnace and new hydraulic engine by Lee Smith & Son, Pittsburg; presentation of dental curios, Dr. W. H. Scholl, Reading.

These officers were chosen for the ensuing year: President, Dr. H. W. Bohn, Reading; Vice-President, Dr. R. J. Wall, Harrisburg; Recording Secretary, Dr. H. J. Herbine, Pottsville; Corresponding Secretary, Dr P. K. Filbert, Pottsville; Treasurer, Dr. C. B. Wagner, Lebanon.

The next convention will be held at Pottstown or in Reading. A number favor meeting in Reading again, as the most central point.

A vote of thanks was tendered to the members of the Reading society.

NORTHERN IOWA DENTAL SOCIETY.

THE tenth annual meeting of the Northern Iowa Dental Society will be held at Waterloo, Iowa, July 26, 27, and 28, 1904. The officers are William Finn, President, Cedar Rapids; A. W. Beach, Vice-President, and Superintendent of Clinics, Sheldon; C. L. Topliff, Secretary, Decorah; H. W. Riser, Treasurer, Lansing.

WISCONSIN STATE DENTAL SOCIETY.

THE thirty-fourth annual meeting of the Wisconsin State Dental Society will be held in Manitowoc, July 19 to 21, 1904. A cordial invitation is extended to all ethical practitioners to meet with us.

A. G. FEE,
President.
W. H. MUELLER,
Secretary.

SUPREME CHAPTER, DELTA SIGMA DELTA.

THE twentieth annual meeting of the Supreme Chapter, Delta Sigma Delta Fraternity will be held Wednesday, August 31, 1904, at St. Louis, Mo. George E. Hunt, 131 E. Ohio Street, Indianapolis, is chairman of the Committee on Arrangements.

CANADIAN DENTAL ASSOCIATION.

THE Canadian Dental Association will hold its next meeting at Toronto, Ontario, September 6, 7, and 8, 1904.

W. CECIL TROTTER,
Secretary.

THE

International Dental Journal.

VOL. XXV. . AUGUST, 1904. No. 8.

Original Communications.[1]

A METHOD FOR REPRODUCING THE NATURAL CON-
TOUR OF ARTIFICIAL TEETH ON THE LINGUAL
AND PALATAL SURFACES OF ARTIFICIAL DEN-
TURES.[2]

BY WILLIAM MIDDLETON FINE, D.D.S., PHILADELPHIA.

MR. PRESIDENT AND MEMBERS OF THE ACADEMY OF STO-
MATOLOGY,—In describing this method for making and finishing
dentures, particularly vulcanite work, I shall refrain from going
into detail regarding the best methods for taking impressions,
running models, etc., but I will state at once that a good plaster-of-
Paris impression is positively essential for the attainment of a good
result.

At the thirty-third annual meeting of the New Jersey State
Dental Society, held at Asbury Park, N. J., July, 1903, I had the
pleasure of meeting Dr. George H. Wilson, Professor of Prosthesis
and Metallurgy, Department of Dentistry of the Western Reserve
University, and while watching one of his demonstrations, the idea

---

[1] The editor and publishers are not responsible for the views of authors
of papers published in this department, nor for any claim to novelty, or
otherwise, that may be made by them. No papers will be received for this
department that have appeared in any other journal published in the
country.

[2] Read before the Academy of Stomatology, Philadelphia, January 26,
1904.

of carving the wax to obtain the natural contour of the teeth on the lingual and palatal surfaces came to me.   Therefore this method is not entirely original.

Dr. George B. Snow, of Buffalo, N. Y., published an article in the *Dental Advertiser,* April, 1899, relating to the Lingual Conformation of Dental Plates; but Dr. Snow confines his ideas to the rugæ and the thickness of the plate.   The late Dr. Charles J. Essig also made reference to a method for carving the lingual and palatal surfaces of artificial dentures.   Again let me state that I do not claim priority nor originality in method of applying the rugæ, tinning the models, etc., but from what I have been able to learn from men of prominence in the dental profession, and from examination of our literature, I feel justified in saying that the method of carving the wax to obtain the natural contour of the teeth on the lingual and palatal surfaces, to which I have the pleasure of directing your attention, has not heretofore been published or generally used.

First, we take a good plaster-of-Paris impression, and if a vacuum chamber is used, one should be carved in the impression. The next step is the model, from that the wax bite, then the articulation and the making of the base plate and the trying in of the piece.   Every dentist is familiar with this phase of the work. The teeth are set up in the usual way in wax.   The gums are carved and the whole denture made to reproduce the lost teeth and supporting tissues.   After this operation is carried out in detail, the case is tried in the mouth, when, if found to be perfectly satisfactory in every way, the patient is dismissed and the case taken to the laboratory for finishing.   Here is where we commune with nature; we strive to reproduce the beautiful and natural, the teeth and gums, the rugæ and all the peculiarities of the roof of the mouth.   We try to be artistic and practical at the same time, though it is hardly possible that the dentist will ever be able to make an appliance so near to nature's models that one cannot detect the difference.

In carving the lingual and palatal surfaces to represent the natural teeth, I have a small spatula that I use for this particular work.   It is made from a broken plug finishing file No. 101, S. S. White, and shaped like the diagram.   **(Fig. 1.)**

The end A is the most used in contouring the wax, as I will describe.   Take the articulator in your left hand and open it so that the upper denture is in front of you and at the top; start at the last tooth on the left side and proceed to carve the wax, using

FIG. 1.

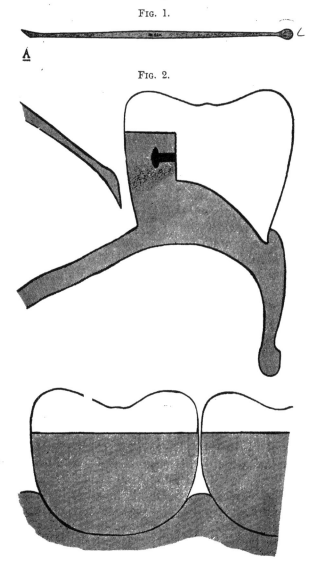

FIG. 2.

point A of the wax spatula, carved downward, using the palatal surface of the porcelain tooth as your guide, and shape up the wax to represent the natural tooth as it stands in the natural gum. (Fig. 2.)

After you have formed the palatal surface of the second molar, proceed to the first, and so on around the arch of the denture until you have completed the work. Then apply the rugæ. The method of technique taught by Dr. A. Dewitt Gritman to the Freshman classes at the University of Pennsylvania is employed. To do this one must have several pure tin or zinc dies; tin is best. Take an impression of your own mouth to start with, or, better still, if the patient has well-defined rugæ, take an impression and make the die; after you have the die, take a piece of No. 40 tin-foil and burnish it over the rugæ on the die, using the rounded end of a lead-pencil eraser to press the foil into contact with the die. If a metal burnisher is used, it will be likely to tear holes in the tin-foil, but a soft eraser or piece of rubber will give a good impression and will not do any damage. A piece of tin-foil should be used large enough to cover the entire palatal surface of the wax denture, and have a free margin of tin-foil one-quarter inch in addition. After the burnishing is completed, remove carefully and fill the impressions in the tin-foil (the side that comes next to the die) with wax, by melting it on a spatula and dropping it on the tin-foil; then heat the spatula quite hot and smooth it down. By this means we have a smooth surface that is brought into contact with the palatal surface of the wax base-plate. After this is done, press the piece, wax side down, into the wax base-plate and finish around the teeth by burnishing very carefully, but do not burnish the edges of the tin-foil down flat, allow it to stand up at right angles so that when the case is invested the free edges will be embedded in the plaster and hold the tin-foil in place. The result is a tin-foil covering to the palatal surface of the wax denture, and after the tin-foil has been applied to the gums, to which it is burnished on in the same way, the case is ready to flask. After the wax has been boiled out, cover the model with very thin tin-foil, No. 4 or 6. We have now a tin-faced matrix in which to pack the rubber. The case is then packed with rubber in the usual way, placing the pink rubber for the gums in around the teeth first, after this is completed pack in the red rubber. Close the flask and vulcanize.

Now, a few words regarding flasking, finishing, etc., etc. Flask the cases in the usual way; any style flask may be used; separate the flask, remove wax, pack in rubber, and place a piece of the waxed cloth (that which comes over the rubber as we purchase it from the dental depots) between the two sections of the flask so that you may separate them and ascertain if you have enough rubber; do not have too much and do not cut too many vents for the surplus material to flow out; if you do, the rubber will not be under the same steady pressure when vulcanizing that it should be. Do not close the flask with too much pressure at first, do this gradually. After the flask is closed, place it in the vulcanizer with cold water, fasten the lid down tight, and proceed to vulcanize. Allow the vulcanizer to run for about ten minutes and then open the safety valve and let the air out. Then take from one-half to three-quarters of an hour to run the vulcanizer up to 320°, and then vulcanize at that point for one hour and a half. This will give you a good substantial plate and one that will take a very high polish. In finishing the cases, it is necessary to scrape but very little if the case has been properly waxed up and tinned. If necessary to scrape, use a very sharp pointed scraper and scrape around the teeth and between them first, the rest of the plate in the usual way. Polish with pumice and felt cone, pumice and stiff brush-wheel, chalk and stiff brush-wheel, chalk and soft brush-wheel, and last a very soft brush-wheel and rouge. If a greater polish is desired, use a chamois wheel and rouge. A still greater polish may be obtained with dry plaster of Paris and oil, using the finger-tip to polish with. Clean the rouge away from the plates with a soft laboratory brush and castile soap.

By this method dentures can be made much thinner and present a more artistic appearance, and they are more natural. They are sure to please those who are unfortunate enough to be compelled to use an artificial appliance. This method may be used in partial cases, and is by no means confined to a full case. I use it in partial cases, both vulcanite and gold with vulcanite attachments. Even in a case of three teeth the patient will tell you how much lighter and thinner the plate feels. They can speak more distinctly and it is easier for them to masticate their food.

Instead of finishing the denture up smooth to the porcelain teeth along the masticating surfaces, as shown in Fig. 3, the case is given a more natural appearance along the gum line on the palatal surface, as shown in Fig. 4. In Fig. 3 is presented the older method of waxing up the case, but in Fig. 4 is given the newer method of carving to represent the natural tooth. One can easily appreciate the " feel" of the denture to the patient and how much lighter the denture is in weight.

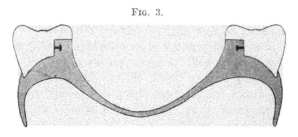

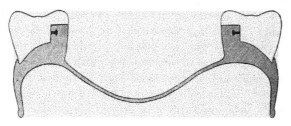

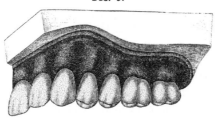

Fig. 5 shows section of a full case finished and ready for the mouth. Sometimes I carve the wax in such a way as to allow of the free passage of floss-silk between the teeth to the gum line. The saliva fills the spaces between the teeth on the denture in the same way that it does in a normal mouth. This doubtless aids in the articulation of words, also in the mastication of food by allowing the saliva to flow down the outside of the plate, over and between the teeth, as it does normally and mixes more thoroughly with the food. The rugæ also aids in the articulation of words and mastication of food. When the palatal surface of the

Fig. 6.

denture is smooth, the tongue has but little power to hold a morsel of food upon it, while with the rugæ the food is easily managed. The importance of the rugæ has been set forth by Dr. Burchard, Dr. Harrison Allen, Dr. Charles J. Essig, Dr. George B. Snow, and others. Some professional men object to the spaces between the teeth on artificial dentures, claiming they are too difficult to keep clean. Is it not the proper thing to clean one's own teeth with floss-silk? Why not a denture? Those who wear artificial appliances should take as good care of them as those who have all the natural teeth in place, using a tooth-brush, floss-silk, tooth-powder, and antiseptic washes.

Articulate speech consists of a modification of the voice by means of the lips, tongue, teeth, palatal arch, and rugæ, and various modifications of the oral cavity and its contents. The true sounds come from the vocal cords. The dome of the oral cavity assists in the modification, and I believe if the spaces are placed between the teeth on dentures, to correspond to the natural teeth, there should

FIG. 7.

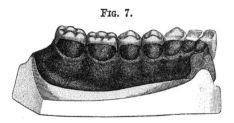

be nearly the same modification of the voice. Of course, a denture, no matter what kind or style, changes the voice slightly. We get nearer to nature by reproducing the rugæ and each tooth accurately.

The peculiar metallic hissing sounds produced by an attempt to pronounce the letter " s," especially in such words as " suscepti-bilities," involving a multiplication of " s " sounds when a smooth surface is given to the denture, is entirely obviated by the use of the rugæ. The sound is broken when it comes in contact with the rugæ and is softened. Or, for example, in singing or talking in a vacant room, the voice has a certain tone. Now, if the room be changed by building off the corners with boards or curtains, the tone of the voice is also changed. This same principle holds good in prosthetic dentistry. Another example: A bridge from the first bicuspid to the third molar, the space between filled with dummies; a singer will tell you that such a piece will change the voice, sometimes to such an extent that it is almost impossible to reach certain notes. It is evident that we must try to reproduce the natural mouth as nearly as possible.

The lower denture should be made in the same way as the upper denture, with the exception of the rugæ, etc. There is a slight depression below the necks of the teeth on the lingual aspect of the lower jaw in the normal mouth. This is reproduced in the lower denture, as is shown diagrammatically in Fig. 6.

Fig. 7 shows a section of a full lower case ready for the mouth.

NON-EXPANDING PLASTER.

BY P. B. M'CULLOUGH, D.D.S., PHILADELPHIA.

WHAT degree of credit for priority attaches to the following original experiments with plaster the writer is unable to state. It would seem that credit for fixing definitely the treatment of the water might be assumed. The writer first saw in a pamphlet advertising Dodel elevators, entitled "Pointers for Dentists," the statement that plaster mixed with lime-water would not shrink.

Following this the writer, as a test to prevent "expansion," used lime-water that had been prepared for domestic use. This water had been filtered, then boiled, and when cold lime had been added to saturation.

A mix of plaster was made with this water and poured in glass tubes; that the tubes did not crack after several months was evidence that the plaster had not expanded. As the stock of lime-water was reduced by its use in the laboratory, water as drawn from the supply pipes was added as required. Later a second test was made, and all the tubes cracked within twelve minutes. That the first tests were made with boiled water and the second with water without boiling made it clear that the water must be boiled to prevent expansion; otherwise the addition of lime makes no perceptible difference. In order to establish definitely wherein the secret lay, the following tests were made. A quantity of water was filtered, then boiled for fifteen minutes, when cold unslaked lime was added in excess of saturation. When the solution had become clear, it was decanted into a smaller bottle, that the sediment might not be stirred up in handling. With this water a mix of plaster was made of the ordinary consistency and placed in a glass tube, tapping the tube on the bench to insure a solid filling. After several hours it was soaked in water as drawn from the spigot, with no change; it was then placed in a vulcanizer resting on a flask above the water and subject to 320° F. for an hour, this test showed the tube without crack.

The second test consisted in adding a little salt to the lime-water. In the third test a little water from the supply pipes was added to the lime-water. For the fourth test plain boiled water, cold, was used. In each case the tubes cracked within twelve minutes.

A solution of gum-arabic, made with plain water, was used, and the test showed the tube without crack. This last experiment was not further tested, because more plaster could be mixed with the lime-water than with the gum-arabic water, hence with the latter the plaster was less dense. It was further thought that the free solubility of the gum-arabic in water might cause the plaster to soften in vulcanizing. The use of lime-water in all of my plaster work, particularly for vulcanite dentures, has been attended with such uniformly gratifying results that I would consider a return to the former practice a retrograde change. For impressions I use "impression plaster." For the model and for flasking I use the "slow-setting." This latter has the advantage of becoming harder than the "medium," these being the three grades of dental plaster with which the writer is familiar. That the reader may have all the information in my possession bearing upon this valuable discovery the following data is submitted:

Doctor X. Dodel,
    San Francisco, Cal.:
    My dear Doctor,—I see in your "Pointers for Dentists," No. 3, 1903, on page 4, "To prevent shrinkage in plaster, mix with lime-water." I will very much appreciate your stating whether there is any special way for preparing the lime-water.
                        Yours very truly,
                                P. B. McCullough.
February 19, 1904.

DR. P. B. MCCULLOUGH,
  Philadelphia, Pa.:
  DEAR DOCTOR,—Lime-water is a saturated solution of calcium hydrate, and you will find its preparation in the American Pharmacopœia. Use it *cold* instead of common water. It is inexpensive and you can get it at any drug store.

Yours very truly,
(Signed)   X. DODEL.

February 24, 1904.

It will be seen that in the " Pointer" referred to the word " shrinkage" is used, and likewise in my letter. This is unsatisfactory, as the problem with the dentist has always been to prevent expansion.

It must be observed, however, that lime-water bought at a drugstore is presupposedly made with distilled water, and when so prepared it would serve the purpose, but as there can be no certainty that bought lime-water is always so prepared, no dentist using it can be said to do so intelligently without the above information, particularly as the writer is informed by a druggist that not one per cent. of the lime-water sold is made with boiled water, and that at most only filtered water is used.

THE FOURTH INTERNATIONAL DENTAL CONGRESS.[1]

BY EDWARD C. KIRK, D.D.S., SC.D., PHILADELPHIA.

WHAT first appeals to us in the consideration of this Congress is the magnitude of its several features and the extent of the interest which the world of dentistry is manifesting in the outcome of the meeting.

There has been called to meet in St. Louis next month a gathering of dentists representing every civilized country on the globe. Each nation having any importance from the stand-point of professional dentistry will be represented by its practitioners and will contribute to the programme the latest development of its dental

---

[1] Abstract of a paper read before the Pennsylvania State Dental Society at Wilkes-Barre, Pa., July 13, 1904.

progress, so that as a whole the St. Louis Congress will constitute an exhibit of the world's dentistry at this dawn of the twentieth century.

To prepare for this great event has been the work assigned to a special committee appointed by the National Dental Association at its meeting in 1902 at Niagara Falls, and confirmed by the Directory of Congresses of the St. Louis Exposition in 1903.

Notwithstanding the comparatively limited time at command since the inception of the movement, the work of organization has proceeded rapidly and upon systematic lines. Committees of publicity and propaganda have been formed in every important country of Europe, as well as in Australia and Japan, so that twenty or more nations are now concerned in this movement and are actively spreading an interest and securing support in every way for the meeting. Contributions to all departments of the programme are rapidly coming in, and to an extent that is causing no small difficulty in regard to their disposal. Each State in our Union is organized by the appointment of State chairmen, who, working with their local committees, are collectively preparing the part which the United States is to perform in this dental congress of all nations.

While it is not possible to give exact figures, it may be safely stated that not less than fifteen hundred committeemen are actively at work throughout the world in preparing for the events which will together constitute the Fourth International Dental Congress. Upward of three hundred clinical demonstrations are being provided for. The ten sectional divisions of the Congress which will hold simultaneous meetings will produce not less than one hundred to one hundred and fifty essays by the leaders of dental thought in all countries, covering all departments of our profession. Dental education, legislation, history, and nomenclature will be the subjects of comprehensive reports made by experts who have for years made these subjects a specialty.

The dealers' and manufacturers' exhibit of dental supplies now includes a larger catalogue of individual exhibits than has heretofore appeared in connection with any dental meeting.

As to the probable number of members who will participate, the indications now point to a larger paid membership than has ever before attended an international dental congress.

The provisions being made by the local Committee of Arrangements for the care and entertainment of members are upon a scale which assures the success of the social features of the Congress,—a feature which, after all, is the most important civilizing influence in our dental meetings, and one which in a great international gathering contributes the most towards harmonizing the different national ideals, thus aiding the progress of dentistry as a whole.

To those in position to watch the growth of this world movement of our profession towards a common object the view is an inspiring one. The conception of our calling derived from a local environment at once loses its significance in the broader aspect which the international feature of this congress presents for consideration. In our local, State, and national associations we meet with differences of opinion as to theory and practice, and out of the multitude of counsel we extract the grist of that wisdom which becomes in time our accepted standard of practice; yet this diversity of opinion is among men similarly trained, speaking the same mother tongue, having the same patriotic sentiments and similar professional ideals. In an international congress are brought together the products of the most diverse systems of training, with corresponding differences of method and theory and the added diversity of language and national characteristics which act as modifying influences in shaping the professional tendencies of each nation towards its own standards and aims. Yet notwithstanding these characteristic national differences, there remains the one professional ideal as the feature common to dentistry in all nations,—the salvation of the human denture and the one animating desire to solve the problems of our calling upon an independent professional basis.

The attitude of mind of our professional organization, if I may so express it, has needed the developing influence of experience to so ripen it that a clearer conception of the position of dentistry among the beneficent callings of mankind might be formulated, and during the past twenty years the needed experience has come with its fruit of ripened judgment as a consequence.

In 1889 France issued a call for the First International Dental Congress. Previous to this the seeds of internationalism in dental associative work were sown by the establishment of a dental section at the International Medical Congress held in London in 1881, and repeated at the International Congress in Philadelphia in 1887. At these meetings the leaders of dentistry of the several nations were brought into contact, and there was born the realization that while all were striving for a common ideal the methods of each were widely different, and that much good would result from a more intimate specialized association that would give opportunity for the comparison and discussion of ideas upon an international and purely dental basis.

The complexity which the international features of the dental professional problem presented were such as could best be worked out upon a basis quite separate from the medical relationship, hence an international congress of dentists dealing exclusively with dentistry was determined upon; and it was France, whose leaders of dental thought were most deeply impressed with this idea, that took the initiative.

The Dental Congress of 1889, held in Paris, was an abundant success, which revealed the fact that the sentiment was strongly in favor of the independence of dentistry as a profession. This first purely dental congress international in scope accomplished the still more important result of practically demonstrating the good which might flow to all concerned by periodically bringing together in harmonious relationship the dental representatives of all nations for the discussion of those problems which are vital to the progress and success of dentistry as a profession throughout the world. In 1893 the Second International Dental Congress was held in Chicago, as the World's Columbian Dental Congress, and the third of these reunions was held in Paris in 1900. Each subsequent congress exceeded its predecessor in importance both as to magnitude of membership, output of work, and general character of results. Especially there should be noted in this connection the growth of the spirit of internationalism in dentistry with each succeeding congress. The active and leading men of all nations have on each occasion been brought into close personal contact, and have learned to regard with respect the efforts which all are making to develop those factors which in each country are placing dentistry upon a higher scientific and social plane.

That type of self-sufficiency and conceit begotten of ignorance which offends decency with its blatant claim of superiority over all others has been made unpopular by these great international meetings, and that higher and nobler spirit of according honor and praise to him who is deserving thereof regardless of his nativity or the language in which he expresses his thought is becoming the dominating principle in these associations; all of which is as it should be.

Dentistry has outgrown its swaddling clothes and is now in the period of a strong and lusty adolescence. It has grown into that independence to which it was from the first destined by virtue of its inherent usefulness to humanity. But it has grown otherwise. In the reaching outward of its spheres of influence it has escaped the geographical bounds which limit the activities of nations, and finding sympathetic response in the touch of the dental professional spirit in other nations has laid the first foundations for the formation of a dental world power which shall know no national limitations, but which shall regard our calling as of that higher order of truth and knowledge that is the exclusive possession of no country, though native it may be to some, yet, withal, a citizen of the world.

It will be seen that the international dental congress fulfils a function with which our State and national organizations are not directly concerned nor are they competent to deal.

We discuss questions of education, legislation, and reciprocity, but in their international aspects these matters develop a much wider significance. Our national pride and our patriotism are touched unpleasantly when, for example, Germany enacts legislation excluding the American graduate from using his doctor title while practising within her territory; yet in all justice there is something to be said in defence of this attitude upon the part of our transatlantic neighbor, and it is the function and purpose of the international congress to develop the kind of attitude and produce the evidence that in the course of time will set such matters straight.

The international congress movement is a movement towards harmony, by comparison and discussion of those conflicting views which interfere with dental progress and bring about a readjustment of relations upon the basis of greatest advantage to our profession throughout the world.

Much has already been accomplished. The spirit of internationalism in dentistry has taken root and is rapidly spreading its influence among the nations, so that already the fruits of its harmonizing tendency are apparent.

Not the least important step which has been taken towards conserving and developing this international spirit of confraternity among dental practitioners the world over is the creation at the Paris Congress of the Fédération Dentaire Internationale, an organization of all the delegates representing the several nations at the Congress of 1900. The purposes of this Federation are to foster the objects for which international congresses are held,— to promote and assist all movements which in an international way can contribute to the advancement of the profession of dentistry. The Federation is represented by an Executive Council, which has power to act upon behalf of the Federation as an *ad interim* committee, to accept invitations to hold international congresses, and to designate the time and place for holding them. The organization of the international movement is thus planned and assured upon systematic lines, and it is at St. Louis, in America, that the first period of organized activity of this great power in dentistry will be terminated and the second period inaugurated.

In all probability it will be many years before such a notable meeting will again be accessible to American practitioners in their own country. We are on the eve of perhaps the greatest event in the history of the world's dentistry. Every professional consideration, every purely selfish interest, alike demands that we should take an active part in this congress. Let the man who claims that American dentistry leads the world go to St. Louis and help to substantiate that claim next month or else hereafter forever hold his peace. America has issued the invitation, you have taken your part in confirming the action of our national association in asking the dental representatives of the nations of the earth to be your guests at St. Louis. The committee has done its work, the feast is prepared, the guests are even now arriving. Let us one and all embrace the opportunity to show them in the best sense our qualities as hosts, and at the same time learn something in a practical way of the good which must accrue to our profession from the development of the international idea, and then give it practical furtherance by our individual efforts.

A PLEA FOR THOROUGH DENTAL EDUCATION.[1]

BY LEO GREEN, A.B., D.M.D.

THIS paper presents at its inception a rather discouraging aspect. The subject is so broad that it is difficult to limit it to a short paper, and yet the omission of a single phase would seem to disturb the sequence of ideas. I expect to bring up some questions that have caused no little difference of opinion in the past, but yet I want to make it clear that I am not bringing an indictment against any one institution or individual, but am merely trying to indicate the faults in the general system of dental education as I see them.

The first part of my paper will deal with the preliminary education of the student and his preparation for entrance into the professional school. I will then pass to the instruction in the dental schools and examine the methods there in vogue, both as to the theoretical and clinical training. We will then discuss the examinations for State licenses, and some professional ideals (or want of them).

But to return to the preliminary education of the dental student, and by that I refer to his mental and manual training prior to his entrance into the professional school. I regret to say that the present method of preparation for our professional career is entirely inadequate, and that the average dental student has no better education than the average clerk. In fact, a large proportion of our dental students have been unsuccessful in a mercantile career and start in, quite late in life, to study dentistry as a last resort. Hurried preparation in a cramming school, or with a tutor, enables them to pass the entrance examinations for the dental schools, or to satisfy the requirements of the State Board of Regents. Or, on the other hand, we find our material in the short course students of the high schools.

Since I wrote this paper, it was my good fortune to be presented with a copy of an article written by Dr. Harry Carlton, dean of the Dental Department of the University of California. I quote from his article as follows:

[1] Read before The New York Institute of Stomatology, April 5, 1904.

" How few professional schools have entrance requirements that amount to much; they may have requirements that look well in the catalogue or annual announcement, but most accept without question or investigation certificates from teachers or obscure preparatory schools, and the like. There are approximately sixty dental schools in America. To quote from a recent compilation, three have no express admission requirements; eighteen have purely grammar-school subjects for entrance; eighteen more, first year standing in high-school work; eleven have requirements covered by two years of high-school work; and six require a three years' high-school course; none of them, as much as is required for admission to any reputable college."

A man undertaking the study of any profession with such a foundation is very much handicapped, unless he is an exceptionally capable student. No officer enters the united service with so little training as our own students exhibit, unless he is on very friendly terms with the administration. No engineer, or lawyer, or teacher prepares for his life's work by the short route. We cannot erect a building on a soft foundation, and cannot turn out an educated, liberal-minded man, be he lawyer or dentist, with a professional education imposed upon mental unfitness. For our average student the study of anatomy, physiology, chemistry, and bacteriology presents a difficult and disagreeable problem, and a lack of respect for the laws of hygiene and pathology remains with him in later years of practice.

The higher classes of professional schools are beginning to demand a college degree as a requisite for admission, and we must soon fall in line. The advantages of this standard must be evident. At present our schools require only what the law demands, and in the case of foreigners or man intending to practice abroad, many concessions are made. A man is prepared, in a measure, to study any profession when he has received a college education. He is all the more prepared to study any one profession when his education has to some extent been shaped to that end in view. If his fingers as well as his mind have been trained, then has the prospective dental student received an almost ideal preparation. When a student enters Columbia University, for instance, with the ultimate intention of studying medicine, he takes the prescribed college courses and chooses such elective subjective as will be helpful to him in his medical course. At the end of three years, he is ready to enter the medical school, with a good education, ability to study and grasp new facts, and, if he has chosen his electives wisely, with a fund of information that will lead up to his medical training. The future dental student could likewise take up such elective courses as would assist him in his dental studies, and, furthermore; apply himself faithfully to manual training, to educate his fingers. Dr. Maurice Richardson, the famous Boston surgeon, attributes his skill to early training at the forge; and I have frequently heard surgeons attribute their dexterity to training in wood work, carving, painting, etching,—in short, to various forms of manual training.

You will say that this long college training entails too heavy a burden and expense upon the poor student. For the benefit of the multitude, the individual must always suffer; and yet, with the many scholarships and opportunities for self-support that our colleges offer, the ambitious student is rarely barred from an education because of his lack of means. For a simple dental operation no great learning or manual skill is necessary, but to keep in touch with the progress of dental knowledge, and to maintain dignified relations with the medical profession, a higher mental standard for our students is imperative. The lack of courtesy, or recognition (so called), from the medical profession of which dentists so frequently complain is due largely to a lack of confidence. Laymen as well as professional men are wont to look upon us as mere skilled mechanics. It is only within the past few years that the government has added dentists to the military service; and the rank of these contract dental surgeons, as compared with the collateral branches of the service,—the medical, the legal, and the clerical,—is not one to be proud of. We have been slow in making the public see the importance of our services, because we have been slow in educating ourselves. The greatest enemies to our professional progress are those men whose slogan is, "Too much theory and too many lectures." If their theory is correct, our schools are unnecessary; an apprenticeship in the office and mechanical laboratory would suffice. We must sooner or later realize that so long as our educational standards are low, so long shall we fail to attract a superior class of men to our ranks. Dr. Carlton, in referring to a paper written by Dr. Kirk and printed in the *Dental Cosmos,* says,—

" He also refers to the demand now being vigorously made from many quarters, that dentistry be classed as an 'independent' profession and given equal status in the specialties of the healing arts. I quite agree with him that much, aye, very much, remains to be done before that recognition, as such, can be accorded. If we would have the respect and regard of other professions we must first respect ourselves. Dentistry should be a full profession and recognized as such, but it only will be when the character of the men who comprise it bring its recognition up to what it should be. The conferring of the dignified degree of Doctor upon men of deficient culture is wrong, and for this reason we fail of recognition not only abroad, but at home. I have said that any increase in dignity and professional status must come from within the great body of the profession itself. To gain these ideals and make the profession what it should be a high grade of young men must be attracted to its ranks. As soon as the best men are attracted, excellent work will really be done, and the development will then be a natural one."

The announcement of a four years' dental course looks imposing in print, but does it really indicate an *advance* in dental education? Until recently, a "year" in most dental schools consisted of five or six months; and terms of more than seven months are still rare. The course of instruction and corps of instructors as represented by many schools in their annual announcements are a delight to the eye; but how different is the reality. Some few schools there are whose faculties plan out a nine months' course, and faithfully carry out this schedule. But is it not natural that students will flock to those institutions making the least demands of them in the way of time and effort? The history of our dental schools during the past twenty-five years has had its full measure of scandal. The disclosure of fraud and the sale of diplomas have incurred for us, from time to time, the distrust of foreign authorities. Less than ten years ago the State authorities were called upon to admonish the officials of one of our local institutions for neglect,—a neglect which nearly resulted disastrously for the interests of the students. Of course, exposure and official prodding have accomplished much in the way of reform, but there is still much to be desired.

An unwise feature in some of the courses is the unnecessary repetition of lectures. Men are called upon to listen to the same sets of lectures several years in succession. A lack of interest and a tendency to cut hours are the inevitable results. Such courses seem to be designed to prepare men up to the hour to pass examinations, which is not the ultimate end of education; it should be merely a feature. And yet the lectures in operative and mechanical dentistry are far superior to the clinical training in these departments. The demonstrators are for the most part inexperienced, recent graduates, for whom the ridiculously small salary is some inducement.

Furthermore, the students are wont to look upon the lecture course as a necessary evil, and as independent of and unessential to the clinical training. If this is not a fault of the system of education, at whose doors shall we lay the blame? The requirements in the actual practice of operative and mechanical dentistry are for the most part inadequate. There are other faults of the system of education to which I could call attention, but time and space prevent me from going into details. I must, however, take advantage of this opportunity to call attention to the questionable practice of permitting students to substitute apprenticeship instruction in operative and mechanical dentistry for the regular college courses in these departments.

Now, as to the annual examinations; the number of failures in the last year is so large, as compared with those of the previous years, that we naturally look for an explanation. The trouble seems to be that the examinations of the first two years are conducted in too loose a manner, and that the weeding-out process occurs only at the eleventh hour. College authorities should indicate to the impossible student, at the earliest opportunity, that his sphere of usefulness lies elsewhere.

Under the present condition of varied efficiency of our dental schools the addition of a fourth year will not produce a new era in dental education. We see in the rulings of the National Association of Dental Faculties the same error that underlies the workings of the labor unions. If all men were of equal ability, the labor union system would be fair; but it is manifestly unjust to be obliged to pay the poor workman at the same rates as the skilled, or to require the sluggard to work only as many hours as his more diligent brother and for the same hire. As it is with men, so it is with colleges. The National Association classifies the thorough institution with the lax one, and lays down a general rule for them all. It is fair to presume that you can learn more about dentistry in nine months than you can in seven; and you must expect better results from an institution which maintains a high standard equally to all, than from one which lets down the bars so that the lame sheep can pass through. Besides, the entrance requirements of some institutions produce a body of students capable of learning and thoroughly assimilating more in one year than those of another institution in two years. I am not opposed to a four years' dental course; under certain conditions I believe such a course would be admirable, and I will attempt to outline these conditions. Start with students *properly qualified to study a profession.* Insist upon their preliminary education being of a high standard and in a measure preparatory to their prospective training; this will enable the college faculties to eliminate such courses as chemistry and physics, which now form part of the dental curriculum. At the end of three years examinations for the degree may be held and successful applicants rewarded accordingly. For the fourth year I would outline a course of clinical work. You may ask, What will be gained by dividing the course in this way? After the student has received his degree, he is relieved of the worry of examinations and attendance at lectures, which, in a measure, must conflict with his clinical work. His opportunities for observation will be broader than before, and unhampered; and any taste for original research can be fostered. The results altogether will be for the good of the public, as well as of the individual.

One of the features peculiar to our form of government is the sovereign right of the State to make laws for its own government. While this has many advantages, it likewise has its disadvantages. A notable instance of the latter is the conflict of the divorce laws, which has brought both trouble and ridicule. The lack of uniformity of the laws regulating the practice of medicine and dentistry in the various States is also to be regretted. This difficulty could be remedied by a national standard of examination, which should be no less exacting in its requirements than the most rigid tests now in force. The English system, whereby a licentiate under the home law is permitted to practise in the colonies, seems eminently fair and is certainly consistent.

Too many of our practitioners suffer from a want of self confidence and individuality, which in itself is a confession of poor training. Men are too apt to accept, unquestioned, the results that others offer; new drugs or patent preparations are readily accepted as a panacea for all ills. Moreover, we have been afraid in the past, to cry out against the commercial tendency in our ranks. We have failed to distinguish the men who labor for the benefit of the profession above those who work only for their personal profit through the dental supply houses. We are either too indifferent to this condition, or else too many of .us are involved in these commercial transactions. It is difficult to make many of our men understand that, while they may have a legal right, they have no moral right to conceal from the profession any useful ideas expressed in the form of new drugs, formulas, instruments, or methods of operation, or to market out the products of these ideas after having secured them by patents. Do these men ever stop to consider how slow would have been the advance of our professional knowledge, and how little they would know to-day, if all progressive thought had been veiled in secrecy or inventive genius had invested its products with patents?

The worst feature of the commercial tendency—and the most degrading—is the rapid growth of the advertising dental companies. A representative of one of our local newspapers recently asked me what form of legislation could be invoked to drive these parasite growths out of existence. Legislation alone could take care of present conditions, but the bright hope for the future lies in education. Education will take care of this and other degrading tendencies in our profession.—that I have already indicated. As regards legal enactments, I would like to quote the English law. Every candidate on being admitted as a licentiate subscribes to the following declaration:

" I do solemnly and sincerely declare that I will exercise the several parts of my profession, to the best of my knowledge and ability, for the good, safety, and welfare of all persons committing themselves or committed to my care; and I hereby promise as a Licentiate in Dental Surgery, that I will not advertise or employ any other unprofessional modes of attracting business. nor will I allow my name to be connected with any one who does so; and that I will loyally obey all by-laws of the Faculty made or to be made for the Licentiates in Dental Surgery."

" Any Licentiate who may be proved, to the satisfaction of the Council, to have violated the obligations in the foregoing declaration shall, if the Faculty so decide, render himself liable to the forfeiture of his diploma and to his name being erased from the list of Dental Licentiates."

Some such legislation might be enacted to advantage in this country.

In closing I wish to pay tribute of my respect and admiration to those institutions which have stood for higher dental education, and to those men of the present and past generations who have devoted their best efforts for the benefit of their profession and mankind.

THE VALUE OF SYMMETRY IN EDUCATION AND CHARACTER.[1]

BY GEORGE F. EAMES, M.D., BOSTON, MASS.

In the contemplation of any subject, be it animate or inanimate, the pleasure and satisfaction derived therefrom is dependent in a great degree on its symmetrical proportions; indeed, asymmetry, as seen in many objects, and especially in the human form, is a positive disfigurement, and is often repulsive.

But symmetry as I wish to discuss it will be considered in connection with the mind and soul. It will be noted at once that lack of symmetry in the mind is not so readily observed as a similar condition of the body, although they are vastly more common, and the deviations from what might be considered typical in the former would be altogether hideous if the same disproportion were exhibited in the physical system. Imagine a nose, which by a slight aberration of development has continued to grow until it is twelve inches long; or one eye eight inches in diameter and the other a mere pinhole! Such an extreme in physical deformity has probably never been known, yet similar disproportions, or greater, may easily be conceived to exist in the different powers of the mind. In the dental profession we should not expect to find excessive abnormalities or great deficiencies in intellect, but there are many indications that the majority of practitioners might de-

---

[1] Chairman's address before the Section on Stomatology at the fifty-fifth annual session of the American Medical Association, at Atlantic City, June 7 to 10, 1904.

velop their mechanical and intellectual powers in certain directions with great benefit to themselves and patients, and everlasting good to all people over whom they have any influence. This means that there are many defects in symmetry to be observed among dentists, and even among stomatologists.

While some defects may be found in the best of men, those which we have now under consideration are such that they, in many instances, ruin the man as a practitioner, and in nearly all the other cases mar his brilliancy and seriously handicap his professional progress. Take, for example, the life of the late P. D. Armour, the great capitalist of Chicago; his strict devotion to business, at the expense of all social life and entertainment, and his abstemious habits were still kept up even after his financial worth was counted by millions. While his business ability was increasing, other faculties of mind and heart were weakening, and when this hypertrophic condition, in the shape of an enormously enlarged business capacity, became pathologic, and the discrepancy between this and other bodily and mental functions became so great that he began to suffer from the strain, he was urged to rest and go to Europe. He went, but he had lost all capacity for the enjoyment of travel and change of scene, and he died in the harness which he had himself constructed. The following quotation from Charles Robert Darwin shows still further the effect of asymmetrical development:

"I have said that in one respect my mind has changed during the last twenty or thirty years. Up to the age of thirty, or beyond it, poetry of many kinds, such as the work of Milton, Gray, Byron, Wordsworth, Coleridge, and Shelly, gave me great pleasure, and even as a school-boy I took great delight in Shakespeare, especially in the historical plays. I have also said that formerly pictures gave me considerable pleasure, and music very great delight. But now for many years I can not endure to read a line of poetry. I have tried lately to read Shakespeare, and found it so intolerably dull that it nauseated me. I have also almost lost my taste for pictures or music. . . . This curious and lamentable loss of the higher æsthetic tastes is all the odder, as books on history, biographies and travels (independently of any scientific facts which they may contain), and essays on all sorts of subjects, interest me as much as ever they did. . . . Why this should have caused the atrophy of that part of the brain alone on which the higher tastes depend I can not conceive. . . . If I had to live my life over again, I would make it a rule to read some poetry and listen to some music at least once every week, for perhaps the parts of my brain now atrophied would have thus been kept active through use. The loss of these tastes is a loss of happiness, and may possibly be injurious to the intellect, and more probably to the moral character, by enfeebling the emotional part of our nature."

Professor Charles Eliot Norton says, " Whatever your occupation may be, and however crowded your hours with affairs, do not fail to secure at least a few minutes every day for refreshment of your inner life with a bit of poetry."

A few weeks ago I met a physician in the suburbs of Boston. He was apparently taking a walk for pleasure, and was observing some birds by the way. My first thought was one of surprise that this physician, in full practice, the author of a large work and in many ways one who must meet numerous demands, could and would find time for such a purpose, but a moment's reflection convinced me that such use of time was very wise and judicious—that it was necessary, not alone for diversion and recreation, but that it served to cultivate the mind, to broaden the view, and to render more sensitive and acute the artistic and moral sense. In many other ways a study of the lower animals increases, by comparison, our knowledge of the higher; and this is, as we well know, of essential value to the physician. It is a grave mistake to neglect the cultivation of the artistic and æsthetic sides of our nature, of a love of the beautiful, of sympathetic feelings and of all that is delicate and refined, whether one is fitting to become a physician, a general, or a special surgeon.

Away with the idea that the surgeon needs no feelings of delicacy and sympathy; that, devoid of all sense of feeling, he cuts across nerve and artery, or that he administers an anæsthetic which suspends nearly all the functions of life without giving a thought to the real condition in which he places his patient—without feeling the full weight of responsibility in holding a precious life in his hands! It is true that a surgeon should not allow his feelings— his emotions—to be uppermost when he is performing an operation. To all appearance he must be devoid of sensibility, and even sympathy—yet the world knows that the greatest delicacy of perception, the keenest appreciation of possible pain are a part of his equipment, and that it is only the well-being of the patient which demands apparent indifference to suffering. If he can not, for the time at least, lock up his "feelings" so that they will disturb neither his patient nor himself, he loses something of his dexterity and physical poise. But sensitiveness—mental as well as physical —is a very important characteristic of a great physician, and this same sensitiveness is cultivated or lessened, as the case may be, by a man's daily living and his attitude towards life. He may harden and blunt his perceptions as he may, dull his tools if he will, but good work demands the keenest edge of which he is capable.

The practical and important issue before us, in view of the conditions to which reference has just been made, is this: What are the more important defects in our professional life, and what are the remedies? The first consideration in seeking to correct a diseased or any undesirable condition is to discover the cause, and here it is to be sought in the early years of child-life, although, indeed, causes may exist generations before. Manifestly, the suitable preparation of body and mind for the duties of life may be included in the broad term, education. Asymmetry due to lack of development, then, of the body or mind is due to faulty education. Many of our college graduates are like statues, carved to be placed in a frieze. The side towards the public gaze defies criticism, but the rest is of rough, unhewn stone.

It is evident that life is too short to pursue studies in every direction available at the present time, therefore a choice must be made; on this choice may hang future success or failure, and to it we may look for the cause of many deficiencies in development of both body and mind. The writer believes that much is taught in all departments of education which has no vital and practical value in the life work to come. With innumerable subjects for study, with the many subdivisions of these subjects and the almost unlimited extent to which they may be pursued, the great need is shown of weeding out, and also the serious difficulty of doing so. Everything which is taught at the present time has a certain value, and one reluctantly strikes out of the list anything which is worth while, but it is a choice between greater and lesser values. From early childhood it should become a matter for serious consideration, not only as to what shall be taught, but also as to what needs curbing, and what should be strengthened. Mere intellect, as some one has said, is as hard-hearted and as heart hardening as mere sense. We need to remember this in our schemes of education. A little child, instead of being confined in a room for hours, where he is taught the alphabet or spelling, would be far better off were he out in the fresh air and sunlight, becoming familiar with the colors and flowers and the facts of nature.

Later in life, in the preparatory schools, no one will question that mathematics is an essential item in the curriculum, yet even here we may make an improvement in the old methods by substituting something more useful and practical for the higher mathematics, leaving these until later, or until the life work is chosen.

The writer has in his school-days spent much time over mathematical problems or catch-traps which had no value beyond the discipline and exercise which it gave the mind, and he believes that something else might have been substituted which would have given the necessary discipline and exercise, and at the same time would have educated me in a useful and practical way. On the other hand, overindulgent parents and unthinking teachers may allow a child to follow his bent too closely, and the very danger is precipitated which we wish to avoid. In order to produce a symmetrical figure, the pedestal or foundation must be strong and well rounded, so that however elaborate the decoration of the capital or head of the column may be, there shall be no incongruity between it and its base. A school course which should fitly train mind, heart and body in the right degree would be the ideal one.

It would seem to be a wise procedure if exercises were introduced at an early age with the object of ascertaining the prominent characteristics inherent in each child; for instance, even in kindergarten life, a talent, or the ability to do one thing better than another, is often shown, as are the inventive and constructive powers. Equal attention should, of course, be given to finding out and strengthening weak points. This, if systematically carried out during school life, and a record made and kept for future reference, would be valuable. For example, a young man, with the help of his friends, wishes to determine in what direction his life work shall be. In coming to this decision he not only considers what he thinks he would like to do, what he is most interested in, and how he could obtain the most money, but he should by no means neglect to take into consideration the direction in which his greatest talents lie, the things which he has done with the most marked ability, the work which by nature he is best adapted to do. For this purpose recourse may be had to his school record, which is on file at the schools which he has attended. This record will show, from child life up, the individual's proficiency in drawing and other work which shows artistic ability, also the student's aptness in a mechanical and manipulative way. The inventive powers are often shown even in kindergarten life in the various shapes and ways in which blocks may be arranged, etc.

These and other items of the student's school record should be of great assistance in the choice of a vocation. To take up the life work to which one is best adapted, means the greatest possible usefulness to mankind, the happiest and most harmonious life and the most symmetrical growth. Again, this system of recording should be of great service to those who have charge of the entrance of candidates into colleges of dentistry, law, medicine, and others. This record should stand not only for the applicant's ability as a student, but for his special adaptability to a given profession, and no other entrance examination should be needed. Why should any second examination be made if the first is satisfactory? Is it not a declaration that the first is not to be depended on if the record is made? What a comment on the learning and teaching ability of our esteemed professors in the dental colleges, that their graduates with a diploma bearing their signature and the seal of the college should fail to satisfy a State board of examiners, or be debarred practice in another State! Surely, there is a great lack of symmetry in the results of our modern college work; if not, then the work of the state board of examiners is unnecessary, for no one should be allowed to practise as a stomatologist without a diploma, and that diploma should stand as the best passport to practice. Regarding the standard of entrance to colleges of stomatology, it should undoubtedly be high, but even this may be overdone and ill-advised. To the writer's knowledge, many who have entered the dental college as graduates of a high school have been among the worst specimens of graduate practitioners, and far below in quality those who had been received without having had such a course. Graduation from a high school as a minimum standard may be used as a basis, but this alone is not sufficient. If symmetry be wanting, the high school graduate is of poor promise and his entrance to the dental college should be postponed or discouraged. If a degree is required for entrance, and it undoubtedly should be, still it is necessary to look for other qualifications, especially if degrees may still be obtained from some sources for money and while it shows nothing of the candidate's manipulative dexterity.

By lack of symmetry in such cases is meant a deficiency in mechanical ability or literary culture, for instance, to such an extent that it would be unwise to receive the candidate. On the other hand, a young student who, for some good reason, has not graduated from the high school, may have such a symmetrical record as far as he has gone, and shows such qualifications of promise, that it would be very unwise to reject him. Of course, desirable candidates do not need an entrance examination; they do not need a four years' course or one of two years; they would reach the high places in the profession in spite of the entrance examination and the college courses, and they are so well endowed, mentally and physically, that they are able to decide as to their own fitness for a certain profession. Their own desire and ambition is for the best things, and they are not limited by years in a college; they would even get on without the college, and no ordinary hinderance could prevent their success. A friend of mine, a physician, now one of my listeners, was with me a few years ago in the Tower of London, and we stood on the spot where Anne Boleyn, Lady Jane Grey, and Katherine Howard were beheaded. My friend the doctor remarked, "If they'd let them alone they would have died themselves long ago." So with the most desirable men of our profession; they are such that if we let them alone they will go on with their professional development without regulations as to entrance standards and length of college courses that we spend so much time in talking about. The problem is to keep out incompetents, and the unworthy, even if they may have in a fashion "gone through" some school or college with the required standard. We might have a ten-year course for Jack Blunthead, and he would still be unfit, while Joseph Sharp has passed all the requirements of the ordinary graduate in two years. A matter of years alone, or even the administration of thyroid extract, will not always qualify, and there is nothing that will qualify if there be not inherent in the individual the incentive and the genius to succeed. Quality, not quantity, is the essential requirement, and if this be attained, what can it matter whether the student has achieved it in one year or four, although the preference should be given to the one-year man? Therefore, when it is proposed to extend the dental course to four years, I am opposed to it; but this should not, by any means, convey the impression that anything but the highest standard is advocated.

Time is too precious to compel such men as we have pronounced worthy to enter the dental college, to give four years of their life in it. Three years is enough time to give to that part of the student life which is spent within the college walls. To all right-minded graduates, the end of the college course is but the beginning of studentship in earnest. Out of college the student, now also a practitioner, has entire management of his education and the development of his talents, and his success and future degree of symmetry, the nearness with which he comes to the finished product in man, is limited only by himself.

Among practitioners many defects in symmetry may be observed. There are some practitioners who have developed their mechanical powers to such an extent, and have become so absorbed in some mechanical specialties, so-called, that they are unable when they look at the human mouth to see anything but a possible bridge, crown, or plate; others have a clear vision as to dollars, their other sense perceptions being weakened from disuse. In fact, atrophy is often associated with hypertrophy, and the former may be an indirect result of the latter, both physically and mentally.

Specialties and specialists have done much to advance their particular lines of work, and this is greatly to be commended, but there are disadvantages as well, and these consist in the neglect of general considerations, which, if given some attention, would help much towards a more symmetrical condition.

In the enthusiasm and interest which is taken in certain lines of work in our profession, many of us forget that there are other departments of our work which should also receive attention ; that, in many directions, our mental and bodily capacity is weakening through loss of function; that we are better dentists by being better citizens; that we are the best stomatologists when we have cultivated our hearts, minds, and bodies in all possible directions around the one central object which draws us all together with a common interest and a common purpose.

DENTAL EDUCATION: A RETROSPECTIVE AND PROSPECTIVE VIEW.[1]

BY JOHN S. MARSHALL, M.S., M.D., SAN FRANCISCO, CAL.

" We will not anticipate the past, our retrospection will be all of the future."

IT is my purpose in this short paper to take a hasty retrospective glance at the history of dental education in the United States, that I may hold before you for a moment a picture of progress that has seldom been equalled in the history of educational advancement, and then to change the view and hold before you another picture, a prospective view, the realization of which will be no more difficult to us and our children than was that of the first picture to our fathers and ourselves.

" Past and to come seems best; things present worse."

Shakespeare never wrote a truer line than this, for, if we were satisfied with the present, there would be no progress in the future. Satisfaction with the present brought decay and ruin on the ancient Egyptians and on the Roman Empire.

A RETROSPECTIVE VIEW.

We learn from history that the art and science of surgery is an outgrowth or evolution of the tonsorial art. Two hundred years ago the barber was also the surgeon. His functions were to shave and cut hair; to bleed the prince or the pauper; to bind up wounds and set broken bones. The striped red, white, and blue pole which stood before his shop indicated that he was ready on occasion to bleed his patron, bind up his wounds, or set his broken bones. The term applied to him was barber-surgeon. His social position was that of a barber, a person to be petted on occasion, or insulted or kicked at the caprice of those of higher social position. To-day his learning and skill have placed him on the highest pinnacle of fame by reason of which kings and emperors

---

[1] Read at the fifty-fifth annual session of the American Medical Association, in the Section on Stomatology, Atlantic City, June 7 to 10, 1904.

have made him their confidant, and freely and without fear have placed their lives in his keeping.

Dental surgery was likewise evolved from the art of the barber, the tinker, and the village blacksmith. A little over sixty years ago there was no such institution as a dental college, no such organization as a dental society or even a journal devoted to the interests of dental surgery. At that time the only means of education in dentistry was by the old system of apprenticeship. The dentist in those days had no social or professional standing; he was envied by the barber and looked down on by the doctor of medicine. To-day he is regarded as a member of a noble profession, standing shoulder to shoulder with the physicians and surgeons and dividing with them the honor of adding to the comfort and longevity of the human race by reason of their learning and technical skill.

The evolution of the surgeon, from the barber to the scientist, required several centuries, while the evolution of the dentist from his low degree to his present honorable position has been accomplished in as many decades. This has been wrought partly by the energy and forethought of the pioneers in the profession, but principally by the more favorable environment which surrounded the infant profession.

In these days of the rapid spread of knowledge and learning, the development of the arts and sciences and of the inventive faculties, the ignorance, prejudice, and bigotry of the race have been swept away and all men and all movements, either social, political, or scientific, are given an opportunity to develop, each standing or falling according to its merit. Surgery in its early struggles had to fight against the ignorance of the people, the prejudice of the scholars, and the bigotry of the church, and little progress was made until the beginning of the last century. The discovery of the microscope, of vaccination, anæsthesia, and antiseptics made it possible for medicine, surgery, and dentistry to reach their present high development, which is still progressing and must continue to advance in the future.

Dental education may be said to have had its beginning in the organization of the first dental college. This institution, as we all know, was incorporated and established in the city of Baltimore, Md., in the year 1840. Its entrance requirements were simply a desire to learn. Its curriculum was anatomy, physiology,

23

chemistry, development of the teeth, principles of operative and mechanical dentistry, and laboratory instruction; yet with this meagre course of instruction, it developed some of the brightest minds that have been found in the ranks of the profession. Its requirements for graduation were for practitioners of five years' standing, one course of lectures of about four months; for students, two courses.

A reference to the text-books of this period will show how circumscribed and narrow was the field of study, when compared with the text-books of to-day and the requirements for entrance and graduation from our best dental colleges.

With the organization òf other dental colleges in various parts of the country, a rivalry sprang up between them, and as the profession advanced in scientific knowledge the curriculum was broadened and the courses extended to five months in each year.

For many years thereafter little or no advancement was made either in the course of instruction or the length of the college year. Hydraheaded commercialism had entered into the schools, taken them by the throat, and well-nigh strangled them, for the great aim in most of them had become large classes and a substantial dividend at the end of the year to be divided among the incorporators.

The organization of dental societies, local, State, and national, and the establishment of dental journals, which followed very soon after the incorporation of the Baltimore Dental College, and through the succeeding twenty years, were the most potent elements in arousing the colleges from the stagnation into which they had fallen through the commercial spirit. The might and power of these influences are still exerted for the uplifting and stimulating of the best impulses in education, professionalism, and ethics. To the dental societies and the dental journals the colleges and the profession at large owe much of their success and scientific advancement.

The regulation of the practice of dentistry by the passage of laws for this purpose, by several of the older States, was an advance step of great moment to the interests of higher dental education. These laws recognized dental surgery as a department of medicine, and for the first time in history it was raised to the dignity of a professional calling. The public had heretofore looked on the dentist as a mechanic, spoke of the trade of dentistry, referred to his office as his shop and his operations as jobs. And, although the dental surgeon was the possessor of the honorable degree of D.D.S., conferred *en course,* many persons addressed him by his title in the same spirit that they spoke of the barber as " professor," or the chiropodist as " doctor."

Time, however, changed all this, and the public, by degrees, came to look on dentistry as a professional calling worthy of the best minds and greatest talents. As a result of this change of status in the minds of the public, the dental colleges of this period were overcrowded with students. The demand for more schools seemed imperative, and, as a natural result, many were organized, too many for the best interests of education. Competition of a commercial character, even more strenuous and active than before, took possession of many of the colleges, and some of the weaker schools, feeling that they were being crowded to the wall, opened their doors to any who could pay the fees, promising to graduate them at the end of two courses of lectures. In many instances students were graduated after one course of lectures, and, to our shame be it said, diplomas were issued in some instances to men who had only attended a sufficient number of lectures to identify themselves with the graduating class.

The courses of instruction in the dental colleges of this period were so diverse in subjects and study requirements that students had great difficulty in passing from one college to another, as the faculties of the different colleges often refused to give credit for work done in other institutions. This state of affairs became so unsatisfactory to the colleges and students that several of the leading schools issued a call for a conference of all the dental colleges, for the purposes of harmonizing the courses of study and arranging for comity between the schools and such other matters as should be of mutual benefit to all concerned. This conference resulted in the organization of the National Association of Dental Faculties.

The organization of this Association marked a great epoch in the history of dental education, for through its deliberations and established rules it has exerted a tremendous moral influence over the colleges, both within and without the Association. It has kept the colleges within the Association up to its prescribed standards for the admission and graduation of students, while those on the outside have been compelled by the State examining boards to seek admission to the Association and place themselves in harmony with the requirements of its educational standards. It has brought order out of chaos, in dental teaching; it has harmonized the courses of instruction and has stopped the practice of granting degrees *in absentia*. It has made it possible for students with proper credentials to finish their course of instruction in any college that they may elect. It advanced the requirements for graduation from two to three years. It established an educational entrance requirement and gradually raised this requirement from nothing to a certificate of having passed the examination of the second year in high school. It has introduced technic teaching in operative and prosthetic dentistry. It has improved and extended the curriculum from time to time by adding such important subjects as physics, embryology, general materia medica and therapeutics, general pathology, bacteriology, comparative dental anatomy, orthodontia, general and oral surgery.

Up to one year ago the minimum preliminary requirements for entrance to our dental colleges was a certificate of having passed the studies of the second year in high school, and for graduation, three full courses of instruction of from seven to nine months in each year.

Until three years ago this was the same standard as that required by the medical colleges. At this time the medical courses were extended to four years and the minimum entrance requirement was advanced to a diploma from a four-year high school. A few of the better class of medical schools now require that the student shall have passed the studies of the sophomore year in liberal arts or natural science, while one insists on the bachelor's degree.

At the present time the minimum preliminary requirements for entrance to the dental colleges having membership in the National Association of Dental College Faculties is a certificate admitting the student to the third year of a high school or its equivalent, while that for graduation is four annual courses of instruction of not less than seven months in each year. This, it seems to me, is a record of which the dental profession need not feel ashamed, and yet it should not felicitate itself too much over its progress, for much greater advancement might have been made in educational matters if the colleges could have been united in their work from the beginning.

A PROSPECTIVE VIEW.

The second picture, or the prospective view, must necessarily be one made up largely of personal opinions and impressions, but nevertheless opinions and impressions bred of many years of experience and general observation. The great need of the profession to-day and for the future is, in my opinion, higher preliminary education and broader and fuller instruction in those fundamental sciences which make up the sum total of a dental education. The profession has done well in the past, but it cannot afford to relax its efforts or to take a backward step, now or ever.

For many years the minimum preliminary educational requirements for entrance to the dental colleges were the same as for matriculation in the medical schools, but at the present time they have fallen somewhat behind. This, in my judgment, is a mistake, and it should be rectified at the earliest opportunity.

The requirements for matriculation and graduation in dental surgery should be in no way inferior to the requirements of the medical schools. The courses of instruction in the fundamental sciences should be the same, and during this period the medical and dental students in the great universities should be taught together, and no distinction made between them. By this plan better and more thorough work can be done and at much less expense. This saving of expense would make it possible to employ teachers, at an adequate salary, who would give their whole time and attention to teaching and original investigation, and as a consequence the teaching would be of a higher grade and the work of the student would be more enthusiastically performed.

What we need to-day and in the future is wide-awake teachers for the fundamental sciences, teachers who are full of their subject and who can impart knowledge in such a fashion that the student cannot help being interested in these, to him, otherwise dry subjects. If the teachers of anatomy, physiology, chemistry, etc., are not enthusiastic in their work, the student soon loses interest in them, and turns to the more practical subjects to which he often gives time that could be spent to better advantage on the fundamentals, as he finds, to his chagrin, in after years.

In my work as an examiner for the Dental Corps of the United States army, I have found that the majority of the candidates who have presented themselves for these examinations were deficient in preliminary education and in those subjects usually denominated as the fundamental sciences. In the practical departments they were, as a rule, quite well prepared. The best marks were usually obtained in operative and prosthetic dentistry, crown- and bridge-work, and orthodontia. In fact, many of them were good jewellers, but lacking in that knowledge which marks the truly professional dentist. This is not the fault of the curriculum, for with the subjects that now comprise the courses of study in our better dental colleges the conscientious, hard-working, well-prepared student will receive an excellent professional education.

The most serious difficulties which the teachers of the fundamental sciences experience in their work is the lack of time properly to cover the subjects and mental deficiency on the part of a large number of students in every class, whose minds have not been sufficiently trained and disciplined by previous study readily to grasp or comprehend the sciences which they are endeavoring to teach. As a consequence, the instructor is obliged to suit his teaching to the comprehension and ability of these students, while those of higher educational requirements, who could progress much more rapidly had they the opportunity, lose interest in the subject for want of a stimulus to study. This fault can only be corrected by insisting on a higher grade of preliminary educational requirements, and I most sincerely hope that the Faculties Association will not only raise these minimum requirements to graduation from a four years' high school or its equivalent, at its next session, but will recommend the completion of the sophomore year or a full academic training in the liberal arts or natural sciences as the proper preparation for the study of dental surgery. It is possible at the present time for students of medicine to procure the bachelor's degree in natural science and the degree in medicine by combining the two years' work of the junior college with the four years' work of the medical school. The University of Chicago, the University of Michigan, the University of California, and Cornell University now offer such courses, both degrees being conferred on the candidate after the completion of his full medical course.

This is a movement in the right direction, and I can see no reason why the universities having dental colleges should not offer the same inducements to their students in dental surgery. With such a class of students the work of the instructor would be a joy, while the profession would gain very greatly by the addition to its ranks of a class of more highly educated practitioners.

A young man who has received a college training has usually been taught the principles of social and political ethics, and is therefore better prepared to understand and appreciate professional ethics. Such a young man is generally imbued with higher standards of conduct and of living. He recognizes the ethical rights of others and demands that he be accorded the same rights. Such men are seldom guilty of conduct that brings reproach on their profession. They are seldom found in the ranks of the advertising quacks or those who selfishly patent a remedy, an instrument, or an improvement in methods, which would be of benefit to suffering humanity, forgetting, or not caring, that nearly every remedy they employ for the cure of disease, every instrument they use, or operation they have been taught to perform was thought out and perfected by some member of the profession who preceded them, and who freely and unselfishly gave these to their brethren for the benefit of suffering humanity. The profession needs more of this unselfish, better-educated, truly professional class of men. It needs to stamp out the commercial idea and install in its place the true professional spirit which places our duty to our patients and the State first, leaving the question of the fee for future consideration.

The lengthening of the college course from three to four years will call out many differences of opinion as to how the extra year shall be employed. Those who teach the practical branches will want to extend instruction in operative and prosthetic technics, while those who teach the fundamental sciences will ask for more time and more thorough courses. The latter, to my mind, is at present the most important side of the question, and it should be given careful and conscientious consideration, for the future of the profession depends on how it is decided.

To obtain the highest degree of instruction the teacher must be a specialist in his department, and with the financial inducements that can be offered by the average dental college such teachers for the fundamental sciences are difficult to obtain.

Specialists in the practical subjects of dental surgery are plentiful and, as a consequence, this part of the training of students leads the theoretical and the scientific.

The student is naturally attracted to those subjects on which he thinks he can see that his future financial success as a practitioner depends. He is, therefore, inclined, through mental shortsightedness and inexperience in the profession, and from his inability to comprehend its responsibilities and his duties to his patients and the State, to neglect those subjects which are of the greatest importance in the development of scientific dentistry, and hence to the welfare of his patients and the best interests of the State. He therefore devotes his energies to those departments which appear to him to promise the largest and most speedy returns in money for the time and study spent on them.

We are a nation of buyers and sellers. Commercialism dominates our people. Trade and trade interests rule the nation. How, then, can we find fault with the student if he partakes of this spirit of commercialism that he can see everywhere around him, that he reads in the newspapers, hears talked on the streets and in the parlor, sees in the bitter competition of some professional men, and cannot help but know exists in the management of many institutions of professional learning?

The best interests of higher dental education demands that the management of these schools should be taken out of the hands of the individual or the teaching faculties and placed under the control of the State, or of the trustees of our great universities, for the reason that the majority of the dental schools to-day are still per force commercial institutions, dependent on the fees of students and the profits of the infirmaries to maintain them and pay the teachers and demonstrators. Just as long as commercialism exists in our system of dental education the best results can not be obtained. The interests of the students should be paramount, but this interest is often obscured by holding the dollar too close to the eye. It is marvellous how small an object will obscure our vision if we but hold it close enough.

The first dental college was organized on the commercial basis, and I do not know of a single dental school, even those under State control, that are entirely free from some form of commercialism, for in all of them the fees of the students, or the receipts of the clinics, bear a more or less important relation, either to the salaries of some of the professors or demonstrators, to the buildings they occupy, or to the apparatus or furnishings.

In most of the State institutions the appropriations are too small properly to conduct the schools, while in the colleges con-

. nected with the large endowed universities no endowments have been made to the dental schools. They are thus left in a measure to " work out their own salvation," in many cases " with fear and trembling," as I know from personal experience.

We could wish that the legislators of the States having professional schools in their universities would appropriate for their support with a more liberal hand; and that good people with fortunes they cannot spend and do not know where to bequeath, would endow the dental colleges and place them above the degrading necessity of catering to the commercial spirit, and entering students who have not a proper educational qualification to begin the study of dental surgery, or who are deficient in that peculiar aptitude for a professional life, through which alone they can hope to develop practitioners who will be an honor to the institutions that are responsible for their education.

I have confidence to believe the day is not far distant when all of the dental schools will either be liberally provided for by the State or abundantly endowed through the munificence of a Rockefeller or a Carnegie. The American people are liberal and just towards all educational efforts, and whenever they are convinced that the best interests of the citizen and the State demand that they render financial assistance to any individual enterprise, it is usually forthcoming.

Another serious drawback in our system of education is the failure to provide advanced standing in the dental course for students who have taken the bachelor's degree in liberal arts and sciences.

These students have had a sufficient amount of didactic teaching and practical laboratory instruction in chemistry, botany, morphology, physiology, zoology, comparative anatomy, etc., to more than equal the work of the freshman class in the dental schools, and under these circumstances their higher preliminary qualifications should be recognized by advancing them to the sophomore class of the dental course. By adopting a policy of this character ambitious students would be encouraged to complete their academic training before entering on the study of dental surgery.

As the matter now stands, the college graduate is placed on the same footing as the student whose qualifications are only those of a second year course of a high school, and the extra six years of study pursued by him in the languages, mathematics, literature, history, and the sciences count for nothing. This is placing a premium, I was about to say, on ignorance, but I will modify the statement and say, on the minimum requirements for matriculation, and thereby turns away many young men from the doors of the dental schools who would have been an honor to the profession.

I am constrained, also, from my sense of justice, to make another suggestion,—namely, on the matter of advanced standing for medical graduates. Since the adoption of the four-year course for medical and dental colleges there would seem to be no good reason why medical graduates who have taken a full four years' course should not be advanced to the junior grade of the dental colleges.

The four years of training of the medical graduate, preceded by a full four years' high school course as a minimum matriculation requirement, is certainly equal to the freshman and sophomore courses of study in the fundamental sciences as taught in the dental schools, preceded by only two years of the high school course as a minimum entrance qualification. It would therefore seem no more than a just recognition of the scientific work performed that he should receive such advanced standing in a dental course. If such students, devoting their full time and energy to the study of the purely dental subjects for two years, cannot make as good operators as their fellows who entered with the minimum qualifications and have spent four years upon the dental course, then the value of higher education as a prerequisite for professional study is a myth and a snare.

Let us look at this matter in a reasonable light and place ourselves on record as favoring the proposition of giving due credit for scientific work performed by candidates for matriculation who hold the B.A., B.S., or M.D. degree from colleges and universities of recognized repute. Scientific knowledge is of as much value to the dental surgeon as it is to the physician and the surgeon, for without the employment of this knowledge in his profession, the dentist is nothing more than a handcraftsman.

Reports of Society Meetings.

THE NEW YORK INSTITUTE OF STOMATOLOGY.

A REGULAR meeting of the Institute was held at " The Chelsea," No. 222 West Twenty-third Street, New York, on Tuesday evening, April 5, 1904, the President, Dr. Brockway, in the chair.

There being no communications on theory and practice, the paper of the evening, " A Plea for Thorough Dental Education," was read by Dr. Leo Green.

(For Dr. Green's paper, see page 585.)

Dr. Eugene H. Smith.—I am in full sympathy with that part of Dr. Green's paper relating to more thorough preliminary training. I would like first, however, to say a few words relative to his criticism of the conduct of the dental schools. The errors he points out are in the main true, but there is a good reason for these errors. First, as to the repetition of lectures. I find this repetition is necessary with the present class of students. I have had a chance to study this question thoroughly, having had to deal with students presenting widely differing degrees of preliminary education, from the minimum requirement to the man who has his college degree. I have asked these different men as to the wisdom of repeating lectures. In every instance the college man has replied it was unnecessary,—that he did not need to have the same thing told him twice. The poorly trained man invariably says, " I was unable to properly grasp the subject at first." I think, however, that there are very few colleges to-day that repeat lectures three years in succession. Most colleges repeat the junior and senior lectures. The correction of all this is a higher preliminary education.

The essayist speaks of the substituting of apprenticeship in an office for college work. This does not exist in any of our colleges, so far as I am aware; certainly not in Harvard. He also speaks of annual examinations, and the large number of failures in the last year as compared with other years. I can only say that this

is not so in my experience. We generally register a class of fifty
members. The first year is their Waterloo, because they are taking
anatomy, physiology, histology, bacteriology, and physiological
chemistry along with the medical students in the Harvard Medical
School. Of this number as many as thirty per cent. fail in a majority of their examinations. If a student successfully passes his
first year he is a very good man.

Another criticism was that of employing young teachers. I
think every dean who has the selecting of instructors will bear
me out in saying that the average graduate of twenty years ago is
not a fit man for an instructor in the present dental school. While
it is desirable that we should have men more experienced in practice, still such a man is apt to have many hobbies. He is set in his
methods, and is apt to be a dangerous man for the young student
to meet, but a most valuable man after the student has become
more matured. Then again it is difficult to get the older men
as teachers. They are busy men, and every hour they teach is a
financial loss to them, more so in dentistry than in medicine. The
dental man who gives his time to charity or to teaching does it at a
greater cost to himself than does the medical man.

The essayist says that the college authorities should make it
plain to the impossible student, at the earliest possible moment,
that his sphere of usefulness is elsewhere. I think the majority
of men who have charge of the education of students do this very
thing. It is a difficult matter, however. to determine. Many men
who do discouraging work to begin with turn out to be first-class
men. So a teacher takes a great deal upon himself who says to a
young man, " You have missed your calling; your field of use- ·
fulness is elsewhere." Again, the student may think otherwise.

The essayist speaks of the habit of practitioners concealing
useful ideas. The men with whom I have had the honor to be
associated have been perfectly free with their ideas, and their laboratories and operating-rooms have not been locked to their fellow-
workers.

A proper preliminary education is essential to any professional education. There certainly can be no question about that.
The only difference of opinion that can exist is as to what that
preliminary education shall be. Some go so far as to say that
the practitioner in dentistry should receive the same education as
the specialties in medicine; that the dental practitioner should

have a medical degree. There is strong logic in their arguments, and it may come to this. On the other hand, we will find other men, like our essayist, who will argue for a college training. I feel that I can enter upon the discussion of this subject without prejudice, as I hold but the one degree, that of dentistry. As far as my experience as a teacher goes, I have invariably found that the man with the right kind of a college training makes the best dental student, and can do more work in a given time than the man can whose preliminary training is represented by two years' work in a high school. This being true, it follows that with high preliminary requirements, and a college course of three years of nine months each, much more can be done in the way of advancing our professional standing than can be accomplished in a four years' course with immature and improperly trained men.

Dr. B. Holly Smith.—There are some misstatements in the paper as to the actual facts, unless the essayist has inside information of which I am not possessed. I have been a teacher for twenty-one years and am a member of the Association of Dental Faculties, and I stand here to-day to say that the system of dental education in this country is not faultless, but it is in every way far above that described by your essayist. I know of no lax treatment of foreign students. Do not we have associates appointed in all the countries of Europe, and are not we more jealous of the good behavior of men who go abroad than of any other class of students? So it seems unfair that we receive this statement as an absolute fact.

As to our preliminary training. Why does not this organization appoint a committee to formulate a proper plan? Do we not resolve too much? Do we not discuss too much? Let us *do* something. Every one of us knows that the dental student should have a special preliminary training. What we need to determine is what that special training ought to be. It would seem desirable that instead of the language courses now necessary for college entrance, a course in manual training be substituted for those students contemplating entering the profession of dentistry. It seems to me here in your Columbia University such a course might be given, not unlike the course for students in medicine. A kind of manual-chemical-physical course. We do want more finger-work. We want training along certain special lines. Now, instead of discrediting those who hold for a four years' course, why not

allow anybody who has secured an A.B. degree in the chemical-
biological course a credit of one year of that four years' course?
The proposition of the essayist as to a nine months' school year does
not at all meet with my approval. I would say broadly that there
are two distinct propositions made in the paper that I should
oppose. First, I do not favor an A.B. degree, excepting one along
the lines of the student's life work. Otherwise it is wasted time.
Secondly, I am opposed to a nine months' course. I grant that in
Boston, where pupils are not subjected to any great changes of
temperature, they can manage to work for nine months. But
this cannot be done in the Southern States. Take Atlanta, Louisville, or Nashville. It is simply impracticable. Then again, many
of our dental students are self-supporting, and it is necessary for
them to have the interval between sessions to secure the where-
withal for a return to college. I do not at all agree with the essayist when he says that a greater part of our dental students are men
who have tried mercantile pursuits and failed. It is not so in
Baltimore, and I do not believe it is so anywhere. A large percentage are men who are much more capable than the average
salesman or clerk. I have never heard of any credit being given a
student for laboratory or office work. Certainly it is against the
rules, and I rather think the essayist is mistaken. Dr. Smith says
that the time is not yet ripe for an A.B. degree. It never will be
ripe for such an A.B. degree as many of the colleges are granting.
Is it not some evidence of education to have secured the degree of
D.D.S.? Is it not necessary that a man should study, should
read, should think, should experiment; that he should use his
hands? Certainly this all-around training makes him a larger
man than would development of the mental faculties alone. I have
known college graduates who could not take the bridle from a
horse, who did not know how to open a gate. The dentist is to-
day in my judgment the most resourceful man in the world. So
far as recognition is concerned, it bothers me not at all. It depends upon the individual whether he is recognized or not.

   Dr. Edward C. Kirk.—I wish to speak about some things that
have been touched upon and also about some things that have not.
I know very little about the majority of dental schools, but I am
surprised to learn what I have to-night,—that they are in such a
state of degeneracy. I was very much interested in the suggestion for a definition of what constitutes a high educational stand-

ard. I have written something about that and said something about it, and I would like to get in the minds of my professional colleagues this idea that there is a difference and a great big one between the quality and the quantity of an educational standard, and its adaptability to a given purpose. I quite agree with Dr. Holly Smith when he says that any old A.B. degree will not do. It must represent a certain kind of training adaptable to the purpose of preparing a man for entering upon the study of dentistry. The question of a Latin requirement has been touched upon. I hold that a year or two years of Latin is insufficient except for the discipline which any study affords. Other than the discipline common to all education, Latin is valuable for two purposes, either for the study of Latin literature or as a side-light upon the study of English. On the theory of Goethe, that he who does not know a foreign language does not know his own, how much does a student get out of one or two years of Latin? Of how much value is it as a preliminary training for admission to the professional study of dentistry? I wish to quote some extracts from a correspondence with a well-known gentleman regarding the uses and purposes of Latin as taught in our schools. " So far as I have ever seen, the training of Latin in the preparatory schools is as bad as it can be. It was bad in Milton's time, and the faults that existed then seem to exist now." I was present at a commencement when the president said, " Qui gradum doctores dentarii accedunt," but not one of the students knew enough of Latin to go up and get his diploma. That might have happened in any dental school under the present entrance standards. If a man does not know enough Latin to come up and get his diploma v hen he is asked to do so in Latin, of what use is it to him. In order to get the use of Latin a student should have a dozen years of it; he would then be in a position to read Latin literature and would understand his English better. I heartily agree with Dr. Smith, of Harvard, that the man with the college training is the better man all round, and personally I am sorry that the opportunity was not given to Harvard University to try this experiment which they are determined to try independently of the Association of Faculties. The objection that I have to the position as expressed by Dr. Smith is that this is the ideal which he thinks ought to be attained by all colleges. I want to have this recognized, that we are not making soldiers. We have no such thing as a system of dental education. We have,

instead, systems of dental education. We are not duplicati
multiplying men of the same caliber or apacity. S me m
come strong in certain ways, and in   necessarily
in others. I believe there is r om t~um f r an institut
will try just this experiment that Harv u University means
but on that account it sho n t be said that as it is g
certain number, th rei re everybody must d the ame thing
special training will be aut t r d int that thing cal
ture. and ther is u u uu i m u n
vated men. But do V

instead, systems of dental education. We are not duplicating and
multiplying men of the same caliber or capacity. Some must become strong in certain ways, and they will necessarily be weak
in others. I believe there is room to-day for an institution that
will try just this experiment that Harvard University means to try,
but on that account it should not be said that as it is good for a
certain number, therefore everybody must do the same thing. This
special training will be manufactured into that thing called culture, and there is undoubtedly room for a great body of such cultivated men. But do you suppose they are the best men to serve the
public everywhere? I do not think so. Such a man will naturally
gravitate to the cities where culture abounds, and where he will
be in sympathetic touch with those of his own class, and he would
be unhappy in any other environment. From this class of men
will doubtless be produced investigators and teachers, and of both
these we need many. But there is room for a much larger number
of men who will be empirics. The average medical practitioner,
when asked why he treats a case thus and so, will give you an
answer based on the rule of thumb. There is room in my judgment for that larger class of men who have only the preliminary
education furnished by the State to practise among that class of
people commonly spoken of as the " common" people. A man
who is in sympathy with them. Then again there is a great class
of men who are unable, because they are brought face to face with
the bread-and-butter problem, to go into the field of education beyond that which the State furnishes. Indeed, the high school furnishes a very good training to-day. Who made dentistry; was it
college graduates? I think not. Or if some of our dental pioneers
were college men, is it not true that the average A.B. of thirty-
five or forty years ago is no better educated than the high-school
graduate of to-day? So I think it is a wrong method to make
an A.B. degree a necessary qualification for entrance into the
dental profession.

The essayist, with a wave of his hand, dismisses the whole
subject of State sovereignty, saying that this difficulty about interchange of licenses could be overcome by the creation of a national
standard. Certainly it could, but that involves an amendment to
the Constitution of the United States, and that is a question affecting State sovereignty, which is a very difficult problem. The last
time that State sovereignty was practically considered in this

country was in the early youth of most of us, when several hundreds of thousands of able-bodied men laid down their lives in the discussion of it. I do not believe there can be any such amendment making an obligatory national standard possible, however desirable it might be.

As to the question of commercialism and what the essayist has designated as English law, I doubt if it is English law. What he has quoted is merely a contract. It might hold under English law, but I doubt if it would hold here.

Dr. Faneuil D. Weisse.—I am an optimist in the full sense of the word and especially so with regard to what the dental institutions of this country have accomplished in establishing dentistry as a profession. I look upon all plans as regards preliminary education as unnecessary, as it has had and is going through its natural evolution, in spite of sporadic spurts by individual institutions. In New York State preliminary educational requirements to enter the profession have been steadily progressive since 1894, and every step forward has been conservative and permanent, with the exception of the experience of 1897, when it was realized that the advance to a 48-count requirement for dentistry was premature.

The way of the dental institutions of the United States has been hard, indeed, as they never have received from contributors to the dental journals any encouragement or commendation for their work. On the contrary, the dental journals of the country give us periodical freshets of articles criticising straw-like shortcomings in the general work.

Turning from the minor details of college work criticised by the author of the paper, let us realize that the present status of dentistry as a profession is due to the aggregate results of the work of our dental institutions.

The calling of the practice of dentistry has been a profession little more than sixty years; before that it was only a handicraft. *No calling is a profession until institutions have been established with a defined scientific curriculum for education and training for its practice.* Surgery was at one time a handicraft, and the surgeon was the servant of the physician and only became his peer after medical institutions had made provision in the medical curriculum for his education as a surgeon.

The birth of the calling of dentistry as a profession was at the sending forth, with the degree of D.D.S., of the first class of the Baltimore College of Dental Surgery, in 1841. Since that time the other dental institutions of the country have been established to educate for a profession.

Some critics have held that the creation of the degree of D.D.S. was a mistake; that all practitioners of dental surgery should be practising under the degree of M.D. To my mind the phenomenal growth of the dental profession is due to the fact that the degree of D.D.S. was created, and that a scientific curriculum for education to enter its ranks was evolved independently of the M.D. degree, thereby enabling the dental student to concentrate his energies within definite lines of his special education unincumbered by subjects which have no bearing on his specialty of general medicine.

Under these advantageous conditions the dental institutions of the United States have made the D.D.S. degree the evidence of special professional education and skill throughout the world where dental surgery is practised.

To-day the D.D.S. degree has won its peerage of the M.D. degree, and that from the hands of the mother profession, in that the American Medical Association has recently voted the D.D.S. degree to membership.

To-day European and Pan-American institutions are organizing along the lines of those of the United States. Only the other day I received a letter from a member of the Parliament of New Zealand asking for information as to the organization of the New York College of Dentistry, in view of the establishment of a dental department of the University of New Zealand.

With the above work achieved by our dental institutions before them, the dental profession of the United States have reason to be proud of the results accomplished by their professional institutions during the short life history of their profession—as such —of only sixty years. When the history of the nineteenth century is written it will record the fact that in the United States, during the last six decades of the century, the handicraft of dentistry rose to the dignity of a profession, by the establishment of special institutions with a specialized scientific curriculum for its education and training, and under the *ægis* of the D.D.S degree.

Dr. Hopkins.—I certainly am very grateful to the society for bringing this subject up for discussion, and while the essayist has come in for a great deal of criticism, I think he may console himself in the thought that he is a martyr to the cause of advanced dental education, and may congratulate himself that he has created a greater interest in the subject than has ever been expressed before at any dental meeting. I am delighted that this dual experiment of a three and a four years' course is going to be tried, and I am not at all sure what the result is going to be. I am not sure but that men equipped as will be the men who enter the Harvard Dental School will be able to accomplish as much or more in their three years than can the ordinary students in four. However, I do not agree with the essayist that any A.B. degree would be a suitable preliminary training. I think that anything which retards the taking up of the technical part of dental work retards the practitioner in the acquirement of manipulative skill. It may have been a faulty observation, but it has been my experience that men who have obtained their academic degree from institutions where they have received no manipulative training, do not acquire skill in practice as early nor as surely as those students who begin their dental work when they are four years younger. It is a question if the academic degree will be altogether helpful until it is changed so that technical requirements may be substituted bearing upon the professional training which is to follow.

Aside from this, I think most of the improvement in preliminary examinations should be upon the subject of English. I believe I can tell, after a student has written an essay of five hundred words, and after I have had fifteen minutes' conversation with him, whether that student is going to be able to understand the lectures in his course and the subjects in his text-books. I think the greatest failing in preliminary education to-day is in English. If a man, no matter whether he comes from the high school or from college, has a correct knowledge of English, it indicates a capacity to understand the theoretical work of his course in dentistry, and is a better preparation than any amount of Latin. There is great encouragement to the profession in the fact that so many representative men are interested in this question of higher dental education, and that each one is seeking for the greatest good of the profession, although perhaps there is lack of agreement as to how it can best be accomplished.

Dr. E. A. Bogue.—It seems to me that the statement has not yet been made as to what the dentist's education should be, though

I have heard some good English, some bad English, and precious little Latin. A good many years ago there were two or three medical men who took up the study of the mouth and its associated parts.

I do not think that a committee from this body could formulate a practical plan for dental education, nor any other committee. The ordinary dentist's work is to prevent pain or loss, or to replace lost parts. The craft began with the mechanical side. It has been enlarged until the medical branch includes prophylaxis. It has become, in the hands of the colleges and practitioners, a liberal profession. As a mechanical art there was very little to study, but as a liberal profession it has opened up the same field for study and observation as the other professions. The question now comes up as to whether Dr. Eggleston was right when he said that the best way of instructing a man in doing anything that his hands could do was to set him doing it. Dr. Holly Smith tells us that the climate of the country is so varying that we must have varying systems. Dr. Eugene Smith tells us that in certain States technical education is compulsory. We may infer that such States furnish the best preliminary education for dental students. Anyway, we shall undoubtedly find that when the dental instructors of this country shall have perfected their organization, and when they decide what they consider for the best for the students, they will adopt it, and that in the end we will come to a system applicable to the students of the entire country and the teaching will be such as will result in the giving to the profession such a body of men as will administer to the needs of their fellows in the most successful and advantageous manner. I have no doubt that hints from any of us will be thankfully received.

Dr. Ottolengui.—I have been delighted to hear with what perfect frankness this subject has been discussed this evening. The points seem to have all been covered by the gentlemen connected with the colleges. While I am a dentist, I have devoted a number of years to the study of entomology, and consequently the story of the "humbug" was familiar to me. I am going to risk another. A professor once asked one of the boys in his class to tell him what a moth is. The boy told him that a moth is an insect with a head, a body, from one to four eyes, one or two antennæ, and from one to four feet, with a pin through the middle of it. The professor said, "Where did you get that idea of an insect?" "From a study of the college collection," was the reply. The essayist's impression of the colleges of the country has been acquired more from similar papers and criticisms than from a study of the colleges themselves. As I have gone about the various cities I have made it my business, wherever there was a college, to visit that college, and I have, without exception, been impressed with the fact that, whether the college was a large college or a small college, the evident intent to do the best that could be done was conspicuously present in all of the schools. I entirely agree with what Dr. Weisse has said. It is well for us to bear in mind that whatever we are, we are the product of our educational institutions, and instead of berating them we should be proud of them and praise them. So far as I myself am concerned, my sympathies are entirely with the schools and what they are doing.

Dr. Kirk brought out the idea that one particular kind of dentist will not suffice for this broad American continent. There is no question but that the system to be adopted by Harvard will be eminently successful and will produce men of the highest attainments, but another class of dentists also is required,—dentists who will be willing to work for the lowly and for lowly fees. We have here in New York a very cosmopolitan centre, and we need men here not only of the highest culture, but also men who will be willing to work among the lower classes and for small stipends. For Thursday night I have accepted an invitation to address a society down in the Bowery, known as the Eastern Dental Society of New York. What litttle I know about these men has interested me. They are practising among an ignorant and cosmopolitan people who understand very little or nothing of the English language. These men are evidently not graduates of Harvard, but are not they doing a good work in this world, and was it not worth while that they were graduated from some school?

So I want to say, with the kindliest spirit in the world to the essayist, that this subject is much larger than his paper has covered or could cover. At the same time, it is in the hands of the very best men capable of solving it, the men who have charge of the colleges. Suppose the schools were all closed. Do you think the men who are criticising them could do better?

Dr. Green.—I feel very much like Daniel in the lions' den, for more than one reason; in the first place, because I do not know whether I am alive or not, and in the second place, because I am about as well able to defend myself as Daniel was. There are just one or two points that I wish to go over. The gentlemen who have discussed my paper to-night represent, with one exception, the side of the Associated Faculties, and necessarily their discussion is one-sided. I want to quote once more from Dr. Carlton's paper, not only because it is apropos, but also because, contrasted with the remarks of some of the previous speakers, it indicates that even the Associated Faculties (to whom Dr. Holly Smith so frequently referred) are not entirely agreed in their " ideas" for dental education.

" Higher education is not a question alone of preparing great men for great things; it must also prepare little men for greater things than they would have otherwise found possible. As a good beefsteak disappears in a man and reappears as energy and vigor, so is education absorbed, and reappears as mature judgment, mental balance, keen, acute, grasping intellect. Is there a practitioner among us not holding the degree of Bachelor of Science, Bachelor of Arts, Doctor of Medicine, or otherwise, who does not bitterly regret opportunity slighted or unavailable? He would indeed be glad to possess them, not for the mere degree's sake alone, but for the education's sake. . . . I trust I have said enough to prove to you that the opportunities of modern dentistry are so new and vast that an ampler education is needed by the practitioner of the future. We cannot give them that education in a four years' course at a Dental College. Let him take ten, if necessary, with the preliminary; it will be worth the while, and his place in the professional world will wait for him. The four-year courses in our dental schools will be well and completely filled with good instruction and practical work."

Now, gentlemen, my motives in presenting this paper have been entirely misunderstood. I did not come here to try to teach the men who are in charge of the various dental colleges of this country how to run their institutions; but, on the other hand, I do not agree with Dr. Ottolengui that we must leave the faults where we find them. I am perfectly willing to take all the fair criticism I have received to-night, if I have provoked an honest discussion of this subject. I think Dr. Kirk was disposed to jest with my paper. Some of the indictments he brings against dental education in his various articles are almost as severe, if not more so, than mine. In his article in the January, 1904, *Dental Cosmos,* on the "Scientific Method in Dentistry," he deplores the empirical methods in our instruction, etc., and regrets the "attitude of downright contempt" towards scientific methods. This is somewhat at variance with his attitude and remarks this evening. I quote from his article as follows:

"There seems to be a widespread feeling that the scientific method in dentistry is a sort of mental jugglery by which certain men find diversion in mystifying others who have no task for that kind of entertainment. I do not think I have overdrawn the situation, for the belief seems to be quite general that there are two aspects to dentistry,—one denominated 'theory' and the other denominated 'practical.' It is voiced generally by State boards of dental examiners; it is the current belief of dental students. Dental college faculties are by no means blameless in this connection. . . . We must understand always that the school is its corps of teachers, and that everything else in the institution is merely accessory thereto. No man should be permitted to teach, to form the habits of mind, the ideals, of the recruits of our profession who has not in some way obtained that breadth of training which means not only knowledge of the data of science, but scientific culture as well. It is not what he teaches so much as how he teaches that indicates his fitness and determines the type of practitioner he creates. In proportion as the teacher uses the scientific method does he eradicate from the minds of his students the empirical method and improve their mode of practice by putting it upon a rational basis."

Empirical methods, as I understand them, are those which depend upon isolated experiments and observation without due regard to scientific principles. I find our educational methods empirical in that they neglect the first principle of scientific procedure,—a lack of preliminary training.

Most of the criticism here to-night has been directed against my suggestion for a baccalaureate degree as a preliminary requirement. All who have discussed the paper have either ignored or forgotten the fact that I distinctly stated what I considered to be a proper baccalaureate degree, and not "any old degree," as stated by Dr. Holly Smith. I am afraid that Dr. Kirk referred to an amendment of the constitution in a spirit of ridicule. I think it would be possible for an understanding to exist among the organized boards of examiners, whereby an interchange of licenses might be effected without a national calamity.

Dr. Holly Smith has mentioned the fact that the climatic conditions in many States makes a nine months' course impracticable. I would like to ask the doctor if in these same States the climatic conditions prevent a man from working more than nine months of the year.

A great many misstatements are charged against this paper. The only reason that I did not mention specific incidents was, that I desired to avoid all personalities. I regret that some of the men who discussed my paper should have accused me of misstatements. To any of these men I shall be very glad indeed to give specific instances in proof of what I have stated.

I am very grateful to you, gentlemen, for having given me so much of your attention.

Adjourned.

FRED. L. BOGUE, M.D., D.D.S.,
Editor The New York Institute of Stomatology.

AMERICAN MEDICAL ASSOCIATION, SECTION ON STOMTATOLOGY, ATLANTIC CITY, JUNE 7 TO 10, 1904.

DISCUSSION ON PAPERS IN SYMPOSIUM ON DENTAL EDUCATION BY DRS. EAMES, CHITTENDEN, BALDWIN, AND MARSHALL.

Dr. Eugene S. Talbot, Chicago.—Anticipating that something might be said in the Chairman's Address in regard to the length of term in the dental colleges, and the position that would be taken at the meeting in Washington, I wrote letters to Professor Eliot of Harvard and to President Harper of the University of Chicago, asking them to prepare papers for this section. President Harper was unable to comply with my request, but I have a letter from Professor Eliot, which I will read at this time:

" DEAR SIR,—I shall not be able to attend the meeting of the Section on Stomatology of the American Medical Association at Atlantic City, June 7 to 10, 1904. The proper person to state the position of Harvard in regard to the future policy of its Dental School is the dean of that school, Dr. Eugene H. Smith, 283 Dartmouth Street, Boston.

" The policy of the Harvard School is not commercial in the least. It is steadily endeavoring to raise the standard of dental education, and has in a good degree succeeded. Just now it is trying to raise the standard of the admission examinations to the school, and is finding that a difficult task. It can not add, at the same time, to the length of its own course. Moreover, the school has been struggling for several years to maintain a close connection with the Harvard Medical School. The task has proved difficult because of the rapid improvement of the Medical School consequent on its admitting none but the persons who already hold a degree in Arts or Science. The Dental School must accomplish both the tasks to which it has set itself before it can lengthen its course to four years. The Section on Stomatology may rest assured that the Harvard Dental School will continue to do what it always has been doing—namely, contribute to the improvement of the preparatory course for the dental profession.

" Very truly yours,
" CHARLES W. ELIOT."

I am sorry to say that Dr. Smith can not be present, but Dr. Briggs will give us some idea of what the school will do.

Dr. E. C. Briggs, Harvard Medical School.—I am sorry that Dr. Smith can not be here to give you the best idea, and as it was only a few days ago that he told me he could not be present, I have not been able to make any real preparation or collect any special data. I can, however, point out one or two things and state a few facts which I hope will impress on your minds the idea that Harvard is not blocking in any way dental education. In fact, it seems ludicrous that others should have placed her in such a position, when she has always been struggling quite the other way, and, I may say, struggling against her own commercial interests. We have decimated our classes time and again by the advances we have made over other schools.

The question is, What elevates the profession? We speak about the progress we have made, but we lose sight of what really elevates the profession as a whole. There are plenty of men in the profession to-day who have elevated themselves as high as any one could wish, who have not had any particular preliminary training. They have had the genius and have made the geniuses, but that does not raise the profession as a whole. That is the feeling that we have at Harvard. To set the profession right before the world, attention must be given to the character of the men and their scholarly attainments, and that is the reason we have paid so much more attention to preliminary requirements than we have to the length of the course. The length of the course is a little misleading. It is four years of seven months; Harvard already has three years of nine months. We are only one month short. With that, and with our entrance requirements, we do not feel that we could wipe out our school altogether. We have about cut it in half now, and what better evidence can you have that we are not commercial? If we were commercial we would take in some of the men who come from other colleges who write to know what their position will be on coming into our school. Not one has accepted, because we say, we will give you time allowance, but you must pass every examination before you can graduate. That is not what they want, and they do not come. For the post-graduate our terms would be entirely different. That does away with the suggestion that our line of thought is due to any commercialism. I wish that you would send, as we have done, for purposes of comparison, to the different colleges, and see what their examination papers are and compare them with ours. Not one man out of ten with a high-school education can come into our school. He must pass the examination with ability to go into college—not twenty-four points, but as many points as he goes. He has got to pass just as good an examination as if to enter Harvard or Yale—I speak of them because they are nearer. So it seems to me that Harvard has been put in an unfortunate light, diametrically opposite to what she really is at heart. The time that a man is in a professional school is of great value to him; we appreciate that as much as anybody else—I do not believe ten years would be too much, if you wish to reach the highest ambition of life. The idea is, that having provided a certain amount of good training, which we think we do in three years, the next step is to have the man who comes into the school one who is already a scholar and fitted to take up any of the liberal professions. You and I are helped just as much by that uplift. We can not stand back and say we did pretty well and that we only had " reading, writing, and arithmetic." If the standard is raised by making it necessary to have something more than that, you will get professional standing. The profession will not make its highest success until the men who come into it are men of education and scholarly attainments.

Dr. Williams, Boston.—One of the things which I thought I would object to in teaching in Harvard was that I would have to teach with men who were not prepared to learn. I am glad to know that the standard of the examination has been advanced so that the students are better able to learn. The preliminary preparation is necessary in order to know how to learn to the best advantage.

Dr. James Truman, Philadelphia.—I feel in a somewhat embarrassing position, coming down here as if I were inspired to attack Harvard. That is not my purpose. So far as I am concerned, I want to advance dental education along the best line possible. In 1884 we organized the Association of Faculties, and for twenty years we have worked steadily to bring up the standard of education to four years. At Asheville last year, when we supposed we had established that, without any prospect of its being changed, we received a blow from the very highest educational centre in this country,—Harvard. It requested that it should be given the privilege of three years, because it intended to advance the preliminary standard to the A.B. degree eventually, and for that reason and for the higher standard which it claims at present, it believes that it had a right to a three years' course. I was chairman of the committee which took that matter in charge, and we could not, under the circumstances, agree to the proposition, because other universities in this country had practically the same standard and the same length of time. Now the action of Harvard on that occasion was an encouragement to the commercial schools. I know very well that Harvard has never been a commercial school. No one can charge Harvard with that. It has always been exactly the contrary, and that is why I was astounded at that time at its action. After they left the Association of Faculties we heard that we were to be met, first at Buffalo and in a day or two at Washington, with the commercial idea of going back to three years because the schools could not maintain themselves. Now, Harvard may not have meant this. Harvard did not mean it, but at the same time that influence has been an injury to general dental education in this country, and I do not see how Harvard can explain it.

We have had this afternoon a good deal that is of value in these papers, and, as a rule, I am in unity with them, especially with the paper of our chairman. I agree with the proposition that the higher in a general way you can educate a man the better, but you must have that education properly arranged in order to be of value. The idea to me is pre-eminently absurd to suppose that because a man has an A.B. degree that he is better qualified thereby to become a dentist. It is a fallacy. The high-school degree is equally fallacious. What we need in dentistry is an education that will fit a man to become a dentist. To accomplish this he should come up from the mechanical school, through the higher schools, and then reach a point where he can be of value to himself and the community at large. There is probably not a man here in this room who ever had more than two years of four or five months' study in the professional schools. I do not believe that we can make dentists out of all men, whether they have the A.B. degree (and we have a number of them) or whether they have the high-school degree; that is not the point. We must go deeper if we expect to have symmetry in our educational effort. My own idea has been that the poor dentists we have turned out have, as a rule, been men of higher education—not the fault of the higher education, but the fault of a lack of proper symmetry in that education. Let me illustrate: I had two boys to educate. One was my own son, the other a nephew. My own son I insisted should take a six years' course to acquire a proper classical education. After several years' preparatory training in a German gymnasium, he graduated with the highest honors of the university and with nothing in anything else. The other boy was mechanical. I insisted on his going through the manual training and from the manual training school to the university, and from the university to a post-graduate department in one of our large manufacturing establishments, making nearly eight years in his particular direction, and at the present time, at thirty years of age, he is superintendent of motive power in one of our largest establishments in Philadelphia. My own son became a teacher. That is what I mean by symmetry in education; training the men from the very beginning so that they can practise whatever they expect to adopt as their calling, and not supposing that because a man has an A.B. degree or any other degree of that character, that he can enter a dental school and become a dentist. This very day I have before me numbers in our own university who are in degree unfit to practise dentistry, and it is a source of tribulation to me that I have to meet that sort of thing. They have not been properly trained from the beginning. They have not the manipulative ability that ought to come with good practice, and they will never get it, because they have reached an age when it is impossible that that shall be perfected in the individual. If we are to advance education we must look at it intelligently. Let us come down to practical matters. Let us take our experience; the experience with me covers nearly half a century. In the old laws regulating mechanical work in my own State, young men had to go into apprenticeship, working for four or five years until they reached their majority at twenty-one, before they could practise any of the mechanical trades. Then they were skilled in their work. Now we are trying to turn out men in three years in one of the most complex mechanical professions that I know anything about in this world, that of dentistry. We would turn them out with a fundamental knowledge of anatomy, bacteriology, histology, etc., and the mechanical training almost entirely ignored. Is that what we are here for? Are we here for that purpose alone? If we are, then I am not a dentist.

Dr. Williams, Boston.—Dr. Truman is right in his views regarding the manipulative qualifications of a dentist. It is necessary that they should be trained properly and early. I have known some of the best manipulators to be the greatest failures in their operations from not knowing when and how to exercise their manipulative skill. I have known of one or two instances of fatal results, from very high skill misplaced.

Editorial.

THE DISSATISFIED DENTAL COLLEGES.

WHEN the Association of Dental Faculties met at Washington, D. C., June 9, as narrated in our last number, the vote to a return to a three years' course stood twenty-one in favor and twenty-four against any change. This was supposed to be final, and yet there was a feeling that possibly certain colleges, in the

minority, might hold that their financial interests were so deeply
involved that some effort might be made to weaken this decision.

Those who thus felt had not long to wait to see a realization
of their prophetic feelings. We now hear of several resignations
from that body, and rumors of more to come. One school, that
failed to vote either way, is so much disturbed by the outlook that
the Dean feels compelled to seek advice as to the propriety of calling a special meeting of the "Faculties" late in August.

The dissatisfaction expressed at Washington, and since, is the
natural outcome of the financial stress the four years' course
brought to many of the dental colleges, and it was generally predicted that if the four years was insisted upon many of the colleges
would be forced to close. If this should be the result, it may be
a question whether this would, or would not, be detrimental to
dental education.

It is not the purpose at present to discuss this phase of the
subject, but rather to call attention to the fact that, if the entire
number of twenty-one should resign, it would not affect the integrity of the Association of Faculties. Its work is not dependent on numbers. It has had a distinct mission to perform ever
since Dr. Winder and his colleagues called the educational bodies
together, in 1884, to legislate, that eventually a higher standard
of dental education might be established in all the dental schools
of the country.

A dean of one of the dental colleges recently resigned had the
honesty to assign as a reason for its act that the very life of the
school depended upon its freedom from control and ability to be
its own judge of whom to admit and whom to reject, and, further,
that financial interests governed its action. Whether this is the
motive of all is not at present known, but behind other ostensible
reasons will be found the necessity of the self-sustaining treasury.

That resignation is the only dignified course for those schools
entertaining this view is admitted, but in taking it they write
down each school as an enemy to advanced dental education and
must bear whatever odium falls to the lot of the school that serves
mammon rather than the higher ideals.

The mistake these schools are making, in the opinion of the
writer, is to suppose that this course will be to their financial interests. This portion of the subject is not pleasant to dwell upon,
for nothing can be more distasteful to the true lover of a high edu-

Ω

minority, might hold that their financial interests were so deeply involved that some effort might be made to weaken this decision.

Those who thus felt had not long to wait to see a realization of their prophetic feelings. We now hear of several resignations from that body, and rumors of more to come. One school, that failed to vote either way, is so much disturbed by the outlook that the Dean feels compelled to seek advice as to the propriety of calling a special meeting of the " Faculties" late in August.

The dissatisfaction expressed at Washington, and since, is the natural outcome of the financial stress the four years' course brought to many of the dental colleges, and it was generally predicted that if the four years was insisted upon many of the colleges would be forced to close. If this should be the result, it may be a question whether this would, or would not, be detrimental to dental education.

It is not the purpose at present to discuss this phase of the subject, but rather to call attention to the fact that, if the entire number of twenty-one should resign, it would not affect the integrity of the Association of Faculties. Its work is not dependent on numbers. It has had a distinct mission to perform ever since Dr. Winder and his colleagues called the educational bodies together, in 1884, to legislate, that eventually a higher standard of dental education might be established in all the dental schools of the country.

A dean of one of the dental colleges recently resigned had the honesty to assign as a reason for its act that the very life of the school depended upon its freedom from control and ability to be its own judge of whom to admit and whom to reject, and, further, that financial interests governed its action. Whether this is the motive of all is not at present known, but behind other ostensible reasons will be found the necessity of the self-sustaining treasury.

That resignation is the only dignified course for those schools entertaining this view is admitted, but in taking it they write down each school as an enemy to advanced dental education and must bear whatever odium falls to the lot of the school that serves mammon rather than the higher ideals.

The mistake these schools are making, in the opinion of the writer, is to suppose that this course will be to their financial interests. This portion of the subject is not pleasant to dwell upon, for nothing can be more distasteful to the true lover of a high educational standard, than to weigh it in the balance with money. This, however, is their standard of valuation, not the writer's. Viewing it, then, from their side it seems certain that, in the end, they will find they have simply dug the pit for their own destruction, and from this there can be no resurrection. The world, at no period in its history, has been kind to those who have attempted to turn the wheels of civilization backward. If these schools were a law unto themselves, there might be a period of limited prosperity coming to them, but they are not now, or ever can be, in the position occupied by the dental schools of this country in 1870. The system of control has altogether changed, and the tendency is to bind the professional schools more and more to law, and from this there is no escape.

Aside from this, there is a sentiment among the people that demands the best in education, and will not be satisfied to patronize those schools that play fast and loose with the higher standards established for the best in collegiate and professional training.

The schools that have resigned and those that propose to follow in this direction will, probably, painfully recall the work, anxiety, and expense entailed in securing membership in the Association of Faculties. The door out is always wide open for those who seek greater freedom, but it will be securely bolted and barred to prevent their return to the fold. Higher professional education has no use for prodigal sons.

The National Association of Dental Examiners will now have a duty to perform. It is not a duty devolving upon this journal to point out the way. It recognizes that this Association possesses only a moral power, but if that be used properly it can meet this crisis in dental education effectively. It will accord with the wishes of those who have stood firmly for the highest available standard, if the Association of Examiners demands all that the Association of Faculties has stood for, and also make it impossible for graduates from the schools outside of the Association to be examined by the State boards. While this may or may not have legal strength, it will, at least, place the bodies that control dental education in the best light possible before a critical world.

Dental education in America is in no danger of a collapse. In the view of the writer, at no period in its history has the view been more encouraging. Some light may become dim, some will expire, but the effulgence will be continually greater with those who maintain that dentistry needs and must have a standard of training that looks to the future and not that which revolves round the crudities of a century, good in itself, but wholly unfitted for the necessities of that future that lies before the new men and the new time,—the eternal progressive march of ideas.

"THE LAST CALL."

To those familiar with vestibuled trains and long distance travel this ominous sound will be recalled as the last warning to belated feeders due in the dining-car. The writer has,. however, no gastronomic idea connected with the title to this article. It belongs to a more important issue,—the last call to the hosts of dentistry in America to be stirring themselves to meet our colleagues from distant lands in St. Louis and, in Congress assembled, devise ways and means to make a standard of excellence for the profession of dentistry.

There is always an uncertain number who delay deciding whether to take part in a great movement or let the opportunity slip by forever. The close of this month will find three important conventions assembling at St. Louis,—the International Dental Federation, the International Dental Congress, and the National Dental Association. Before the September issue of this journal reaches our subscribers these great meetings will have concluded their labors.

It is supposed that it is scarcely necessary to remind our intelligent circle of readers that they have a duty to perform in this connection, and that duty lies not in the direction of an exposition, great as that undoubtedly is, but in a concentrated effort, shoulder to shoulder, to make such a representation of American dentistry that, in numbers, at least, the occasion may be made impressive. We would not be misunderstood here, for while numbers carry force, they cannot bear, in any convocation, a close relation to quality. The mob in science is to be deprecated as much as the mob in misrule. Dentistry, however, should not be a mob, in the ordinary acceptation of that term. The time has arrived when all who claim the title of stomatologist, and all dentists do so claim, have received a training that warrants the expectation that they are all drilled soldiers in the army of dental science and will fall into the ranks as naturally as the German or French reserve will enter into active service with his regiment.

The doubtful man will argue with himself, " Of what use will I be there among the thousands? Every one cannot prepare papers of scientific value, and for myself, as I cannot write or speak, it will be time and money wasted for me to be present." This, in effect, is the personal argument with many. It is the self-depreciation that multiplies the dead weight in all the active work of the world. Every man, in the generic sense, has a work to do, and to shirk it without good reason is but little short of a crime. The common thief takes that which he has never earned. The man who is willing to accept an improvement that advances his profession without returning an equivalent is simply absorbing that which does not by right belong to him. While it is true that all are not equally gifted, and some cannot, or, perhaps, think they cannot, aid in organized effort, no one is so incapable as not to be able to give the light of his countenance to the labor, and thus encourage others to do the work he professes his inability to accomplish.

There is another and, possibly, a selfish side to this subject. The man or woman interested in dentistry cannot afford to miss any of the conventions, and especially those that will meet at St. Louis. He or she who feels that all the good of these meetings can be gathered from the journal reports lives in a " fool's paradise." The visual, the objective, is the training of value, and that many never avail themselves of this is evidenced all around us in a practical inability to become masterful in their calling.

Now, therefore, is it the last call to you, wherever you may be, to send in your membership fee. It means ten dollars of personal responsibility. You are, to that extent, a stockholder in the last great convocation that will meet in many years on this side of the Atlantic. The present generation will have become grizzled with age before the world of dentistry will again gather in our country. In all human probability the last of the great expositions in America will have been held when that at St. Louis closes its doors. The cost, which has gradually grown to such enormous figures, precludes the possibility of another of similar proportions. *Then grasp the present opportunity.*

From indications the membership list will exceed anything heretofore known of international dental congresses. This one

24

promises to be an exposition in itself, for our dental manufacturers are making every effort to give an exhibit worthy the occasion. Dentistry in America will be on trial. Whether we have anything new to show or not may not be so important, but let the best be shown, and whether it be on the scientific or the practical side, may that be worthy of our people. Therefore, let every practitioner heed the last call to duty, and during this month, August, find the ways and means to reach St. Louis and to then actively enter into unison with the host that will gather there from all the civilized centres of the world.

THE RETROGRADE FRACTIONAL MEETING AT ST. LOUIS.

In an article in this present issue, written some time previous to the meeting of a number of the members of the National Association of Dental Faculties at St. Louis, the views of the writer were given up to that time, but the meeting of the dissatisfied has now been held, and its action on July 18 is open to the support or condemnation of the dental profession. Twenty-seven colleges were represented out of a total of fifty-three members. How many of these had a legal right to sit there and vote is not known, as the number or names of colleges having resigned was refused when the request was made. This, as it stood, represented half the colleges connected with the Association.

No forced construction could make this body a meeting of the National Association of Faculties, but it was a special gathering of those who suffered defeat at Washington, D. C., in June, with a few additional interested observers.

It is difficult to treat of this meeting with that calm consideration due the serious results that may follow its deliberations. It marks one of the most important departures from a correct standard of dental education that has been experienced in fifty years. To treat, therefore, its retrograde action with complacency is impossible. It carries the dental profession in these United States back to a period in the sixth decade of the last century, when chaos reigned and every educational man's hand was against every other man, a condition not changed until the National Association of Faculties was organized in 1804. All that that organization has patiently and persistently worked for has been cast to the four winds, and unless there be a courageous effort made to withstand this sudden wave of commercialism, it is feared the last state will be found worse than the first.

That our readers may know exactly what was done by this retrograde faction, we give the following resolutions:

Resolved, That the minimum time for dental teaching required by this Association to qualify students for examination for graduation shall be thirty weeks of six days each, in each of three separate academic years, exclusive of holidays. This resolution to take effect at once; and be it further

"*Resolved,* That all rules, or parts of rules, in conflict with this resolution be and are hereby repealed."

That these resolutions were passed by and at a meeting convened without any semblance of authority under the constitution need not be stated to any one conversant with the rules and usages of the Faculties Association, but this article is for the enlightenment of the profession generally, and not especially for the members of that organization. That a body of men could come together and unitedly agree to violate all the rules in order to carry out their predetermined plan is beyond the comprehension of the writer. An organization containing such a membership is a rope of sand and unworthy the respect of the intelligent thinking portion of the dental profession.

The past year has witnessed three meetings called without authority, and each one naturally led to the succeeding as a wilful violation of the rules governing the organization. The following bear directly upon what shall constitute a quorum. It was not to be expected that such a body would pay much attention to the slight matter—to them—of a quorum.

"Article IV. Two-thirds of the colleges belonging to this Association shall be necessary to constitute a quorum. In all matters not in conflict with Article VIII. of the constitution, a majority of the colleges belonging to this Association shall constitute a quorum."

Turning to Article VIII., it reads: "Any contemplated change involving the interests of the schools represented, or of the Association, shall require one year's notice before any action is taken." Compare this constitutional provision with the action at this St. Louis meeting, where the resolutions adopted directly affected the interests of all the schools, and should, in a properly regulated body, have been held over for action next year. But this body went farther than this and ordered that " all rules and parts of rules in conflict with these resolutions be and are hereby repealed." Lawlessness could go much farther, and the resolutions seemed to give great satisfaction.

There was one slight sign of sensitiveness to what the world might say, for this peculiar body passed a resolution that hereafter all proceedings should be held sacred and nothing should be permitted publication until the official sanction had been given. This spasm of sensitiveness was the result of the publication of the vote at Washington adopting the four-year rule. We are not surprised that such a resolution was passed, but if these educators expect that the profession will close its eyes and ears to their doings, or that this journal will cease to make note of their proceedings, they have misjudged the temper of the profession and the character of the editor of the INTERNATIONAL DENTAL JOURNAL.

The result of such work is not easy to determine, but if the history of dental education in this country counts for anything, we must expect that when these schools are a law unto themselves, there will be, as a result, a violent competition, that will end in the destruction of all the weaker schools and, in the end, the survival of the stronger. If this were all, it might be contemplated with serenity, but it means more than this,—a body of unqualified men forced into the dental profession unless these are halted at the portals of the State boards. What will be the action of these final arbiters of ability it is not difficult to determine. In those States lacking a law requiring four years they will eventually be passed into the ranks of the qualified.

It is probably true that all the dental schools will experience a period that will try them to the uttermost, but out of this chaotic condition, the writer feels assured, will come the golden period of stability in educational methods. The weeds in our educational garden will all have been dug up and cast into the ash-pits of civilization, and the refreshed garden will yield a thousand-fold more to the glory of the dental profession than at any period of the past.

Whether the Association of Faculties as originally organized will survive this blow remains to be seen. Confidence in it and its proceedings will be entirely shattered. It will require years to build up the confidence lost by the action at St. Louis. It is to be hoped that there will be a remnant, with courage unshaken, who will take up this work and leave those who passed that resolution at St. Louis to flounder in the mire of their own creating. The true Association of Faculties has stood for the highest in dental education, and by the help and encouragement of all that are loyal to the faith it will still work on through the twentieth century until the commercial taint in our profession is entirely eradicated.

Bibliography.

A GROUP OF DISTINGUISHED PHYSICIANS AND SURGEONS OF CHICAGO. Compiled by F. M. Sperry. Illustrated. J. H. Beers & Co., Chicago, Ill., 1904.

This is a handsome volume of two hundred and forty pages, and worthy of the men and women who are embalmed within its covers. While books of this character abound, from " Who's Who ?" to smaller specimens of the personal glorification order, this book seems to be free from the usual criticism, and is really what its title indicates,—a history of the prominent physicians of Chicago.

It is eminently proper that Dr. N. S. Davis should occupy the frontispiece. While Chicago has a due proportion of men with national and international reputations, no one of these better represents the broad, liberal medical thought of the day than Dr. Davis. Dentistry holds him in grateful remembrance for his many kind words and deeds in its behalf. Not that our profession needs special aid and encouragement, but that out of the mists of medical prejudice that have beclouded the mental horizon of that profession since the days of Harris and Hayden there could be found one man who could see beyond this into the clearer life and hygienic value of the work of dentistry and its intimate relation to the healing art. While dentistry is perfectly able to maintain its independent position, forced upon it by Dr. Davis's predecessors, it nevertheless feels that the appreciation of such a man means added honor to its work.

Among the illustrations of this book are several of prominent women in medical practice in Chicago. The writer has not to go back very far in medical history to recall a period when the medical men of that day would have felt themselves humiliated to have been embalmed in a volume with medical women. The fact that this generation has outgrown the narrow professional bigotry of the past is an encouragement to believe that that profession is steadily outgrowing the swaddling clothes of medical infancy.

Dentistry finds an honorable place in this volume. Very excellent portraitures of Eugene S. Talbot, M.D., D.D.S., and Truman W. Brophy, M.D., D.D.S., LL.D., are among its illustrations.

It is interesting to read in the history of Dr. Talbot traces of the beginning of the active life of this renowned thinker, investigator, and voluminous contributor to the scientific side of medicine and dentistry. It is well sometimes to recur to these personal histories of distinguished men, as they furnish valuable lessons and are oftentimes corrective of narrow conceptions and conclusions. Dr. Talbot was born in Massachusetts, and received a public school education, " followed by academic training at Stoughtonham Institute until the age of sixteen years." He apprenticed himself to the South Boston Locomotive Works, and was trained to work on marine engines. He became a master mechanic at nineteen, and was, subsequently, foreman at the Pennsylvania Railroad Repair Shops. He subsequently graduated in dentistry and medicine, the former at the Pennsylvania College of Dental Surgery, and the latter at Rush Medical College, Chicago.

In the very strenuous demand for higher preliminary education, it may be well to recur occasionally to the fact that the future of a young man does not depend so much on the degree secured as upon the determination to build upon that which has been obtained. The lesson of Dr. Talbot's life is, therefore, instructive in this direction, and should be an encouragement and incentive to higher work throughout the graduated body in dentistry of recent years.

Dr. Brophy's career is of very similar character to Dr. Talbot's. Like the latter he received his education in the public school and academy at Elgin, Ill. His professional education was carried on in the Pennsylvania College of Dental Surgery and Rush Medical College of Chicago.

His achievements as a dental educator and surgeon are well

known. His one contribution, among many, to oral surgery, that of the radical cure of cleft palate, known as the "Brophy operation," has made his name known throughout the surgical world.

These facts are recalled here that the young men entering dentistry may not be unmindful that energy and persistent cultivation of the mental forces will insure a place in the world's regard, and this can be accomplished in no other way. It is through just such efforts that dentistry has been recognized at its true worth,—one of the most important professions of modern life and superior to some in its hygienic relations and its possibilities in the prolongation of human life. What is of greater importance, however, is the continuance of the mental powers to an indefinite period in the life of the individual through its advanced practice in the treatment of the oral cavity, the vestibule of the entire organism.

Domestic Correspondence.

NEW HAVEN DENTAL CLINIC.

[THE following account of the. recently organized Dental Clinic at New Haven, Conn., will be read with interest. While it is not the first attempt of the kind to render service to the poor, it has features superior to other attempts preceding it.—ED.]

" The latest addition to the New Haven Free Dispensary, and one of the most important, is the dental clinic which is now in operation under the direction of the New Haven Dental Association. The dispensary is, of course, under the direction and management of the Yale Medical School, but the physicians and students who have been doing work there have not been able to do any dental work, and need for a department of this kind has been felt for some time. During the winter it was proposed to the New Haven Dental Association that a clinic of this sort be established under its direction. The matter was brought before the Association and was almost unanimously decided upon. Dr. William H. Carmalt, the director of the surgical clinic at the dispensary, immediately appointed Dr. E. S. Gaylord, Vice President of the Dental Association, director of this new clinic. It was through

his efforts and those of Dr. George E. Nettleton that the room
has been furnished and completed for operation.

" The room itself, with its tile floor, white painted walls, and
white enamelled furniture, is an example of cleanliness and purity.
The furniture was especially made for this purpose, and a hose
might be turned into the room without injury. The furniture
consists of two operating-chairs, the upholstery of which is dark
red leather, two ordinary metal chairs, a metal chest of drawers,
and a metal and glass case for instruments; also two electrical
engines. An interesting feature of the furnishing of the room
is the fact that it was donated to the society by Mr. Clarence R.
Hooker, Mr. Donald R. Hooker, and Miss Elizabeth R. Hooker,
the children of the late Frank H. Hooker of this city. It was a
purely unsolicited donation, and for that reason all the more valuable. The furnishings of the room are practically the property of
the dispensary, whose duty it is to care for them, furnish new
pieces if necessary, and replace lost or broken articles.

" This is to all practical purposes the first clinic of its kind
in New England. It furnishes the dental profession of this city
an opportunity to do charitable work for the worthy poor who are
unable to pay for such services. And only that class of poor who
can prove that they are unable to pay for this work are admitted.
The fact that this clinic was needed has been proved by the number
of people who have availed themselves of this opportunity up to the
present time. The room is open two afternoons a week,—namely,
Tuesday and Thursday,—from two until four o'clock, or until all
who apply for help have been cared for. There are two operators
in attendance each afternoon, who have been appointed by the
director. Dr. Gaylord has made out the appointments for six
months, giving each dentist four afternoons in that time. It has
been so arranged that two strangers will not be there the same
afternoon, that is, when a man goes for the first time, there will
also be an operator in attendance who has been there before, and
who can instruct the new man to a certain extent. If the number
of applicants increases, so that the two afternoons will not be
sufficient, additional time will be given and other operators assigned. The members of the dental society have been very enthusiastic about the work and very ready and willing to do their
part towards carrying out the plans. It is to be hoped that this
enthusiasm will not decrease, as it is a good and important work,
and one that ought to be carried out.

" The card system is used in keeping record of the work done, and a complete record of each case is kept, including name, age, and address of the patient, date of operation, character of operation, and name of operator. Although the work has only been going on about three weeks, it has been running along very smoothly, and everything promises a very successful future."—*Saturday Chronicle,* New Haven.

DR. BLACK'S CORRECTION.

To the Editor:

SIR,—In your editorial on the " Meeting of the Faculties at Washington, D. C.," on page 548, in the last paragraph, you say, " Upon motion of Dr. Black, it was decided, by a vote of colleges, to give the weaker schools some relief, and the final vote was cast for four years with a six months' course." I wish to say that you are mistaken in attributing that motion to me. I not only did not make the motion, but I opposed it as sharply as I knew how at the time the motion was made and voted against it. I would be very unwilling that this go uncorrected. The whole outcome of the meeting was extremely unsatisfactory to me. The vote by which the four-year course was maintained was too small, and I felt so at the time, but I was opposed to a course of six months in any case or for any purpose.

Very truly,

G. V. BLACK.

[REMARKS.—It is with regret that the writer failed to understand whence the motion originated to make the time four years with a course of six months. The " Foster Resolution," covering the same ground, had been under consideration, but the question had become much confused, and it was supposed the meeting was acting upon a new motion and that Dr. Black was its originator. He gave the impression to many that he favored such a change, and it seemed to the writer that this was a very creditable course to take, hence there was no hesitation in making use of his name. Dr. Black's repudiation of the statement made in our last issue, and also his opposition to the change adopted, came as a surprise, but he certainly ought to know his true position, and we, therefore, very willingly make the necessary correction.—ED.]

Current News.

FOURTH INTERNATIONAL DENTAL CONGRESS, ST. LOUIS, MO., AUGUST 29 TO SEPTEMBER 3, 1904.

Committee of Organization.—H. J. Burkhart, Chairman, Batavia, N. Y.; E. C. Kirk, Secretary, Lock Box 1615, Philadelphia, Pa.; R. H. Hofheinz, Wm. Carr, W. E. Boardman, V. E. Turner, J. Y. Crawford, M. F. Finley, J. W. David, Wm. Crenshaw, Don M. Gallie, G. V. I. Brown, A. H. Peck, J. D. Patterson, B. L. Thorpe.

The Department of Congresses of the Universal Exposition, St. Louis, 1904, has nominated the Committee of Organization of the Fourth International Dental Congress which was appointed by the National Dental Association, and has instructed the committee thus appointed to proceed with the work of organization of said Congress.

Pursuant to the instructions of the Director of Congresses of the Universal Exposition, 1904, the Committee of Organization presents the subjoined outline of the plan of organization of the Dental Congress.

The Congress will be divided into two departments: Department A—SCIENCE (divided into four sections). Department B—APPLIED SCIENCE (divided into six sections).

DEPARTMENT A—SCIENCE.

I. Anatomy, Physiology, Histology, and Microscopy. Chairman, M. H. Cryer, 1420 Chestnut Street, Philadelphia, Pa.

II. Etiology, Pathology, and Bacteriology. Chairman, R. H. Hofheinz, Chamber of Commerce, Rochester, N. Y.

III. Chemistry and Metallurgy. Chairman, J. D. Hodgen, 1005 Sutter Street, San Francisco, Cal.

IV. Oral Hygiene, Prophylaxis, Materia Medica and Therapeutics, and Electro-therapeutics. Chairman, A. H. Peck, 92 State Street, Chicago, Ill.

DEPARTMENT B—APPLIED SCIENCE.

V. Oral Surgery. Chairman, G. V. I. Brown, 445 Milwaukee Avenue, Milwaukee, Wis.

VI. Orthodontia. Chairman, E. H. Angle, 1023 North Grand Avenue, St. Louis, Mo.

VII. Operative Dentistry. Chairman, C. N. Johnson, Marshall Field Building, Chicago, Ill.

VIII. Prosthesis. Chairman, C. R. Turner, Thirty-third and Locust Streets, Philadelphia, Pa.

IX. Education, Nomenclature, Literature, and History. Chairman, Truman W. Brophy, Marshall Field Building, Chicago, Ill.

X. Legislation. Chairman, Wm. Carr, 35 West Forty-sixth Street, New York, N. Y.

COMMITTEES.

Following are the committees appointed :

Finance.—Chairman, C. S. Butler, 680 Main Street, Buffalo, N. Y.

Programme.—Chairman, A. H. Peck, 92 State Street, Chicago, Ill.

Exhibits.—Chairman, D. M. Gallie, 100 State Street, Chicago, Ill.

Transportation.—(To be appointed.)

Reception.—Chairman, B. Holly Smith, 1007 Madison Avenue, Baltimore, Md.

Registration.—Chairman, B. L. Thorpe, 3666 Olive Street, St. Louis, Mo.

Printing and Publication.—Chairman, W. E. Boardman, 184 Boylston Street, Boston, Mass.

Conference with State and Local Dental Societies.—Chairman, J. A. Libbey, 524 Penn Avenue, Pittsburg, Pa.

Dental Legislation.—Chairman, Wm. Carr, 35 West Forty-sixth Street, New York, New York.

Auditing.—(Committee of Organization.)

Invitation.—Chairman, L. G. Noel, 527½ Church Street, Nashville, Tenn.

Membership.—Chairman, J. D. Patterson, Keith and Perry Building, Kansas City, Mo.

Educational Methods.—Chairman, T. W. Brophy, Marshall Field Building, Chicago, Ill.

Oral Surgery.—Chairman, G. V. I. Brown, 445 Milwaukee Avenue, Milwaukee, Wis.

Prosthetic Dentistry.—Chairman, C. R. Turner, Thirty-third and Locust Streets, Philadelphia, Pa.

Local Committee of Arrangements and Reception.—Chairman, Wm. Conrad, 3666 Olive Street, St. Louis, Mo.

Essays.—Chairman, Wilbur F. Litch, 1500 Locust Street, Philadelphia, Pa.

History of Dentistry.—Chairman, Wm. H. Trueman, 900 Spruce Street, Philadelphia, Pa.

Nomenclature.—Chairman, A. H. Thompson, 720 Kansas Avenue, Topeka, Kan.

Promotion of Appointment of Dental Surgeons in the Armies and Navies of the World.—Chairman, Williams Donnally, 1018 Fourteenth Street N. W., Washington, D. C.

Care of the Teeth of the Poor.—Chairman, Thomas Fillebrown, 175 Newbury Street, Boston, Mass.

Etiology, Pathology, and Bacteriology.—Chairman, R. H. Hofheinz, Chamber of Commerce, Rochester, N. Y.

Prize Essays.—Chairman, James Truman, 4505 Chester Avenue, Philadelphia, Pa.

Oral Hygiene, Prophylaxis, Materia Medica and Therapeutics, and Electro-therapeutics.—Chairman, A. H. Peck, 92 State Street, Chicago, Ill.

Operative Dentistry.—Chairman, C. N. Johnson, Marshall Field Building, Chicago, Ill.

Resolutions.—Chairman, J. Y. Crawford, Jackson Building, Nashville, Tenn.

Clinics.—Chairman, J. P. Gray, 212 North Spruce Street, Nashville, Tenn.

Nominations.—Chairman, A. H. Peck, 92 State Street, Chicago, Ill.; W. E. Boardman, 184 Boylston Street, Boston, Mass.; M. R. Windhorst, 3518 Morgan Street, St. Louis, Mo.; Wm. Conrad, 3666 Olive Street, St. Louis, Mo.

Ad Interim.—Chairman, G. V. I. Brown, 445 Milwaukee Avenue, Milwaukee, Wis.

The officers of the Congress, president, vice-presidents, secretary, and treasurer, will be elected by the Congress at large at the time of the meeting, and will be nominated by the Nominating Committee.

The Fourth International Dental Congress, which will be held August 29 to September 3, inclusive, 1904, will be representative of the existing status of dentistry throughout the world. It is intended further that the Congress shall set forth the history and material progress of dentistry from its crude beginnings through its developmental stages, up to its present condition as a scientific profession.

The International Dental Congress is but one of the large number of congresses to be held during the period of the Louisiana Purchase Exposition, and these in their entirety are intended to exhibit the intellectual progress of the world, as the Exposition will set forth the material progress which has taken place since the Columbian Exposition in 1893.

It is important that each member of the dental profession in America regard this effort to hold an International Dental Congress as a matter in which he has an individual interest, and one which he is under obligation to personally help towards a successful issue. The dental profession of America has not only its own professional record to maintain with a just pride, but, as it is called upon to act the part of host in a gathering of our colleagues from all parts of the world, it has to sustain the reputation of American hospitality as well.

The Committee of Organization appeals earnestly to each member of the profession to do his part in making the Congress a success. Later bulletins will be issued setting forth the personnel of the organization and other particulars, when the details have been more fully arranged.

H. J. BURKHART, *Chairman.*

E. C. KIRK, *Secretary.*

Approved:

HOWARD J. ROGERS,

Director of Congresses.

DAVID R. FRANCIS,

President of Exposition.

COMMITTEE ON STATE AND LOCAL ORGANIZATIONS.

(J. A. Libbey, Chairman, 524 Penn Avenue, Pittsburg, Pa.)

The Committee on State and Local Organizations is a committee appointed by the Committee of Organization of the Fourth International Congress with the object of promoting the interests of the Congress in the several States of the Union. Each member of the committee is charged with the duty of receiving applications for membership in the Congress under the rules governing membership as prescribed by the Committee on Membership and approved by the Committee of Organization. These rules provide that *membership in the Congress shall be open to all reputable legally qualified practitioners of dentistry.* Membership in a State or local society is not a necessary qualification for membership in the Congress.

Each State chairman, as named below, is furnished with official application blanks and is authorized to accept the membership fee of ten dollars from all eligible applicants within his State. The State chairman will at once forward the fee and official application with his indorsement to the chairman of the Finance Committee, who will issue the official certificate conferring membership in the Congress. No application from any of the States will be accepted by the chairman of the Finance Committee unless approved by the State chairman, whose indorsement is a certification of eligibility under the membership rules.

A certificate of membership in the Congress will entitle the holder thereof to all the rights and privileges of the Congress, the right of debate, and of voting on all questions which the Congress will be called upon to decide. It will also entitle the member to one copy of the official transactions when published and to participation in all the events for social entertainment which will be officially provided at the time of the Congress.

The attention of all reputable legally qualified practitioners of dentistry is called to the foregoing plan authorized by the Committee of Organization for securing membership in the Congress, and the committee earnestly appeals to each eligible practitioner in the United States who is interested in the success of this great international meeting to make application at once through his State chairman for a membership certificate. By acting promptly in this matter the purpose of the committee to make the Fourth International Dental Congress the largest and most successful meeting of dentists ever held will be realized, and the Congress will thus be placed upon a sound financial basis.

Let every one make it his individual business to help at least to the extent of enrolling himself as a member and the success of the undertaking will be quickly assured. Apply at once to your State chairman. The State chairmen already appointed are:

General Chairman.—J. A. Libbey, 524 Penn Avenue, Pittsburg, Pa.

Alabama.—H. Clay Hassell, Tuscaloosa.

Arkansas.—W. H. Buckley, 510½ Main Street, Little Rock.

California.—J. L. Pease, 1016 Clay Street, Oakland.

Colorado.—H. A. Fynn, 500 California Building, Denver.

Connecticut.—Henry McManus, 80 Pratt Street, Hartford.

Delaware.—C. R. Jeffries, New Century Building, Wilmington.

District of Columbia.—W. N. Cogan, The Sherman, Washington.

Florida.—W. G. Mason, Tampa.

Georgia.—H. H. Johnson, Macon.

Hawaii.—M. E. Grossman, Box 744, Honolulu.

Idaho.—J. B. Burns, Payette.

Illinois.—J. E. Hinkins, 131 East Fifty-third Street, Chicago.

Indiana.—H. C. Kahlo, 115 East New York Street, Indianapolis.

Iowa.—W. R. Clark, Clear Lake.

Kansas.—G. A. Esterly, Lawrence.

Kentucky.—H. B. Tileston, 314 Equitable Building, Louisville.

Louisiana.—Jules J. Sarrazin, 108 Bourbon Street, New Orleans.

Maine.—H. A. Kelley, 609 Congress Street, Portland.

Maryland.—W. G. Foster, 813 Eutaw Street, Baltimore.

Massachusetts.—M. C. Smith, 3 Lee Hall, Lynn.

Michigan.—G. S. Shattuck, 539 Fourth Avenue, Detroit.

Minnesota.—C. A. Van Duzee, 51 Germania Bank Building, St. Paul.

Mississippi.—W. R. Wright, Jackson.

Missouri.—J. W. Hull, Altman Building, Kansas City.

Montana.—G. E. Longeway, Great Falls.

Nebraska.—H. A. Shannon, 1136 " O" Street, Lincoln.

New Hampshire.—E. C. Blaisdell, Portsmouth.

New Jersey.—Alphonso Irwin, 425 Cooper Street, Camden.

New York.—B. C. Nash, 142 West Seventy-eighth Street, New York City.

North Carolina.—C. L. Alexander, Charlotte.

Ohio.—Henry Barnes, 1415 New England Building, Cleveland.

Oklahoma.—T. P. Bringhurst, Shawnee.

Oregon.—S. J. Barber, Macleay Building, Portland.

Pennsylvania.—H. E. Roberts, 1516 Locust Street, Philadelphia.

Rhode Island.—D. F. Keefe, 315 Butler Exchange, Providence.

South Carolina.—J. T. Calvert, Spartanburg.
South Dakota.—E. S. O'Neil, Canton.
Tennessee.—W. P. Sims, Jackson Building, Nashville.
Texas.—J. G. Fife, Dallas.
Utah.—W. L. Ellerbeck, 21 Hooper Building Salt Lake City.
Vermont.—S. D. Hodge, Burlington.
Virginia.—F. W. Stiff, 2101 Churchill Avenue, Richmond.
Washington.—G. W. Stryker, Everett.
West Virginia.—H. H. Harrison, 1141 Main Street, Wheeling.
Wisconsin.—A. D. Gropper, 401 East Water Street, Milwaukee.
    For the Committee of Organization,
                    EDWARD C. KIRK,
                            Secretary.

PROGRAMME OF THE FOURTH INTERNATIONAL
DENTAL CONGRESS.

DEPARTMENT A—SCIENCE.

Section I.—Anatomy, Physiology, Histology, and Microscopy.
(*Chairman, Dr. M. H. Cryer, 1420 Chestnut Street, Philadelphia, Pa.*)

Florestan Aguilar, Madrid, Spain, " General Anæsthesia by
Somnoform."

G. G. Campion, Manchester, England, " Determining the Actual
Path and Extent of Movement of the Mandible Condyle in the
Living Subject."

D. E. N. Caush, Brighton, England, " Is there Uncalcified
Tissue in the Enamel?"

M. H. Cryer. (Subject to be announced.)

W. T. Eckley, " Phylogenetic Evidence regarding the Function
of the Accessory Sinuses in Man."

John E. Grevers, Amsterdam, Holland, " Anatomy of the
Facial Skull—Normal and in Mouth-Breathers."

————, " Geometrical Construction of the Mandible."

————, " Behavior of the Teeth under Polarized Light."

A. Hopewell-Smith, London, England. (Subject to be
announced.)

Eugene S. Talbot, Chicago, Ill. (Subject to be announced.)

A. H. Thompson, Topeka, Kan., " Ethnographic Odontography: The Mound-Builders and the Pre-Indian Peoples of the Mississippi Valley."

J. G. Turner, London, England. (Subject to be announced.) Arthur S. Underwood, London, England. (Subject to be announced.)

O. Walkhoff, Munich, Germany, "Concerning the Crania of Diluvial Peoples." (Illustrated with lantern slides.)

Section II.—Etiology, Pathology, and Bacteriology. (Chairman, Dr. R. H. Hofheinz, Chamber of Commerce, Rochester, N. Y.)

C. F. W. Bödecker, Berlin, Germany, "Percussion in Dental Diagnosis."

G. W. Cook, Chicago, Ill., "The Effects of Chemical Agents on Bacteria with Relation to the Saliva."

Samuel A. Hopkins, Boston, Mass., "Application of the Results of Research Work to Daily Practice."

W. H. G. Logan, Chicago, Ill., "A Consideration of Some of the Etiological Factors that produce Tissue Changes of the Alveolar Process and Overlying Soft Parts."

Jos. P. Michaels, Paris, France, "Sialology: Differential Analyses; Elements of Value in Medical Diagnosis."

W. D. Miller, Berlin, Germany, "Researches relating to Various Pathological Processes in the Teeth."

Louis Ottofy, Manila, P. I., "Observations on the Causes of Erosion: (a) Erosio Areca (betel erosion); (b) Erosio Orientalis."

J. D. Patterson, Kansas City, Mo. (Subject to be announced.)

M. L. Rhein, New York, N. Y. (Subject to be announced.)

Oskar Römer, Strasburg, Germany, "Some Patho-histological Observations on Pyorrhœa Alveolaris."

D. D. Smith, Philadelphia, Pa., "Pericemental Abscess."

Eugene S. Talbot, Chicago, Ill., "Constitutional Causes of Tooth-Decay."

F. Vicentini, Chieti, Italy, "Leptothrix Racemosa."

Section III.—Chemistry and Metallurgy. (Chairman, Dr. J. D. Hodgen, 1005 Sutter Street, San Francisco, Cal.)

J. P. Buckley, Chicago, Ill., "Chemistry of Pulp-Decomposition."

H. C. Carel, Minneapolis, Minn. (Subject to be announced.)

J. D. Hodgen, San Francisco, Cal., " Chemistry and Dentistry."

Hof-Zahnarzt W. Pfaff, Dresden, Germany, " Das Aluminium und seine Anwendbarkeit in Allgemeinen."

R. W. Simon, Boston, Mass. (Subject to be announced.)

Herbert L. Wheeler, " The Chemistry of Porcelain."

Section IV.—Oral Hygiene, Prophylaxis, Materia Medica and Therapeutics, and Electro-Therapeutics. (Chairman, Dr. A. H. Peck, 92 State Street, Chicago, Ill.)

Samuel Taylor Bassett, St. Louis, Mo., " Application of Electro-Therapeutics to Dental Surgery."

L. P. Bethel, Columbus, Ohio, " Some Results from Dental and Oral Prophylaxis."

Julio Endelman, Philadelphia, Pa., " Contribution to the Therapeutics of Post-Extraction Accidents."

Richard Grady, Annapolis, Md., " Oral Hygiene: Mastication."

J. E. Hinkins, Chicago, Ill. (Subject to be announced.)

Edward Hoffmeister, Baltimore, Md., " Materia Medica."

Prof. Dr. Jessen, Strasburg; Dr. Loos, Vienna, and Zahnarzt Georg Schlaeger: I. " Zahn-hygiene in Schule and Heer." II. Eine Wandtafel für den Ausschauungsunterricht in der Schule in Farben, " Gesunde und Kranke Zähne." III. Eine Wandtafel, ii. Auflage auch farbig, " Die Zähne und ihre Pfläge."

Weston A. Price, Cleveland, Ohio. (Subject to be announced.)

E. Sauvez, Paris, France, " Study of the Various Means of inducing Local Anæsthesia for Extraction of the Teeth."

Zahnarzt Dr. Schaeffer-Stuckert, Frankfort-on-Main, Germany, " Paranephrin Bitsert: A New Preparation of Kidney Atrabilarian in Connection with Local Anæsthetics in Dentistry."

Edward Schlinkmann, Baltimore, Md., " Electric Absorption in Therapy."

C. R. Taylor, Streator, Ill. (Subject to be announced.)

DEPARTMENT B—APPLIED SCIENCE.

Section V.—Oral Surgery. (Chairman, Dr. G. V. I. Brown, 445 Milwaukee Street, Milwaukee, Wis.)

Chairman's address, G. V. I. Brown, Milwaukee, Wis., " Oral Surgery: Its Relations to General Surgery and Dentistry."

T. W. Brophy, Chicago, Ill., "Necessity for Early Operation for Cleft Palate."

T. L. Gilmer, Chicago, Ill., "The Teaching of Oral Surgery in Our Dental Schools."

H. H. Grant, Louisville, Ky., "Solid Tumors involving the Body or Ramus of the Inferior Maxillary Bone."

J. G. Kiernan, Chicago, Ill., "Embryogenetic, Congenital, and Acquired Stomato-Neurologic Relations."

A. H. Levings, Milwaukee, Wis., "Importance and Methods of Early Diagnosis of Malignant Growths affecting the Maxillary Bone."

J. S. Marshall, San Francisco, Cal., "Fractures of the Mandible and their Treatment."

E. S. Talbot, Chicago, Ill., "Etiology of Cleft Palate and Harelip."

Section VI.—Orthodontia. (*Chairman, Dr. Edward H. Angle, 1023 North Grand Avenue, St. Louis, Mo.*)

Edward H. Angle, St. Louis, Mo., "Malocclusion: Class II. and its Divisions."

G. V. I. Brown, Milwaukee, Wis. (Subject to be announced.)

L. C. Bryan, Basel, Switzerland, "Nature as a Regulator, and our Duty as her Assistants."

Calvin S. Case, Chicago, Ill., "Principles and Methods of Retention in Orthodontia."

M. Chiwaki, Tokyo, Japan. (Subject to be announced.)

Wm. Slocum Davenport, Paris, France, "Contribution to the Treatment of Short Bite and Jump Bite Cases."

Robert Dunn, San Francisco, Cal., "Mesial Position of the First Molars in Class I."

John E. Grevers, Amsterdam, Holland, "Proposal for an International Nomenclature for the Various Forms of Malocclusion."

Chas. A. Hawley, Columbus, Ohio, "Method of determining the Normal Arch, and its Application in Orthodontia."

Francisque Martin, Lyons, France, "The Correction of Deformities in Fractures of the Nose."

R. Ottolengui, New York, N. Y., "Spreading the Maxillæ *versus* Spreading the Arch."

W. Booth Pearsall, Dublin, Ireland, "Irish Types of Malocclusion."

Herbert A. Pullen, Buffalo, N. Y. (Subject to be announced.)

Jose J. Rojo, Mexico City, Mexico, "Study of the Etiology of Anomalies in Human Teeth."

Dr. Schroeder, Greifswald, Germany, "Prognathous Forms and their Orthopædic Treatment."

A. Hopewell-Smith, London, England. (Subject to be announced.)

J. Sim Wallace, London, England, "Nasal Obstructions and Mouth-Breathing, with Special Reference to Malocclusion of the Teeth."

S. Merrill Weeks, Philadelphia, Pa. (Subject to be announced.)

Edmund Wuerpel, St. Louis, "Art."

Franz Zeliska, Vienna, Austria. (Subject to be announced.)

Section VII.—Operative Dentistry. (Chairman, Dr. C. N. Johnson, Marshall Field Building, Chicago, Ill.)

E. A. Bogue, New York, N. Y. (Subject to be announced.)

Jas. M. Magee, St. Johns, N. B., "The Instrumentation and Filling of Crooked Root-Canals." (Illustrated.)

Sylvester Moyer, Galt, Ont., "The Enamel and its Consideration in Cavity Preparation."

C. G. Myers, Cleveland, Ohio. (Subject to be announced.)

Garrett Newkirk, Los Angeles, Cal., "The Whole Question of Matrices and their Uses."

Frank L. Platt, San Francisco, Cal. (Subject to be announced.)

Geo. C. Poundstone, Chicago, Ill., "The Cement Problem in Inlay Work."

M. L. Rhein, New York, N. Y. (Subject to be announced.)

Arthur Scheuer, Teplitz, Austria, "Tin-Cement, Sponge Tin: Two New Filling-Materials and their Uses."

E. K. Wedelstaedt, St. Paul, Minn., "Gold-and-Tin."

H. L. Wheeler, New York, N. Y. (Subject to be announced.)

Section VIII.—Prosthesis. (Chairman, Dr. C. R. Turner, Thirty-third and Locust Streets, Philadelphia, Pa.)

L. W. Baker, Boston, Mass. (Subject to be announced.)

George Brunton, Leeds, England. (Subject to be announced.)

Reuben C. Brophy, Chicago, Ill., "Rationale of the Use of Materials for Base-Plates in the Construction of Artificial Dentures."

Calvin S. Case, Chicago, Ill., "The Mechanical Treatment of Cleft Palate."

Edw. G. Christensen, Drommen, Norway, "Which is the Ideal Crown,—the Banded Crown or the Crown without Band?"

B. J. Cigrand, Chicago, Ill., "Facial Guide Lines as taught by Artists."

Bernard Frank, Amsterdam, Holland, "A New Articulator on Anatomical Principles."

Hart J. Goslee, Chicago, Ill., "Porcelain Crowns."

F. H. Mamlock, Berlin, Germany, "(a) Ueber Porzellanstiftzähne. (b) Ueber Magnalium Prothesen und ihre Herstellung nach Dr. Eug. Müllerschen Gummidrucksystem."

Francisque Martin, Lyons, France, "Immediate Prosthesis after the Method of Dr. Claude Martin."

Joseph Nolin, Montreal, Canada, "The Decline of Æstheticism in Prosthesis."

B. Platschick, Paris, France, "(a) Influence de Fauchard sur la Prothèse dentaire. (b) Les dents à tube en général et leur emploi special pour les pièces à gencive continue. (c) Contribution à l'étude des Couronnes."

Jas. H. Prothero, Chicago, Ill. (Subject to be announced.)

Rudolph Weiser, Vienna, Austria, "Some Cases illustrating the Possibilities of Prosthetic Dentistry."

E. Lloyd Williams, London, England. (Subject to be announced.)

Geo. H. Wilson, Cleveland, Ohio. (Subject to be announced.)

Section IX.—Education, Nomenclature, Literature, and History. (*Chairman, Dr. Truman W. Brophy, Marshall Field Building, Chicago, Ill.*)

M. Chiwaki, Tokyo, Japan, "Dentistry in Japan."

Charles Godon, Paris, France, "Educational Standards of Europe."

S. H. Guilford, Philadelphia, Pa., "Nomenclature."

A. W. Harlan, New York, N. Y., "Dental Literature."

A. O. Hunt, Omaha, Neb., "The Count System of Students' Credits."

Chas. McManus, Hartford, Conn., "International Character of the Early Development of Dentistry in America."

Louis Ottofy, Manila, P. I. (Subject to be announced.)

Jose J. Rojo, City of Mexico, Mexico, "Historical Annotations and Present Condition of Dental Education in the City of Mexico."

B. L. Thorpe, St. Louis, Mo., "History of American Dentistry."

James Truman, Philadelphia, Pa., "Dental Education from the View of Experience."

Section X.—Legislation. (Chairman, Dr. Wm. Carr, 35 West Forty-sixth Street, New York, N. Y.)

(Not received.)

CLINICS.

(Reports for the East and South have not yet been received.)

Porcelain.—C. C. Allen, Kansas City, Md.; W. V.-B. Ames, Chicago, Ill.; E. H. Ball, Tama, Iowa; F. E. Cheeseman, Chicago, Ill.; W. A. Coston, Fort Scott, Kan.; W. H. Cudworth, Milwaukee, Wis.; A. W. Dana, Burlington, Iowa; S. F. Duncan, Joliet, Ill.; Adam Flickinger, St. Louis, Mo.; V. H. Frederick, St. Louis, Mo.; H. J. Goslee, Chicago, Ill.; F. B. James, Wilton Junction, Iowa; Robt. LeCron, St. Louis, Mo.; L. A. Meyer, Oconomowoc, Wis.; J. E. Nyman, Chicago, Ill.; W. T. Reeves, Chicago, Ill.; W. H. Taggart, Chicago, Ill.; C. N. Thompson, Chicago, Ill.; J. E. Wait, Superior, Neb.; C. M. Work, Ottumwa, Iowa.

Gold Inlays.—F. T. Breene, Iowa City, Iowa; O. H. Simpson, Dodge City, Kan.; C. N. Thompson, Chicago, Ill.; W. F. Whalen, Peoria, Ill.; C. H. Wright, Chicago, Ill.

Surgery.—T. W. Brophy, Chicago, Ill.; T. L. Gilmer, Chicago, Ill.; G. D. Moyer, Montevideo, Minn.

Gold Fillings.—A. G. Fee, Superior, Wis.; F. O. Hetrick, Ottowa, Canada; J. G. Pfaff, St. Louis, Mo.; C. H. Seeger, Manitowoe, Wis.; F. G. Van Stratum, Hurley, Wis.; J. W. Wick, St. Louis, Mo.; (G. V. Black Club) S. Bond, Anoka, Minn.; K. E. Carlson, St. Paul, Minn.; W. R. Clack, Clear Lake, Iowa; J. V. Conzett, Dubuque, Iowa; Wm. Finn, Cedar Rapids, Iowa; S. R. Holden, Duluth, Minn.; A. M. Lewis, Austin, Minn.; J. B. Pherrin, Central City, Iowa; G. A. Rawlings, Bismarck, N. D.; A. J. Schlueter, Aberdeen, S. D.; A. C. Searl, Owatonna, Minn.; J. F.

Wallace, Canton, Mo.; E. K. Wedelstaedt, St. Paul, Minn.; R. B. Wilson, St. Paul, Minn.

Gold Crowns.—J. G. Hollingsworth, Kansas City, Mo.; C. M. Work, Ottumwa, Iowa.

Pyorrhœa Alveolaris.—W. H. G. Logan, Chicago, Ill.; O. H. Manhard, St. Louis, Mo.; G. R. Richter, Milwaukee, Wis.; C. R. Taylor, Streator; Ill.

Extracting.—J. W. Slonaker, Chicago, Ill.

Miscellaneous.—H. F. Cassel, St. Louis, Mo., " Striking up partial gold plate with swaged enforcement single thickness gold."

W. L. Ellerbeck, Salt Lake City, Utah, " Electric furnace construction."

Otto J. Fruth, St. Louis, Mo., " Replantation with porcelain restoration."

R. R. Johnson, Great Falls, Neb., " Artificial velum and obturator."

Elgin MaWhinney, Chicago, Ill., " New drugs; valuable old ones; with therapeutics and indications for uses."

T .W. Pritchett, Whitehall, Ill., " Bonwill method of articulating full dentures."

J. B. Ridout, St. Paul, Minn., " New method of backing facings for Richmond crowns; new method of making continuous gum plate; method of putting gold corner or filling in porcelain tooth."

H. A. Shannon, Lincoln, Neb., " Æsthetic crowns and dummies."

C. O. Simpson, St. Louis, Mo., " Demonstrating strength and durability of amalgams and cements."

G. O. Sitherwood, Bloomington, Ill., " Soldering bands and fixtures; gold plating and adjusting."

W. R. Smith, Pawnee City, Neb., " Prosthetic."

Richard Summa, St. Louis, Mo., " Practical application of Angle fracture band."

S. H. Voyles, St. Louis, Mo., " Saddle bridge; pinless teeth."

E. R. Warner, Denver, Col., " Masticating force of human jaws, demonstrated by appliances."

Subjects not given.—C. S. Case, Chicago, Ill.; W. D. James, Tracy, Minn.; F. E. Roach, Chicago, Ill.; Jas. Weirick, St. Paul, Minn.

EXHIBITORS.

The following manufacturers and dealers have reserved space up to date:

The S. S. White Dental Manufacturing Company, Claudius Ash & Sons, Limited, H. D. Justi & Son, Kress & Owen Company ("Glyco-Thymoline"), J. W. Ivory (Specialties), Oakland Chemical Company, American Cabinet Company, Ransom & Randolph Company, Ammonol Company, John T. Nolde Dental Manufacturing Company, Hisey Manufacturing Company, E. De Trey & Sons, Johnson & Johnson, Detroit Dental Manufacturing Company, Harvard Company, Lee S. Smith & Son, Sanitol Chemical Laboratory Company, John T. Milliken Company, S. Eldred Gilbert Dental Manufacturing Company, Ritter Dental Manufacturing Company, Young Dental Manufacturing Company, McKesson & Robbins Chemical Company, Dentists' Supply Company, Pinches & Ely (Specialties), Frink & Young, W. V.-B. Ames, A. C. Clark & Co., Horlick's Food Company, Chas. H. Phillips Chemical Company, Whiteside Dental Manufacturing Company, Klewe & Company (Jenkins porcelain), R. C. Brophy, L. O. Green, L. D. Caulk, Dutro & Hewitt, Blair Dental Manufacturing Company, Peroxident Chemical Company, Goldsmith Bros., Adrian Rutherford.

NOTE.—The United States government will make an exhibit consisting of a complete dental outfit as furnished to the members of the Army Dental Corps.

FOURTH INTERNATIONAL DENTAL CONGRESS BANQUET.

THE Fourth International Dental Congress Banquet will be held on September 1, 1904, at 8 P.M., in the Coliseum Building adjoining the Congress Hall. The price per plate is three dollars. It is requested that all who expect to attend will send their names and money to Dr. A. H. Fuller, P. O. Lock-Box 604, St. Louis, Mo., at once, and not later than August 20. Arrangements to pay can be made with Dr. A. H. Fuller at the time of registration, provided notice is given before August 20.

G. A. BOWMAN,
A. H. FULLER,
ADAM FLICKINGER,
Banquet Committee.

UNIVERSAL EXPOSITION—HOTEL RATES.

FOURTH INTERNATIONAL DENTAL CONGRESS.

(Saint Louis, August 29 to September 3, 1904.)

THE Local Committee and Bureau of Information wish to dispel from the minds of the profession and all persons that labor under any misconception that the rates of St. Louis Hotels are extortionate.

We have investigated the conditions and rates of the leading hotels of St. Louis, and notwithstanding the fact that this city is entertaining a World's Fair, the hotel rates are no higher than in other cities.

We will append a number of the leading hotels and rates of same, and call your attention that it is not required of you to put up at any of the hotels mentioned, as there are many hotels and boarding-houses in the city where rooms can be secured for from fifty cents to two dollars per day. The exact date should be stated in securing rooms.

We append a list of hotels and rates of same as follows:

Southern Hotel.—The American plan rate is $5 per day for room without bath and $6 a day for a room with bath. The rate is $10 per day if two persons occupy the room.

Planters Hotel.—Room without bath, occupied by one person, $3 to $4 a day. Same for two persons, $6 to $7 a day. Room with bath for one person, $4 to $5 a day, and for two persons $7 to $8 a day.

Jefferson Hotel.—Room without bath, for one person, $4 a day; when occupied by two persons, $6 a day. Room with bath for one person, $5 a day and up; when occupied by two or more persons, $7 a day and up.

St. Nicholas Hotel.—Room without bath, for one person, $2.50 to $3.50 a day; for two persons, $4 to $5 a day. Room with bath, for one person, $3 to $5 a day; for two persons, $5 to $7 a day.

Lindell Hotel.—Room without bath, for one person, $2 a day; for two persons, $3 a day. Room with bath, for one person, $3 a day; for two persons, $4 a day.

Washington Hotel.—Room without bath, for one, two, or three persons, $5 to $7 a day; room with bath, for one, two, or three persons, $8 a day.

Laclede Hotel.—Room without bath, for one person, $1.50 to $2 a day; for two persons, $3 a day; room with bath, for one person, $3 a day; for two persons, $5 a day.

Terminal Hotel.—Room without bath, for one person, $2 to $3 a day; for two persons, $4 to $5 a day. Room with bath, for one person, $5 a day; for two persons, $7 a day.

Mosier Hotel.—European plan, $1 to $3 per day, with Silver Moon Restaurant attached at very reasonable rates. Located at Ninth and Pine Streets.

Hotel Rozier.—Opposite Exposition Building, Olive and Thirteenth Streets. Rooms without bath, $1 to $2 a day.

Mammoth Hotel Company.—S. E. Corner Olive and Twelfth Streets. Can accommodate two thousand five hundred guests per day at rates from fifty cents to $1.50 per day.

The Inside Inn.—With a capacity for five thousand five hundred people, is within the Exposition Grounds, erected under a contract with the Exposition Management, stipulating its rates.

This Hotel offers five hundred rooms at $1 per day, five hundred at $1.50 a day, five hundred at $2 a day, and the remainder, which are larger, with baths, at higher rates. The Napoleon Bonaparte, the Forest City, the Fraternal, the University, the Kenilworth, the American, the Epworth, the Grand View, the States, the Oakland, the Iowa, the Guaranty, the West Park, the Christian Endeavor, the Visitors, and others, with a capacity of from five hundred to five thousand guests, are within easy walking distance of the World's Fair gates. In fact, we have hotels, boarding-houses, apartment houses, and rooming-houses, all over the city, of respectable character and on the street-car lines.

An impression prevails that there may be lack of accommodation at reasonable prices. Not only will there be sufficient room for all who come, but the rates will be reasonable. We appeal to the profession of the country to give information respecting the accommodations in a spirit of fairness and justice to St. Louis based upon the above facts.

St. Louis is prepared to care for and welcome all comers and to show them the grandest Universal Exposition of the world's resources and products in the history of man.

The Fourth International Dental Congress is now an assured success. Many foreign nations have signified their intention to take part in this Congress. The Islands of the Pacific Ocean will be well represented. Their assembling in the centre of this great republic should stimulate every American dentist to action, and each individual of this great profession should feel under obligations to help to push the Congress to a successful issue. We have our professional record to maintain and act the part of host. As a consequence we should endeavor to sustain the reputation of American hospitality.

Here is the birthplace of the Dental College, the most of the inventors, the mechanical geniuses, and the men who have brought about the wonderful advances in our great profession.

We trust the profession of America will take hold with their accustomed vigor, let nothing be undone that will be for the good of the profession, and carry it out with a most liberal spirit to a surprising conclusion.

A list of hotels, boarding-houses, rooming-houses and private homes, with their rates appended, will be furnished by the Committee to all asking for same. Any other information will be freely given by corresponding to any of the following committee:

D. O. M. LeCron, *Chairman*, Missouri Trust Building.

Max Fendler, *Secretary*, Missouri Trust Building.

H. F. D'Oench.

George H. Gibson.

S. H. Voyles.

Orme H. Manhard.

Joseph G. Pfaff.

G. L. Kitchen.

FOURTH INTERNATIONAL DENTAL CONGRESS, SECTION VI., ORTHODONTIA.

The programme of the Section on Orthodontia of the Fourth International Dental Congress is as follows:

" Irish Types of Malocclusion," W. Booth Pearsall, Dublin.

" Nasal Obstructions and Mouth-Breathing, with Special Reference to Malocclusion of the Teeth," J. Sim Wallace, London.

" A Contribution to the Treatment of Short Bite and Jump Bite Cases," William Slocum Davenport, Paris.

" Nature as a Regulator and our Duty as her Assistants," L. C. Bryan, Basel, Switzerland.

"A Proposal for an International Nomenclature for the Various Forms of Malocclusion," John E. Grevers, Amsterdam, Holland.

"The Study of the Etiology of Anomalies of Human Teeth," Jose J. Rojo, Mexico City.

Essay, M. Chiwaki, Tokyo, Japan.

"The Correction of Deformities in Fractures of the Nose," Francisque Martin, Lyons, France.

"Prognathous Forms and their Orthopædic Treatment," Dr. Scroeder, Greifswald, Germany.

Essay, Franz Zeliska, Vienna.

Essay, Hopewell Smith, London.

"Malocclusion: Class II. and its Divisions," Edward H. Angle, St. Louis.

"Mesial Position of the First Molars in Class I.," Robert Dunn, San Francisco.

"Principles and Methods of Retention in Orthodontia," Calvin S. Case, Chicago.

"Spreading the Maxilla *versus* Spreading the Arch," R. Ottolengui, New York City.

"Art," Edmund Wuerpel, St. Louis.

Essay, Herbert A. Pullen, Buffalo.

Essay, S. Merrill Weeks, Philadelphia.

Essay, G. V. I. Brown, Milwaukee.

"A Method of determining the Normal Arch and its Application in Orthodontia," Charles A. Hawley, Columbus.

EDWARD H. ANGLE, *Chairman.*
MILTON T. WATSON, *Secretary.*

NATIONAL ASSOCIATION OF DENTAL EXAMINERS.

THE National Association of Dental Examiners will hold their annual meeting in the Coliseum Building, corner of Thirteenth and Olive Streets, St. Louis, Mo., on the 25th, 26th, and 27th of August, beginning promptly at 10 A.M. Telephone and telegraph offices in the building. Hotel accommodations will be secured for the members. Special railroad rates will be secured for those in the East desiring to attend, trains leaving on the 23d from New York.

The Committee on Railroad Accommodations for the East have made arrangements for fast through Pullman service to St. Louis from New York with the Delaware and Lackawanna Railroad. Two special Pullman cars will leave New York Tuesday, August 23, at 10 A.M. The cost of our excursion including berth each way will be $35.50. A proportionate reduction is made for those going from Buffalo, Toledo, Fort Wayne, and cities on the line connecting with the Wabash Railroad. To those desiring to go on the special cars, send notice to Charles A. Meeker, D.D.S., Secretary of the National Association Dental Examiners, or to Guy Adams, General Passenger Agent of the Delaware and Lackawana Railroad. Accommodations have been secured for the National Association of Dental Examiners at the Franklin Hotel, northwest corner of Sarah and Westminster Place, with rates from $1.50 to $6.00 per day, European plan. Hotel first-class. Secure rooms by writing to E. C. Dunnavant, St. Louis Service Company, Seventh and Olive Streets, St. Louis, Mo.

CHARLES A. MEEKER, D.D.S.,

Secretary.

"F. D. I." FÉDÉRATION DENTAIRE INTERNATIONALE.

THE next (fourth annual) meeting will be held in the Coliseum Building, St. Louis, Mo., August 26 and 27, 1904. The first session will convene under the presidency of Dr. Charles Godon, at 11 A.M. There will be a meeting of the Executive Council on Thursday, the 25th, at the Hotel Jefferson, at 10 A.M.

The Section on Education will meet at 3 P.M. Friday; the Section on Hygiene and Public Dental Service, at 3 P.M. Friday; the Section on International Dental Press, at 4.30 P.M. Friday.

The officers of the Sections are:

Education.—President, Dr. T. W. Brophy; Vice-Presidents, Dr. E. C. Kirk, Dr. W. B. Paterson, and Dr. O. Zsigmondy; Secretaries, Dr. M. Roy and Dr. R. B. Weiser.

Hygiene and Public Dental Service.—President, Dr. W. D. Miller; Vice-Presidents, Dr. Cunningham, Dr. Forberg, Dr. Jenkins, and Dr. Rose; Secretaries, Dr. R. Heide, Dr. Sauvez, and Dr. R. B. Weiser.

Commission of the International Dental Press.—President, Dr. E. Forberg; Dr. A. W. Harlan; Secretary, Dr. E. Papot.

Executive Council.—President, Dr. Charles Godon; Vice-Presidents, Dr. A. W. Harlan, Dr. W. D. Miller; Secretary, Dr. E. Sauvez; Treasurer, Dr. F. Aguilar.

Members.—Dr. George Cunningham, Dr. E. Forberg, Dr. R. B. Weiser, Dr. J. E. Grevers, Dr. F. Heisse, Dr. Klingelhofer.

On behalf of the Federation,

A. W. HARLAN,
Vice-President.

1122 BROADWAY, NEW YORK CITY.

SUPREME CHAPTER, DELTA SIGMA DELTA.

THE twentieth annual meeting of the Supreme Chapter, Delta Sigma Delta Fraternity will be held Wednesday, August 31, 1904, at St. Louis, Mo. George E. Hunt, 131 E. Ohio Street, Indianapolis, is chairman of the Committee on Arrangements.

RESOLUTIONS AMERICAN DENTAL TRADE ASSOCIATION.

WHEREAS, In the estimation of our Association, which is composed of the representative manufacturers of and dealers in dental supplies in the United States, the amendment to patent laws introduced in Senate Bill 4256, House Bill 6771, will remove a class of patents which have long caused annoyance to the dental profession; therefore, be it

" *Resolved,* That the American Dental Trade Association heartily endorse the amendment and urge favorable action thereon, and that the Secretary be instructed to notify the Committees having the amendment in consideration of such action.

" But no patent shall be granted upon any art of treating human disease or disability, or attached to be used in the treatment of human disease, or attached to the human body and used as a substitute for any lost part thereof, or upon any art of making such device unless such device is adopted to be put on the market and sold."

LEE S. SMITH,
Secretary.

THE INTERSTATE DENTAL FRATERNITY.

THE Interstate Dental Fraternity will hold its annual meeting at St. Louis on Tuesday, August 30, 1904. The business meeting will be at 3 P.M., to be followed by a banquet.

The committee in charge are Dr. Burton Lee Thorpe, Chairman; Dr. Edward Everett Haverstick, and Dr. Ernest P. Dameron. Members may procure their banquet tickets in advance by remitting to Dr. E. E. Haverstick, 346 N. Boyle Avenue, St. Louis.

R. M. SANGER,
National Secretary.

PROGRAMME OF THE F. D. I.

THE International Dental Federation will carry out the following programme, in the Coliseum, St. Louis, on Friday, August 26, at 11 A.M., Dr. Charles Godon presiding.

Address of Welcome, by Dr. William Conrad, of St. Louis.

Response by Dr. Godon.

Address by a representative of the Louisiana Purchase Exposition.

Address by the Mayor of St. Louis.

Response by Dr. H. A. Smith, of Cincinnati, Ohio.

Short addresses by the representatives of the Foreign Countries present; after which the President's Address, by Dr. Charles Godon.

Report by the Secretary-General, Dr. E. Sauvez.

Adjournment, subject to the call of the President.

Commission on Education.—Professor Truman W. Brophy, of Chicago, presiding. Will meet in the Coliseum Building, St. Louis, Mo., August 26, at 2 P.M.

Address by the President, Dr. Brophy.

Dr. Charles Godon will give a *résumé* of the status of Dental Education in France.

Dr. Mitchell, of London, will make some observations on technical education.

Dr. Gordon White, of Nashville, Tennessee, will make a short address on the present status of Dental Education in the United States.

Dr. R. B. Weiser, of Vienna, Austria, will give an address on education.

Drs. H. L. Banzhaf, of Milwaukee, C. N. Johnson, of Chicago, M. W. Foster, of Baltimore, and W. E. Boardman, of Boston, will also read papers.

Commission on Hygiene and Public Dental Service.—Professor W. D. Miller, of Berlin, presiding. The meeting will convene Friday, August 26, at 2 P.M.

Address by Professor Miller, on Dental Hygiene in Germany.

Dr. George Cunningham, of Cambridge, England, will present a report on Public Dental Service, by the late Dr. J. Franck, of Vienna, Austria, with comments.

Dr. E. Forberg, of Stockholm, will give a paper on Hygiene and Public Service.

Other papers will be presented by members of the Commission.

Commission on International Dental Press.—Dr. E. Forberg, of Stockholm, Sweden, presiding. The meeting will convene Friday, August 26, at 4.30 P.M. in the French Building at the Fair Grounds.

Address by Dr. E. Forberg, President.

Paper by Dr. A. W. Harlan, New York, " The advantages of an International Review."

The programme for Saturday will be published and distributed early Saturday morning.

Dr. Conrad has secured the use of the French Building for the members of the F. D. I., from 4 to 6 P.M., Friday, August 26.

The Executive Council will meet at 6.30 P.M. in the Hotel Jefferson.

Members of the dental profession affiliated with the dental societies of the United States, or in foreign countries, are cordially invited to join any or all of the sections of the International Dental Federation.

On behalf of the Federation.

A. W. HARLAN,
Vice-President.

1122 BROADWAY, NEW YORK CITY.

THE

International Dental Journal.

VOL. XXV.   SEPTEMBER, 1904.   No. 9.

Original Communications.[1]

RECENT METHODS IN THE ADMINISTRATION OF ANÆSTHETICS.[2]

BY FREEMAN ALLEN, M.D., BOSTON, MASS.

MR. PRESIDENT AND GENTLEMEN OF THE NEW YORK INSTITUTE OF STOMATOLOGY,—It is a great pleasure to speak to you upon this subject, because members of your branch of the profession have always been prominently associated, not only with the discovery of anæsthetics, but with promoting the scientific use of them.

You know that Horace Wells, a dentist living in Hartford, Conn., first used nitrous oxide as an anæsthetic in 1844, and that in 1864 Dr. Colton, a New York dentist, continued the use of gas, which had practically ceased with the death of Wells in 1848.

You know also that Dr. Morton, a Boston dentist, first administered ether in 1846 at the Massachusetts General Hospital, and the names of Carlson, a German dentist, and Billeter, a Swiss dentist, are associated with the first considerable use of ethyl chloride as a general anæsthetic in 1897.

---

[1] The editor and publishers are not responsible for the views of authors of papers published in this department, nor for any claim to novelty, or otherwise, that may be made by them. No papers will be received for this department that have appeared in any other journal published in the country.

[2] Read before The New York Institute of Stomatology, May 3, 1904.

Since the discovery of these various agents very many of the improvements in method and apparatus for administering them have come from members of the dental profession.

During the ten years that followed the discovery of gas by Wells, and of ether by Morton, no progress in method and apparatus was made; but in 1858 Dr. John Snow, of England, did some work on the physiological action of chloroform and ether and devised inhalers for their administration.

Still more important work was that of Mr. J. T. Clover, of London, who in 1862 invented a regulating chloroform inhaler, and in 1876 demonstrated the advantage of using gas as a preliminary to ether.

In recent years Dr. Frederick W. Hewitt, of London, has done much to promote the scientific administration of anæsthetics. His most important work, begun in 1886, was the administration of nitrous oxide with definite percentages of oxygen, and in 1894 he perfected an excellent apparatus for this purpose.

So, although Americans discovered gas and ether, yet it appears that since 1858, until very recently, most of the literature of anæsthesia and many of the improvements in methods and apparatus have come from England.

I think the reason for this is the discovery of chloroform by Sir J. Y. Simpson in 1847. Chloroform was found to be a valuable but dangerous anæsthetic, requiring more caution in its administration than gas or ether. The English investigators began by inventing methods and apparatus for the safe administration of chloroform, and, in so doing, their attention was attracted to similar improvements in gas and ether. It became evident to professional men in England that the administration of anæsthetics was too important to be intrusted to inexperienced persons, and men began to devote themselves entirely to this work, with the result that anæsthesia became more systematized than in America.

Since the days of Clover the number of professional anæsthetists in England has greatly increased. To-day in the dental and general hospitals of London anæsthetics are administered almost entirely by professionals. Anæsthesia is systematically taught in the medical schools, and students are required to pass examinations and receive practical training in this line of work before graduation.

Different anæsthetists hold different appointments, just as do surgeons; thus Dr. Frederick W. Hewitt is Anæsthetist to His Majesty, the king; anæsthetist and Instructor in Anæsthetics at the London Hospital; Anæsthetist at the Charing Cross Hospital and at the London Dental Hospital.

There are societies of anæsthetists who hold regular meetings devoted to the science of anæsthesia; thus Dr. Dudley Buxton is Ex-President of the Society of Anæsthetists; Administrator of Anæsthetics and Lecturer in the University College Hospital; Consulting Anæsthetist to the National Hospital for Paralysis and Epilepsy; Senior Anæsthetist to the Dental Hospital of London.

Many London anæsthetists are men well advanced in years. Dr. Buxton, for instance, is fifty or fifty-five years old, with gray hair and beard, but well preserved and active; and I remember well at the Middlesex Hospital in London a Mr. Norton, who must have been sixty-five or seventy years old, but a careful and skilful anæsthetist, equal to any emergency.

So, although the most useful and important anæsthetics were discovered in America, they were elaborated in England.

In recent years, however, American investigators have taken up this line of work. In 1889 Dr. Thomas L. Bennett, now of New York, but then of Denver, Col., began to investigate the subject of anæsthesia. He used a Clover inhaler for several years, but finally invented his combined gas and ether inhaler, which is far ahead of anything any country has produced for this purpose. He was, I think, the first professional anæsthetist in this country, and has been practising this line of work in New York since 1897. Dr. Bennett has had many imitators, of whom I am one, and interest in anæsthesia has gradually increased; as yet, however, the anæsthetist's profession in this country is not an overcrowded one.

SECTION II.

The anæsthetics in common use to-day are nitrous oxide, ether, chloroform, mixtures of chloroform and ether, and ethyl chloride. In considering these agents in detail, the most important thing is the question of their safety, which it can do no harm to review.

Of all agents, nitrous oxide, as ordinarily used, is the safest. Considering the innumerable times that it is given, both in this country and in England, exceedingly few deaths are reported. It is considered so safe that most writers make no attempt to estimate its safety in figures. I have seen somewhere its death-rate given as one in two hundred and fifty thousand.

Nitrous oxide and oxygen is a still safer form of anæsthesia, when limited to short operations, but lately anæsthetists, especially in this country, have undertaken to use gas and gas and oxygen for the longer major surgical operations, and have reported administrations of from thirty minutes to two hours and a half.

When thus used the danger of gas, or gas and oxygen, is very materially increased. I have seen very alarming symptoms occur, and, on one occasion, almost lost a patient under this form of anæsthesia. In certain special cases of advanced renal and cardiac disease, however, it gives the patient the best chance, especially if the operation is one which does not require muscular relaxation. My longest case was one of forty-five minutes, the operation being dilating and curetting, ventral suspension, and appendectomy. For long operations, however, I have come to regard this form of anæsthesia as treacherous and as less safe than chloroform.

Ether.—Next in safety to gas comes ether. Excepting in people who are distinctly feeble or diseased, ether is perfectly safe. In ether accidents respiration always fails before the circulation, so that, if taken in time and persisted in long enough, artificial respiration will almost always save such cases. The most reliable statistics give the death-rate from ether as one in sixteen thousand.

Chloroform.—Chloroform is the most dangerous of all anæsthetics. Besides being a direct cardiac depressant, it has a tendency to cause irregularities in respiration which react upon the heart. These irregularities are seen mostly in the lighter degrees of chloroform anæsthesia, and may be produced by reflex causes. During the stage of excitement the respiration is especially irregular and the patient may suddenly, with a deep inspiration, inhale an overdose; any interruption of respiration during chloroform anæsthesia is therefore dangerous, as the chloroform already in the lungs becomes incarcerated and reacts upon the heart. Reflex causes, such as operative procedures, are apt to produce temporary arrest of breathing and consequent danger, and, as reflexes are more active during a light anæsthesia, a deep chloroform narcosis is, in some ways, safer than a light one; for this reason, too, chloroform is particularly dangerous in mouth, nose, and throat operations, since respiration is very apt to be interfered with in these cases.

Chloroform is especially unsafe when given to a patient who is sitting upright, because, besides being a cardiac depressant, it is a vasodilator, and allows the blood to gravitate from the great centres in the medulla into the dilated splanchnic vessels. Again, although a deep chloroform narcosis is, as I have said, in some ways preferable to a light one, it has the danger of overcoming the heart by an overdose, so chloroform is dangerous from any point of view. Its death-rate is estimated as one in three thousand.

Mixtures.—I consider mixtures containing ether and chloroform just as much safer than pure chloroform as they contain more ether than chloroform, provided they are administered with certain precautions which tend to produce an even evaporation of their ingredients; thus Schleich's Mixture No. 3, containing—

> Petroleum ether, 15 volumes;
> Chloroform, 13 volumes;
> Ether, 80 volumes,

is comparatively safe if given with ordinary precautions, owing to the preponderance of ether in it. When a house officer at the Massachusetts General I gave this mixture for two months as a routine anæsthetic, having two or three accidents, but no deaths.

The English A. C. E. Mixture, containing—

> Alcohol, 1 part;
> Chloroform, 2 parts;
> Ether, 3 parts,

is safer than pure chloroform, though not so safe as Schleich's No. 3.

The best and safest mixture that I know of is the " Anæsthol," recently introduced by Dr. Willy Meyer, of New York. This contains approximately—

> Ethyl chloride, 1 part;
> Chloroform, 2 parts;
> Ether, 3 parts,

and is said to be a true molecular mixture, having a boiling-point of 40° C. (104° F.); this secures the almost simultaneous evaporation of the three drugs, and adds materially to the safety of the mixture. Mixtures are not used enough for valuable statistics to be prepared in regard to them. I think they are safer than pure chloroform, although not so safe as ether.

Ethyl chloride has lately become popular as an anæsthetic. The most reliable statistics place its death-rate as one in sixteen thousand, but as it has not been used nearly as long as other anæsthetics, statistics in regard to it have not much weight. It is analogous in its action to gas, and my limited experience with it leads me to believe that it is safe if restricted to short operations. It does not produce cyanosis, but seems at times to have a slight depressing effect upon the circulation, especially during the first part of the administration. If we accept its death-rate as one in sixteen thousand, we find it safer than chloroform, as safe as ether, but not so safe as gas.

This gives the following order of safety of the anæsthetics we have been reviewing:

1. Nitrous oxide and oxygen (if limited to short operations).
2. Nitrous oxide.
3. Ether.
4. Ethyl Chloride.
5. Mixtures.
6. Chloroform.
7. Nitrous oxide and oxygen, when used in long operations.

Deaths occurring under anæsthetics should always be reported promptly and in full detail, as this is the surest way of determining the safety of any anæsthetic.

But simply because one agent is statistically safer than another, it should not be arbitrarily used in preference to that other, nor should any one method, such as giving morphine and atropine, be recommended as a routine procedure. As in other branches of medicine, different patients require different agents and methods, and the anæsthetist, having carefully examined his patient, must select and vary his treatment according to age, sex, disposition, habits, condition of the heart, lungs, etc.

To meet the indications of various cases anæsthetics are administered in sequence, as it is called; for example, we use the gas-ether sequence, the ethyl-chloride-ether sequence, the anæsthol-ether sequence, and the gas-ether-chloroform sequence.

Besides the proper selection of the anæsthetic the anæsthetist must concern himself with many details, such as the influence of posture upon the respiration and circulation, the proper protection of the patient during operation against drafts, pressure paralyses, etc., and must attend to the proper stimulation of the patient in case of necessity. He should be held entirely responsible for the safety of the patient as regards the anæsthetic. Ether pneumonia and other sequelæ may also be said to be due to lack of care on the part of the anæsthetist.

SECTION III.

I will now speak of some practical points in the administration of these agents.

Gas.—Gas is so easily eliminated that in order to be effective it must be made to replace the residual air in the lungs, and the access of fresh air must be cut off for the time being. In other words, to produce the best results pure gas and no air must be given, at least for the first part of the administration. The practical difficulty that we encounter in giving gas is not from giving the patient too much gas but from giving too much air, thus delaying anæsthesia. Therefore, in order to be effective, the gas machine must be so made as, first, to keep out air; secondly, to replace residual air in the lungs with gas; and thirdly, to keep a certain amount of gas constantly in the lungs.

The simplest and most effective form of apparatus for this purpose is the one ordinarily seen in the dentist's office where much extracting is done. Gas is liberated from a cylinder and enters a long tube of large caliber which ends in a mouth-piece. This is placed in the patient's mouth and the lips are closed over it. If the nose is also closed the patient inspires pure gas; if the nose is not closed he inspires gas plus a small amount of air; during expiration air plus a certain amount of gas passes through the nose; thus with each inspiration the patient gets more gas; with each expiration he loses more air, so that gas gradually replaces air in the lungs and anæsthesia rapidly results. When the inhalation is stopped there results an anæsthesia of varying duration, which is called the " available" or working anæsthesia. This apparatus is simple and effective, but is not portable, and is suited only for dentistry.

The same result is accomplished in other forms of apparatus which have closely fitting face-pieces to exclude air and inspiratory and expiratory valves; the best form of such an apparatus is Bennett's gas inhaler. Gas is liberated from a cylinder and conducted by a rubber tube to a distensible rubber bag of about two gallons capacity; the closely fitting face-piece is accurately applied, gas is liberated from the bag, and is inspired by the patient through the inspiratory valve; the patient expires through the expiratory valve, the expirations going into the surrounding air and no fresh air entering the lungs during inspiration, the expiratory valve being closed. In this way gas is made with each inspiration gradually to replace the residual air in the lungs. When signs of approaching anæsthesia occur, the gas may be shut off and the valves thrown out of action by turning the stop-cock; the patient breathes back and forth into the bag. The result of this, however, is not asphyxiation, but delaying of asphyxiation, because the patient is breathing a mixture of gas plus what residual air there is left in the lungs, whereas, if he had been permitted to go on breathing gas through valves the gas would have replaced all the air in the lungs and asphyxia would result, so this manœuvre of throwing the valves out of action delays asphyxia and also results in a longer available anæsthesia, because, as a rule, the longer the inhalation the longer the available anæsthesia.

For dentistry, perhaps, this form of apparatus presents little advantage over the simpler form that I at first described. For the longer surgical operations it presents distinct advantages: in the first place, the bag, being near the face-piece, offers no mechanical impediment to respiration; in fact, by keeping the bag well filled, a constant positive pressure is kept up which keeps a steady stream of gas flowing into the lungs without much inspiratory effort on the patient's part. The vents for the admission of air enable us to keep the patient under, and, at the same time, to admit such small definite quantities of air as are necessary to prevent too much cyanosis. In using this machine the most essential point is to select an accurately fitting face-cushion, as even very small amounts of air admitted during the first part of the inhalation will spoil a good gas administration.

It is possible to give gas with suitable proportions of air for long operations, but it usually produces an unsatisfactory form of anæsthesia, owing to the lack of muscular relaxation and the asphyxial symptoms that occur with it. Without discussing the physiological reason for this, the clinical fact is, that it is not possible to give enough air with gas to dispel these asphyxial symptoms and, at the same time, to control the patient. My longest case of gas and air anæsthesia was a nephrectomy lasting thirty-five minutes.

Other methods of giving gas in which you may be interested are (1) Dr. Flux's open method; (2) Dr. Patterson's apparatus for giving gas in long operations on the mouth.

In Flux's method an open cone made of glass or celluloid, with an accurately fitting inflatable rubber-cushion, is used. Gas is allowed to flow into the top of this cone during inspiration only, and, being heavy, sinks at once to the bottom of the cone and is inhaled. In timid persons and children this method is said to produce a tranquil and satisfactory anæsthesia without cyanosis; it consumes a great deal of gas, however, and does not seem to me practical.

Patterson's apparatus I have seen used at the London Dental Hospital. It consists of a gas-cylinder with a foot-key by which gas is liberated through a long rubber tube into a rubber bag of four gallons capacity; at the top of the bag is a stop-cock which turns on gas or air as needed. From the stop-cock two tubes lead to the nose-piece fitted with an inflatable rubber cushion to permit of closer approximation. This is closely applied over the nose and the patient breathes gas. Anæsthesia takes a little longer by this method, owing to the air inhaled through the mouth; if more rapid anæsthesia is desired, there is a separate mouth-piece fitted with an expiratory valve, by which the patient gets no air and the anæsthesia results more rapidly. With the nose-piece only, in about fifteen or twenty seconds; eight or ten gallons are used for an ordinary administration and twenty or thirty gallons last ten or fifteen minutes.

An important advance was made in 1894 when Hewitt perfected his apparatus for the administration of gas with definite percentages of oxygen. You know that nitrous oxide is a pure anæsthetic and is not dependent upon asphyxia for producing its results; this is proved by the fact that by admitting definite percentages of pure oxygen it is possible to keep patients deeply and quietly anæsthetized for long periods of time without any asphyxial symptoms. A suitable patient under this form of anæsthesia appears to be sleeping peacefully, with normal or slightly improved color and tranquil or gently snoring breathing: it gives a longer available anæsthesia in dentistry than does pure gas. (Describes apparatus.)

Ether is commonly administered in one of two methods,—the semi-open method and the closed method. The semi-open method is the one ordinarily seen in hospitals, and consists in giving ether on a cone made of tin or paste-board. The paste-board cones are the best, as they can be accurately fitted to the face. This method is the best for persons who are not experts, but it requires large amounts of ether unless the cone is accurately moulded to the face so as to exclude air.

The principle of air limitation in giving ether was expounded by Clover in 1876 when he invented his inhaler. This is known as the closed method, and in experienced hands is much better than the open method, because it requires very much less ether, and the proportions of air and ether-vapor are under perfect control. The result is that patients are less apt to become " soaked" with ether, and recoveries are much more rapid and free from nausea and vomiting. Bennett's ether inhaler is the best type of the closed inhaler; with it suitable patients can be comfortably and safely anæsthetized with ether in from two to five minutes, and the entire apparatus can be boiled and sterilized without damaging it.

A third, and exceedingly useful, method of giving ether is by the apparatus invented by Dr. Fillebrown, of Boston, or the Harvard Dental School. In dental and oral surgery it is necessary to give ether with the mouth open in order that the surgeon may work while the anæsthesia is being continued. Ether, as ordinarily used, could not control the patient in the presence of so much air; nor is chloroform safe for such cases owing to the danger connected with giving this direct to patients in the sitting posture. Dr. Fillebrown's apparatus heats the ether, thus doubling the rate of its evaporation and intensifying its strength so as to make it effective with large amounts of air. His original apparatus was modified by his assistant, Dr. Rogers, and still further improved by Mr. Lockwood, of Boston. It is exceedingly practical in head cases of all kinds, and will control very difficult subjects. (Demonstration of apparatus.)

Gas and ether, or the gas-ether sequence, is much used in surgery. When properly administered it is a great comfort to both patient and surgeon. Instead of ten or fifteen minutes of struggling, shrieking, coughing, retching, and vomiting the patient may be safely plunged in a profound anæsthesia in two minutes. English statistics estimate the safety of gas and ether as greater than that of ether alone. When gas is used there is much less nausea and vomiting and a more rapid recovery; the patient is spared all the suffocating sensations so often produced by ether alone. This method is useful in dentistry because it is safe in the sitting posture and will give an available anæsthesia which may be anywhere from four to ten times as long as that resulting from gas alone, and a recovery which is often unattended by nausea and vomiting. (Demonstration of Bennett's combined gas and ether inhaler.)

The principles of giving chloroform are exactly the opposite of those for ether. It must, under all circumstances, be administered with large amounts of air, as it is easy to give an overdose. Chloroform is best given on an Esmarch or Schimmelbusch mask, using a drop bottle and the constant drop method. It can also be satisfactorily given on a small, square piece of folded gauze, by the so-called " Scotch" method, which consists in shaking on comparatively large doses of chloroform at intervals. For dental and oral surgery, tracheal chloroforming, etc., many regulating chloroform inhalers have been devised. A good one is Krohner's regulating inhaler. (Demonstration of Krohner's regulating inhaler.)

Mixtures, according to the amount of chloroform they contain, should be given with more or less air; thus the English A. C. E. mixture, having two parts of chloroform and three of ether should be given as chloroform, while Schleich's mixture No. 3 can be given on a cone or other form of semiopen inhaler. As I mentioned before, the danger in mixtures is the different rates of evaporation of their ingredients, but if the mixture has a definite boiling-point and is administered by the drop method, this danger is practically nil.

I have had considerable experience with mixtures, and consider them safer than chloroform.

Much has been written lately about ethyl chloride, which until 1897 was used only as a local anæsthetic. Ethyl chloride is exceedingly volatile, has a low boiling-point,—that is, 12.5° C. (55° F.), —a slight, rather oniony odor, and is inflammable. It is sold in graduated glass vials with patent stoppers under various proprietary names. The commonest kinds are " Antidolorin," " Anæstile," " The Cleveland Gas Company's Agent," " Kelene," and " Narcotile." Of these, I have found that kelene and narcotile give the best results, and I have used narcotile more than any other.

Ethyl chloride is analogous in its action to gas, producing its effects more rapidly and being very rapidly eliminated. It must be

given on the same principles as gas,—namely, with almost complete
exclusion of air. Ethyl chloride is useful, and I believe safe, in
slight operations that do not require muscular relaxation nor a
deep anæsthesia. I believe it has been found by American practitioners to be unsatisfactory in dental surgery, on account of the
short available anæsthesia that it produces. Dr. Thomas D. Luke,
of Edinburgh, however, reports a series of dental cases in which the
available anæsthesia varied from one to five minutes, which is
longer than that produced by gas. It does not produce cyanosis,
but it will not abolish the higher reflexes nor produce muscular
relaxation. My longest case with it was one of forty minutes,
given for an orthopædic operation on the ankle-joint. This anæsthesia was very ragged, and was followed by intense and persistent
nausea and vomiting. My experience with this drug is limited to
about sixty cases, which, I regret to say, I did not record systematically, but many of them were followed by nausea and
vomiting.

Since many writers, carried away by enthusiasm for ethyl
chloride, have claimed that it is superior to gas and will supplant
gas, it may be profitable to compare the two. Ethyl chloride,
although it seems to be safe, is not so safe as gas, and has not
been put to anything like the test for safety that gas has, only
having been used since 1897. Ethyl chloride is not so agreeable
to inhale as gas; gas has more of a taste than an odor, and patients
who have taken both have assured me that they preferred gas.
Recoveries from ethyl chloride are much less satisfactory and much
more often attended with headache, nausea, vomiting, and a dazed
condition of the mind than are recoveries from gas, in which the
patient is usually free from nausea and vomiting and perfectly
normal at once. So, although ethyl chloride produces no cyanosis,
is perhaps less expensive, is more portable, and requires less skill
to administer than gas, yet these trifling advantages should have
no weight in the face of the three facts I have just mentioned. It
may be used to precede ether, but in this respect, also, is inferior
to gas. (Demonstration of Ware's and Ash & Sons' inhalers.)

PATHOLOGICAL IRREGULARITIES.[1]

BY M. H. FLETCHER, D.D.S., M.D., CINCINNATI, OHIO.

ENUNCIATION.

THE terms orthodontia and irregularities of the teeth conventionally carry with them the idea of irregular teeth in children and youth, connected with their treatment for correction. The causes are usually hereditary, but may be acquired. One could quote from writers from Etruscan days down to the present time and give the opinion of more than fifty authors, but their definitions of the etiology would most likely each differ somewhat from the other.

There have been handed down to us such explanations as " She inherited large teeth from one parent and small jaws from the other," or " His baby teeth were not extracted soon enough," or " were taken out too soon." " Lack of absorption of the roots of the temporary teeth, while the growth of the permanent set is rapid," etc. One author thinks " the development of the hind end of the jaw does not keep pace with the absorption of the front end."

Then there are a lot of platitudes, such as " The teeth are too large for the jaw," " Too many teeth for size of the jaws," " Projecting jaws," " Sleeping with the mouth open," " Enlarged tonsils," " Want of room in the jaws," etc., etc.

In summarizing the above opinions it would seem that symptoms, or results, have been given in place of the real cause. Nevertheless, this is only another opinion.

ETIOLOGY.

Guilford divides the causes into hereditary and acquired, and Colyer into general and local.

" Talbot has shown that irregularities of the teeth were often due to two factors. Those of constitutional origin, which develop with the osseous system, and those of local origin." " The deformity always commences at the sixth year and is completed at

---

[1] Read at the fifty-fifth annual session of the American Medical Association, in the Section on Stomatology, Atlantic City, June, 1904.

the twelfth." " Forward movement of the posterior teeth produce the same result as arrest of development of the maxillæ. It was also shown that the vault is not contracted by mouth-breathing. That contracted dental arches are as common among low as in high vaults and that they simply appear high because of the contraction. That mouth-breathing due to hypertrophy of the nasal bones and mucous membrane, deformities of the nasal bones, adenoids, or any pathologic condition producing stenosis, does not cause contracted jaws, but all these conditions are due to neuroses of development."

EFFECTS.

The ill effects of these deformities must be apparent to such an audience as this with a mere suggestion. The degree and extent of the ill effects have not only to do with the unsightliness of the patient, but Talbot has done much to prove the connection of extreme cases with idiocy and crime.

Aside from uncomeliness, irregularities undoubtedly interfere with the proper care of the teeth and gums, and in this manner are a large factor in fostering diseases of the alveolar process, including the surrounding tissues; many times involving other parts of the jaws, the nose, eyes, and ears, often inducing chronic disorders of digestion and fostering the causes of zymotic diseases. Neuroses of many varieties may have their origin in diseased alveolar process and teeth.

TREATMENT.

As to treatment, our best men differ in their procedures. Cleft palate and harelip are of course dealt with from a surgical standpoint. Prognathic cases, showing atavistic tendencies, with diastoma behind the canines, are sometimes treated surgically by removal of bone from these spaces, but such treatment is rare. In the treatment of lesser deformities mechanics are almost entirely relied on. Some operators resort to the removal of one or more teeth in order to accomplish the desired end. On the other hand, Dr. Angle says, " The best balance, the best harmony, the best proportions of the mouth in its relation to the other features, require in all cases that there shall be the full complement of teeth, and that each tooth shall be made to occupy its normal position. And if we accomplish this we shall have satisfied the demands of art, so far as they are concerned in the relation of the mouth to the rest of the face."

To restore the features to harmony and the teeth to perfect position and usefulness requires .mechanical skill of the highest order, coupled with an æsthetic sense and artistic eye.

PATHOLOGIC IRREGULARITIES.

Definition.—In contradistinction to the above, there is a class of irregularities not treated of in works on orthodontia, nor have they been considered under the head of dental orthopædia. In fact, these cases seem in a way to be " the stones which the builders disallowed."

They are in many particulars the exact opposite of the others. 1. They do not appear until the age of mature years. 2. They are purely acquired. 3. They are entirely pathologic, in the sense that they are the result of disease, localized in the alveolar process. 4. They are only amenable to mechanical treatment by first removing the causes of the disease producing them.

Name.—In order to distinguish these from those previously described, the writer has called them pathologic irregularities.

Etiology.—To describe all the causes of pathologic irregularities would be to give a treatise on interstitial gingivitis, known also as pyorrhœa alveolaris and Riggs's disease.

To make the matter plain from my stand-point it will, however, be necessary to briefly describe the anatomy, the pathology, and the causes, with treatment other than mechanical.

Anatomy.—An intimate knowledge of the anatomy is of course necessary in order to comprehend the pathology, or to apply treatment intelligently. It is presumed this is understood.

Now, when we consider that a hard, unyielding substance like a tooth is not only supported and held in place by, but entirely dependent on, the thin, bony walls of the alveolar process, it is a marvel to realize what hard usage it withstands, and what enormous pressure and lateral strain it is continuously subjected to without displacement or injury. Let this bone become diseased, however, and ere long the teeth become tender and unusable, and vast numbers are finally lost without the least defect in the tooth itself.

In the last decade these diseases and their treatment have engaged the attention of the profession to a marked degree, much to its credit.

Terminology.—To Talbot is due the credit of having classified the various phases of this disease and described its different stages. He has given the name "interstitial gingivitis" to inflammation of the gums, alveolar process, and peridental membrane. The term Riggs's disease and pyorrhœa alveolaris were formerly applied to any or all the stages and conditions.

The term Riggs's disease is indefinite and is to-day obsolete. Pyorrhœa alveolaris now indicates a flow of pus from the sockets about the roots of the tooth, and is a terminal stage of inflammatory action. It is the result of previous inflammation known as interstitial gingivitis. Inflammatory action may continue, however, and exfoliation of the teeth result without pus infection. One termination of the inflammatory action is the tendency of the teeth to be expelled from their sockets, with the result that they become elongated, tilted to one side, or pushed in or out of the normal arch.

To give a plan of arresting this process before it has gone too far and to replace the teeth into their normal position is the object of this paper.

Causes.—In order to arrest or eradicate a disease, its causes must first be found and removed. Talbot says, " The local causes which produce interstitial gingivitis are an accumulation of tartar about the necks of the teeth, decayed teeth producing hypertrophy of the gums, unfinished fillings, gold crowns and bridge-work, artificial dentures, rapid wedging of the teeth, collections of food and everything that will produce irritation of the gum margin, setting up a chronic inflammation or gingivitis. This in turn extends to the deeper tissues (the peridental membrane and alveolar process), where it becomes interstitial in character. The constitutional causes which act locally, producing interstitial gingivitis, are the toxic effects of mercury, lead, brass, uric and other acids, potassium iodide, and other agencies acting in a similar manner, such as scurvy," etc.

He further says, " Autointoxication (meaning self-poisoning due to a faulty metabolism) is the great cause of interstitial gingivitis resulting in pyorrhœa alveolaris."

In contradistinction to investigators who hold that the disease is often entirely systemic, the writer's opinion is that the disease must have a local cause, this cause producing a point of least resistance for the localization of systemic disorders, which general disorder or condition of autointoxication increases the local symptoms.

There seems no reason to believe that drug poisoning or other morbid systemic conditions can produce interstitial gingivitis unless a lesion of the gum pre-exists. This lesion may be the merest break in the mucous membrane, caused by the smallest deposit of calcareous material, this local mechanical irritation being one requisite of the etiologic moment. On the other hand, there may frequently be found in gingivitis the systemic disorders accompanying cases of sapræmia and septicæmia.

The continual pressure against the gum tisssue of rough, irritating calcareous deposits, which continuously increase in quantity and insinuate themselves deeper and deeper beneath the soft tissues, are accompanied with all the products of repair by granulation or second intention, and may be accompanied by surgical fever. These deposits may be found wherever saliva can penetrate. It has never been my privilege to see deposits of tartar about the necks of teeth that were innoxious, but they are always irritating to some degree, and usually greatly so. This condition may exist in all stages, from that of being imperceptible to the naked eye up to a complete state of pyæmia, and may result in death.

On the other hand, there is abundant evidence to show that autointoxication, or a low state of health from any cause, greatly favors the progress of the disease, and with this state of affairs present a chronic pus-forming condition may soon be found about one or more of the teeth where the local exciting cause exists, but that autointoxication or other systemic disorders cause this disease, without local irritation, does not appeal to the writer's reason any more than to say that the same disorders cause inflammation of the pleura or conjunctiva without a local point of least resistance from local cause.

Degeneracy or faulty development may bring the etiologic moment at a very early stage of the local irritation. This might be almost coincident with the initial lesion, whereas in normal and healthy individuals the pyorrhœal stage, even in its mildest form, may be deferred indefinitely or never appear even where calcareous deposits are excessive.

The fact that the tissues involved are transitory in nature does not seem an adequate factor in accounting for the disease, as suggested by Talbot, since they are as transitory in cases where the disease does not exist as where it does, and these tissues recover as readily as other structures which are not transitory.

There seems no question but that calcareous deposits about the teeth should be looked on as noxious foreign bodies, and that the constant effort on the part of nature to extrude them results in the progressive death of the surrounding tissues, with the malposition of the teeth as one result. We find in this disease zones of granulation tissue with the result of destructive metabolism, in the soft tissues and the creation of sequestra in the bone. This condition, however, is changed to constructive metabolism the moment the tartar, sequestra, or other local irritants are removed.

The sinus in the pyorrhœal stage of this disease is between the root and alveolar process, unless the lesion be so deep in some place on the outside of the process that a gingival abscess is formed. In either event the alveolar process is continually bathed in pus, which results in its destruction. So long as the tartar is present as a foreign body the irritation is continuous and sequestra are formed which are a second source of irritation until they are removed or absorbed.

All these cases will heal by removal of the deposits and sequestra or by the loss of the affected teeth. The removal of the teeth invariably results in recovery, and a patient without teeth, either young or old, cannot have the disease, regardless of transitory structures, degeneracy, heredity, drugs, environment, or systemic disease. If lesions of the gums or maxillary bones appear where there are no teeth, it is not interstitial gingivitis, but something else.

Of all the causes mentioned, the writer believes that ninety per cent. of cases of interstitial gingivitis are due to hard deposits about the teeth.

Treatment.—As to treatment, I believe that all authorities are agreed that absolute removal of all deposits about the necks and roots of teeth is the first requisite to recovery. In my own hands this requires from three to ten sittings, approximately a week apart, washing out the socket each time with hypodermic syringe, using fifty per cent. alcohol, saturated with boracic acid, painting the gums with iodine or iodide of zinc. They must then have constant care thereafter from one to six times a year in order to preserve a good state of health, or a "healthy stump," as surgeons say. Dr. W. A. Price, of Cleveland, has had good results by local treatment with the X-ray after having removed the deposits.

As to instruments, each one capable of doing the work will adopt his own methods and choose his own instruments and remedies for local treatment. If the diagnosis has been correctly made the practitioner will be the judge as to whether systemic interference be necessary. If constitutional treatment is called for, abstinence from excess of nitrogenous and acid foods, with the necessity of ten to twelve glasses of pure water daily and the addition of lithia for a period is usually indicated.

Much can be learned about the condition of the system by examination and analysis of the saliva and urine; neither should be more than slightly acid and both should be normal in other particulars.

Talbot says, " In the severer types of disease, such as tuberculosis, asthma, chronic indigestion, kidney disease, etc., very little curative effect is to be expected from treatment. Constitutional treatment is tentative, since autointoxication will continue in most cases until death. The chief treatment of such cases will be removal of local irritation.

" The system excretes forty ounces of water daily. If this amount be not taken into the system, or if it be not eliminated every twenty-four hours, autointoxication will follow. Every drop of water taken into the stomach enters the blood. It is one of the best purifiers which we possess. From five to seven pints of pure water should be taken each day to flush the blood and kidneys and thus cleanse the system."

Mechanical Treatment.—The causes having been determined and treatment carried well along, the malposition of the teeth should begin to have attention. This is usually begun before healing of the tissues is complete. The writer has had the most satisfactory results in these cases by straightening out their defects in the same manner that ordinary irregular teeth are treated. A description of the mechanical devices contrived and used for the purpose of regulating teeth would fill large volumes; yet in addition to all these the inventive powers of the operator are continuously called on in carrying these cases to satisfactory completion. In my own hands cumbersome regulating appliances have largely given way to a most simple plan,—namely, that of a simple bow of heavy German silver wire on the outside of the dental arch, so adjusted that the teeth are drawn to it by the use of ligatures of German silver or platinum instead of silk or rubber. Torsion is produced by putting on a band to which a tube is soldered; in this tube is inserted a spring lever, the outer end of which is ligated to the bow. The use of the bow on the outside of the arch is one of the oldest devices known, but the manner of its handling is varied, being susceptible of a great variety of uses.

The resiliency of the heavy bow is such that its steady pull or push moves the teeth out or pushes them into line. Its resiliency can also be utilized to expand or contract the strongest arch. It has nearly done away with jack-screws, Coffin plates, and many other intricate and annoying appliances where they were formerly used, and simplifies the treatment to a very great degree, and has done so in my hands for the past ten or more years.

This bow and its accessory appliances being entirely on the outside of the arch are much less annoying than appliances inside, and are very much more effective. It will be found that pathologic irregularities yield to pressure more readily than in younger persons because of the partial loss of alveolar process; then there are no short, partly erupted teeth to be dealt with.

Regarding the imaginary difficulty of changing the shape of bones in mature adults, it may be said that live bone never becomes so old that it will not yield to continuous pressure, and teeth are more easily replaced into a former position than moved into a new one. Nevertheless, two of these cases here presented show where adjoining teeth have been brought together and occupy spaces where a tooth had been extracted or lost from disease, both in patients fifty years of age.

As to changing the shape of bones, Dr. M. H. Cryer says, " After the birth of the child muscular action and various forces have direct influence over the change of the bones, according to the following general laws: The normal application of forces in developing bone results in the normal development of the form of the bone. The abnormal application of forces under the same circumstances results in the development of an abnormal form. Abnormal applications of forces to bone in adult life will also change and modify the shape and character."

These pathologic cases, like the others, must be retained in their new position for a period of months, may be years, or until the bony arch has become thoroughly ossified again. This is usually done by ligating them with platinum ligature. Sometimes a heavier platinum wire is fitted to the lingual surfaces and ligated to the teeth with the light platinum. The German silver and platinum ligature is No. 25 B. & S. gauge.

In November, 1893, I presented one of these cases, giving this plan of treatment, and read a paper on the subject before the Cincinnati Odontological Society. Since that time I have treated several additional cases with most satisfactory results.

DISCUSSION.

Dr. Eugene S. Talbot, Chicago.—I appreciate highly the new term coined by Dr. Fletcher, "pathologic irregularities" of the teeth. It is an important and common condition, and classified under this head defines the pathologic state. The tooth itself is to a great extent a foreign body in its relation to the alveolar process. The teeth, from want of antagonism, constantly move in the alveolar process due to interstitial gingivitis. This is particularly true of the old method of separating teeth by the rapid process for filling. An interstitial gingivitis was set up, because of this the teeth separated, and in later years a space resulted between the teeth. Because of the transitory nature of the alveolar process, an interstitial gingivitis always occurs after the second teeth have obtained their position. There is what may be called an inflammatory process continually going on in the alveolar process. This is the reason why a dental arch which has lost one or two teeth is always more or less out of order. This " inflammatory process" starts an absorption of the alveolar process, because of which the teeth move in different directions. How far such an alveolar process can be restored is an open question. Some operations of Dr. Fletcher, beautifully performed, bring the teeth back into place and hold them in position until the alveolar process is restored to partial health. It is never restored to complete health. This last is a physical impossibility. Local treatment is all right, so far as it goes. It is very essential that the deposits should be removed; that the roots of the teeth should be thoroughly cleansed, but besides that there is considerable to be done in regard to draining the system. It is necessary to restore the excretory organs to their function. Autointoxication is the great determining factor, no matter what the systemic condition may be. The greatest cause of this is intestinal fermentation.

HYPNOTISM.[1]

BY CHARLES GILBERT CHADDOCK, M.D.

GENTLEMEN,—In a lecture which I had the honor to give before the Senior class of this school about a year ago, I discussed the subject of " Pain," [2] in its physiologic and psychologic relations. In that discussion I had much to say about the mental aspect of pain and the ways in which consciousness of pain could be modified by influencing the state of mind of the individual suffering it. In the cases cited as demonstrating the variability of pain with the variations of the state of consciousness, I made no direct reference to hypnotism, and attempted to show the effects of suggestion alone to induce insensibility to pain. It seems, then, appropriate to continue the discussion, to some extent, of the influence of suggestion as it is shown in the practice of hypnotism.

Hypnotism is a term derived from the word " hypnosis," which was first introduced by an English physician, Braid, in 1841. It is a word of Greek origin, which signifies sleep, and was used by Braid to cover a peculiar state of somnolence which he induced in certain individuals by means of certain procedures. Braid was the first observer who attempted to investigate scientifically certain peculiar states of mind of spontaneous or induced origin, which had previously been regarded as due to animal magnetism, but he never went so far as to deny the existence of animal magnetism.

A French charlatan, Mesmer, in the latter part of the eighteenth century, made himself famous by the wonders he performed with the aid of so-called animal magnetism, and so celebrated did his work become that his name became attached to the procedures which he employed and the state of mind which he induced. Until Braid's work was published these phenomena were classed under the term Mesmerism; thus animal magnetism, Mesmerism, Braidism, and hypnotism are terms for the same phenomenon; the name has been changed with variation of the conception of the nature of the phenomenon.

---

[1] A lecture delivered to the Senior Class of the Marion-Sims Dental College.

[2] INTERNATIONAL DENTAL JOURNAL, August, 1903.

Notwithstanding the scientific spirit in which Braid approached the subject, it did not emerge from the realm of mystery until more light was thrown upon it by the studies of Charcot and the School of Nancy in the seventies. Even under the search-light of a scientific mind like that of Charcot, the mysterious subject of hypnotic phenomena was only elucidated after years of study and observation, and even at the present time there are striking differences of opinion between rival observers; which only serves to emphasize the difficulties the human mind has to encounter in forming just opinions about the phenomena of life.

It would be unjust to omit reference to an earlier observer who clearly explained the nature of hypnotic facts. In 1784 the subject of animal magnetism was brought before the French Academy of Sciences for discussion at the time when Mesmerism was at its zenith of popular interest. Many were the occult and mysterious explanations offered for these remarkable manifestations. In reference to this animated search for supernatural causes, an extract from a report of Bailly before the French Academy of Sciences is worthy of citation: "In searching for an imaginary cause for animal magnetism the actual power that man exercises over his fellow-beings without the immediate and evident intervention of a physical agent, is recognized." By this you will see it is meant that the mental state of one man is influenced by the mental state of another or others, and it is a fact that it is not necessary to appeal to the supernatural to explain it. Bailly in support of his assertion had shown "that the power of man over the imagination can be elaborated to an art, at least in relation to such persons as believe in the possibility of such things." In this statement Bailly explains perfectly the phenomena of Mesmerism, which was, in fact, only the art of suggestion, exercised upon those who were by belief or faith or prejudice in awe before the supernatural.

Mesmerism, Braidism, and hypnotism are not new. The phenomena to which these terms have been successively applied are as old as humanity itself. You all know that for centuries the fakirs of India have practised upon the credulity of a fanatical and ignorant people by means which to-day we speak of as suggestion; and we have no farther to go than to our immediate neighbors to realize the potency of the wonder-worker. The travelling quack, the painless tooth-puller of the country district, is practising in our day what the fakir of India has practised for ages.

In discussing a subject it is necessary to define, if possible, its limitations; in other words, we must attempt to understand what is meant by hypnotism, hypnosis, hypnotic suggestion, etc.

Hypnotism is a general term applied to all phenomena which characterize the state of hypnosis; therefore it will be understood if a satisfactory limitation can be given to the term hypnosis. Hypnosis is a peculiar state of consciousness which manifests itself under certain circumstances, characterized by a limitation of ideas to a narrow circle within which the subject acts and out of which he cannot pass without the aid of extraneous ideas or influences which have no immediate relation to the series or circle of ideas which dominate consciousness. It should be added to justify the term hypnosis that the individual manifests during the time of limitation of consciousness a certain state of sleep or somnolence but remains more or less subject to the influence of others.

The first observer who clearly stated the theory of suggestion, as it is understood to-day, was Liebeault, in 1866. He refers all phenomena of animal magnetism, so-called, to the influence of suggestion reaching the subject through physiologic avenues. His views became the starting-point of the School of Nancy, which maintains that the phenomena of hypnosis are normal, and claims that eighty per cent. of human beings can be hypnotized.

In contradiction to the Nancy School arose that of the Salpêtrière or the Charcot School, which claimed that the phenomena of hypnotism were abnormal and presented certain somatic or bodily symptoms which were characteristic and pathognomonic. While the Nancy School regarded all the manifestations of the hypnotized subject to be due to the effect of idea, the Charcot School maintained that certain physical means exercised a direct influence upon the patient without the intervention of the mind.

There flourished at the same period a belief in the power of medicines to exercise their effects at a distance. These views were maintained until his death by Luys, notwithstanding the scientific demonstration that his ideas were entirely false and that the phenomena he attributed to the influence of medicine were the result exclusively of suggestion.

At the present time the contradictions between the School of Nancy and the Charcot School continue to exist, though some of the early elements of dispute have been eliminated, and the question has now become narrowed to the discussion as to whether hypnosis and hypnotic manifestations form a part of the disease known as hysteria, or are without pathologic significance.

In my lecture of last year, I pointed out the efficacy of suggestion as a means of overcoming pain, and showed how almost universally human beings are open to suggestion and persuasion; how our habitual beliefs and our manner of thinking are the result, in a large measure, of suggestion.

The efficacy of an idea given to another depends largely upon the mental training and habits and beliefs of the individual, as well as upon the nature and source of the idea which is intended to influence him; thus there must be great variability in the susceptibility of individuals to suggestion, though all probably are more or less subject to its influence. Probably the extravagant claims made for hypnotism by the Nancy School, in the belief that the vast majority of human beings can be hypnotized, is based upon this general fact of almost universal suggestibility; but it is a long step from mere suggestibility to true hypnosis, and in reality the persons in whom a true hypnosis can be induced make up but a small portion of humanity in general.

Before attempting to explain the nature of hypnosis, and before making any statement of its uses or abuses and possible injurious effects, it will be well to give you some idea of the means by which the condition may be induced in certain susceptible persons.

In the practice of Mesmerism, so-called, sleep is induced by the belief that some supernatural indefinable influence (fluid) leaves the operator and effects the subject in such a way as to induce in him the conditions which have been predicted; for example, the operator makes certain passes in the neighborhood of the subject, all the time stating that the result will be sleep, and that in this state he will become subject to the will of the operator, performing all that he is commanded to perform and with inability to resist the commands. In order to place a subject in a receptive state of mind, certain procedures are also employed, such as fixing with the eyes a bright object, with the command that the subject is not to wink and that sleep will follow. The natural result of fixing the eyes on a given object is a burning of the eye-lids that induces heaviness of the eyes, which naturally suggests sleep, even though the idea of sleep has not been otherwise imparted to the subject. In this way susceptible persons pass into an hypnotic state. Braid was accustomed to use such means with verbal suggestion, though he believed that fixation was an essential element. Later, as has already been explained, Liebeault discovered the essential element in the idea imparted, and that all that was essential was verbal suggestion. The method now generally employed is to place the subject in a position of repose and suggest that the eyes are heavy and that drowsiness is creeping over the individual. Certain external circumstances lend weight to these ideas. It is especially effectual to place the subject to be operated upon in the presence of hypnotized or sleeping persons for the aid lent by subconscious suggestion. If a subject be influenced, he apparently sleeps, but is in relation with the operator, and may be induced to act in accordance with ideas communicated to him by the operator. In this condition, however, the subject is rarely, if ever, *absolutely* in the power of the operator. There is a certain limit beyond which suggestions have no power to influence the individual. Thus it is very easy to induce the hypnotized person to perform silly acts or those which are without special moral meaning, or which are not in opposition to his moral training; but even in the most susceptible hysteric patients it is practically impossible experimentally to induce them to attempt acts which are manifestly criminal, providing that such acts are out of harmony with their training and habitual attitude of mind. However, it is true that in the hypnotic state, the subject accepts ideas more readily than in the waking state, and on account of this, during hypnosis, ideas may be imparted to the subject which overcome ideas that are habitually active during the moral waking state. This makes it possible to remove or overcome certain mental or bodily symptoms which are dependent upon idea. Thus psychic pain may be removed by suggestion, and paralysis, anæsthesia, contracture, etc., that have as their basis an idea, conscious or subconscious, frequently may be overcome and permanently cured by suggestion in the hypnotic state. On the other hand, by the same means (suggestion) similar phenomena may be made to appear in the hypnotic state; so that after waking from the hypnotic state the subject presents pain, paralysis, tremor, contracture, anæsthesia, etc.

The hypnotic state of consciousness is peculiar in this, that it is a secondary state, or a state differing from that of moral consciousness, so that the person that has been repeatedly hypnotized comes to have a double consciousness in a sense. During hypnosis memory of the events of the normal waking state is quite obliterated; and on the contrary, in the normal waking state memory of the events during the continuance of the hypnosis is wanting, but with repetition of hypnosis there is memory for the facts of previous hypnotic states. In certain individuals this doubling of consciousness is so marked, and the two states are so distinct, that actually two personalities are created.

Since many of the writings on hypnosis still refer to the original conception of Charcot, it may be well to review the phenomena which were regarded by that observer as essential in so-called " Grand Hypnotism."

It should be stated at once that grand hypnotism as understood by Charcot was observed only in persons subject to hysteria in its most marked form. The procedure employed in general was to suggest to the patient that she would fall asleep, at the same time the operator pressed with his fingers on the eyeballs after the patient had closed the eyes. The patient passed into a somnolent state which lasted indefinitely, and in which she was not open to verbal suggestion. Owing to the apparent state of relaxation, with resemblance to sleep, this condition was called lethargy. Without interference from the operator this state would last indefinitely. In the state of lethargy, however, certain procedures produced peculiar phenomena. If the operator stroked a limb, for example the forearm, the muscles touched would become forcibly contracted. This contracture would continue indefinitely, and remain after the patient had been wakened, if pains had not been taken to remove it by some procedure—either by forcible pressure on the muscles or by blowing lightly upon them. This phenomena of contracture could also be induced by approaching a magnet to the patient.

If now (during lethargy) the patient's eyelids were raised by the operator, they remained open and the gaze fixed. The raising of the eyelids induced a secondary altered state. In this condition the patient remained fixed in the attitude which she happened to be at the moment the eyelids were raised, but this attitude could be altered by the operator, and whatever position was given to the limbs or body was maintained indefinitely; in other words, this condition was one of catalepsy. In this cataleptic state the patient was more open to suggestion, but still seemed to be dominated by a single fixed idea, or in a state of suspension of mental activity. Mainly suggestion exercised its effect through attitude, for the facial expression changed in harmony with the attitude (prayer). The phenomena of contracture evocable in the state of lethargy could not be induced here. If the eyelids were mechanically closed the patient immediately passed again into the state of lethargy, from which she could again be changed by suggestion into an apparently normal waking state, but which is an exceptional mental condition in which she is entirely subject to the will of the operator. This condition the Charcot School called somnambulism, for the reason that the patient walked, talked, and acted without special abnormality, and accepted all possible ideas from the operator; thus a hypnotized patient in a condition of somnambulism may be made to believe that she hears or sees anything which the operator suggests, and many of the bodily functions may be influenced in the same way; thus all the symptoms of hysteria may be brought into being by suggestion, such as anæsthesia, paralysis, contracture, and attacks of grand hysteria (convulsions).

Charcot's study of these three states was at fault in that he failed to recognize that all three states were equally the result of suggestion; for he believed that they were characteristic of hypnosis, and that stroking, pressing, blowing, and magnets exercised a direct physical effect to induce the changes observed. However, he admitted that there were certain cases in which these phenomena did not occur, or could not be induced in their fully developed form. The similarity between lethargy, catalepsy, and somnambulism, as manifested in his patients, and certain phenomena characteristic of hysteric persons, led at once to the view that these conditions were identical; in other words, that grand hypnosis and grand hysteria were the same thing.

Out of the error which led the School of Charcot to regard certain phenomena of hypnotism to be due to the specific physical effect of certain procedures on hypnotized subjects, and the probable truth that the characteristic conditions of hypnosis are identical with those observed in certain persons subject to hysteria, resulted the controversy which has waged for years between that school and the adherents of the School of Nancy. On the one hand, the influence of suggestion was in part overlooked; on the other, namely, by the adherents of the School of Nancy, the identity of hysteria and hypnosis has been entirely ignored. This controversy has been waged especially around the therapeutic value of hypnotism. The School of Charcot has from the first been very sceptical as to the therapeutic value of hypnotism in the treatment of disease, whereas the School of Nancy has gone to great lengths in its advocacy of suggestion and hypnotism as means of cure of all forms of disease. The Parisian school (Charcot) has at no time underestimated the value of *waking suggestion* as a possible means to cure all disease of psychic origin, and in this respect it would seem to an unprejudiced observer that the diversity of views between the two schools under consideration were one of name rather than of nature; in fact, the School of Nancy has gradually abandoned the use of hypnotic suggestion *per se* and advocates the use of suggestion given in the waking state merely, claiming that results can be obtained which compare favorably with those which were formerly said to be possible only as a result of suggestion given during hypnosis. To-day the adherents of the School of Charcot hold practically the same view with regard to the therapeutic uses of suggestion, but they maintain the view that hypnosis, which in itself represents only the highest degree of suggestibility, is only a manifestation of hysteria, and can be induced only in those subject to hysteria; and further, that all the cures that have been reported as due to hypnotic suggestion are due to the fact that the symptoms or conditions that have been cured or changed by hypnotic suggestion are hysterie in nature.

Probably much of this difference of opinion arises from lack of identity of understanding of what is meant by hysteria.

It would take me too far to go into detail regarding the pathology of this mental disease, but it may be stated that the phenomena of grand hysteria and grand hypnosis are practically the same; in the one case the symptoms arise spontaneously; in the other they are artificially or secondarily induced.

What are the uses of suggestion in general and the uses of hypnotic suggestion in particular?

Waking suggestion, as we see in every-day life, exercises a profound influence upon the mental state of individuals, and is perhaps the most important aid to the physician in his treatment of patients, whether they are suffering with physical ailments or those due to idea. To the patient suffering with actual physical disease, it lends hope and faith, and thus enhances or favors the action of drugs that have been administered with the view to cure physical disease. Oftentimes it assists the patient through a crisis, thus giving time for material remedies to act. Such cases are not instances of hysteria in any true sense of that term.

Hypnotic suggestion can only be employed in relation to conditions that are actually hysteric; in other words, in conditions that are the result of idea—psychic. By means of hypnotism or suggestion given in hypnosis, it is possible to overcome accidents or symptoms which have not yielded to waking suggestion; in other words, this procedure is only practicable with hysteric persons; and the fact that hypnosis in a strict sense can be induced is practically a demonstration of the hysteric condition of the individual. However, not all hysteric individuals can be hypnotized, and therefore the range of application of hypnotism is necessarily limited; furthermore, hysteric patients presenting hysterie symptoms of the gravest nature, even though it be possible to hypnotize them, cannot always be improved or cured. In many cases of this kind the symptoms can be removed during the continuance of the hypnotic state, but they return and persist after awakening from hypnosis.

The wide range of application of hypnotism, suggested by the writings of the School of Nancy, does not find support in the facts of experience; for to obtain results by this means it must be applied to hysteric persons, and only a certain portion of hysteric individuals can be benefited by it.

In addition to this limitation, there must be mentioned the possible dangers which attend the indiscriminate use of hypnotism. Since those in whom hypnosis can be induced are essentially hysteric, there is the danger of grave hysteric accidents or conditions arising during or as a result of hypnosis. In particular, a person predisposed may be so affected that she become thereafter subject to periodic attacks of grand hysteria, which remain refractory to all means of treatment. It has also been observed that persons frequently subjected to hypnosis become more and more easily influenced by others, until finally they become subject to auto- or self-suggestion, and thus an original condition of hysteria has been intensified or a latent hysteric predisposition has been developed into fully developed grand hysteria.

Popular and public exhibitions of wonders of hypnotism are to be most emphatically condemned; indeed such theatrical travesties should be prohibited by law. In the first place, the hypnotist who practises the art for the amusement and mystification of the public is but rarely acquainted with the nature of the instrument he wields, and in nowise responsible for the lasting harm he may cause. But the ignorant hypnotist who plays upon the credulity of the people is no more to be condemned than the ignorant newspaper writer or reporter, and the more cultivated writer of modern novels, who employs the mysteries of hypnotism to heighten interest in his impossible. I have no doubt that many educated persons entertain ideas of hypnotism gathered solely from reading such popular novels as " Trilby" and the supernatural effusions of Marie Corelli. Such popular and unscientific presentations of a subject which at first sight seems so mysterious only serve to foster in the minds of the masses a belief in the supernatural, with all the errors and mental aberations which spring from ignorance. Whether it be in the uncultured or in the educated, false ideas concerning the nature of Mesmerism and hypnotism are in a measure responsible for many prevalent errors that afflict the world to-day. The hypnotism of the Indian fakir, which can be traced back to Persia in the person of the celebrated Zoroaster, is doubtless in large part responsible for the occultism that reigns and has reigned for centuries among the Hindoos, and which has found acceptance among some of the brightest, though misguided, minds of the Occident.

Spiritualism, as it is understood to-day, was born in hypnosis (autosuggestion) and developed through suggestion.

Christian Science is perhaps the most remarkable monument ever erected by the human mind to celebrate the powers of autosuggestion. It goes without saying that were the true nature of the means by which the very remarkable results of practical Christian Science understood by its adherents, such results could not in the nature of things be obtained. All depends upon faith in the supernatural nature of the means which bring about the end. If these remarkable and sometimes exceptional results had not a reverse, it would not seem absolutely necessary to attempt to destroy the delusion of which they are the consequence. Unfortunately, the devotee of an idea or theory that is believed to be of universal application must come in conflict with actual conditions and physical obstacles. Thus great harm results. The Christian Scientist, in his ignorance of the natural limits of his " science," applies his theory to physical disease, and thus throughout our country many innocent lives are sacrificed yearly to blind and unreasoning bigotry.

When one walks the streets to-day or glances over the advertising pages of the daily newspapers, he is almost forced to the conviction that the superstition and ignorance of the Middle Ages have come down to us unchanged. Fortune-tellers, clairvoyants, mind-readers, and palmists seem to have their signs in every available window. The advertising hypnotist has now developed the school of hypnotism, which does not confine its instruction to the student in attendance, but teaches the art of hypnotism by letter.

In the same category are to be reckoned certain writers on so-called mental science, who very plausibly present the thesis, convincing to the mind of one unschooled in physiology, of the actuality of mind-reading, thought transference, and mental suggestion.

I make these cursory allusions with a view merely to point out the dangers which attend the spread of errors concerning the mind and its nature; and especially because I consider that the erroneous views still prevalent with regard to hypnotism are in some measure responsible for the facility with which these errors are accepted and propagated.

In conclusion permit me to emphasize one fact which I wish you to retain. Hypnotism is a natural, though abnormal, phenomenon. It does not depend upon supernatural influences. All the symptoms and conditions of mind which characterize the hypnotic state are subjective; that is, they belong exclusively to the individual presenting it, and its fundamental cause lies not in the influence of a second person, but in the peculiar state of the person presenting the phenomenon. If a second person can excite in a susceptible subject the phenomenon of hypnotism, it is only by means of the communication of ideas to that person by actual physical means, exactly like those we employ daily in our communication one with another.

SOME PHASES OF DENTAL EDUCATION.[1]

BY A. E. BALDWIN, M.D., D.D.S., LL.B., CHICAGO.

In order to realize that we are living at a very rapid rate, we have but to look backward to see the progress that has beeen made in almost all lines within the memory of even the younger men of the profession. By observation we are shown that the educa-

---

[1] Read at the fifty-fifth annual session of the American Medical Association, in the Section on Stomatology, Atlantic City, June 7 to 10, 1904.

tion required to enable one to call one's self an educated artisan, scientist, or professional person was very meagre as compared with the demands and the requirements of to-day.

The question often arises in my mind whether or not stomatology, as a specialty, has kept pace with the march of progress in other lines, and especially in coincident professional lines. Much has been written, much is being written, and much more is being thought, as to the proper lines of progressional development in education in our specialty. Within the past few years we have seen that the National Association of Dental Faculties has, after long discussions, extended the requirements, preliminary and graduating, until now the time required in our most progressive schools is nothing less than a four years' course, with more strict preliminary requirements. However, by noticing the actions of some of our educators, we fear that there is a movement on foot—especially in the schools which are conducted by private ownership—because of a fear that with these added requirements the collegiate expenses will be increased, with a corresponding decrease in receipts; consequently these schools—which are conducted, if you please, for financial gains incidentally—look on the matter as a strictly mercantile transaction, and I fear that there may be a retrogressive move lessening the preliminary requirements, and also lessening the amount of time necessary to be spent in schools in order to graduate.

It has been my observation for a score of years that there are many people practising with us who seem to have a fear of acquiring too broad and comprehensive an education; indeed, a short time ago a paper was read before the Odontological Society of Chicago by Dr. H. T. Carlton, San Francisco, in which he advocated a radical advance in not only the preliminary requirements for entering our colleges, but also an emphatic advance in the requirements which must be met before graduation is allowed. This paper was read before the largest assemblage of dentists ever gathered in the world, and, much to my surprise, many men who had been classed with those who were in favor of advanced education showed by their discussion of this paper that apparently they were afraid that the young men entering our field might be too broadly educated and too well grounded in knowledge, not only of the whole human frame, but in all other scientific directions. It was convincing to a reasoning and observing mind that the only hope

26

for rapid and thorough educational progress in our field lies in the schools which are maintained and conducted otherwise than for financial ends. In other words, the hope of dentistry, in its progressive advance, lies more largely than we will admit, first, in the schools which are founded and conducted in connection with our great colleges and universities, and, second, in the gradual elimination of the schools which are conducted by organized capital for the income which it produces, or by the organized professional band who, for notoriety or gain, organize and conduct schools which apparently are more anxious for numbers than for intellectual prominence. This is said with regret and with no intention to belittle or attack any school or college in particular, but with recognition of the fact that if the teachers or the organization have a direct financial interest in the income, gross and net, it must hamper or modify the influence which the school and teachers may exert over the student and the requirements demanded of him.

A great movement in advance can be forced if our national organization of the several State boards unify and exact constantly advancing requirements for entering our chosen field.

THE EVOLUTION OF STANDARDS IN DENTAL EDUCATION.[1]

BY CHARLES C. CHITTENDEN, D.D.S., MADISON, WIS.

IN a paper read before this Section one year ago I reviewed the various steps by which dental educational standards had been slowly and laboriously advanced from a mere shadowy pretence of individual schools to the establishment by the National Association of Dental Faculties of a minimum educational requirement for admission to all schools, which was equivalent to two full years of high school, and also the adoption of a full course of instruction for graduation of four years of seven months each.

The four years' course was proposed by resolution in that body in 1899. Action was laid over for one year, and at Mil-

---

[1] Read at the fifty-fifth annual session of the American Medical Association, in the Section on Stomatology, Atlantic City, June 7 to 10, 1904.

waukee, in 1900, the Faculties' Association deliberately and after careful consideration decided on its adoption, setting forward the time for its inauguration to the autumn of 1903, thus reserving three years more in which it would be possible to change their decision in case it should develop that the time was not ripe for such advance. Thus at the annual meeting of 1903, held at Asheville, N. C., the subject came up for final irretrievable action, which was precipitated by Harvard University Dental Department.

That school informed the Association that it would "not at present extend its course to four years," assigning as its reason that it was engaged in contemplating the raising of its educational requirements for entrance at some time in the future.

A special committee had the matter under advisement for three days as to whether the Association should "concede that Harvard is entitled to one year less time than other schools having an equal standard of admission, with the exception, it may be, of analytical chemistry and physics." The committee reported recommending that Harvard could not be granted such concession, and after a free discussion the report was unanimously adopted on a roll-call of colleges. Harvard then resigned its association membership, and the resignation was promptly accepted. In all this the National Association of Dental Faculties deliberately, unanimously, and finally placed itself on record as standing firmly for the four years' course.

Simultaneously at Asheville an attempt was made in the National Association of Dental Examiners to have rescinded the following standing resolution, adopted at Milwaukee in 1900 as a treaty of peace and good faith between the colleges and the examiners,—viz.:

Resolved, That no college not an acceptable member of the National Association of Dental Faculties be placed on or continued on the recommended list of this association.

This attempt to rescind failed, and the two associations adjourned in full accord and with the mutual conviction that the four years' course was established for all time, and that the two associations would stand firmly together for its maintenance as a criterion of the reputability of dental colleges.

Thus it transpired that every dental college in the Faculties'

Association, and, in fact, every dental college in the United States, save one, opened up the school year of 1903-04 with the four years' course inaugurated and advertised to the world as the established standard deemed necessary by the educators themselves for the proper preparation of the dental student for graduation and practice. It was a brave move,—a grand achievement,—and the profession at large gave a great sigh of satisfaction that the schools had made this advance step towards removing the stigma which had been cast in foreign countries on the educational methods and standards of the schools of the United States.

It seemed that there remained only the necessity to secure the further requirement of high-school graduation for matriculation (which step had been practically promised by most of our universities and actually inaugurated in some of them) to place this country in the forefront of the nations, with practically no peer. The dream of raising up a generation of educated, scientific professioual gentlemen to serve as the standard bearers of dentistry for the near future seemed about to be realized.

The school year for 1903-04 opened with the new order of things, but to the great disappointment of many deans, whose freshman classes were much smaller than the year previous. This condition was largely accounted for by the fact that prospective students had hastened to take advantage of a last chance to graduate in a three years' course and had flocked to the schools the year before in large numbers. This fact also made the first four years' freshman classes seem abnormally small. Of course, the income to the schools was correspondingly small. To the older-established and the endowed schools and departments of universities this did not so much matter, as the check was, of course, only temporary. But the smaller proprietary schools at once took alarm at the decrease in income, and without regard, it would seem, to what effect such a course would have on their standing and reputability in the eyes of the public, began, within a month after the opening of the school year, to devise some plan for inducing the National Association of Dental Faculties to return to the old course of three years for graduation. An effort (which finally proved successful) was made to hold an extra meeting of the Association at Buffalo during the Christmas holidays to act on such a proposition. At this meeting it was held and ruled by the president that no action could be taken or business transacted until the next regular annual meeting, but much time was spent in discussing the situation. Sentiment was divided about as follows: One factor, consisting of about one-third of the Association membership and representing almost exclusively the proprietary schools struggling for existence, were avowedly for an unequivocal return to the three years' course of seven, or even six, months each. Another smaller fraction favored a high-school diploma for matriculation and a three years' course of nine months for graduation. And, lastly, those schools having adequate financial foundation on which to bank in conducting their work on any reasonably advanced standards, those schools representing about one-half the membership in the Association, stood and pleaded for professional honor and professional unity—stood firmly for no retrograde of standards and requirements. When the meeting adjourned it seemed reasonable to believe that no further attempt at lowering standards would be made.

When the national body adjourned at Asheville in 1903 it was with the general understanding that the next annual session would be held at St. Louis at about the same time in August, 1904, as would be held the International Dental Congress,—that is, the latter part of that month.

It has been the rule of the schools to issue their annual announcements for the coming school year course some time in June, as the business for the coming year begins immediately after the old term closes. Had the National Association of Dental Faculties held to the plan laid out at Asheville as to the time of the annual meeting, these announcements would all have been issued on the basis of a four years' course before the meeting could occur, and a change in the course would have been practically impossible; but for reasons best known to themselves the majority of members have recently decided to hold the meeting in the city of Washington, June 9. Such a change in programme is so unusual that it is but natural to seek a reasonable explanation. At this early date the annual announcements will not have been issued, and it would be entirely reasonable to infer that another attempt may be made to lower standards. Should such an attempt prove successful, there are a great many things likely to happen. It is not conceivable that the endowed and independent schools will tamely submit (even should they be in the minority) to a retrograde educational movement. They could in no sense afford it, nor would it be in accord with any of their traditions. They have for years submitted to being held back by the inability of the weaker schools to move forward rapidly on account of their financial handicap. It is but reasonable to expect that the Faculties' Association would either go to pieces or become divided into two separate organizations with separate standards.

The question at once presents: What would be the attitude of the legally appointed examiners in the States which hold their boards responsible as to the judging of the reputability and standing of the colleges from which their applicants for license have graduated?

What would be the attitude of the profession at large? Will the men who are out in the open, bearing the heat and burden of the day before the public, tamely submit to the open discredit that would be cast on their chosen calling by a national lowering of its educational standards?

It seems impossible that such a calamity as a division of college forces on this question could occur, and still more impossible that a decided retrograde movement can possibly receive the sanction of a majority of the schools. But should this happen, it is safe to predict that the rank and file of dentists will put their stamp of disapproval on such a transaction in no uncertain manner. The prediction is reasonable that schools of the trimming and retrograde type would be allowed to fall back out of sight and be forgotten in the onward march of the development and evolution of dental educational standards.

AN INSTRUCTIVE CASE OF HYPERTROPHIED PULP.

BY LEONARD C. HALES, D.D.S., WELLINGTON, NEW ZEALAND.

Miss B. became a patient of mine in December, 1903. After making a careful examination of the teeth I noted that although most of the anterior teeth were free from caries, the molars, both first and second, on both the upper and lower jaws, and on either side of the mouth, were badly decayed.

The patient, being about twelve years of age, naturally had her permanent teeth in position. After a thorough cleansing of the organs of mastication, I took the lower left first permanent molar, which was badly decayed and seemed to be giving the most trouble, the cavity of decay taking in the greater part of the occlusal surface and the mesial wall, along with the lingual wall, on which side the cavity extended well under the gum margin.

The shell that remained was filled with a large bulbar mass of pulp-tissue, and which I recognized at once to be a far-advanced case of hypertrophied pulp.

Contrary to my expectations, I found the tissue to be abnormally sensitive, and suffused with blood, which seemed to gush out when the part was touched. I tried cocaine in the dry crystalline form, but it had no effect, as the pulp did not seem to absorb it. I then made an application of trichloracetic acid, but its action, apart from being exceedingly slow, gave the patient intense pain, so I removed the agent; and as I noticed that the patient was fast arriving at an unpleasant nervous condition, I at once resorted to Dr. Maercklen's suggestion, and, packing the parts with iodine crystals, I made a cap of base-plate gutta-percha, closed the cavity, and told the patient to return in two days' time.

Two days later the patient returned; the pulp was less sensitive, but still bled profusely. I was enabled, however, to remove the larger portion of it with a sharp excavator, and, making another application of the iodine crystals, I closed the cavity and dismissed the patient for two days.

When the patient came again I was enabled, with the aid of a hypodermic syringe, to inject the root-canals and pulp-chamber with a cocaine solution with comparatively little pain to the patient. I then extirpated the remainder of the pulp-tissue, thoroughly cleansed the canals, inserted a dressing of oil of eucalyptus in the canals, and again dismissed the patient, this time for a period of four days.

When the patient returned I removed the dressing and filled the canals with oxychloride of zinc, and after allowing the tooth to remain stopped with gutta-percha for several weeks, with no signs of trouble, I inserted an amalgam filling. The tooth has remained comfortable ever since, and to all appearances will continue to do so.

ROOT-FILLING.[1]

BY T. WILSON HOGUE, D.M.D., VERMONT, BOURNEMOUTH, ENGLAND.

Mr. President and Gentlemen,—I have such an exalted opinion of American dentistry that it is with the greatest diffidence I lay this short paper before you.

It seems like sending coals to Newcastle to send a paper on dentistry to America. Nevertheless it may interest some of the younger members of the Harvard Dental Alumni Association to hear the experience of one who has tried not to work in a groove, but fairly to try all new methods of practice that at all promised success, and has done so during many years.

When the pulp of a tooth is exposed, whether by decay or an excavator, my practice is not to cap, but destroy. Capping has such an element of uncertainty about it that I favor extirpation of the pulp, and use S. S. White's devitalizing fibre, sometimes incorporating with it a minute quantity of S. S. White's nerve-paste, being most careful that the application is properly sealed in the cavity.

Excelsior, or Donaldson's pulp-canal cleansers, are in my hands the best instruments for removing the pulp, and I only use the finest size. In a large canal I insert two of the cleansers and sometimes, say in a large upper canine, three, rotating them together.

Mummifying pastes I have not found reliable, and I have given them up for a better and more certain treatment.

Free and easy access to the canals must be made, however much tissue has to be sacrificed, and very small canals sometimes slightly enlarged with suitable drills,—Gates-Glidden and Bentelrock's are excellent.

My experience is that the apex of the root should not be perforated, and I am very careful to avoid perforation.

For disinfecting septic canals I use perchloride of mercury or oil of cloves.

Oxychloride of zinc I have found by far the best material for filling canals, as it remains sweet and pure indefinitely.

[1] Read before the Harvard Dental Alumni Association. " Alumni Day," June 27, 1904.

Stiffened paper points for drying pulp-canals I use extensively, and find useful.

Gutta-percha in every form has proved with me very inferior to oxychloride of zinc; if the former filling is removed from a root, it always smells nasty, although it may only have been there for a few weeks.

It is a great help to have a large assortment of suitably curved instruments for inserting dressings, as well as for permanently filling the canals of roots.

Although charcoal has only been used by me for a few months, yet in concluding this short paper I wish to say that I have found it an exceedingly valuable filling, and as it is practically insoluble it ought to prove a permanent one also.

This paper will, I hope, be the means of leading to an interesting discussion.

I do not know exactly how it is in America, but I believe that in England no operation is so often imperfectly performed as the filling of roots. It seems to me no operation in dentistry— I had almost said in surgery—demands more time, skill, and care.

PYORRHŒA ALVEOLARIS: A CASE IN PRACTICE.

BY H. C. FITZHARDINGE, D.D.S.

Miss R., aged twenty-nine, a stenographer by occupation, presented for treatment during the latter part of November, 1903. On examining her mouth I found that she was wearing a full upper plate. She said all her upper teeth had become loose and had been extracted. The gum had receded from her lower six anterior teeth, which were very loose. The teeth had a dense, opaque appearance, the gum was puffy, of a bluish livid hue, and had a shiny, polished appearance on the surface. Pus was exuding from pockets around the teeth. I diagnosed this as a case of so-called pyorrhœa alveolaris. Considering the age of the patient, and also the fact that she was most anxious to have these teeth saved if possible, the prognosis was favorable. I removed the accretions of calculus from the roots very carefully, washed out the pockets with hydrogen dioxide, cauterized the necrosed tissue with fifty per cent. sulphuric acid, washed out with a stream of warm water, and followed with the Truman method. With the exception of the sulphuric acid, this treatment was continued once a week (the patient could not come oftener) until April, 1904, using the sulphuric acid about every second visit and reducing the strength to twenty-five per cent. I prescribed a mouth-wash, No. 1 (see below), to be used three times daily, and she is now using the mouth-wash No. 2, as it is a little more palatable, to be continued all the time. The teeth are now firm and the gums, though re-ceded, are healthy.

No. 1.

Hydronaphthol, gr. xv ;
Sp. vini rect.,
Aquæ dest., āā ℥ii. M.

Sig.—Two to ten drops in a glass of water. Use with a brush as a mouth-wash.

No. 2.

℞ Hydronaphthol, ʒii ;
Ol. cinnamomi, ♏xv ;
Ol. menth. pip.,
Ol. gaultheriæ, āā ♏v ;
Sp. vini rect., ℥iss ;
Aq. dest., ℥iv. M.

Sig.—Twenty drops to a tumbler of water twice daily with a brush as a mouth-wash.

THE INTEREST OF THE DENTIST *VERSUS* THE IN-TEREST OF THE PUBLIC.[1]

BY R. ANEMA, D.D.S.

UPON receiving the kind invitation of the Chairman to read a paper before your society, I felt very much pleased, and gladly accepted it, because I know there are among you many men who are more learned and more able than I am to give valuable sug-gestions upon a subject in which I am very much interested. The subject, to which I hope you will give some thought, is " The Interest of the Dentist *versus* the Interest of the Public." The main feature, which makes the title less arbitrary than you at

---

[1] Read before the thirty-sixth annual session of the Pennsylvania State Dental Society, July 12, 13, 14, 1904.

first might have thought, and of which I am going to present you as a study, is "professional egotism." I say *study* purposely to let you know that my paper, instead of being a well-designed and nicely framed picture, is merely a sketch.

Problems such as we have to consider here may be called in some ways sociological problems. In trying to resolve such questions, it seems next to impossible to leave out the mental factors called moralizing and preaching, as well as the fiercer one of condemning. These factors are dangerous friends when we earnestly wish to probe a sociological question to its bottom. In endeavoring to come as near to the truth as possible, let us therefore leave those three passionate friends at home and look upon things as the German philosopher, Nietzsche, would do, from a point on the other side of good and evil.

I am unable to give you a synthesis of professional egotism, by which you might see at once its whole spiritual body, with its clear outlines and distinct limits. The method I shall follow is the one of analysis and the study of symptoms as I see them or mean to see them.

Perhaps it is unnecessary to say that this way of treating the subject will occasionally show a hiatus on the road on which the essayist leads you, or, in other words, will occasionally give the essay a somewhat incoherent character.

In my language, the Netherland language, there are two words for your one word "profession," both words being almost equally common in use. The one gives the concrete signification of profession, meaning the number of class of men that practise the same art; the other gives the abstract signification, and means vocation or calling. With these two words in mind, it is easier to make one's self understood than with one. The concrete word class for dental profession is a rather unfamiliar word in American society, because class differences are not as distinct as in older countries, and perhaps, also, because the atmosphere in the younger world is oftener and more heavily attacked by idealistic storms. When one keeps in mind only the abstract signification of profession, professional egotism is a *contradictio in terminis,* but when one thinks of the concrete the new term becomes more familiar.

To my mind there is no more doubt of the existence of professional egotism that there is of a certain kind of patriotism, called jingoism, that says, "My country, right or wrong," or of that egotism which, by instinct and brute force, extinguishes weaker races. Of the latter, we have in the history of mankind many instances. Of the former, I hope to give you an instance later on. All these forms of egotism are brought about by instincts of the individual becoming active in the mass at certain times and intervals of its existence. In seeking the genesis of professional egotism, allow me to tell you first something of the instinct of self-preservation, and then of what I call self-preservation of the class.

In our days when education and civilization are overestimated, perhaps it needs some courage to declare that even a dentist is an ordinary human being, with instincts giving active power to his mind and body.

One of your best authors says that " Of all animals, man has the most instincts." Among the strongest instincts of man is the one of self-preservation. It is a common truth that instincts are hard to deal with, if, indeed, they can be dealt with at all. They may become concealed to the inexperienced eye, covered by so-called civilization, which oftentimes is nothing but a social veneer, or by an amiable self-deceit of good people, which makes them believe that at least among the higher classes instincts, and especially the one of self-preservation, are rudimentary. If, however, these good people believe that those higher classes look out merely for the interests of others, they are mistaken. The lesson given nearly two thousand years ago, " Love thy neighbor as thou lovest thyself," is still generally applicable, which means that man, as a rule, loves himself more than his neighbor and more than any other man. His instinct of self-preservation dominates his altruistic feelings. I will not say, however, that there are no such people as martyrs, in which this instinct seems almost lost, but this specimen is very rare.

When a man joins a profession he brings his instinct of self-preservation with him. It brings him quite often in closer contact with the profession, as he hopes that the profession may at some time be of some use to him. Notwithstanding man's idealistic feelings and the almost overwhelming influence of them, as is the case after long solitary contemplation, or transferring thoughts to others in enthusiastic gatherings. it cannot be denied that the average professional man not only possesses this instinct of self-preservation. but that he needs it wherewith to earn his daily bread.

When we take the dental profession as a class, each man making a living through dentistry, to protect himself and his family from starvation, should it be at all surprising that there exists such a thing as self-preservation in this class? Again, our professional family may be compared with the still larger family of nation or race, in which the instinct of self-preservation is always present, being especially awake and active in times of rude competition, called war, but dormant at times where no attacks are to be feared. The following, I think, is an example of professional self-preservation: In a certain country a society of dentists, forming the editorial staff of a dental journal, desired to change the rules. One of the members proposed the following as the principle on which the new structure should be erected:

" The society intends to serve the public by promoting dentistry, dentistry in the most remote sense of Art and Science." His obvious reason, as he explained at the time, was to have as the leading motive the " interest of the public." After having been carefully considered, the proposition was rejected almost unanimously. So far as the thoughts of the opposition could be understood, the men who voted against the " public interest" proposition, feeling themselves representatives of their profession, considered it their duty not to look out—at least not in the first place—for interests other than those of the body of men represented. The new rules were now based upon a foundation which can easily be laid bare and understood by looking upon the flag and emblem of one of our best dental journals, which says " Devoted to the interests of the profession."

As dental journals are leaders and at the same time the voice of the profession, I consider these two facts as very valuable ones and as a proof that the dental profession needs devotion to its own interests; and as devotion to one (the profession) excludes devotion to another (the public),—otherwise it is no devotion,—what else can be the cause for the demand of this highest form of affection than the instinctive self-preservation of the class? But as an instinct acts without consciousness of the purpose, its purposive action may not be generally observed, and therefore my conclusion that we have with these two journals also two instances of self-preservation of the class may not be generally accepted.

Judging from these cases and comparing them with similar ones in other countries, I think I am right in saying that the dental profession, as all young bodies, has a strong instinct of self-preservation, and at the same time is limited in its motive power, handicapped as it is on its way to the general ideal, "the interests of the public," by its class instinct, "the interest of the profession."

After this I may give you at once my definition of professional egotism as the *aggressive self-preservation of the class.* This potent inner prompting becomes fully awake and highly active in times and places where attacks are to be feared by competition, in the same way as wars are brought about by collision of the interests of nations.

Here follows an instance of professional egotism: In a certain country a body of dentists use their power to prosecute respectable foreign dentists for using legally acquired but foreign degrees of doctor. As their country does not furnish a dental doctor degree, the dentists claimed that the foreigners gained an undue reputation by the use of that title, thus doing harm to the interests of the local dentists.

Here I might have finished my paper on the "interest of the dentist *versus* the interest of the public and professional egotism," but as I feel somewhat in debt to the original title, especially to the last part, "the interest of the public," I hope you will allow me to make a few more remarks.

If it is true that the profession as a body is limited in its motive power (being devoted to its own interests), an interesting question to treat, especially from the public point of view, is, "Who looks out for the interests of the public in the case of dental legislation?" Dental legislation, according to some, exists to protect the public from malpractice, and, according to the same, is necessary for that purpose.

However, it cannot be according to this principle that a law is made which debars a foreigner from practising his art, no matter from which reputable school he comes or how many years of reputable practice he may have had, but compels him to pass through all the preliminary examinations and to spend at least two years in the local dental school, after which he must pass the dental examinations. And yet there is such a law in France.

And what shall we think of the legislation of many of the American States, as cited by Dr. Kirk in his paper on "The Unification of Dental Legislation," when he says, "Much of our dental legislation owes its existence to the effort of those who make the protection of the dental practitioners against the competition of his unqualified neighbor his primary and leading motive"?

And to think of the professional legislation of Austria, Belgium, and Italy where only medical men are allowed to practise dentistry, and that, too, without the necessity of passing any dental examination at all!

And when all the European countries give to their physicians a right to practise dentistry, do you think that all this legislation is made in the interest of the public, or merely to satisfy a class that at the time has the most influence upon the legislature? The leading motive in all these cases may have been protection of the public from malpractice, but if it was, in my opinion the object has not been gained.

It may surprise some of you that in Germany the healing art is free. Every one who likes may practise medicine and also dentistry. It has been a long time an open question to me why this should be, but in looking back upon professional legislation, perhaps we may come to the conclusion that Germany is not so wrong after all. Anyway, we know that Germans are a philosophical race, and think a long time before they act. Is it merely accidental that in Germany the philosophical thought originated that the main desire in man was the desire for power?

These were the suggestions I owed to the "interests of the public."

At the end I apologize for what moralizing I have done. Notwithstanding I have endeavored to hold back my friends, the preacher and the condemner, I know that I have not fully succeeded.

Now, when I am free again, I hope you will allow me a few moralizing remarks. That I have not spoken more for "the interest of the dentist" I hope will not be a reason for accusing me of criminal neglect, as there is sufficient proof that the dentist can look out for his own interests. Still, I fear that some of you will condemn me for talking so much of professional egotism and for exposing the profession as I have done, and, as I dislike to be censured, I promise that, at some future time, I will write a still longer essay on "professional altruism," in that way turning my critics into friends. Because, with Plato, I am a firm believer in the absolute good, a spirit which is also largely represented in our profession. However, the sun does not always shine, neither does the good.

Reviews of Dental Literature.

THINGS OF SPECIALISM AND OF THIS SOCIETY THAT MAKE FOR OPTIMISM.[1]   By William M. Beach, A.M., M.D., Pittsburg, Pa.

The specialist must be gifted in letters sufficiently to reduce to writing a correct description of a case, and be possessed of an analytic mind to the end that he may be able to philosophize upon disease in its most minute details. It has been a lamentable fact that the medical profession, skilled as it is in management of patients, and learned in the science of medicine, neglects that literary qualification which is a requisite to success among our leaders and authors of the day.

To be proficient, certain fundamental principles must be comprehended and appreciated. Since the ideal man is rare enough, and would probably be an expensive article could we find him, it must needs be we should get our work done by special hands, and as we employ separate men for classics, mathematics, and modern languages, in educational affairs, so we should find one who has made physiology, pathology, etc., his province in medical matters.

It is obvious that a man's character has at least two sides, and that his temperament may be separated into two opposing factors, —viz., the active and the reflective principles. The exercise of the one to the neglect of the other will produce opposite conditions,— the active will be a poor student but good in business, whereas the reflective characteristic will reverse the order.

It is also obvious that the perfect man should be a compound in the same degree of these two temperaments, and that neither element should gain more than a temporary advantage over the other. Among most men of wide sympathies there is always something of a contempt for the man who makes a study of but one subject.

---

[1] Abstract of an address before the Proctologic Society, Atlantic City, June 8, 1904.

I would not argue that segregation of effort be tolerated to the exclusion of general knowledge, but would rather teach that our professional ship should have that ballast secured by a mastery of the elementary principles upon which all true specialism is based. There is great power in division of labor. In diagnosis, the omniscient person is good enough, but for treatment it were perhaps wise to call in a dentist, laryngologist, gynæcologist, or proctologist.

It seems to me that for personal enjoyment to the highest degree the individual should aim at a moderate excellence in many subjects, but for the highest good to the world at large he will do better to devote himself exclusively to one. The man who is moderately conversant with many things has a more pleasant life, but to the specialist alone is given to make new discoveries and inaugurate new eras in his profession. The man who stands askance, criticises, and views with doubt the utility of new procedures should have breadth of view and high attainments in order to differentiate the wheat and the chaff, and being thus equipped he becomes no less a hero by practising the idea that he once criticised than the one who promulgated it. A less subtle mind is incapable to occupy a seat and dispense opinions from the judicial citadel.

Having thus briefly defined the specialist in the abstract, this leads us to consider,—

Secondly: That specialism makes for optimism in that it insures greater skill in technique by virtue of frequent intercourse with similar diseases, and enables the physician to institute research in given lines.

Some one has said that there is a widely spread idea that the man who knows the most about one thing is not very likely to know much about most things. Conversely, there is an idea that the man who knows something about most things is not very likely to know any one thing thoroughly. It is argued by some that to limit one's field of action his mental horizon becomes narrow. If, perchance, mental concentration on a given subject does contract, does not the possessor gain a deeper knowledge, and is not science the gainer? Again, does not the amusing subdivision of "Entomologist and Scarabœist," by Dr. Holmes, contribute to the boundaries of science even though their intellectual stature be stunted? It is a physiologic principle that the exercise of one muscle or group of muscles contributes to the health and vigor of the entire muscular system. Then, is it not reasonable to claim that mental concentration on one thing will have a salutary effect on all the faculties, and that therefore the resultant skill will redound to the enlargement of science and the highest good to the public? For example, is it not obvious that the physician who sees a large variety of diseases in one line is more skilful in diagnosis and the right selection of treatment? Does not his philosophic range of vision establish the various relations between his special field and the general system? That co-ordination and dexterity that comes from frequent handling of the same instruments in the examination and treatment of special diseases vouchsafes superiority and adds immeasurably to the public welfare.

To illustrate further, in the great Waltham watch factory each wheel or part of the watch is placed by as many different individuals trained in the one thing in order to insure despatch and perfection in construction. How much more important that the physician who has to deal with complex organic structures be skilled in his operations!

The groundwork of a specialist in any field should consist of that skill and experience that emanates from general surgery; in short, he should be a skilled general physician and surgeon, and develop into a special branch by evolutionary methods. Progress is a law of evolution. The advance in knowledge has produced a rather formidable list of instruments,—namely, the ophthalmoscope, laryngoscope, microscope, spirometer, pleximeter, proctoscope, sigmoidoscope, etc.,—and should deter any one from aspiring to master the use of all. Each instrument represents several ideas, more or less exact and precise, rendering the skilful use of them a *sine qua non* in diagnosis and treatment, reducing discomforts of the patients to the minimum.

Therefore, is it not pertinent to claim that the man who is thoroughly familiar with the construction of his instrument, the principles involved therein, and their frequent use in a given line of diseases is more competent to apply them than the man who occasionally has an applicable case? Cannot the same conclusion be made with reference to direct operative procedures and subsequent care? I think we must admit that specialists and specialism are necessary, and make for optimism in medical practice. In this connection I wish to state that it is not my object to detract one iota from the high regard we must all have for the general physician and the general surgeon. All honor to the family doctor whose conservatism, varied experience, and sublime judgment we all delight to emulate, and whose council we cherish. It is upon these men the specialist must depend, these men whose honesty of purpose has made specialism possible, and whose confidence we seek.

Third: Specialism makes for optimism in the fact that most discoveries are made by specialists, which results are incentives to the best efforts.

It is interesting to observe how evolution has made specialism possible, and a subject of speculation how much further the process may develop. It was a primitive maxim that a man should be self-sufficing, and in certain frontier localities this may be true to-day, but in advancing civilization and knowledge, *pari passu,* the necessities of the public multiply, new conditions arise, diseases are more complex in their nature and become more difficult to treat, and the public more exacting. The result was that more professions sprung up and subdivided. The common illustration of the tree and branches as given by thinkers and writers on evolution is very apropos in medical history and development.

From Tubal Cain there descended not only blacksmiths, but all artificers in brass and iron, so it may be said that from the leech there came a progeny of medical specialists that number a score or more. The idea of subdivision tends to place man in the position of a part of the great machinery of human activity, and that he is coherent to the main body, and well it is for the skilled artisan, should he become detached, to be of sufficient equilibrium by previous experience to sustain himself.

Subdivision in medicine has installed such vigorous methods in research and invention as are of incalculable value to humanity. By it Harvey discovered the circulation, Koch the bacterial pathology, Morton anæsthesia, Priestly oxygen, then the clinical thermometer, another the ophthalmoscope, and a long line of discoveries and inventions by specialists, the product of careful study and experience. To the man who limits himself, there is more time for thought, and if endowed with sufficient ingenuity he is able to contribute to the armamentaria for the exact diagnosis and treatment of disease. He can also add to our knowledge of pathologic states which forms the basis of all legitimate and rational medicine.—*Louisville Journal of Medicine and Surgery.*

THE USE OF ETHYL CHLORIDE AS A GENERAL ANÆSTHETIC.—
To the *Edinburgh Medical Journal* of November 3, 1903, Dr. Luke
contributes his views as to the use of this drug. He believes that the
dose of ethyl chloride is a variable quantity, varying with the patient, the nature of the operation, and the length of anæsthesia.

It is seldom necessary to employ more than ten cubic centimetres, and seldom possible to use less than three cubic centimetres; but with this latter amount, properly administered, an
anæsthesia of seventy to ninety or more seconds can be obtained
even in adult patients. With young children, one and a half to
two and a half minutes can be reckoned on. If the administrator
fails to get anæsthesia with such an amount in seventy to ninety
seconds, it is due far more probably to air being unknowingly
admitted than to an insufficient dose.

The rapidity with which anæsthesia is induced in some cases
is very remarkable, and even startling. If the patient takes deep
breaths from the start, consciousness is sometimes lost after the
first three or four breaths, stertor commences, and the patient is
ready for the knife in twenty-five to thirty seconds.

M'Cardie finds the average time of induction to be 50.9 seconds, and the average length of anæsthesia 71.3 seconds.

In his own practice the author has found the average of induction a few seconds longer, but the duration of anæsthesia has
been correspondingly long.

Luke's longest period of available anæsthesia, after complete
removal of the inhaler, was five minutes.

After-Effects.—Headache and nausea or vomiting are the most
common. Anything further is extremely rare, and any faintness
or syncopal tendency which is seen is probably due to loss of blood
or *vertigo a stomacho* than to any action of the anæsthetic on the
cardiovascular system.

Of patients anæsthetized for short dental extractions during
the early part of the day,—from ten to two o'clock,—the author
has found that not more than about one in twenty suffers from
sickness. Patients anæsthetized in the afternoon seldom do so
well as those narcotized early in the day. Sickness is more common
where the anæsthetic has been pushed, or where some blood has
been swallowed. There are some types of patients who are frequently sick or upset after any anæsthetic,—namely, people suffering from chronic digestive disorder, and school-boys who eat questionable articles of diet at odd times.

An interval of two, and if possible three or four, hours is desirable between the last meal and the taking of the anæsthetic. Sickness does not recur, at most, in more than thirty per cent. of cases, and this is considerably less than we see after chloroform or ether. If troublesome, the patient should be directed to lie down in the supine position, and albumin-water, or chloreton (ten grains), administered, and toilet vinegar may be sniffed at. Headache, if it occurs, generally passes off soon, but if not is best treated with a cup of tea or some acetanilid, five to ten grains.

Both during the early stage of anæsthesia and the recovery stage, the thoughts or dreams of patients are not infrequently of an erotic nature, and this may lead to complications. The same, of course, is known to occur with nitrous oxide.

The Death-Rate under Ethyl Chloride.—Patients seem to vary a great deal as to their susceptibility to the vapor. Alcoholics and those addicted to cocaine and morphine require a great deal of the anæsthetic, and are scarcely affected by a strong vapor. On the other hand, those who are anæmic and weakened by disease are frequently very soon influenced, and as small a dose as three cubic centimetres has been followed by violent tonic spasms, opisthotonos, and cyanosis. Any toxic effect of the drug seems to make itself first felt in the patient's respiratory system. The action there seems to be supplemented by the onset of muscular spasm, which most frequently commences in the masseter muscles, but may spread to the muscles of the tongue, larynx, and thorax. The cyanosis is much accentuated, if not primarily caused, in many cases, by this spasm of muscles at the base of the tongue. This spasm, and also laryngeal spasm, can readily be relieved by tongue traction, supplemented by artificial respiration for a few moments in some cases. The appearance of the patient is extremely unpleasant, and very similar to that of a person deeply under the influence of nitrous oxide. Clonic spasm is usually seen with this anæsthetic, and the retraction of the head and opisthotonos is very similar to that produced by laughing-gas. The patient's face looks very swollen, the eyes are usually open, the pupils dilated and fixed, but the pulse usually beats quite well.

Seitz, of Constanz, a dental surgeon, has gone very carefully into the question of safety. He has collected an account of over sixteen thousand cases, with only one death recorded. This occurred at Innsbruck in 1889. The patient was a laborer, aged forty-one, and died of respiratory syncope, apparently. At the necropsy he was found to have an enlarged and fatty heart and sclerosed coronary arteries. No other case has actually been published, except that of a child, aged one and three-fourths years, suffering from diphtheritic croup, who died during a tracheotomy. There is no record of a death during a dental operation.

There have been cases recorded in which asphyxial symptoms have appeared and been promptly relieved by suitable treatment.

Luke's general conclusions in regard to ethyl chloride are as follows:

1. It is very rapid in action, and pleasant to inhale.

2. The duration of anæsthesia compares very favorably with that afforded by nitrous oxide.

3. It causes no change of color, or cyanosis, under normal conditions.

4. The administration is very simple in technique.

5. Its lower rate of mortality, more agreeable odor, and method of administration, and the possibility of repeating the dose and continuing the anæsthesia, make it greatly preferable to ethyl bromide, which cannot be safely readministered at one sitting.

6. The after-effects are slight, if there are any.

7. It is by no means inexpensive, but cheaper than nitrous oxide.

8. It is especially useful when the patient is very young, very old, or anæmic.

9. It is extremely portable—a flask with sufficient for ten to twelve cases being readily carried in the breast pocket.

10. It is much safer than chloroform, as safe as ether, and much better adapted for brief operations than either.

New anæsthetics are like a new horse, and one is inclined at first to go very gently with them. When the writer first began to try ethyl chloride, about three years ago, he used it "with fear and trembling;" but though familiarity has not bred contempt, he now uses it with confidence, as a tried friend. He has personally administered it in over three hundred cases, and has had no reason to regret doing so. One or two patients have given some trouble, from the onset of marked spasms and cyanosis; but as we not infrequently experience both when using nitrous oxide, if one is accustomed to that anæsthetic these symptoms are not so disconcerting. He is convinced that ethyl chloride is an anæsthetic which needs great care and watchfulness in its adminstration; and the great rapidity of the onset of anæsthesia is calculated to catch napping the uninitiated and inexperienced. But, bearing in mind the rapid elimination, and the fact that, when trouble has occurred, it has always been of an asphyxial and not syncopal character, one realizes there is a fair margin of safety. And if we meet difficulties, as we are practically bound to do from time to time whatever anæsthetic we are giving, a cool head and the precise and methodical carrying out of the usual restorative measures are in all probability all that will be necessary to bring about the happiest results.—*Therapeutic Gazette.*

Reports of Society Meetings.

THE NEW YORK INSTITUTE OF STOMATOLOGY.

A REGULAR meeting of the Institute was held on Tuesday evening, May 3, 1904, at the " Chelsea," No. 222 West Twenty-third Street, New York, the President, Dr. A. H. Brockway, in the chair.
The minutes of the last meeting were read and approved.

Dr. E. A. Bogue presented the model of a combined bridge and retaining appliance for lower and upper teeth loosened by pyorrhœa. The patient had been requested to call by Dr. Barnes, of Cleveland, one of our fellow-members, the work having been done by Dr. Phillips, of Los Angeles, Cal. It consisted briefly of a lingual and buccal plate accurately fitting the teeth, screwed together, with cement between them and filling all interstices. It took sixteen days to make the upper, and nine days to make the lower, apparatus. The pyorrhœa had stopped as soon as the fixture was in place and there had been no recurrence so far as the patient could perceive.

Dr. F. Milton Smith.—The case presented by Dr. Bogue reminds me of an article written by Dr. William I. Fish, of Newark, nearly five years ago, and published in the INTERNATIONAL DENTAL JOURNAL, upon this subject of bracing loose teeth. That article prompted me to make a brace after this plan for the lower incisors and canines, which proved very useful; I think it would have proved more so had the patient come to me regularly to have the tartar removed. As it was, he came in after three years with the piers very loose.

Dr. H. S. Sutphen.—Five years ago I inserted a similar apparatus for the lower, and have seen that patient every six months since. The whole thing is somewhat loose now, because the cuspids are somewhat loose.

Dr. L. C. LeRoy.—A patient came into my hands for whom Dr. Fish had made a similar appliance to brace all of the upper and lower incisors and cuspids. There was also a condition of cleft palate, and consequently these upper teeth were necessary to hold the plate which was worn for its correction. The appliance strengthened the teeth to such an extent that to-day they are still doing good service after about five years. The lower ones are also doing well. I think Dr. Fish should receive all credit for giving us this excellent method.

Dr. H. W. Gillett.—Dr. Fossume has described a process which is often valuable in these cases. The bar is attached to incisors by dowels, the lingual portions of the cutting edges being removed to permit of so applying it that it shall be inconspicuous. This device interferes with the process of cleaning the teeth than any other I have seen mentioned.

Dr. Freeman Allen, of Boston, read a paper entitled " Recent Methods in the Administration of Anæsthetics." Dr. Allen illustrated his paper with the various apparatus used in the different methods.

(For Dr. Allen's paper, see page 665.)

(For Dr. Allen's paper, see page 665.)

DISCUSSION.

Dr. Emil A. Rundquist.—The safety of anæsthesia depends upon a great many things, not the least important of which is the skill and resource of the anæsthetist. The first factor to be considered is the choice of the anæsthetic with regard to the individual and the nature of the operation. The rapidity of the operation, whether long or short, is also a factor upon which the safety of the anæsthetic depends. The preparation of the patient before the operation and the position of the patient during operation are also to be considered, a sitting position always being avoided except when administering nitrous oxide.

The choice of the anæsthetic is influenced by the climate.

Chloroform seems to be safer in hot climates, probably because it is more easily eliminated, most deaths from chloroform occurring in the cold season of the year.

Age also influences the choice. Generally speaking, children take ether more satisfactorily, while in old people chloroform is preferable. The normal adult should be given ether instead of chloroform. The pathological adult should be handled with more caution. If the blood-pressure is low, ether is indicated. In diseases of the arteries it should be borne in mind that chloroform diminishes the strain on the blood-vessels. Hence in an old person with brittle vessels chloroform is often the safer. In cases of fatty heart and myocarditis ether is indicated, but it should be administered with care. With regard to the *lungs,* chloroform is indicated in cases of chronic bronchitis or chronic tubercular lesions. In pneumonia, with poisoned heart, or empyema, ether should be given the preference. For the removal of foreign bodies in the larynx or trachea, or for the removal of tumors in these localities, chloroform is the better. Anæsthetics should be given with great care in cases of profound anæmia and blood-changes of that type. In general diseases, diabetic patients require ether. In alcoholism chloroform is better, chiefly because a person addicted to the excessive use of alcohol will require an enormous amount of ether to produce anæsthesia. In regard to the kidneys, in chronic nephritis, tension is the key note. When there is increased arterial tension, chloroform had better be given, otherwise ether is the safer, as it produces less marked degeneration. However, there is great difference of opinion on this subject. In sepsis, shock, and hemorrhage, the minimum amount of anæsthetic should be used. Ether is probably best, but must be given with care. In fat people with short necks, who generally have mechanical inspiratory difficulty, chloroform is the anæsthetic of choice.

The kind of operation influences the choice of the anæsthetic to be given. For abdominal operations Kelly prefers chloroform, but in New York the majority of men use ether. It is probable that ether is safer and gives just about as good results. In operations about the face of considerable duration, besides the methods spoken of by Dr. Allen, there is the method of administering the anæsthetic by means of a tracheotomy tube; the method of rectal anæsthesia is mentioned only to be condemned. For peripheral operations that do not require marked relaxation, in well-selected cases, laughing-gas and oxygen will do. Ethyl chloride is also used, but is not so safe, as it lowers arterial tension. In obstetrics, chloroform is generally used to ease the labor-pains, but in cases of version or Cæsarean section, ether is better. Chloroform should be avoided in cases where repeated narcoses are necessary, as chloroform is not eliminated as readily as ether, and may cause fatty changes in the viscera.

The dangers of an anæsthetic are remote and immediate. With ether there is danger of sudden respiratory paralysis causing death (rare). The remoter dangers have not been quite so clearly laid before the medical profession, but they are being met with all the time. Remote pulmonary dangers are more marked with ether than chloroform. Renal dangers may occur all the way from acute congestion with little albumin, up to suppression of urine. This occurs less with chloroform than with ether. Fatty visceral degeneration does not occur with ether. Both ether and chloroform have post-operative sequellæ, ether not causing the degeneration that is caused by chloroform. In a typical case of late chloroform death, the patient was negative to examination, but required a great deal of chloroform to produce relaxation. Convalescence went well till the second day after the operation, then jaundice appeared, with albumin and casts in the urine. There was no temperature. The patient died in coma on the fifth day. Autopsy showed fatty degeneration of all the viscera.

Of deaths from chloroform and ether, the best statistics show: ether, immediate, one in twenty-nine thousand cases; chloroform, immediate, one in three thousand cases. Remoter pulmonary deaths from ether, according to statistics from St. Thomas Hospital, London, show one in two thousand four hundred.

The causes of post-operative lung complications are: (1) Direct bronchial irritation with hypersecretion of mucous, washing down the bacteria into the terminal alveoli, setting up a pneumonia. This is worse with ether. Cyanosis distinctly increases the secretion of mucus in the bronchi. (2) Toxic action on the pulmonary blood-vessels. This is a little worse with ether than with chloroform. There is dilatation and exudation of serum. The resistance to infection by direct inspiration, emboli, and through the blood is lowered. (3) The inspiration of vomitus, blood, or infected secretions from the mouth, nose, etc. (4) Infected thrombi from operative wound. In cocaine anæsthesia in German clinics this explained the very frequently resulting pneumonia. The small thrombi were washed over into the mesenteric vessels, thence passing into the pulmonary circulation. (5) Chill, fright, or shock of operation all lower the resistance. (6) Prolonged anæsthesia even with small amounts of anæsthetic. (7) Restricted respiration from pain or tight dressings. (8) Maintenance of one position, especially in old people, may cause hypostatic pneumonia. (9) Operation or infection near pleura. The results of these post-operative lung complications may be enumerated as follows: Pulmonary œdema, acute bronchitis, lobar and broncho-pneumonia, pleurisy, hemorrhagic infarctions, gangrene, abscess and exacerbations of chronic processes, emphysema, and tuberculosis.

Several precautions are used to prevent pulmonary complications: (1) Morphine and atropine are given before an operation with ether. (2) Digitalis and strophanthus before chloroform. These are more for the effect upon the heart. (3) The stomach is washed out, and care is taken that there is not a regurgitation of the contents of the stomach, the patient virtually drowning in the vomited material. (4) Rose's position is used. (5) Interrupted ether narcosis. Sometimes possible in breast cases where complete relaxation and deep narcosis is not necessary; giving one-sixth to one-fourth grain of morphine one hour before operation and combining with local anæsthesia if necessary. (6) Becker in Hildesheimer's clinic adds twenty drops of oil of pini pumilionis to ether before beginning. In five hundred cases it stopped secretion of mucus. It has been used in cases of pulmonary disease. (7) Asepsis both of the wound and of the apparatus used. (8) The minimum amount of anæsthetic should be used. (9) The rapidity of the operation diminishes the likelihood of lung trouble. (10) Avoid undue exposure, fright, etc. (11) The patient's position in bed should be changed as frequently as possible, especially in aged patients.

Regarding the amount of anæsthetic used, out of one hundred personal cases using nitrous oxide and ether the average time of the operation was seventy-five minutes, requiring an average of 4.7 ounces of ether. This would average three and three-fourths ounces of ether per hour. Out of this number of cases the best required five ounces of ether for an anæsthesia of two hours and forty minutes. Regarding the time required for complete anæsthetization with ether used in the ordinary method, thirteen minutes is about the average, while with nitrous oxide and ether complete relaxation can be produced in an average of three minutes, and in some favorable cases in one and one-half minutes.

There is no apparatus that will make chloroform safe. Chloroform is distinctly a dangerous drug, and for the unskilled man ether is much better. I wish to deprecate the habit etherizers have of rubbing the conjunctiva to ascertain the degree of anæsthesia. It is distinctly a bad custom, because of the resulting infection and subsequent conjunctivitis. Care should be taken during operations to avoid pressures which will result often in paralysis of the musculo-spiral, brachial, or popliteal nerves. In pelvic work the anæsthesia can be pushed to stop abdominal breathing. Anæsthesia deepens somewhat in the Trendelenburg posture.

The essayist spoke of anæsthol as a very satisfactory anæsthetic. It is claimed to be a new solution, and not merely a mixture. It consists of ethyl chloride, seventeen per cent.; chloroform, thirty-six per cent.; and ether, forty per cent. It boils at $104°$ F. It is given on a mask by the drop method. Of course, the ideal anæsthetic would be one a certain number of minims of which, injected by a hypodermic syringe, would give a certain definite result. Some work has been done along this line. Scopolamine and morphine have been used. The two act in opposition except in the brain, where they unite to narcotize. Scopolamine is not toxic like atropine. It dilates the pupils, stimulates the pulse and respiration, stimulates peristalsis, and raises the blood-pressure. Morphine is the more dangerous drug of the two. One death has been reported in one hundred and sixty-two cases. A test dose is given the evening before of scopolamine, $1/_{130}$ grain; morphine, $\frac{1}{2}$ grain. In the morning scopolamine, $1/_{65}$ grain, and morphine, one grain. After waiting one and one-half hours, give the evening dose again. This is the maximum dosage. If the pupils are not dilated, give more scopolamine. Blos reports one hundred and five cases, one death, seventy ideal, twenty-nine required little ether, and six could not be narcotized. The danger lies in the respiratory paralysis. The muscular relaxation is not perfect.

Dr. Bryan D. Sheedy.—I feel very grateful to the reader of the valuable paper presented this evening for your consideration. I also thank Dr. Wheeler, your secretary, for affording me the pleasure of hearing the paper, and your chairman for allowing me to take part in the discussion. The subject matter attracted me, though I feel very much like an outsider in taking part in this meeting, made up, as it is, almost wholly of gentlemen of another profession, and in a discussion of subjects that the medical prae- titioner seldom considers. As my work is limited to diseases of the mouth, ear, nose, and throat, almost daily do I come in con- tact with the work of the dentist. It is impossible to divorce your work from that of the rhinologists. I hoped for something in the paper and discussion that would throw light on the subject of anæsthesia of the parts which you are so often called upon to oper- ate. The paper has certainly been a valuable and practical one along the line of general anæsthesia, and I fear the remarks I expect to make will be a little off from the point, as I intend to discuss very briefly anæsthesia as applied to the locality of our daily occupation.

One word in regard to ether and chloroform anæsthesia. In the New York Post-Graduate Medical School and Hospital, where there are probably as many surgical operations as in any other in- stitution in New York, gas and ether anæsthesia is the rule. In London ether is seldom used. It will be a difficult matter for us to explain why most English and continental surgeons consider chloroform a safer remedy than ether, while in America ether is used almost to the complete exclusion of chloroform.

Personally I have had some very disagreeable experiences with both ether and chloroform in operations in and about the mouth, nose, and throat, and I firmly believe that if statistics were pub- lished of the operations in and about these parts under profound ether or chloroform anæsthesia, the percentage of death would be very much higher than that ordinarily given in standard text- books. I know of more than one death that has occurred in New York City during the past few years in connection with operations about the upper respiratory tract that have not been figured in estimating the percentage of deaths from anæsthetics. My personal experience in one case not very long ago will remain with me for some time. I have been teaching the students of my clinic in the New York Post-Graduate Medical School and Hospital that for short operations in and about the upper respiratory tract profound and complete anæsthesia by ether or chloroform is not advisable. I know of the arguments advanced in regard to the dangers of primary chloroform anæsthesia, but these arguments do not hold in regard to primary ether anæsthesia, as I believe the danger from complete anæsthesia in operations about the nose, throat, and mouth, and of infected secretions passing into the trachea and lungs of the patient, are not sufficiently emphasized. I recommend that just enough anæsthetic be used to prevent fright and pain, but not enough to destroy the laryngeal reflex, thereby allowing blood or infected material to gain entrance into the larynx.

I believe, if we bear this point in mind, we will not have the dangerous symptoms manifested in profound anæsthesia where bloody operations are performed in the mouth and upper respiratory tract. We will also save our patients many cases of pneumonia and other infectious diseases of the lungs following the use of general anæsthetics.

Regarding the question of chloroform and ether, I believe the average American surgeon knows very little about chloroform anæsthesia, as it is so seldom used in this country. In New York and other American cities a death from chloroform is looked upon almost as malpractice, while abroad you are immediately picked out as an American if you mention ether. The remote results of ether are far worse than we generally consider, while the immediate effect of chloroform is much better in the hands of experienced surgeons than Americans generally allow.

When we become more familiar with chloroform as it is used in Great Britain, I firmly believe we will use less ether and more chloroform.

With apologies to the essayist, allow me to discuss local anæsthesia for operations about the nose and throat as it is carried on in the clinics of the New York Post-Graduate School and Hospital at the present time. Operations have been done without pain under cocaine anæsthesia during the past four months, in which general anæsthesia was always considered necessary. It is a daily occurrence in that institution for the antrum to be opened, the ethmoid cells curetted, the turbinates excised, septal spurs removed, and cutting operations of other sinuses done under a five or seven per cent. cocaine solution. For the complete antral operation we cocoanize as follows:

We apply the cocaine on a pledget of cotton saturated with an eight or ten per cent. solution, allowing this cotton to remain next the part to be operated upon for from fifteen to twenty minutes while we inject into the antrum a small quantity of a two or three per cent. solution. I believe all the operations that we are called upon to perform about the nose and throat can be done with a five or six per cent. solution, and we will avoid many of the disagreeable toxic effects by confining ourselves to the weaker solutions. The application of adrenalin to the parts at the same time the cocaine is applied reduces the danger of cocaine poisoning. I apply the adrenalin and cocaine to the tissues on the same pledget of cotton, so that the combined effect is obtained. The probable action of adrenalin is the contraction of the smaller lymph- and blood-vessels, thus preventing the too rapid absorption of the cocaine.

Adrenalin is also one of the best heart tonics we have, so that it is barely possible that some of the symptoms associated with cocaine anæsthesia may be avoided by using adrenalin. There is only one feature connected with adrenalin that has proved disagreeable in my hands. There seems to be a great tendency to secondary hemorrhage, which occurs four or five hours after the operation, so that to-day I do not use it as often as when it first came on the market.

I thank you, gentlemen, for allowing me the privilege of this discussion, and the only excuse I make for introducing the subject of local anæsthesia is its common applicability to your every-day work.

Dr. L. C. Leroy.—How much adrenalin do you use?

Dr. Sheedy.—I generally apply equal parts of the one to one thousand adrenalin solution and a seven per cent. solution of cocaine to the parts on a pledget of cotton.

With regard to adrenalin, let me say that it is a drug which deteriorates very rapidly, and should be used within a short time after the bottle is opened, else it becomes acid and very irritating.

Dr. J. Morgan Howe.—I have nothing to say except to express my appreciation for the valuable service rendered us this evening by these gentlemen who have been so kind as to come here and tell us what we have heard, and to express my sincere thanks to them for their kindness. I would at this time move a vote of thanks to the gentlemen who have been so kind as to enlighten us upon the subeet of anæsthetics.

Dr. S. E. Davenport.—It seems to me that considerable advance has been made in the last few years in the manner of producing general anæsthesia. My mind goes back some ten years to the occasion when a lad, especially dear to me, was anæsthetized, and so unpleasant was the experience that the boy ascribed all his subsequent illness during the slow recovery from the condition which had made an operation necessary to the bitter medicine, as he characterized it, that the doctor had forced upon him. I was informed by a lady patient the other day, that her son had recently been operated upon for suppurating mastoid processes, and that she could not say enough in commendation of the method used by the gentleman who administered the anæsthetic. The anæsthetist, evidently fond of children, made himself very agreeable, and gained the boy's confidence in a few moments. He opened his bag and invited the lad to help him take out the things. An apparatus similar to one exhibited to-night was produced, and the boy was asked if he would be willing to help " blow up this bag," and he finally went off to sleep in the midst of the game. While I am told that it is not good form to commend an essayist for what he has done for a society, I really thing that Dr. Allen, by leaving his busy life and taking the pains to bring to us such a complete exhibit of all the paraphernalia of his profession, should receive from us the very highest thanks.

Dr. Allen.—I should like to express my appreciation for the kind invitation and for the cordial reception and the courtesies I have been shown.

Dr. Bogue.—I would like to ask Dr. Sheedy how he is able to get deep local anæsthesia in the manner described, as the anæsthesia from cocaine travels from the centre towards the periphery.

Dr. Sheedy.—I would not attempt to give a physiological answer to the doctor's question. I only know that we do get results.

Dr. Bogue.—I had occasion recently to open down on to the buccal root of a molar, using the chloride of ethyl. I asked my patient if she felt it, and she did not reply. I made my operation and still she did not reply.

Dr. Allen.—I believe the properties of ethyl chloride were discovered while it was being used as a local anæsthetic.

Dr. Bogue.—I have seen it used in Paris very extensively for adenoid operations.

Dr. Allen.—About the dangers following etherization being underestimated, this is the point I have been trying to bring out. Both ether and chloroform have their post-operative sequellæ.

Adjourned.

FRED. L. BOGUE, M.D., D.D.S.,
Editor The New York Institute of Stomatology.

ACADEMY OF STOMATOLOGY.

THE regular meeting of the Academy of Stomatology of Philadelphia was held at its rooms, 1731 Chestnut Street, on the evening
of January 26, 1904, Dr. L. Foster Jack, President, in the chair.

A paper, entitled "A Method for reproducing the Natural Contour of Artificial Teeth on the Lingual and Palatal Surfaces of
Artificial Dentures," was read by Dr. William M. Fine.

(For Dr. Fine's paper, see page 569.)

A paper, entitled, "Lack of Dentition, with Presentation of an
Illustrated Case, and the Exhibition of a Patient with Ankylosis
of the Mandible," was read by Dr. William J. Roe.

(For Dr. Fine's paper, see page 569.)

DISCUSSION OF DR. FINE'S PAPER.

Dr. J. H. Gaskill.—The method described by the essayist is
certainly interesting, and his results are most beautiful from an
artistic stand-point. The question arises whether the plate is not
greatly weakened by cutting away so much of the palatal portion.
According to the diagrams it is brought down very thin and at
a short angle. I would like to ask whether there is not danger of
breaking.

Dr. Fine.—The plate looks much thinner in the diagram than
it is in reality. The joints between the teeth are much stronger
than one would think. I have several patients wearing these, in
both gold and vulcanite, and they say they would not care to change.
The plate is very strong, as you can see by the samples passed
around.

Dr. G. Milliken.—The process described is, from an artistic
stand-point, very interesting, and I should think the results would
be very beautiful. We cannot take too much pains in the making
of fixtures for the mouth, and the nearer we approach to nature
the more beautiful will be the result and the more agreeable to
those who have to wear these appliances.

Dr. R. H. Nones.—While listening to the paper it seemed to me
that the method was an old one, presented in a new form. I do not
mean to detract, but would say that this method, with modifications,
has been pursued for a number of years. The work is beautiful
and artistic, and it is useful, and strength is not sacrificed to
artistic effect when the work is properly done. The apparently

27

weak plate shown in Diagram No. 4 is really much stronger than the one shown in Diagram No. 3. It is surprising how readily some of these thick plates break, because the strength is not put in the proper place.

Some will say they have not the time to do this work. If a man cannot take the time to do prosthetic dentistry, he had better let it be done by the men who can.

Instead of cutting the form of the vacuum chamber in the plaster impression, I prefer to inset the metal form upon the model, as I can judge better of its proper location.

Instead of covering the model with tin-foil, I make, when it is possible, a tin model, preferably a tin shell, which has the advantage of being readily removed from the plate, and is easily fastened to the articulator.

A peculiarity which I cannot explain is that rubber, when vulcanized upon tin, is totally different from rubber vulcanized in contact with plaster. It seems to lose its weight almost one-half.

I think the essayist is to be commended from the stand-point of doing well that which is worth doing at all. Prosthetic dentistry can be made quite as pleasurable as operative dentistry, provided it is well done and an interest taken in it.

Dr. Fine (closing).—I cover all of my models with tin-foil, thick on the outside and thin on the inside, and when possible I use a tin die. I use tin-foil because the latter is not always possible.

DISCUSSION OF DR. ROE'S PAPER.

Dr. Roe.—The anchylosis in this case is almost complete. The condition was recognized when the patient was quite young. I expect to operate in a few days and liberate the mandible.

Dr. Darby.—Did the boy ever have scarlet fever?

Dr. Roe.—No. He has had measles. He eats everything and talks well. The upper and lower gums are in contact in both buccal regions, but are not united, as I have passed a thin pliant instrument between them.

Dr. Arnold.—I cannot tell why there are no teeth in the case exhibited by Dr. Roe. This is a case of arrested development, and, like most of these cases, there is no known reason. I am sure there is nothing in the family history to account for it. Two more healthy, robust-looking people than the parents are not easily found.

Question.—Has a radiograph been taken?

Answer.—No; Dr. Roe has that in contemplation.

Question.—I would like to ask Dr. Roe whether anything is known in this case concerning prenatal maternal impressions?

Dr. Roe.—I made special inquiry, and the mother assured me that she had in every sense as normal gestation as with her other children. There was no abnormal condition during gestation, no fright or other strong prenatal impression.

Dr. S. H. Guilford.—I did not know that Dr. Roe was going to allude to a case which I observed some twenty years ago, but he has given some of the important facts regarding it. It is the only case I know of which was totally edentulous. The man never had any teeth, either deciduous or permanent. I know this, because I took the trouble to travel through the country where he lived and inquired of people who had known him from early childhood. I was unable to trace his ancestry or find out whether his peculiarities were transmitted. When he was in Philadelphia, twenty years ago, he was forty-eight years of age. I have brought with me the models taken from the impression made at that time. They look like those of the mouth of an old person. A strange thing was the ability of this man to eat. His meat was cut in rather small pieces, and these he would press between his tongue and the roof of his mouth and in this way he had developed a very muscular tongue. An aunt on the mother's side had a similar condition. Of the children whom I saw, the boys' dentures were normal. Of the daughters, one had fourteen teeth and one sixteen. They had four or five scattered teeth in the lower jaw, and the balance scattered about the upper jaw.

In collecting the cases for my paper read before the California Congress, I visited dime museums, boarding-houses, etc. Some cases reported as being edentulous turned out not to be.

Another point which interested me was that this boy has been troubled with ozæna. The patient that I had was also troubled with this condition.

In trying to make a scientific investigation of this kind we do not always come out exactly where we expect to. Ten years ago I thought that I was going to prove that where there is absence of hair there is absence of teeth. I found, however, that sometimes there is a deficiency of the one and abundance of the other, and the cases are so confusing that it is difficult to get satisfactory data.

Dr. E. T. Darby.—I have nothing special to say except to speak of models at the University of a case similar to that of this boy. There are, however, two permanent molars in the mouth. The boy had had no temporary teeth at all, but when about fifteen or sixteen years of age he erupted these two molars. From the models they look like second, instead of first, molars. The models were sent to me by a dentist in New York State. He said he had known the boy from the time he was an infant, and had watched the development of his mouth, and that these were the only teeth the boy had had.

Dr. Guilford.—Were they in the same jaw?

Dr. Darby.—No; in the opposite jaws. There was a fine alveolar ridge in the lower jaw. I corresponded with the dentist about the case, and he wanted to send him on, but the boy never came. Artificial teeth were made, but the lad got along so well without them that he did not care to be bothered. He could eat fairly well.

It is said that the absence of hair and absence of teeth are noted together. The man whom Dr. Guilford speaks of I believe never perspired, and he slept in the cellar. I have known one or two persons who practically never perspired, but they were not edentulous.

Dr. G. Milliken.—It seems to me that something might be found out about such cases. An exhaustive examination of the blood, saliva, a section of the skin, or, if possible, a portion of bone, possibly taken from the jaw, might throw some light on the question.

Dr. Roe (closing).—I am gratified with the interest the members of the Academy have taken in this boy's condition; and, following out Dr. Milliken's suggestion, I certainly think that a histological examination of the skin would be interesting. Whether an examination of the blood and saliva would reveal anything is a question.

Much waste product of metabolism is eliminated by the normal skin. If the skin be not capable of this normal function, there must be a very great deal of work thrown upon the other excretory organs, such as the lungs and kidneys.

(Replying to Dr. Milliken.) I have inquired into the family history for evidence of syphilitic infection, tuberculosis, or chronic alcoholism, and have found no evidence of any of the three conditions. The family shows every evidence of normal good health and generally good development.

OTTO E. INGLIS,
Editor Academy of Stomatology.

Editorial.

THE EDUCATIONAL RETROGRADE AT ST. LOUIS.

THE indignation expressed at the action of the—so-called—Association of Faculties at St. Louis has been widespread since the publication in our August number. This is not confined to the residents of this country, but is being voiced by those interested in dental education in other lands, and this will be intensified as time gives opportunity for expression.

The blow fell, and dental education in America suffered a collapse that will require years to overcome and re-establish confidence.

The faction that passed the absurd resolutions at St. Louis were well assured that its action could not be sustained, but there was sufficient intelligence to be aware that, however iconoclastic this might be, it would have the result of creating a panic in the ranks of those favorable to a continuance of four years. The active workers in this faction had, apparently, no higher incentive, and, now that they have accomplished their purpose, they must feel great gratification, and can leisurely proceed to destroy each other without let or hinderance from any organization; for have they not "repealed all rules or parts of rules" interfering with them? The motive that actuated this action on their part may be right from their point of view, but it means, to many of them, college destruction. Those who so enthusiastically adopted these resolutions, in the expectation that they could be a law unto themselves, will assuredly find that the protection of the National Association of Dental Faculties meant something, and was not a mere resolution to be rescinded at pleasure, but a shield that enabled each member to feel that the rules adopted for the protection of each college would be rigidly enforced. This confidence, destroyed at St. Louis, cannot be restored, and while the Association of Faculties may retain a nominal existence, its power for good has ceased, not, however, through a decision of a majority of its members, but through the determination of the minority to rule or ruin. Is it possible to place confidence in the future of such a membership?

The present is full of doubt, and leading dental educators are viewing the prospect with anxiety and with grave uncertainty. The dental colleges of this country will doubtless all accept this retrograde action, and matriculate students this year for three years and postpone further changes until State boards and Legislatures have decided to act.

At this writing it is impossible to determine the influences that may be brought to bear in this direction in the near future. The probabilities are that no positive action will be taken this year, and it is a question whether anything can be suggested that will improve the present chaotic condition.

It is humiliating to feel that dental education in the United States will have nothing to show at the two World's Congresses,— the International Dental Federation and the International Dental Congress. The delegates to these have been invited to see the fruits of a dentistry that has steadily advanced through a century, and they will see some of this, but they will also see a profession incapable of maintaining a standard worthy of their respect, or that of those who sent them, representing all nationalities of the world.

If these iconoclasts at St. Louis supposed that their action would be permanent, they must be convinced by this time that they were positively mistaken. The element in this country solicitous for a more perfect standard will not be thus lightly repulsed. It is an element not governed by mercenary considerations, and, in consequence, possesses a vitality that will long outlast the dollar motive, that, at best, is intrinsically weak and short lived. While the blow dealt at dental education from the house of its supposed friends has been a severe one, it will not be lasting, for the best in professional life cannot remain submerged, but will rise above the temporary deluge of selfishness into the clearer atmosphere of a truer educational work and life.

CORRECTION.

IN the last line on page 634 of last number the types made our editorial say, " The National Association of Dental Faculties was organized in 1804." It should have read 1884.

Bibliography.

MANUAL OF MATERIA MEDICA AND PHARMACY. Specially designed for the use of Practitioners and Medical, Pharmaceutical, Dental, and Veterinary Students. By E. Stanton Muir, Ph.G., V.M.D., Instructor in Comparative Materia Medica and Pharmacy in the University of Pennsylvania. Third Edition. F. A. Davis Company, Philadelphia, 1904.

The first edition of this book was published eight years ago. The object, as stated in the preface, is, " To give to practitioners and students of medicine, in as concise and clear a manner as possible, those points which are of value, without the lengthy detail usually found in text-books."

There is always a danger in this condensing, inasmuch as matter vital to a correct understanding of the character of the drug and its therapeutic use may be practically eliminated. It is a question whether a student can study materia medica through a mere outline of the drugs described, any more than the student of anatomy could confine himself to the skeleton to acquire a knowledge of the human organism in its entirety. The true student will demand, and earnestly seek, other and fuller sources of information. While this defect is apparent in this book, it is not a subject for extended criticism in this respect.

The book will be valuable to dental students, but in a limited degree, as it fails to deal in the dental use of drugs. There is a general opinion prevalent that the therapeutic use of drugs is the same in all diseases of the human organism. While this is true the specialist finds general directions not always available. It is equally true that these special details must be taught by and received from the teacher, but a line or two in this direction would be of decided advantage to a book prepared for dental workers as well as veterinarians.

The real fault of the book is that it fails to notice some of the most used drugs in dentistry, especially of the important antiseptic class. In illustration it is only necessary to mention formalin and naphthol. It can hardly be said that these have not been sufficiently tried as to their value. It would seem that these might be found of decided value in veterinary medicine, in which the author is evidently most at home. They have been so long used in dentistry that the well-trained practitioners regard these, and others, indispensable in every-day work.

Part I. of the book is devoted to Botany, Part II. to Drugs, and Part III. to Pharmacy. This makes an excellent arrangement. The drugs follow each other in alphabetical order. This is much more satisfactory than that adopted in some of the recent works on Materia Medica. While much may be said in favor of other methods of arranging the drugs, it is thought that the method adopted by the author is the best for the average student.

The use of interleaved blanks for memoranda is an excellent aid, and is worthy of adoption in more pretentious publications. Aside from the criticisms made, the book, as a whole, must be regarded as superior to the ordinary manuals and of distinct value as an aid to the study of the subject.

Domestic Correspondence.

DR. PEIRCE ON DENTAL EDUCATION AND THE ST. LOUIS MEETING.

To the Editor:

Sir,—I have read your several editorials in the August number of the INTERNATIONAL DENTAL JOURNAL, and as usual have read them with interest and pleasure, but what came close to my idea were the practical remarks you made in the American Medical Association, Section on Stomatology, when you state that " the higher in a general way you can educate a man the better, but you must have that education properly arranged in order to be of value. The idea to me is pre-eminently absurd to suppose that because a man has an A.B. degree he is better qualified thereby to become a dentist. It is a fallacy. The high-school degree is equally fallacious. What we need in dentistry is an education that will fit a man to become a dentist. To accomplish this he should come up from the mechanical school, through the higher schools, and then reach a point where he can be of value to himself and the community at large. . . . I do not believe that we can make dentists out of all men, whether they have the A.B. degree or whether they have the high-school degree; that is not the point. We must go deeper if we expect to have symmetry in our educational effort. My own idea has been that the poor dentists we have turned out have, as a rule, been men of higher education—not the fault of the higher education, but the fault of a lack of proper symmetry in that education."

I should say a lack of mechanical ability and cultivation of the same. You are not alone in your knowledge of men with the dental degree, who are unfit to practise dentistry. They may pass a satisfactory examination and comply with the requirements for a degree, but for a thorough knowledge of the manipulative skill essential to the successful practice of their profession they are deficient, and sadly so; hence we have in the profession men who would have been brilliant in other industries, but in dentistry they are a failure. It was the recognition of this fact that induced me at Washington to throw what little influence I possessed in favor of three years of eight months. I felt that this period was long enough to test ability, and, if qualified, to make successful practitioners. To this time and qualifications attained, the graduate adds his experience, which makes his reputation and his living.

I must unite with you as to the action of the St. Louis meeting. It certainly had no authority to do more than consider and express its views in certain resolutions; beyond this their action cannot be binding. To say that all rules and parts of rules in conflict with these resolutions be and are hereby repealed, is simply wind. While it may encourage schools to do what they desire, it cannot make legal their action.

C. N. PEIRCE.

PHILADELPHIA, August 4, 1904.

Obituary.

DR. EDGAR ROSE RUST.

DIED, Thursday, June 2, 1904, at Coronado Beach, Cal., Dr. Edgar Rose Rust, in the forty-fifth year of his age. Dr. Rust had recently left his home in Denver, Col., and was visiting, with his family, places of interest on the coast of California, when an acute middle-ear disease, followed by erysipelas, caused his death. Dr. Rust was the son of John and Elizabeth E. Rust, and was born at Waverly, Westmoreland County, Va., which for more than two hundred years was the home of his paternal ancestors, who were of English origin. In early life Dr. Rust acquired a good education through private tutors at home, and later in the schools of the neighboring city of Baltimore. Soon after leaving school he entered upon the study of dentistry under the perceptorship of his brother, Dr. David N. Rust, of Washington, D. C., then located in Alexandria, Va. He graduated from the Baltimore College of Dental Suregry in the year 1882, and shortly thereafter became associated on very favorable terms with the court dentist of Madrid, Spain. This association continued but a few months, when the death of the latter left Dr. Rust under the disadvantages of a brief acquaintance with his associate's clientele and a limited command of the language of the country; but these disadvantages soon disappeared and a lucrative practice was readily acquired. The climate of Madrid was, however, found so unsuited to Dr. Rust that he was compelled to relinquish his promising professional career there and return, in 1885, to the capital of his native country, where he was again successful in establishing a large practice among the more desirable of the resident and official classes of Washington. But more than mere business success, which he seemed quite able to attain anywhere in the world, Dr. Rust's genial and sociable nature found a greater degree of gratification through the large measure of social advantages which he enjoyed at the nation's capital. He was an honored and active member of the old Washington City Dental Society, and was regarded by its members as an exceptionally skilful operator, having been one of the few who operated with equal facility according to the higher ideals of both the cohesive and non-cohesive gold advocates. Among his numerous Washington friends were numbered the best type of his own and other professions, and the trial of his life came when, acting on the advice of his physicians, he was compelled to sever these relations and seek to maintain health in a more suitable climate. It was under such circumstances that he resigned the presidency of the Washington City Dental Society in 1891, gave up his social and professional connections in Washington, and removed to Denver, Col., where he continued in professional labors for three years, when he retired from active practice and spent his remaining years in country life near Denver. While he continued actively and successfully several business enterprises, he took an especial pride in owning and raising fine stock, some of his horses being among the most valuable in America.

Dr. Rust married, in 1894, Miss Stella Hoyt, a member of an old and highly respected Denver family. His wife and their three children survive him.

At a meeting of the District of Columbia Dental Society, formerly the Washington City Dental Society, held June 21, 1904, a resolution was passed instructing the undersigned committee to furnish the dental journals with the above sketch and to convey to Dr. Rust's family suitable expressions of the Society's sympathy and sorrow.

WILLIAMS DONNALLY,
W. E. PAIRO,
G. F. SIMPSON,
Committee.

NORTHERN OHIO DENTAL ASSOCIATION—RESOLUTIONS OF RESPECT TO DR. JONATHAN TAFT.

WHEREAS, In the death of Dr. Jonathan Taft, which occurred at Ann Arbor, Michigan, October 15, 1903, the dental profession has lost a most valuable member; one who gave generously of his knowledge for the advancement of his ideals; a noble manhood, ideal operations, and faithful services; a man, unselfish, gifted, kind, and true, using his God-given talents for a noble purpose,—

serving man; and one whose fidelity and Christian character must ever be an example, to the coming generations, of an ideal dentist; be it

Resolved, That we, his followers and members of the Northern Ohio Dental Association, in annual convention assembled, at Cleveland, June 7 to 9, 1904, express and record our appreciation of his noble life and generous contributions to the dental profession, and urge upon every member to live the life this gifted man lived, in order to bring to pass his conception of an ideal dental profession.

C. R. BUTLER,
CORYDON PALMER,
F. S. WHITSLER,
Committee.

C. D. PECK,
    Recording Secretary.

Miscellany.

POISONING BY CORROSIVES.—Important as is the employment of a chemical antidote, there is something more important in view of the power of the concentrated poison and the rapidity of its action. For, in order to apply the chemical antidote, it must be ascertained just what poison has been taken. This will consume time and delay treatment during the period of greatest danger to the tissues. The important thing to do at once is to limit the corrosive action of the poison. The author believes that the most important thing, which can always be done most readily, is to dilute the poison largely by a copious draft of water, and this without reference to the character of the poison. By this means we stop further corrosion by converting the strong acid, alkali, or salt into a comparatively harmless dilution of it. The selection and use of the chemical antidote can then follow as a matter secondary in point of time.

The poison having been diluted, it should then be neutralized as quickly as possible by the chemical antidote. Corresponding closely to the three groups of poison under consideration, the chief antidotes of practical value comprise the following three groups: (1) Dilute alkalies; (2) dilute acids; (3) albuminous substances.

For the group of caustic alkalies the proper antidote would be a dilute acid, preferably vegetable acids such as vinegar or lemon-juice, but any acid largely diluted may be employed. In case the poison is stronger water of ammonia, a volatile acid is needed in addition to neutralize the irritating vapor in the air-passages. Strong acetic acid by inhalation will answer this purpose.

The coagulant group will all be neutralized by egg albumin, or, as substitutes for it, by milk or flour paste. In addition a mild alkali is indicated in order to neutralize the liberated acid, except in case of carbolic acid poisoning, which requires special treatment, in addition to the use of albumin. The special antidotes for agents of this group in addition to albumin will be here noted: For carbolic acid alcohol has come to be employed, its effect being probably more upon the tissues than upon the poison itself. Soluble sulphates are also employed and continued for some time in order to avert within the system the formation of the products which are irritating to the kidneys. For silver nitrate, sodium chloride is an excellent additional antidote.

A marked peculiarity of carbolic acid poisoning is the rapidity of systemic effect, seemingly out of proportion to the injury done to the tissues. Death from carbolic acid will very frequently ensue within an hour's time, showing that either severe shock to the nervous system or very rapid systemic poisoning becomes a factor.

After the proper chemical antidotes have been administered emesis should be favored, unless already excessive, by copious drafts of warm water. When the poison or its compounds have been removed, demulcents should be employed freely to soothe the corroded and irritated tissues, and they should be allowed to remain within the stomach in sufficient bulk to prevent further damage to its walls by friction. Either of the ordinary classes of demulcents may be employed, which include the oils, mucilages, and albuminous substances. These measures will constitute the immediate treatment of poisoning by corrosives and the attendant damage to the tissues. In addition it may be necessary to employ morphine hypodermically in order to relieve pain and lessen peristalsis, and to employ stimulants judiciously. Perfect rest in

bed for a number of days is enjoined, with attention to details as
each case may require.

Although arsenic does not belong to the class of corrosives, its
destructive action permits reference here to its antidotal treatment. Its chemical antidote is easily prepared, and the process
should be indelibly fixed in every practitioner's mind, as it must
be fresh when needed. The usual antidote is the hydrated oxide
of iron, obtained by mixing any solution of a ferric salt with water
of ammonia, both having been previously diluted. Either tincture
of the chloride or Monsel's solution may be employed for the purpose, and the water of ammonia may be substituted by hydrated
magnesia, in which case the product is the equally valuable hydrated oxide of iron with magnesia. The antidote, suspended in
water, may be given freely.—*Therapeutic Gazette.*

A MODIFIED NEEDLE FOR PRESSURE ANÆSTHESIA.—I have
modified the form of the ordinary long, re-enforced hypodermic
needle, so that with it the local anæsthetic used by me in extracting is made to do all and more than I could do with the saturated
solution following the common method. In this manner I use
analgine, which contains but one-half of one per cent. of cocaine.
I dare say any similar solution would give the same result. I
find this method especially adapted to the treatment of children's
teeth, for, as a rule, the dam cannot be used, and all danger from
the solution escaping into the mouth is eliminated. Every dentist
will find in his cabinet abundant material with which to make the
points to which I have referred and now will describe.

From the base of an old point make a section which will be
bell-shaped. Selecting another needle, remove the steel point and
thread the end of the re-enforcement to screw into the bell-shaped
point just described, and the instrument is complete. Three of
these points have answered in the majority of cases. The angles
may be changed at will by slight bending of the stems. It is
unnecessary to say that these points are used with the regular
syringe. In using this instrument apply the dam where possible,
as an aseptic precaution. Dry the cavity as well as permissible
and apply sanguestine chloride [lily] or adrenalin, wiping the
cavity with carbolic acid. Now from a sheet of unvulcanized

rubber cut a disk large enough to amply cover the point of exposure. With rubber-dam punch make a small hole in the centre of this disk of rubber, which you will now slightly coat with cavitine varnish or chloropercha and place over exposure so that the central opening is directly over the point of exposure. It only remains now to make application of the bell-shaped point over the hole in the disk and gradually get the pressure necessary to force the solution through the entire pulp. It is now almost a year since I adopted this method, and trust that others of the profession may have as good results as I have had in its application.—DR. J. A. JOHNSON.

TEMPORARY FILLING.—Absorbent cotton saturated with cement which has been mixed to a creamy consistency makes an excellent temporary filling-material. It will last for months. If only required for a short time, nearly fill the cavity with dry cotton before inserting the plug. This will facilitate the removal of the filling when it becomes necessary.—R. E. SPARKS, Kingston, Ont.

Current News.

MISSISSIPPI VALLEY MEDICAL ASSOCIATION.

THE thirtieth annual session of the Mississippi Valley Medical Association will be held at Cincinnati, Ohio, October 11, 12, and 13, 1904, under the presidency of Dr. Hugh T. Patrick, of Chicago. The head-quarters and meeting places will be at the Grand Hotel.

The annual orations will be delivered by Dr. William J. Mayo, of Rochester, Minn., in Surgery, and Dr. C. Travis Drennen, of Hot Springs, Ark., in Medicine.

Request for places upon the programme, or information in regard to the meeting, can be had by addressing the Secretary, Dr. Henry Enos Tuley, Louisville, Ky., or the Assistant Secretary, Dr. S. C. Stanton, Masonic Temple, Chicago, Ill.

The usual railroad rates will be in effect.

HENRY ENOS TULEY,
Secretary.

HARVARD DENTAL ALUMNI ASSOCIATION.

THE following officers were elected June 27, 1904, at the thirty-third annual meeting of the Harvard Dental Alumni Association, held at Young's Hotel, Boston:

President, Harry S. Parsons, '92, Boston; Vice-President, Ned A. Stanley, '84, New Bedford; Secretary, Waldo E. Boardman, '86, Boston; Treasurer, Harold De W. Cross, '96, Nashua, N. H.

Executive Committee.—Waldo E. Boardman, '86, chairman, *ex officio,* Boston; Samuel T. Elliott, '01 (for one year), Boston; Walter A. Davis, '01 (for two years), Boston.

The council is composed of the above-named officers.

WALDO E. BOARDMAN, '86,
Secretary.

NORTHERN INDIANA DENTAL SOCIETY.

THE date of our next annual meeting, to be held at Huntington, Ind., has been postponed to October 18 and 19, 1904.

A programme of unusual interest has been completed, a synopsis of which will be announced in the next issue of this magazine.

Don't forget to read it.

OTTO U. KING,
Secretary.

KING BUILDING, HUNTINGTON, IND.

SOUTHWESTERN IOWA DENTAL SOCIETY.

THE eighth annual meeting of the Southwestern Iowa Dental Society will be held October 11 and 12, 1904, at Osceola, Iowa.

J. A. WEST,
Secretary.

CRESTON, IOWA.

THE

International Dental Journal.

VOL. XXV.   OCTOBER, 1904.   No. 10.

Original Communications.[1]

PULP DEGENERATION.[2]

BY EUGENE S. TALBOT, M.S., D.D.S., M.D., LL.D., CHICAGO.

THERE are two forms of pulp degeneration,—physiologic and pathologic. The physiologic is along the line of evolution and under the general law of economy of growth or use and disuse of structures. Physiologic degeneration was discussed in a paper, " The Evolution of Pulp."[3] It was shown that structures nourishing the placoid scales were larger than the scales themselves. Later, in some sharks, toothed birds, elephants, etc., the circumscribed pulp is as large as the tooth; in the horse and cow it is smaller, while in the anthropoid apes and man the pulp grows smaller and smaller until, in adult life, the apical end is so small that only one or two small arteries and nerves enter the root of the tooth. I demon-

---

[1] The editor and publishers are not responsible for the views of authors of papers published in this department, nor for any claim to novelty, or otherwise, that may be made by them. No papers will be received for this department that have appeared in any other journal published in the country.

[2] Read at the annual session of the American Medical Association, Section on Stomatology, Atlantic City, June 7 to 10, 1904.

This paper is one of a series read before this Section for a number of years, and was referred to in my paper on " The Constitutional Causes of Tooth-Decay."

[3] Journal American Medical Association, August 2, 1902.

strated the vasomotor system of the pulp with nerve-endings in a
paper on the " Vasomotor System of the Pulp," [1] still later in
" Constitutional Causes of Tooth Decay." [2]   I also demonstrated
nerve degeneration and inflammation resulting in abscess of the
pulp by disease of the body in connection with the vasomotor system and nerve degeneracy.

A pulp with such a record as I have demonstrated could hardly
avoid pathogenic degeneration. Scarcely a pulp is exempt from
influences of this, due to diseases of the body, external violence, or
pathologic changes. In the very nature of events, physiologic degeneration must necessarily result in pathogenic degeneration under the law of economy of growth and the struggle for existence
between organs, influence by bodily defects. Before taking up the
different degeneracies, the nature of the pulp must be briefly considered.

The number of nerves, arteries, and veins entering the apical
foramina depends on the age of the individual and the tooth itself.
A larger number enters early in tooth development than later in
life, when the foramina is exceedingly small. Age and exostosis
naturally reduce the size of the opening. Only one or two arteries
enter the pulp-chamber from the main trunk. These divide and
subdivide, forming many branches and loops.

Because of the small opening at the apical end of the root,
collateral circulation is impossible; hence, with end nerves and
arteries, the pulp is an excellent illustration of an end organ. This
constitutes its susceptibility to disease. The pulp enclosed within
bony walls is without an opportunity for expansion in arterial dila-
tion and sclerosis; it has only one or two small trunk arteries and
veins for supply and waste. The blood likewise increases disease
susceptibility. The vasomotor system makes the pulp to respond to
any disease to which the general system may be subjected. Diapedesis follows. Thermal changes from without also modify the circn-
lation of the pulp. Sudduth, and later Miller, are of opinion that
there are no lymphatics in the pulp. If they be not present, still the
pulp has great predisposition to degeneration, since Wedl, Tomes,
Smale and Colyer, and many others, as well as myself, have found
large spaces, without walls, whose lymphatic nature has not been

---

[1] Journal American Medical Association, December 19, 1903.
[2] Dental Digest, December, 1903.

determined. That débris and waste products may be carried from the pulp through the veins seems probable.

One influence but little considered in relation to pulp degeneration or tooth-structure in general, and one that exerts a marked consequence on tooth-decay, is the factor of interstitial gingivitis, abrasion, and erosion, which are degenerative conditions that take place at the fourth period of stress, at the senile stage or period of evolution at from forty to forty-five years of age. Not infrequently the senile stage occurs prematurely in neurotics and degenerates. At this period all excretory organs are weakening, faulty metabolism results, and the vasomotor system does not respond quickly. Marked disturbances take place in all the structures of the body, including the alveolar process as well as the pulp. Wedl in 1872 first called attention to the senile condition of tooth-structures shown by their discoloration.

Morbid change in the pulp other than nerve-end degeneration, inflammation resulting in abscess, as already discussed, may be summed up as arteriosclerosis, endarteritis obliterans, thrombosis, and embolism, cloudy swelling, fatty degeneration, mucoid, colloid, hyaline, and amyloid degeneration, pulp-stones, neoplasm, and fibroma. Some of these have been discussed by Wedl, Tomes, Smale and Colyer, Hopewell-Smith, Black, Bödecker, Arkövy, Andrews, Römer, Morgenstern, Caush, Latham, and many others, and can be studied more at length in the original monograph.

Here it is not my intention to study each morbid condition, but to show that the pulp is susceptible to them (individually and collectively), resulting in tooth degeneration.

Among vascular changes and circulatory disturbances, thrombosis in the blood-vessels of the pulp is not uncommon. From the present knowledge of pathology and the pathogenic condition of the pulp, it is evident how thrombosis must occasionally result. The pulp, an end organ without anastomosis and collateral circulation, the blood returning through a single vein, creates an anatomic predisposition for formation of a thrombus. The many degenerations and retrogressive changes which take place in the pulp make it susceptible to this morbid state. The spontaneous death of the pulp which sometimes follows disease can be thus accounted for. Formation of different calcic deposits causes the current to become slower and the leucocytes to be retarded in their progress from and to the apical end of the root-canal. In time the blood-plates separate from the blood-current and are caught at the apical end of the pulp-canal.   Sudden blindness occurs under similar conditions. The vessels become injured or abnormal, due to calcic deposits, and other retrogressive changes and stasis take place, eventually furnishing a basis for future thrombosis and inflammation (Fig. 1).

FIG. 1.

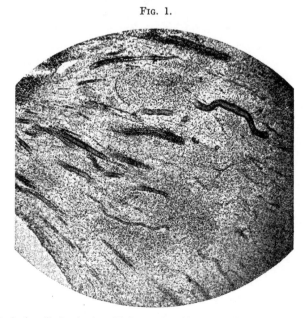

Thrombosis of capillaries of pulp and inflammation. × 137. Arteries and capillaries closed. Thrombus. Acute inflammation, showing there has been a hyperæmic condition.

A thrombus may be located in any part of the arterial system, but more especially the heart.   Simple or septic fragments may become dislodged and carried through the blood-streams to or into the pulp of the tooth.   Having entered this cavity, its return is almost impossible.

Embolism consists of various structures, such as fat drops, tissue fragments, tumor-cells, air, etc.   These follow the blood-current. The size of the body regulates the distance to which an embolus may travel.   It stops in vessels whose lumen prevents its passage.   More frequently it is arrested at the bifurcation of the artery.   The pulp is especially adapted for this purpose, since it is an end organ, with numerous loops terminating in one or more veins for exit.

Emboli, according to Hektoen, act in two ways, mechanically, clogging the circulation, and specifically, depending on the nature of the embolus, whether infected or sterile, whether composed of dead or living cells, capable of further proliferation. The circulation may be mechanically obstructed. If septic material has lodged in a

FIG. 2.

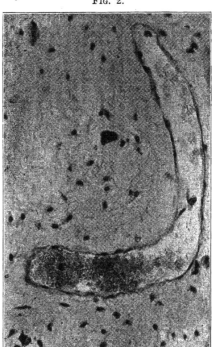

Dilated vessel. Diapedesis and embolus. × 280.

blood-vessel, inflammation may extend to the surrounding tissues (Fig. 2).

Endarteritis Obliterans and Arteriosclerosis.—Inflammation of the arterial coats in the pulp is very common. This is due, in a degree, to pulp embryogeny, anatomy, environment, and to its end-organ nature, as already stated. The diseases most commonly observed are endarteritis obliterans and arteriosclerosis. While it is not uncommon for each coat of the artery to take on a special type of inflammation, yet all frequently become involved.

Original Communications.

Endarteritis obliterans is an inflammation of the inner coat of the artery, usually of a chronic type. The inflammation may arise from an irritant in the blood-current from the main current, through the vaso vasorum, or through the lymphatics. The first is the most usual; in the alveolar process all three may occur. In the pulp, irritation in the blood-stream is the most common method. Proliferation of the endothelium results. Bands of fibrous tissue develop. The blood-vessels become obstructed and finally obliterated, impeding the circulation (Fig. 3).

FIG. 3.

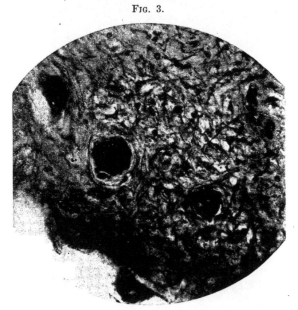

The wall in one artery is thickened (endarteritis) and almost occluded by inflammatory products. In the smaller artery the intima contains round-celled infiltration almost occluding it. The pulp-tissues show the myxomatous character very well, branched spindle and round nucleated cells in many places. × 225.

The structure pulp, made up of loops of blood-vessels and situated within bony walls, with only one or two arteries and veins for the passage of blood, renders it a unique end organ, and its arteries susceptible to arteriosclerosis. This, together with endarteritis obliterans, predispose the arteries to degeneration and necrosis. This is a thickening of the arterial walls, especially of the intima. It is secondary, according to Hektoen, to certain inflammatory or degenerative changes in the media. This is seldom observed early in life. It is commonly found after puberty, but more frequently at the senile stage, from forty years on. The causes producing arteriosclerosis in other parts of the body produce it in the pulp arteries.

The causes are usually autointoxication and drugs taken into the system, which likewise become irritants. Besides the distensive force and change in composition of the blood, local irritation on the

FIG. 4.

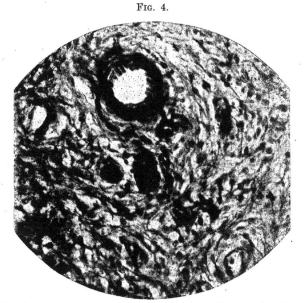

An enlarged artery in an early stage of thickening, the small vessels plugged up, well-marked myxomatous pulp-tissue. × 225.

arterial wall is an active cause. In diseases such as syphilis, gout, rheumatism, Bright's disease, alcoholism, and chronic mercurial, lead, brass, arsenic, and bromide poisoning, the walls become irritated, resulting in thickening of the arterial coats.

"The inebriate, whose brain and body after death exhibit a confused mass of wreckage, which the pathologist is often unable to trace back to the exact causes and conditions, has, according to Crothers, always sclerotic conditions of the large and small arteries, together with atrophic and hypertrophic states of the heart, kidneys, and liver, with fatty degeneration and calcification of the

coats of the arteries.   These organic changes are so frequently
present in inebriates that they constitute a marked pathology which
is traceable to the use of alcohol."

These irritants, acting through the vasomotor system and increasing the arterial pressure, finally cause paralysis and diminution of the caliber of the arteries and capillaries, producing stasis
of blood (Fig. 4).   This morbid state of the arteries tends to produce any or all of the other degenerations previously referred to.

Fig. 5.

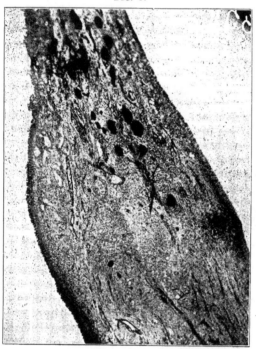

Pulp-stones scattered throughout, here and there a form of round-celled infiltration,
longitudinal nerve-trunks, few degenerated vessels surrounded by hyaline degeneration in
the middle of nerve-trunk.   Early sclerosis and cloudy swelling or granular degeneration.
Odontoblasts *in situ.*   × 21.

The inflammatory process of the intima was first charged to
direct irritation of material floating in the blood.   Rokitansky and
Thoma are of opinion that it is secondary and dependent on the
degenerative changes of the middle coat.   This view I cannot accept,
since autointoxic states produce irritation in the blood-streams.

Many degenerations of the pulp are the result of arteriosclerosis, endarteritis obliterans, and nerve degeneration. These degenerations occur in connection with each other; in other words, sometimes two, three, and even more are to be found in the same pulp. The causes producing these degenerations are not understood.

Retrogressive Changes.—One direct result of arteriosclerosis and endarteritis obliterans is cloudy swelling and fatty degeneration. These conditions are observed in connection with such diseases as typhoid fever, septicæmia, and other acute infections and toxic diseases. The tissues present a whitish or shiny appearance, without fibrous structures. Under the microscope the tissues present an opaque mass and do not take stain. The cells are quite large and swollen (Fig. 5).

"When a tissue, as for instance the heart-muscle, receives a diminished quantity of blood on account of the narrowing of the

FIG. 6.

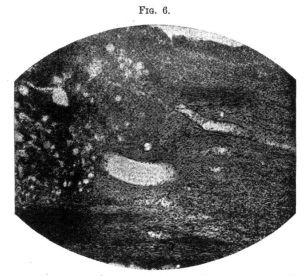

Fatty degeneration, acute pulpitis, sclerosis of nerves. Nerve degeneration, dilatation of vessels, faint outline of degenerated odontoblasts. × 137.

lumen of the arteries due to thrombosis, embolism, or disease accompanied by thickening of the intima, albuminous and fatty changing, remarks Hektoen, usually result. In the case of the different forms of anæmias, degenerations with fat production are found in the liver, heart, kidneys, and muscles. In such conditions there is not

754   *Original Communications.*

enough oxygen and other nutritive material to maintain the function of the cells. In actual starvation there is first absorption of all the fat in the bódy, accompanied by a marked diminution of the structure. In the later stages, albumin and fatty degeneration take place. Albuminal and fatty changes are very common in febrile diseases. They occur in practically infectious diseases and in a large number of the intoxications, such as the drug poisons. They are also found in abnormal metabolism, due to direct action of poisons and the abnormal process of oxidation." Owing to the pulp's peculiar structure and environment, fatty degeneration is commonly found in its tissue (Fig. 6).

Amyloid degeneration is a peculiar degeneration of the connective tissue, causing an albuminous substance to be deposited in

FIG. 7.

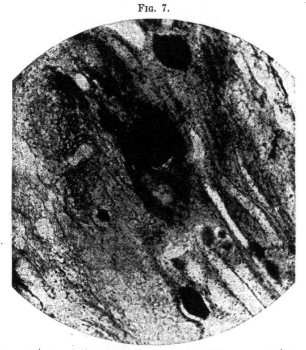

Shows pulp-stones and their close relation to the vascular channels. Dilated vessels with amyloid deposit. × 62.

the surrounding tissue. The walls of the blood-vessels also become involved. It presents a shiny appearance and differs from other tissues in that it turns a dark red color with iodine. The morbid state is found in syphilis, tuberculosis, chronic dysentery, etc. (Fig. 7). Almost every structure in the body may be involved.

Hyaline degeneration (Fig. 8) is, according to Stengle, closely allied with amyloid, mucoid, and colloid degeneration, and all can

FIG. 8.

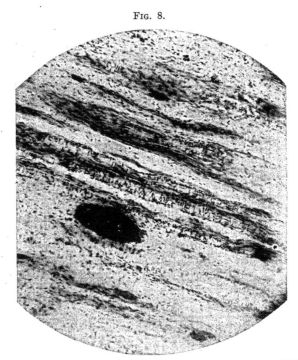

Calcareous deposit, medullary nerve. Early connective cell formation. × 225.

pass into each other. It can occur in tissues during infectious and septic processes, following traumatism, in autointoxications such as drug poison, hemorrhages, in cicatrices, in senile blood-vessels, arteriosclerosis, endarteritis obliterans, and in the nervous system. It can also occur in connective tissue which has undergone a change by inflammation. This morbid state depends for its action on local or general nutritive disturbances. The pulp, therefore, is susceptible to it. The intima, as well as the entire walls of the small blood-vessels in the pulp, easily becomes involved. Some investigators believe that fat connective tissue cells so arrange themselves as to undergo a change into myelin substances (Fig. 9). These ultimately lead to calcification. This raises the question of calcic deposits or so-called pulp-stones. Pathologists know that tissues elsewhere in the body (which have necrosed or degenerated) are the localities where lime salts are deposited. Dying tissue which has undergone more or less change possesses, according to Ziegler, a kind of attraction for the lime salts in solution in the body. The tissues, to which attention has been called, are especially susceptible

Fig. 9.

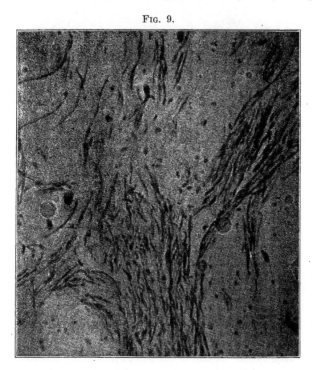

This shows medullary nerve-fibres and internodes, axis-cylinders, myelin degeneration.
× 280.

to calcic changes; hyaline and fatty degeneration, tissues involved in disease or drug poisoning, already mentioned here and elsewhere. Regions affected by slight degeneration and in structures like the pulp, a constricted end organ, are predisposed to deposits of lime salts. Calcic deposits have different shapes and location in the pulp-tissue. Circumscribed structures which appear solid under the microscope, to the naked eye, or to the touch, are not pulp-stones or calcic deposits, but in a large percentage of cases belong to other retrogressive changes. These deposits (Fig 10) are, no doubt due to degeneration of pulp-tissue, especially in structures undergoing hyaline or fatty degeneration. Large masses of deposits in the form of spherules often occur. Bone formations are sometimes observed.

FIG. 10.

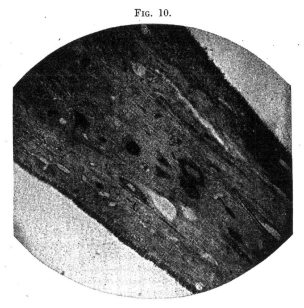

Shows medullary nerve-fibres slightly thickened. The connective tissue is degenerating, and hyaline odontoblasts show well on both surfaces. × 156.

These deposits, both in pulp-stones and spherules, take on a dirty, bluish-violet color, with hæmatoxylin. These Dr. Latham and I have observed many times. Crystals may sometimes occur.

"This applies, however, as Ziegler remarks, only to deposits of lime carbonates and phosphates, and not to those of lime oxalate." These deposits may take place at any time, but are most likely at the senile or fourth period of stress.

I shall not consider neoplasm at length in this paper, since Dr. Latham has this subject under discussion, but will now refer to fibroid degeneration in closing. Fibroid growth of the pulp may be both rapid or slow. Inflammatory reaction in fibrous pulps is rare, although when followed by infection or exposure, it may take place. Various degeneracies like those already mentioned are liable to occur, especially those in which connective tissue in general is predisposed. The fibres are observed in bundles, closely packed

together, with many connective tissue corpuscles shown at intervals.
Fibroid degeneration is easily distinguished from the other degeneracies of the pulp (Fig. 11).

FIG. 11.

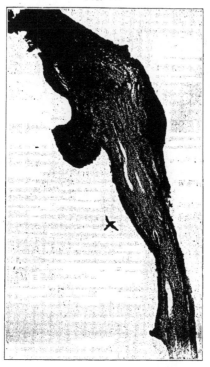

Shows interstitial fibrosis with acute inflammatory cells. Odontoblasts have been
destroyed.   ×22.

In these cases, the blood-vessels and nerve-tissue are relatively
few. The blood-vessels remaining usually have thickened walls,
especially in the external and middle coats. This, of course, nar-
rows the lumen. Not infrequently the blood-vessels are entirely
obliterated. These fibromas, very common in exposed pulps, are not
now under consideration. In nearly if not all of these degenerations the blood-vessels are first involved, later nerve-tissue.

All these degenerations, including the pathologic processes of
evolution, are the direct constitutional causes of tooth-decay, erosion
and abrasion brought about by diminution of tooth vitality.

THE VITAL ACTION OF·THE DENTAL PULP.[1]

BY R. R. ANDREWS, A.M., D.D.S., CAMBRIDGE, MASS.

I HAD the honor, several years ago, of reading a paper before this Section on " The Embryology of the Dental Pulp." This paper gave a minute description of the various processes taking place during the development of the tooth from its formative pulp. I propose in the present essay to consider the nature of the mature pulp, and to call your attention to its vital action after the tooth is formed. I shall consider the pulp within the pulp-chamber and its myriad fibrils, for these fibrils are as much a part of the pulp as any portion of it, and are the channels by which its vital functions are carried on. These canals are slightly undulating, and radiate from the pulp-chamber to the outer surface of the dentine. Each canal contains a fibre bathed in a fluid, and this fibre is an arm of the pulp. Branches from this fibre anastomose with others through the dentine matrix. They form a delicate net-work in the substance of the crown near the enamel.

In the region of the cementum they anastomose with the fibres of the granular layer of the root. When the tooth is fully formed, the principal function of the pulp is for the vitalization of the substance of the dentine by means of its fibrils, which permeate into every portion of the matrix of the dentine. Its function is not only to vitalize, but it may again assume its formative function whenever causes for repair demand this action.

One of the difficulties we find in our research work on the mature pulp is the fact that we can not look on its tissue in life. We can not see these vital processes while they are going on, but must make our deductions on freshly extracted normal teeth and pulps that are as near the life period as possible. But it is always dead tissue that we have to examine. We draw our conclusions from what is shown to have taken place when the tissue was alive; we know that the living pulp, with its blood-vessels and nerves, nourishes the dentine; that vital changes do take place, and that this pulp is the source of vital action. It is a living organ, subject

---

[1] Read at the annual session of the American Medical Association, Section on Stomatology, Atlantic City, June 7 to 10, 1904.

to any physiologic or pathologic process, which may act on any living matter; therefore, we may expect to find its connection with the general economy similar to that of other tissues. It will respond to the action of returning health, and caries which have commenced have been arrested by this vital action. They appear as polished blotches on the teeth and are not uncommon.. Professor miller, in his work on " Micro-Organisms of the Human Mouth," calls this condition a spontaneous healing of dental decay. The dentine, which had become softened, has become hard again, and the decaying process is stopped. This change also takes place in the temporary teeth. The healed dentine retains its discolored appearance, but becomes nearly as dense as normal dentine. These changes have been brought about by vital action, and this action came from the agency of the pulp.

The histologic structure of the normal pulp, at the time of the full formation of the tooth, as has already been described in a former paper, is as follows: At the periphery we have the pear-shaped cells, then the spindle-shaped conjugation layer of cells, then the spindle-shaped and irregularly shaped cells with their anastomosing processes, and lastly, the connective tissue elements in the central portion of the pulp, which seem to be scant in protoplasm. These cells are not very numerous, and are in a jelly-like matrix. The blood-vessels enter at the apex, the trunk-vessels resting near the centre of the pulp. Sometimes as many as three arteries are seen to enter the apical foramen. They then divide into innumerable branches and form an extensive net-work of capillaries near the layer of the pear-shaped cells next the formed dentine. There are numerous veins also found, but these are somewhat larger than the arteries. Black tells us that the blood-vessels of the pulp are remarkable for the thinness of their walls, and that the smaller veins seem to be nothing more than endothelial cells which are placed edge on edge, or margin on margin. The arteries have a circular and longitudinal layer of muscular fibres, but these are very thinly distributed.

There is always an effort on the part of the pulp to protect the dentine from destruction from whatever cause. A microscopic examination shows us how misleading it is to call this organ a nerve. Its matrix is a mass of connective tissue, in the substance of which we find nerve-fibres, medullated and non-medullated. These enter the pulp through the apical foramen in bundles of various sizes. As they pass into the pulp they break into branches and form a rich net-work, a delicate plexus of fine nerve-filaments, next the outer pear-shaped cells. It is not certainly known how they communicate with the fibril. It has been suggested that the finer fibres may pass between the pear-shaped cells, winding themselves around the dentinal fibrils and thus pass into the dentinal canal. There is also a rich capillary net-work of blood-vessels near these pear-shaped cells in the newly formed tooth, and when we inject these and examine them under the microscope there seems to be little room left for other tissues there. When the dentine is irritated by infection or its surface is uncovered by a break, there immediately follows a period of vital activity. If we examine sections of a tooth made when these changes are taking place, we shall see that the formative cells in that portion of the pulp nearest the point of repair are filling up with glistening globular bodies, and the tissue about it is showing an increased vascularity, as though an active formative action were taking place; and in the canals opening towards the area of irritation, within the dentine matrix, we find minute glistening granules, which are being carried outwardly towards the point of lesion. These glistening particles have the appearance of being minute calco-spherites. In studying this condition, some years ago, I satisfied myself that these appearances were the result of the vital action of the pulp in its efforts to repair the tissue, and that the minute glistening particles within the canals were in many ways similar to the minute globular bodies found in the tissues while the dentine matrix was developing. They are being forced into and through the canals of the matrix to the point of irritation, and I have seen long lines of them in the canals, nearly filling them up. In favorable cases the canals against the irritation do become filled and a formative process goes on within the pulp-chamber, until a calcified barrier is formed there, corresponding to the part disturbed or destroyed. When this change takes place the consolidated dentine in this area becomes slightly darker in color than normal tooth-structure, and might easily be mistaken for decay.

In carious pits and fissures of the bicuspids and molars the organisms of infection proceed inward through the dentinal canals towards the pulp. As it nears the pulp this protecting barrier is formed, and under normal conditions the infection is retarded, changes its course, and moves in the next weaker direction towards the approximal surface, usually without exposing the pulp—if taken in time. We also find the protecting consolidation in teeth that are worn down, usually in the mouth of old people, and when this change has taken place these teeth are not liable to decay again, except under very unfavorable circumstances. This protecting process forms that tissue known as the zone of resistance; the hyaline appearance of this zone tissue under the microscope is caused by the lime globules consolidating the canals that are in the substance of the zone. These changes are due, in a large measure, to normal conditions, as regards the vitality of the individual. But in cases where the constitutional condition is below the normal, even where they seem favorable to decay, there is always an attempt made to retard the infection. Under certain conditions of environment and infection, penetrating decay is so rapid that the vital action of the pulp is overwhelmed; and the pulp becomes exposed, and is in a pathologic condition even before the breaking away of the cavity walls.

The pulp is the central and largest source of vitality to the tooth, and it acts through its myriads of fibrils. Sometimes the ends of the fibrils are seen to be running slightly into the enamel substance. In the root portion they anastomose with the fibrils of the granular layer near the cement, and a communication is seen, in many cases, to be continued through the cementum by means of the lacuna and their fibrils, and in a few cases I have traced them out to the pericementum. Pain of the dentine, following the touch of an instrument, or from any irritation, is expressed through the agency of these fibrils, and we become conscious of the sensation through them. When irritation is caused by wear, erosion, or a break exposing the dentine, a section under the microscope will show that secondary dentine has been formed within the pulp-chamber, and this corresponds to the loss of substance of the dentine which has been affected. This secondary dentine is a tissue that has been called dentine of repair, and this is a manifestation of the vital action of the pulp. It is formed within the pulp-chamber, and is always an addition to the already formed dentine. It forms against the portion of the pulp-cavity next to the fibrils which have been affected by the lesion. The enamel might wear or break indefinitely, and we shall find no compensation of any kind occurring until it reaches the surface of the dentine, whereon the vital power of the pulp is aroused and an action of repair progresses in proportion to the extent of the injury. Some have thought these changes occur only in the teeth of old people, but such is not the case. They may occur at any age, and this process of repair has been found to have taken place in the tissues of a temporary tooth. These changes are all characteristic of the vital action of the pulp. The dentine is and was meant at all times to be a living tissue. As I have shown, it receives impressions of injuries and responds by processes of repair. Some of the ablest men in the profession have questioned the further value of the tooth-pulp after the full formation of the tooth has taken place. They look on it as simply a formative organ, and consider its mission closed with the formation of the tooth. It is, therefore, in their judgment quite as well to destroy it, take it out, and fill its chamber. The microscopic appearance of dentine, after the pulp is removed, shows that a large amount of dead organic tissue is left within the canals that cannot be taken out, and this dead tissue is a source of considerable danger to the health and vitality of the pericementum.

The subject of vitality, tissue repair, and compensation for injury on the part of the pulp should suggest a lesson for us all. The whole phenomena of vital action shows that the pulp is, under proper conditions, always helpful in bringing about successful results, if properly attended to. The restoration to a healthy condition of an irritated and troublesome pulp, is among the highest acts of professional skill. It is unfortunate that so many pulps have to be destroyed. It is fortunate that so many teeth remain quiet and apparently healthy after pulp extirpation and treatment. With the death of the pulp we lose not only sensation in the dentine, but also all the changes which vitality give to an organ, such as nutrition and recuperation. These can never by any possible means be revived. The main mass of the dentine of the tooth is dead. Myriads of lifeless fibrils are in its canals. It is true that the cementum, which was not formed from the pulp-tissue, does furnish a limited amount of vitality and nourishment to the root, which is covered by the pericementum; but the health of the pericementum is threatened by the dead tissue which is locked up in the canals within the dentine matrix. In vigorous health pulpless teeth have been successfully treated and remain serviceable for years. In cases of a lessened vitality, we may expect more or less pericemental trouble, a darkening of the tooth, a recession of the gums, and an absorbing of the alveolar processes. The tooth is beyond the influence of any systematic process, and there is no probability of a change for the better. Abscess and necrosis may supervene, and extraction is the last resort. I conclude by quoting an extract from a paper written in 1874 by Dr. J. E. Craven, who says,—

"Here is an organ formed of a delicate tissue, as is the eye, and because some agent of decay threatens its ivory walls, the ruthless hand of a blissful ignorance pours on its devoted head such destroying angels as carbolic acid, creosote, cobalt, and arsenous acid. Poor little pulp, you have been caught, and the destructive genius at the chair wills that you be deprived of your previous life. Why not lay aside those substances that blister and crisp the tissue until its life is enfeebled or lost, and, instead, resort to milder agents whose influence tends to cool the fevered part and allay the pain, reduce the inflammation, and use the food that nature herself would suggest to replace the covering the pulp has lost by decay?"

ANKYLOSIS OF THE JAWS.[1]

BY G. LENOX CURTIS, M.D., NEW YORK.

My present purpose in speaking is to report some causes of the varieties in permanent ankylosis and to show plans of treatment that I have found very successful. I do this in the hope that it will be of service to others. Preparatory to the permanent cases, I will refer to cases of temporary ankylosis that I regard as unique and interesting.

Temporary ankylosis, so commonly found, can be so speedily treated successfully that little new remains to be told. Nevertheless these cases sometimes cause much trouble to both patient and practitioner, when they result in serious complications, which may occur if proper treatment is not given in the early stage. See Garretson, Marshall, and others for recognized methods.

The principal irritating causes of inflammation which lead to ankylosis of the jaws are exposed tooth-pulps, retarded, malposed, or impacted third molars, traumatism, cicatrix, tetanus, alveolar abscess, tonsillar, diphtheritic, and septic injections.

---

[1] Read at the annual session of the American Medical Association, Section on Stomatology, Atlantic City, June 7 to 10, 1904.

Permanent ankylosis is the result of osseous formations within the joint, causing partial or complete displacement or arrest of the synovial fluid, a condition, however, that may not occur for months or years of immobility. Fortunately this is rarely met with, except in cases of rheumatoid arthritis; because of the great activity of the lower jaw its joint is usually the last to become affected. Inflammatory conditions arising from any cause should be corrected as early as possible, in order to prevent cicatricial formations.

In one case of temporary ankylosis which had lasted for several days I found on examination that it seemed to be caused by an exposed pulp. This case was immediately relieved by extracting from the pulp a drop of blood and applying a dressing of campho-phenique.

The cicatricial variety follows suppurations and surgical operations through the face, such as are resorted to for the removal of tumors and necrosis of the jaws. When this condition is found in childhood and continues for a considerable length of time, it is generally followed by an arrest in the development of the face and jaws. In illustration of this are the photograph (Fig. 1) and casts

FIG. 1.

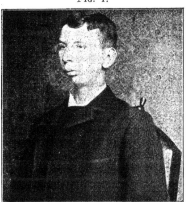

of the face and teeth of a boy, aged sixteen, who, when in his second year, fell from a window, fracturing his femur and also the inferior maxilla at the neck of the left condyloid process. The jaw fracture was not noticed until six months later, when the jaw was found to be ankylosed. The surgeon concluded that the trouble was due to muscular injury at the time of the fall. Thinking that in time the muscles would recover of themselves, he advised no treatment.. Three years later another surgeon found the fractured jaw, but did not suggest any plan of relief. Later, indefinite different attempts were made to force the jaws apart, but were unsuccessful.

On examination, I found the ankylosis and the shortening of the jaws were due to the overlapping of the bones, which had become firmly fixed. The median line of the chin was considerably to the left. Several of the deciduous teeth which should have been cast off were present, and the mouth was in a generally disordered condition. I removed these teeth, reduced the inflammatory condition of the gums, and advised an operation for adjusting the ends of the fractured bones. I was told that several surgeons were consulted by the father, who was told that they would discourage surgical interference, consequently the boy was allowed to grow up in this unfortunate condition. My belief at that time was that the bones could be separated by means of a saw, or bur, and readjusted, and the ends of the fracture freshened and held in position until union of the bones was complete. He is now twenty-eight years of age.

Another case of ankylosis, the cause of which is of more than usual interest, is that of a young woman who for several years had been treated for repeated granular growths in the sockets of the lower left molars that had been extracted. On examination it was found that all of the jaw, including the ramus back of the first bicuspid, was necrosed. To my amazement I found the third molar was malposed and lying at the neck of the condyloid process directly below the condyle. The treatment consisted of opening the periosteum sufficiently to permit the removal of the tooth and the necrosed bone, and treating the wound until bone was reproduced. The periosteum was retained as an interosseous splint until sufficient new bone had formed to hold the jaw in position.

By this plan there was no shortening of the jaw and no deformity of the face. It is obvious that this operation was done within the mouth. I was unable to ascertain whether ankylosis on this side of the jaw was complete or was of the temporary variety. By the use of the screw-jacks a complete and permanent use of the jaw was re-established.

I saw in consultation another case of permanent ankylosis, resulting from a surgical operation made through the face for the removal of necrosed bone in the lower jaw, that resulted from an abscess on a molar. The cicatrix was several inches in length and about an inch in width. The patient told me he had been under treatment in a hospital for more than a year, much of which time his face was bandaged. I advised resecting of the scars, skin induction, and forcible separation of the jaw by means of screw-jacks.

I am now pleased to be able to bring before you here a patient who, at the age of fourteen, was brought to me in June, 1893. At the age of six years the patient had diphtheria, with extensive ulcers in the throat, the soreness from which continued for a considerable time after the disease had subsided. During this period pain was caused in opening the mouth, when the child was per-

FIG. 2.

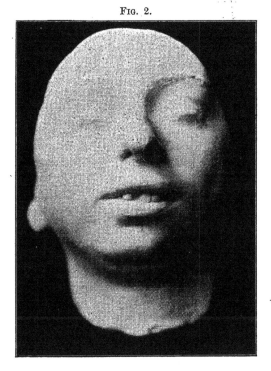

mitted to take liquid food between the teeth. This method of taking nourishment became a habit. Four years later, owing to toothache, she was taken to a dentist, who, finding her jaws were ankylosed, referred her to a surgeon for treatment. Various methods, including the use of the " Grady screw," to pry and keep the jaws apart, were resorted to with slight results. Precaution was not taken, however, to protect the teeth from fracture, and some were broken and abscessed; gingivitis also resulted. Efforts to correct the ankylosed condition were finally abandoned, and the jaws closed and became rigid. At the time the effort was made to force the teeth apart the patient was encouraged to crowd solid food between the upper and lower teeth and crush it with the tongue against the roof of the mouth. This she was finally able to do with considerable success, but in doing this she had forced the lower teeth back and the upper teeth forward, causing some deformity. Fig. 2 shows a cast of the face. Examination showed the patient to be anæmic but otherwise in a fairly good state of health.

By forcing a wedge between the teeth I was able to secure one-eighth of an inch space on the left side. The reason for this was that on the left side there was only cicatricial ankylosis, while on the right side it was osseous. The condition of the mouth was deplorable. General gingivitis prevailed, and several of the permanent teeth were loose, while others were abscessed, and many of the deciduous teeth were present, thus retarding the full eruption of the permanent teeth. The crown of the upper right central was lost. By treatment much of the inflammatory condition of the gums was reduced, but not until the jaws were so far separated that the abscessed and the deciduous teeth could be extracted. My first thought was to devise and construct a mechanism that could force the jaws apart by causing an even pressure on the teeth. Fig. 3

FIG. 3.

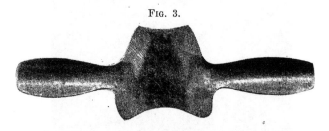

shows the depressor made of steel spring, which I was able to crowd between the jaws while the wedges were in position and while the patient was under profound anæsthesia. While the head was firmly held by an assistant I was able to put sufficient force to the depressor to gain one-eighth of an inch space. With this space I was able to insert a flexible double screw-jack, represented by Fig. 4, that I also devised for this purpose. The surface of the hand-depressor and the blades of the screw-jack were serrated, the object of which was to lessen the danger of slipping. If it is necessary to further reduce this danger, soft vulcanite rubber or gutta-percha may be

FIG. 4.

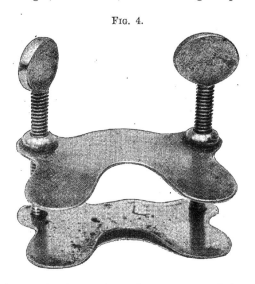

placed on the masticating surface of one or more of the molar teeth on either side of the mouth. The blades of the jack were made of thin spring steel. The object of this was not only to cause even bearing on the teeth, but to prevent undue pressure on the teeth and luxation of the jaws. The screws were purposely made long, so that the patient might tighten or loosen the jack at will. By this simple mechanism the patient was enabled to adjust it and make as slight or as much pressure as could be easily tolerated. This patient was able to wear this jack much of the time both day and night. When three-eighths of an inch space had been secured soft wax was flowed over the blades of the screw-jack and the jack was again put in position. By this means I was able to secure an impression of the antagonizing ends of the teeth, by which casts were made and splints of vulcanite were constructed, the approximating surfaces of which were made flat, so that when in place there was an equal bearing at all points. These splints enabled me to put greater pressure on the screw-jacks as well as eliminating all danger of fracturing the teeth. As the jaws opened, better fitting splints were applied. Chloroform was administered every few weeks, and all possible pressure was made to force the jaws apart. Almost from the beginning of the treatment there was an inflammation established in the right joint. While at times this operation was attended by considerable discomfort to the patient, which prolonged the work, it had much to do with the final success, because absorption of the osseous deposit within the joint was established, and by this constant agitation it continued until a fair action in the joint was established.

One of the things which retarded our efforts was the degenerated temporal and masseter muscles because of years of disuse. These muscles required redevelopment from that condition found in a child of six years to that of a young girl of sixteen. Until this was accomplished there was but moderate benefit derived from opening and closing the mouth. In order to develop the strength of the muscles of the face, as well as to elongate them, I devised a set of springs which were securely fastened in grooves cut in the approximating surfaces of the splints on either side of the mouth (Fig. 5). At the forward end of the grooves there was an opening

FIG. 5.

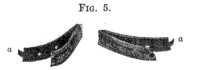

made through the splint of sufficient size to accommodate the studs *a, a,* which were one-sixteenth of an inch in thickness and one-eighth of an inch in length. The principal object of these studs was to prevent the springs from slipping out of place, and to doubly secure them they were also wired to the lower splint. These springs were very stiff, and only with great effort by the patient could be compressed. In order to get the splints into the mouth with the springs in position they were applied while bound tightly together, and when in position these ligatures were cut. At the end of one year's treatment the patient had about one-half the normal opening of the jaw, and for the next year the work of continuing the treatment was intrusted to her, because by personal illness I was absent from practice. On my return I was pleased to find that substantial progress had been made, the space gained was maintained, and that the muscles had materially improved. I took up the work again along the same lines and continued until almost the normal opening of the jaws had been secured, with, however, but little lateral motion, the adhesions which held the left side of the jaw readily giving way to the continued pressure of the jack. In the course of a year the patient's health demanded exclusive attention, and because of tuberculosis further maxillary irritation was at this time discontinued. Within the past six years, however, the patient has seldom found it necessary to make use of the springs; her health also has gradually improved. As you can see, the patient, though not robust, is in fairly good condition.

DISCUSSION.

Dr. G. V. I. Brown, Milwaukee.—I think Dr. Curtis is in danger of being misunderstood, since he evidently describes conditions of true and false ankylosis. He speaks of permanent and temporary ankylosis, and gives as etiologic factors malimposed third molars, pulpitis, and conditions of that character. What Dr. Curtis really means is not ankylosis, but trismus. I think we ought to draw a very distinctive line between a muscular contraction of a temporary nature, as described, due to more or less direct irritation of the nerve-trunks, and a condition caused by inflammatory processes or degenerative conditions of the temporo-maxillary articulation. So far as operative measures are concerned nothing can be said but the highest praise. These cases are extremely troublesome, and Dr. Curtis's results are a warrant that the proper methods were employed.

Dr. Charles F. Allan, Newburgh, N. Y.—I have never had a case of osseous formation in the jaw, and I think they are very, very rare. The coagulation of the secretions as a result of traumatism, which causes the ankylosis, is sufficient to make a strong bar to the jaws closing as they should. I have never found that any application made to cause absorption was in any way effective. Pressure under chloroform and daily use of the screw opener by the patient would be the only means to cause return to normal conditions.

Reports of Society Meetings.

AMERICAN MEDICAL ASSOCIATION, SECTION ON
STOMATOLOGY, ATLANTIC CITY, JUNE 7 TO 10,
1904.

(Continued from page 629.)

DISCUSSION ON THE PAPERS OF DRS. EAMES, BALDWIN, CHITTEN-
DEN, AND MARSHALL, ON DENTAL EDUCATION.

Dr. N. S. Hoff, Ann Arbor, Mich.—I do not believe it will do
any good at this time to discuss the possibility or the probability of
a four years' course of instruction in our dental schools, because the
Faculties Association will do what it pleases, and, naturally, to this
we shall have to submit. The matter of arranging the course of
study in our own school has been my work for several years. Our
institution is not very unlike that of Harvard. We have a medical
faculty with high ideals, and our work in the line of scientific
medical branches is done in the medical school, and our students
are compelled to do that work on the same basis as the medical
students. I can readily appreciate the situation in which Harvard
finds itself. Our school was early forced to go into the four years'
course, not because we wanted to get ahead of anybody else, but because our medical school had taken such advanced ground on the
scientific subjects that we were compelled to have our students instructed in those departments by a proper amount of time. What
shall be the position of our school in view of the position of the
Faculties Association, I am not prepared to say, but I do not see
how it will be possible for us to do our work short of a four-year
basis; and I think that if things go on as they have in the medical
department, we shall be driven to a five years' course. My impression is that by our plan of working we are not developing our
course symmetrically. The scheme that I have been turning over
in my mind is that in the first year our students should take up the
technic work, and as fast as possible they, should be advanced
through the practical courses, at the same time carrying sufficient
of the scientific branches to keep up the mental discipline which

they have already acquired by their high-school training. We admit students from high schools, but they are all examined, and we know what their teaching has been. We require two years of Latin, if the student has had only one language. We prefer that he has one modern language, preferably German. The majority of our students from the high school come at the age of nineteen, which it seems to me is not an excessively mature age for a man to take up technical training. I believe such men will develop their technical training more rapidly if taken up at that age than if it is delayed until later in the course; and, if we can advance them more rapidly at that period, why not do it, and at the same time allow them to carry, not full work in the scientific departments, but only sufficient amount to keep them in mental drill; for instance, the study of chemistry and anatomy may be properly carried along, because they do not need to see the relations of chemistry at the beginning. They will be able to complete the subject of chemistry later on in the course. I was talking with the deans of two medical colleges in the West in which they have dental departments, and who complained of the difficulty in getting dental work done. They asked me how we did at Ann Arbor. I said, "We don't do it; it is a physical impossibility to get a medical man who has never had any dental training to interest a dental practitioner in the subject from a theoretical stand-point. He must know something practical about it that will call the student's attention to the work. I have found this true in therapeutics; the students could answer me according to the text-books, but they had no idea of the relations to practical work. I do not know how they will make that application of their work, unless we first teach them to be practical dentists. Then when they come to these physiologic principles they will see the relation to their own work. I remember that it took me a long while to apply my one hundred per cent. chemistry in my examination record to my dental chemistry. I think the profession recognizes the fact that if there is a standard it must not be dogmatic, for there are different classes, and I do not think it is necessary for the schools in Class A to take into consideration the schools in Class B. The standard is sentimental, and it is the greatest power for the uplift of our profession. It is this unwritten standard, or whatever it may be called, that I am looking for. I think it will be thoroughly discouraging, if the course of study is put back to three years, or if a lower standard is made by the

Association of Faculties. It will take years for us to get back to where we now are. I do not believe the subject has ever been studied from a proper stand-point. I have given you the standpoint from my own view.

Dr. Alice M. Steeves, Boston.—My idea is that the dental student does not work from the idea of benefiting the entire body; he does not see the relationship very often. I think we should impress on him that he is working for the benefit of the whole and not for one individual.

Dr. Bogue, New York City.—The chairman and Dr. Hoff have assisted in crystallizing my incoherent views. My boy, who had promised me he would study dentistry, felt that he wanted to study medicine. I said to him, " I claim the fulfilment of that promise. When you have done that, all you can earn you may devote to the study of medicine." He worked so hard that after graduation in dentistry he had already passed his first year in medicine. He afterwards graduated in medicine, and in that obtained what I had been desiring for years,—that he should know when he began the study of medicine what he wanted to get out of that study. He could not do that until he had graduated as a dentist. He received his operative practice at the University of Pennsylvania, where individual ability I found could be recognized, and got this practice at an earlier age than he could have gotten it at either of the other schools. It has been demonstrated to us how the musician beginning at an early age becomes technically so perfect that his fingers accomplish the thought of his mind almost automatically. Let that musician begin later on in life and it can never be done. From that stand-point I draw a parallel with the dentist's work, and I believe that unless a dentist begins his technical work comparatively·early in life he will never succeed in his profession. Now, what is his profession, gentlemen? Suppose this room-full of practitioners were called in an hour from now to attend a case of broken lower jaw, how many of us are perfectly qualified to take that case in hand? How many of us would treat a case of cleft palate? I am sure I would not dare undertake Brown's operation. Right there is another cause that should call this body into relationship with the great medical body. I allude to these things, because it seems to me they have a bearing on the curriculum yet to be decided on. There are things in dental education which have been left behind which we should have with us, and one is private tutelage before the student ever undertakes to enter college. I have spent some time in the class-rooms in Harvard, and in those of other colleges, and have noted the difference in what I have seen of the students. I do not say that the classes graduated at Harvard would be any better able to do the work that a dental surgeon ought to feel himself called on to do than those from other schools; but I do know all too sadly that the dental graduate as a whole is not the man he ought to be. He is not sufficiently qualified by any manner of means to take charge of the oral cavity and to keep it in health.

Dr. M. L. Rhein, New York City.—These papers and this discussion and all the literature of our profession on this subject are most conclusive evidence of the correct assumption of our chairman in his paper on the crying need of symmetry in general education. My own impression in this matter is that the cause of the trouble is not in the professional education. The source is much deeper. It is in the primary methods, or pretences at methods of education to which the world has been accustomed; the education of youth from childhood up is in a very great progress of evolution at the present time, and has been progressing materially. It is impossible for us to arrive at any of the ideals that Professor Truman or Professor Hoff would like to see at the present time, and the main trouble is at the primary education. I differ entirely with the theory of Dr. Hoff, and which Dr. Bogue advanced, of taking up the general medical education later. That will not cure the trouble. The trouble can be reached if the education of youth is properly conducted. The greatest progress in this direction is the induction of manual training in the primary education. Manual training brought to its proper level is the true solution of this problem. If a child in its primary education has received the proper manual training, so that he becomes deft enough with his fingers as a child to do a piece of wood-carving or the work of the other departments, it will be as impossible for him to lose this deftness as it will be impossible for him to lose his skill on the ice, so easily acquired in childhood and so difficult in later life. Another thought which is uppermost in my mind in this direction is that it is impossible to make dentists. We can aid in the education of different classes of dentists, from very good ones, to certain inferior ones; and yet, out of certain material, we must recognize that it is impossible to produce any sort of dentists. The fact that so much

of that material is brought into the profession with the degree of
D.D.S. attached to the name is not to the credit of the institution
that such men should have passed three years there when it is self-
evident that they are unfit to ever become successful practitioners.
In view of this fact, last year, I was led to say that I was strongly
in favor of getting rid of all the poor colleges at any cost; that I
thought the ultimate interest of the profession would be enhanced
if any means were used to annihilate what is known as the commercial institute in dentistry. It is in these institutions that such
material is allowed to go through. I have no doubt that some of it
gets through the better grade of institution, but in no such proportion. I have stood aghast at the position Harvard has taken in this
matter. It is to me one of the most inconceivable things for an
institution of that character to do. I sympathize with everything
that Dr. Briggs has stated to us as being the position of Harvard,
but it is no excuse for Harvard's action. I agree with Dr. Briggs
that it may be a matter of discussion whether it is better to advance
the preliminary education, or whether it is better to advance the
course, but that discussion should have been entered into long before the actual meeting. There were two years of the discussion
before the meeting of the Association of Faculties, when Harvard
had an opportunity to consider that subject in a way that she failed
to do, or to lead any one to suppose that she would take the position
that would be utilized by the commercial institutions for the degra-
dation of dentistry. No one fails to realize that Harvard is not
allied with them, but they take advantage of the position which
Harvard has taken. As an earnest advocate for the highest advancement of dental education, I do not believe that it would suffer
one iota if at the meeting at Washington a large number of the
colleges would secede from the four years' course. I believe it
would result in the annihilation of the commercial colleges, because
the examining boards are in favor of the four years' course. Another point of interest was that referred to by Dr. Hoff,—the difficulty in securing instruction to the dental student from the medical
men. That is another point where education requires a great deal
of remedying in the future; that is, lack of proper education, not
only of the medical teacher, but of the medical student, because the
medical student must ultimately become the teacher. If he knows
nothing about the mouth he is not qualified to teach the groundwork of medical practice to future dentists or stomatologists.

Another point, and one which has been eloquently dilated on by Dr. Marshall: We know that we are not willing to take a position lower in the scale of the medical men, and yet we are placed in that position, because we have failed to keep up to the trend of evolution in medical education. Is there any reason why our education should be inferior to that of the medical institution? None in the least. Dr. Briggs is right there. That is where Harvard is right, and we are wrong. It is not only necessary for us to stand for a four years' course, but we must not present them with a calling that places dental practitioners on a more inferior basis than the medical men, if we would attract to our specialty the best of the youth of this country. We do that the moment we lower the standard of our entrance examinations in our institutions. I would like to emphasize this on the departments of the universities who are interested in the real uplift of the educational standard. It matters little how many students they may lose in a matter of this kind. It matters much whether they elevate the character of the material that is attracted to us. One of the curses of the general education to-day is that in the lower branches the teaching is uniform. The minds of the children are trained alike, and yet they are all totally different.

It is impossible to satisfy the desire of our friend Dr. Bogue in telling how we shall make the model dental education. I have simply tried to bring up a few of the defects; but I want to say that if the manual dexterity is acquired in childhood, the basic principles which should precede specialization can not fail to be properly acquired. I want to introduce a resolution as part of the discussion of this subject, as follows:

Resolved, The Section on Stomatology of the American Medical Association, in session at Atlantic City, sends its greetings to the National Association of Dental Faculties. We congratulate the Association on the completion of the first year of the advanced four years' course. We sincerely trust that having the honor and standing of the profession in your hands, no action will be taken that will tend to lower the advanced stand that has been taken.

I would like to have this Section send to them this expression and our hope that they will not falter in the position taken.

On motion, the resolution was adopted.

Dr. William Lederer, New York City.—Dr. Rhein said correctly, "Dentists are born." To my mind dentistry is both a science and an art. The man who is a scientist alone or the one who is a craftsman and an artist alone is not a dentist. Whether a course in a school is three or four years, that will not make him a better or a worse man. To have ideal conditions and to further dental education two factors are necessary, just as two factors are necessary to produce a work of art,—the artist and the material which he turns into a work of art. If the most ideal conditions prevail in the institutions, and the material which is entered is not capable of properly imbibing the teachings, the result will not be good dentists. Theory can be taught, but mechanical ability can not be taught, and, therefore, I should think the essential training would be a combination of the practice and the teaching. It is stated that there is only one school in this country whose degree enables a man to practise in Germany, and that is Ann Arbor. I am sure we have other schools in this country which turn out as able men as Ann Arbor. How they place the standard I do not know. Ann Arbor is a State institution. If some movement were started to create State institutions which can not be commercial, perhaps that would solve the problem, and we would have proper material and proper artists to do a work of art.

Dr. Edward C. Kirk.—I agree with Dr. Rhein that the great defect in the mind, in the career, in the qualification of the dental student for acquiring his education is the fault of his training in the kindergarten. I do not believe it is because the method is uniform, but because the method is faulty. You cannot make a mind elective that has not the power of election. That is what parents are for. Education is to be of use. We study arithmetic, and we go on farther with the relations of numbers until we get into higher mathematics. Only those whose calling demands the use of mathematics employ them. There is another use for mathematics,—the mental discipline. That is to get into the mind of that human being an appreciation of the fact that two and two make four—not three and seven-eighths or four and a quarter. It is to develop a respect for precision as an element of character. The great fault in the dental student is that he is not precise and does not reason logically and accurately. I had a talk with my colleague, Dr. Truman, on the bad use of English and the misspelling of these men. I kept in my examination markings a list of terms misspelled by American-born and educated students of our high schools. Dr. Truman tells me that it is a psychic state developed by the examination stress. He is very tender-hearted with his delinquents. I believe the training of the dentist should be begun in the kindergarten. There is room for us to suggest improvement in the methods of preliminary education. I agree also with Dr. Rhein that it is unsafe in the making of a dentist to postpone his manual training, and such manual training should be specific; it must be related to his calling as a dentist. I do not agree that a man should take a medical training as preparatory to dental education. I am of the opinion that we must superadd whatever he needs in the medical training. I also believe it is a mistake for a student to have his preparatory training in a dental office. Such training should be postgraduate. Under the present arrangement of the college curriculum we have the methods for training, which is a better plan than the old apprenticeship system. I think that any one who has looked at this thing conscientiously and who knows anything about the subject will agree that it is impossible to produce a dentist worthy of the name in less than four years under present conditions. I believe the whole reason why there is a desire on the part of the faculties (I except Harvard; I understand her position, and it has nothing to do with my remark; she has adopted a different plan of arriving at the same end) to revert to the three year's course is purely a commercial one. I know that there would have been no opposition to the four years' course had there not been a drop in the Freshmen classes of from fifty to seventy-five per cent. in many instances. That recalls to my mind one point referred to by the essayist,—that as a purely commercial proposition it pays to maintain the highest possible standard. There are enough decent, honest people in the world to back up such an effort, and on the principle that honesty is the best policy, even in the absence of any other moral consideration, it would pay. The main reason is, of course, that the four years' course makes better dentists.

Dr. George V. I. Brown.—I believe I am the real culprit. Mine happened to be the resolution passed in our Faculty Association for the four years' course. I believed in it very thoroughly then, and I believe in it even more now. I believe Harvard's going out last year was a mistake, and I hope that before very long the Association and Harvard will meet on common ground. The criticism of the kindergarten system refers to matters which we can not change. We have to deal with students who have been educated under a system, good or bad, that has been in existence, and it is well for us to help in rearranging the future. I believe we must and will have a four years' course. No matter whether one man who is more highly educated than another can learn more in six months or a year than the other, we must base our standard on the average. There is no question that the more a man trains his fingers in dental work the better, and no one will question that he can do more of that in four years than three. I believe that if we are doing our duty we will have a personal interest in the men under our care, and I believe we can do more to uplift them ethically in four years than in three. I have had to face the proposition of trying to make a dental student do in one year the same work that medical men were doing and do forty hours a week beside, and I found he could not do it. I am hopeful about this Faculty Association meeting. When the final issue has come on any question there have always been enough good men to carry what is right. So far as Harvard's position is concerned, the University of Iowa, Ann Arbor, and I daresay Pennsylvania, will have more than a full year more of instruction than they, but we are willing to suffer that disadvantage—if it is a disadvantage—for the sake of training much better men.

Dr. Eugene S. Talbot, Chicago.—I am glad that Harvard has taken the position she has. I am in favor of the four years' course, and I am sure that there is a great deal of good going to come out of this peculiar condition in which the profession stands. It is only by this friction that we arrive at results. I am going to discuss this subject on a little different plan from what most have spoken. They have been talking along the mechanics of dentistry. The question comes up at the present time, Is there not another side than the mechanics of dentistry? There was not when the first dental school was established. But it seems to me we know a little more along the line of stomatology than we knew sixty-four years ago, and the question arises, Are the dental colleges keeping pace with our present knowledge? We have been talking of the practice of dentistry as it is to-day. What will become of the practice of dentistry sixty-four years from now, if it progresses as it has in the last sixty-four years? Are we going to remain as mechanics and manipulators? It seems to me that there are two conditions at the present time that are uppermost in the minds of the dental profession,—decay of teeth and interstitial gingivitis. We have been studying decay of teeth as a local condition, and we have advanced far enough in the last few years to know that disease of the human body has a great deal to do with decay of teeth. We know that it has much to do with the saliva of the mouth, that it produces a change in the saliva. We know that pregnancy has much to do with decay of the teeth, also typhoid fever and pneumonia. Yet at the present time, although we have been teaching sixty-four years, we have not gotten down to the first principles of decay of the teeth and interstitial gingivitis. There is not a single dental college teaching the principles of the nervous system. What have we to say in regard to interstitial gingivitis? What do we know about intestinal fermentation, the great cause of gingivitis? I want to say to the teachers here that we have yet to learn the first principles of teaching these diseases, and we have got to introduce them in our schools. Until we have educated students we must have educated men in order that we can teach the students the diseases of the human body. We come to the point that some school, and I hope it will be Harvard, will take the lead and will require, first an academic degree; second, two years in pathology in our medical schools, and third, manipulation; and as soon as some university will teach men to become teachers to fill our dental colleges with men who are capable of teaching, we shall have better dental students.

Dr. G. V. I. Brown.—I agree with Dr. Talbot that we should have more of the teaching to which he refers. We have men here who have been teaching for years, and Dr. Talbot has said we do not teach about nervous diseases. I should like to know their statements on this question.

Dr. Talbot.—There are no chairs on the pathology of the nervous system.

Dr. Kirk.—We teach the nervous system, but I understood the secretary to lay down rather dogmatically that the perverted nervous system had as much to do with interstitial gingivitis, if not more than any other factor, except the local conditions. I think that is rather a broad statement, and there comes to the mind the proposition of which came first, the egg or the hen. There is such a thing as faulty metabolism, and that probably has something to do with the perverted nervous system. We have not taught that faulty action of the nervous system is the fundamental error, but we teach fundamentally that faulty metabolism is back of the whole disturbance.

Dr. E. C. Briggs, Boston.—I do not want you to think that
Harvard does not want four years, or that she is standing out
against it. That never has been the point. I think the time is
coming when Harvard will demand four years. The time is coming
when she will demand other things. While we felt that we could
not take every step at once, we felt that the step which we did take
was the next step to take. I can not deny the accusation that Dr.
Rhein made that this thing ought to have been threshed out before
the motion was carried to make four terms the course. It seemed
to me that Dr. Truman's remarks, stating that there were some
students whom he did not like to see go out as dentists, are an
argument for my point. You can not help getting men in who are
not fitted, and the men who go out are safer if they have had a
good preliminary education.

Dr. A. E. Baldwin, Chicago.—The question is not one of degrees; what we want is the education. Dr. Talbot is correct in
his statement that we should pay more attention to the definite
causes of the conditions and not content ourselves with the manipulative end. We have too many men in the profession whose minds
go no farther back than the work and the correction they can give
it. I do not think there is a man practising dentistry to-day or
being prepared for practice who is not the better for the broadest
kind of an education. In the medical school I saw as much evidence of manipulative skill as in the dental college. At the same
time, I do not mean to belittle the manipulative part of the education taught in our dental colleges. We do not occupy a progressive
field when we talk about going back to the pupilage system. That
can not go farther than the men. If the institutions are what we
suppose them to be they are a combination of the teaching of the
best men, and to go from them to the office of some fossilized person—of which, perhaps, I would be one—would be very foolish.
I have seen men of broad education who were failures in their
chosen vocation, but I do not lay it to the broad education. There
are some men who have a wonderful lack of education and who are
yet wonderful successes. Education is not a method of cramming
things in, but it is the drawing out of what is within. We will
have some failures even with four, or a ten years' course, but we
shall have more intellectual work done.

Dr. M. L. Rhein.—I am sure that all the gentlemen who spoke
of the manipulative point in educational acquirements had no in-

tention of objecting to the phase presented by Drs. Baldwin and Talbot. We realize that all the scientific attainment possible is valueless without the manipulative ability in our specialty. The two must go hand in hand. The point is that it is impossible to instil that manipulative ability if it is lacking in the personality of the individual, and one of the defects in our institutions is the absence of a method by which applicants may be received for a probationary period, and if it is found at the end of this time that they are out of their sphere, they may be rejected.

Dr. George F. Eames, Boston.—Dr. Baldwin has stated that education is a drawing out of what is within. My idea would be to ascertain the bent of a child while in the kindergarten and in his later education, taking a broad view to determine his probable choice of professions. Then when he has arrived at the age when he knows what he wants there will be some data of value. It is not a degree; it is not a number of years, but it is the qualification of the individual to be in our specialty, and an American citizen, and when he has developed equally and symmetrically in all of these lines, he has attained the object, and it is for us to decide the time spent in preliminary education, and how much within the college walls. I believe a man who has it within him to be a success, must escape the bonds and rules of an institution by the time he is twenty-five years of age. We have not a lease on life. If we increase the length of the course, we do not have the life in proportion.

ACADEMY OF STOMATOLOGY.

A REGULAR meeting of the Academy of Stomatology of Philadelphia was held at its room, 1731 Chestnut Street, on the evening of April 26, 1904, the President, Dr. L. Foster Jack, in the chair. A paper, entitled " The Superiority of High-Fusing Porcelain for restoring Teeth," was read by Dr. Herbert Locke Wheeler, of New York City.

(For Dr. Wheeler's paper, see page 414.)

Dr. Gardiner.—I have listened with a great deal of interest to the paper, and while I have been using porcelain to a considerable extent for a number of years, I have made no comparative tests, and I do not feel that I am qualified to discuss the paper along the lines the essayist has chosen.

Dr. E. C. Kirk.—This paper seems important in that it represents a stage in the development of our ideas about the use of porcelain which we must necessarily take up and go through before we really know anything at all about the subject of porcelain, which seems quite analagous to that of amalgam. There we have a composite material. Dentists have been using it since 1835 or 1840, and we have been placing amalgam in teeth in an empirical, haphazard sort of way, assuming that amalgam was a uniform thing and that any combination of metals with mercury made an amalgam which for our purposes was the same as any other amalgam. After awhile we experienced many failures as the result of the fact that it was almost as variable in composition, considering the way in which it was manipulated, as the nondescript material served in boarding-houses under the name of "hash." Then we did what should have been done long before, and that was to investigate this material in order that we might obtain a definite knowledge of its properties as data to work upon. So, the profession has taken up enthusiastically the question of porcelain, because the material has qualities that recommend it and offer relief from two things, of which we should have been relieved long ago,—viz., the drudgery of hammering gold into teeth, and the barbaric display of gold in the human denture. We took it up heartily, because of its artistic quality and for relief from amalgam and gold.

We have had dealt out to us a variety of things called porcelain, and the essayist has truthfully directed our attention to the fact that all these things supplied as porcelain are by no means porcelain. We have no right to classify them under such a general term as that.

It is true that the distinction between high- and low-fusing bodies, based upon the melting-point of gold, is an arbitrary distinction. As the essayist says, it is difficult or almost impossible to say where glass begins and porcelain ends, as it is difficult to say where iron leaves off and steel begins. It is true that the tendency of so-called low-fusing porcelains, which are nothing more than modified glasses, to disintegrate in the fluids of the mouth is due to their basic element, potash or soda, on which depends their low-fusing quality. I do not know much about porcelain and glass in relation to inlay work, but there are some data in relation to glass and porcelain which have a distinct bearing on the case. It is not generally known to those who have not investigated the subject that glass will disintegrate even under the action of distilled water, and in contact with certain corrosive fluids, strong alkaline solutions, and strong or even dilute acids; so that in the storing of chemicals and in the production of chemical glassware it is of the utmost importance, particularly in photographic work, to have a special composition of glass that will not disintegrate under this influence and contaminate the contents of the vessels, spoiling them as chemical reagents. The disintegration of glass under these circumstances is well known in chemical laboratories. If this be true of glassware, it is also true of these low-fusing porcelains.

Another item of importance is in regard to the use of felspar and the disintegration of this felsparic rock we speak of as a name for a class of minerals as complex as the alums. The tendency of this material to disintegrate is in proportion to its alkalinity. That is an important question in relation to the manufacture of porcelain. It is undoubtedly true that the composition of this material is one which greatly affects its durability; and it is equally true that the higher the fusing-point, the less tendency is there to disintegrate. We are only finding this out in dentistry by experience. We should have known that in advance from the study of other related facts. It is also true that the question of preservation of color in the inlay under the high temperature of the furnace depends largely upon the composition, and also upon the fusing-point. The more fluid the porcelain glass becomes—the so-called porcelain glass—the more tendency there is for the oxides which form the color ingredient to undergo chemical changes that cause their disappearance.

I am very glad, indeed, that the essayist has brought this kind of a subject before us, because it shows that an effort is being made to solve this problem on lines which will eventually relieve us from the danger of making very serious mistakes in the use of these substances. It is a serious mistake to have these accidents with so-called porcelain materials, because then all we hear is "Porcelain is no good;" "Porcelain has been a failure in my hands," etc., and you will find that the man has not used it intelligently or that he has used an improper material, and he therefore condemns the whole process. If we can know scientifically and practically what we should concerning porcelain, it will take the place it ought to make for itself.

Dr. Hickman.—I have enjoyed this paper, and I have learned a great deal from it. I came here, however, to be converted, and I am still among the lost. I cannot understand why it is that these other Dresden disciples do not speak, because the room is full of them. It does seem to me a strange thing that these failures of the low-fusing porcelain, the decompositions of the low-fusing porcelain, and these accidents on account of which porcelain is condemned, all come through the men who use the high-fusing porcelain. You do not often hear of the man who is using the low-fusing porcelain speak of this continual disintegration.

The essayist speaks of the careless manner in which we use the low-fusing porcelain as being one of the principal things against it. That is just the trouble. It is more difficult to make a good low-fusing porcelain inlay than to make a high-fusing one. Dr. Head is a high-fusing porcelain worker and he has had several men at conventions as exhibitors of the work, and at any angle you can see particles of food between the teeth. There is a gentleman in the room, who is much too modest to speak, who has put in at least a dozen porcelain inlays in one mouth, and at two feet from that patient I will defy any one to tell that the teeth have been filled. That is done with Jenkins low-fusing porcelain. He has done the most beautiful porcelain work in Philadelphia, but he does it with low-fusing porcelain and a gas-furnace. I do not use a gas-furnace entirely, especially when I bake porcelain on crowns. I use the Jenkins porcelain and an electric furnace. When you heat the whole body there is not the danger of fracture spoken of by the essayist, and I have yet to see a fracture of that kind. Only a short time ago while using a tooth made by the Consolidated Dental Manufacturing Company, in baking some Jenkins porcelain upon it, the body of the tooth split. Part of the enamel of the tooth broke off and was left on the porcelain instead of splitting off at the joint. I frequently use the Jenkins body in fitting a porcelain crown to a root, and I have yet to see an accident of that kind.

Dr. Gaylord.—I know from what Dr. Hickman said that the failures of low-fusing porcelain come from the men who are advocates of high-fusing porcelain, and Dr. Wheeler is going to tell him that the reason they are using the high-fusing is because they failed with the low. I do not think that is so. I cannot be a close-communionist, or a hard-shell, but am more of a universalist and so I use both high- and low-fusing. I feel that both have a place in dentistry, that failures are bound to exist in the use of both, but that satisfactory and good results can be produced with either.

I do not think that all of the arguments against low-fusing bodies will stand muster. I have yet to see Jenkins porcelain or any other low-fusing porcelain disintegrate in the mouth. I have had the pleasure of doing work for a family who some five years ago had porcelain work done by Dr. Jenkins himself, and the fillings have certainly stood five years' wear in the most beautiful manner. The surface of the porcelain is as perfect as any one could wish it to be. The lustre is good, and there is not a sign of disintegration. I do not mean to say that disintegration will not occur with low-fusing body, but I have yet to see it. If low-fusing porcelain is properly used it will turn out a good filling-material and one which will last. It is not so much what we use as how we use it. I could not well get on without using porcelain in my office. I am not an enthusiast, but when the opportunity presents itself I put porcelain in; sometimes the high-fusing, sometimes the low-fusing.

I read a little article in a Western dental journal in regard to the swaging of the matrix, which I have tried and found very helpful. The idea is to first make a pellet of cotton and carry the matrix to the bottom of the cavity, then to withdraw the cotton and finish the swaging with gum camphor. It is an ideal material to swage out the matrix. Fill the cavity nearly full before paying much attention to the margins. After the edges are worked down, finally fill the cavity with camphor. Your matrix has a stable material which helps to retain its form while removing it. The camphor burns out, leaving no ash, and the matrix is perfectly clean.

. *Dr. Wheeler* (closing).—Dr. Gaylord very kindly made my answer on one point. I will continue what he had in mind. I have not said that low-fusing porcelain would not serve the purpose for which it was used in any or all cases, but I do know that the first case of disintegration in Jenkins porcelain I ever saw was put in by Dr. Jenkins himself at his office in Dresden. I know a young man in New York who has one of the most desirable practices in America, and he says that Jenkins enamel sometimes disintegrates in his hands and turns black. It does not go to pieces, but it loses any claim to being æsthetic that it may have had when put in. I have sometimes thought that its tendency to be opaque might be an advantage in certain cases, because backing it with opaque cement does not change its shade so badly as high-fusing material.

The question is, there are certain principles that I am sure are true, for instance, phenol sodique, if put into a bottle with a glass stopper, will make it difficult to remove the stopper. This shows you what a strongly alkaline fluid will do against glass. Dr. Kirk says it is hard to tell where glass ends and porcelain begins. I have given a definition something like this, which, to my mind, in a general way describes the situation as clearly as anything I have ever seen. I contend that anything in which all the ingredients fuse in the baking is a glass; but, if proportionate parts of that fusible material are not fused, and remain, as it were, as a sort of matrix or framework, that is a porcelain. It is possible, you must remember, to take silica, and by adding a sufficient quantity of basic alkaline salt, to dissolve the whole thing and make it into glass, because, so far as I know, the compounds are soluble in alkaline solutions.

In the matter of shrinkage, I have this afternoon learned from Dr. Guilford that in some experiments he had made, after a certain temperature there is no more shrinkage. This was never distinctly settled to my mind before. I have often wondered if my first bakes, which I never carry to a thoroughly smooth glaze, would shrink. I find that when you get to the point where it is baked, even though not glazed, the shrinkage ends; that is, in a true porcelain. Of course, you get a great change of shape with a glass. Drs. Hickman and Gaylord spoke about the high-fusing people being the ones who found fault with, or knew of cases of disintegration of low-fusing enamel. I hardly think that is so. I think any one who has kept a careful record of his work with low-fusing material will find cases in which there are marks of disintegration taking place. It is like cement. There may be mouths in which it never occurs, but again there are mouths in which it will occur. The line between high- and low-fusing bodies is an indistinct one, and there are a great many conditions that have a bearing on the question of the length of service of a porcelain inlay. The lower the point at which you get the glaze, the greater the probability that you are going to have the surface affected. All my experiments will bear me out in this.

OTTO E. INGLIS,
Editor Academy of Stomatology.

F. D. I. INTERNATIONAL DENTAL FEDERATION— FOURTH ANNUAL SESSION.

THE International Dental Federation convened on Friday, August 26, 1904, in Music Hall, Coliseum Building, St. Louis, Mo. The meeting was called to order by the President, Dr. Charles Godon, Paris.

He introduced Dr. William Conrad, St. Louis, who delivered the welcoming address on behalf of the dental profession of the State of Missouri and of the city of St. Louis. To his hospitable and fraternal remarks, the chairman, Dr. Godon, responded as follows:

Members of the International Dental Federation, ladies, and gentlemen, the first thought I wish to express here on behalf of the International Dental Federation is one of admiration for your great nation, your mighty republic, to which are bound by so many ties of sympathy and gratitude all citizens, the admirers of liberty, progress, and civilization. Your magnificent exhibition constitutes a new proof of the progressive genius of the American nation and deserves a leading place among the accomplishments of human activity. We acknowledge a debt of gratitude to the American dental profession, to which modern dentistry owes so much, and to its eminent representative members who are here with us.

Hail to the members of the dental profession throughout the world who so kindly responded to our invitation, and who are now with us as members of the Executive Council. While speaking of these devoted fellow-workers in this great international task, let us not forget those who, because of unavoidable circumstances, are prevented from being with us at this time, likewise those who have left us forever.

To-day we inaugurate in St. Louis the session that finishes the work of the first period of the F. D. I. We shall soon have to report to the Fourth International Dental Congress upon the mission intrusted to us by the Third International Dental Congress, and will turn over to them our powers.

I shall not attempt to make a long report of the work of our body during that period of four years. That is the duty of our general secretary and devoted co-laborer, Dr. E. Sauvez, who has from the beginning worked indefatigably for the benefit of the cause. I only wish to recall to your minds the principal phases through which the F. D. I. has passed in its first period of existence. It originated in Paris, in 1900, through the enthusiasm of the twelve hundred congressists from every corner of the globe. It uttered its first lispings in Cambridge the following year—in that old English university, under the presidency of the eminent professor of physiology, Sir Michael Foster, who then determined the real philosophy of education as related to dental training, defining and limiting the sphere of influence of the F. D. I. in order to make of it a great international advisory council of dentistry. The next meeting took place in Stockholm, where, in the midst of discussions which had in view the planning of an international dental curriculum and the determining of the best conditions under which public dental services should be carried out for the greatest and most effective benefits to suffering humanity, it was decided that it should be in St. Louis that the Fourth International Dental Congress should be held. From that decision ensued a long, feverish, and fruitful contention about the interpretation to be given to the powers of the Federation or its representative members, and about the conditions of its participation in different kinds of professional movements. That discussion lasted over two years, and the session of Madrid in 1903 was almost exclusively devoted to it.

I have said feverish, inasmuch as it has caused deep discussions in our profession, especially in the United States, and fruitful also, because thus its existence has been made manifest to every one, and its importance as a factor in the proceedings of professional nature has been made equally evident.

We have therefore been enabled to prepare a constitution and a set of by-laws, which, when confirmed by the next Congress, will assure, I hope, the success of its future work.

In this, the twentieth century, these international federations constitute a new organism necessary not only to dentistry, but to all departments of professional and scientific activity. When men thus meet in great peaceful sessions and universal expositions and congresses, wholly given up to the pleasure of exchanging ideas, and of communicating the result of their works and investigations, they must forget political and geographical limits and think only of the greatest good that may be derived for the benefit of all, regardless of nationality or local susceptibilities.

As new agents in the development of progress in civilization these great federations do not interfere with national questions, for those remain under the safe keeping of political and diplomatic bodies; but their activities take place on the high plane of human science, where territorial divisions have no action, where the end can be only peaceful because the contests are only of the intellect, and where the presiding goddess is like the statue of Liberty in the harbor of New York, having in one hand the torch of truth, and in the other the olive branch—both symbols of true human fraternity.

The President then called on Dr. C. C. Chittenden, Madison, Wis., president of the National Dental Association, who in a few appropriate words expressed his admiration for the work and purposes of the F. D. I.

Dr. H. A. Smith, Cincinnati, Ohio, was the next speaker. He made a short address, in which he referred to the far-reaching influence of the Federation's work and to his pleasure and satisfaction that such an eminent body of men should meet upon American soil.

Dr. Godon then called on Dr. Sauvez, the Secretary-General, who read an able and carefully prepared report, in which he reviewed the work of the F. D. I. from its organization to the present time.

After the reading of the Secretary's annual report, addresses were made by Dr. José J. Rojo, Mexico; Dr. Vincenzo Guerini, Italy; Dr. Florestan Aguilar, Spain; Dr. Alfred Burne, Australia; Dr. John Grevers, Holland; Dr. L. C. Bryan, Switzerland; Dr. N. S. Jenkins, Germany; Dr. R. B. Weiser, Austria; Dr. J. Y. Crawford, Nashville, Tenn.; Dr. J. D. Patterson, Kansas City, Mo.; Dr. H. B. Tileston, Louisville, Ky., and Dr. J. J. Reid, president of the National Association of Dental Examiners.

In the afternoon the several commissions which together constitute the International Dental Federation held separate sessions in the same building. The deliberations of the International Commission of Education were presided over by Dr. Truman W. Brophy, Chicago; those of the International Commission of Hygiene and Public Dental Service by Dr. N. S. Jenkins, Dresden, Germany; those of the Commission on International Dental Press by Dr. A. W. Harlan, New York, in the absence of the regular chairman, Dr. Elof Förberg, Stockholm, Sweden.

At the afternoon sessions and at those held on the following

day papers were presented and read before the respective commissions,—by Dr. Charles Godon, on "Dental Education in France;"
by Dr. William Mitchell, of London, on "Technical Education;"
by Dr. W. E. Boardman, Boston, on "The Necessity for Establishing Libraries in Dental Schools;" by Dr. C. N. Johnson, Chicago,
Ill., "A Brief Consideration of the Grading of Students in Dental
Colleges;" by Dr. H. L. Banzhaf, Milwaukee, Wis., on "International Dental Education;" by Dr. A. H. Thompson, Topeka,
Kan., on "The Development of Dental Education in the West;"
by Dr. Gordon White, Nashville, Tenn., on "The Present Status
of Dental Education in the United States;" by Dr. R. B. Weiser,
Vienna, Austria, on "Education;" by Dr. Charles Godon, on
"Emergency Dentistry and Complete Dentistry for the Poor;" by
Dr. Burton Lee Thorpe, St. Louis, Mo., on "The *American Jour-
nal of Dental Science* and its Influence;" and by Dr. J. Endelman,
Philadelphia, Pa., on the "International Federation Bulletin."

The Executive Council held several business meetings, and at
the last one, held in the Coliseum Building on Saturday, September 3, prior to the closing of the Congress the following officers
were elected:

Honorary President, Charles Godon, Paris; President, W. D.
Miller, Berlin; First Vice-President, Emile Sauvez, Paris; Second
Vice-President, R. B. Weiser, Vienna; Third Vice-President (to
be elected by the British Dental Association); Secretary-General,
Edward C. Kirk, Philadelphia; Assistant Secretaries, Shaffer-
Stuckert, Frankfort, Paul Guye, Geneva, and Burton Lee Thorpe,
St. Louis; Treasurer, Florestan Aguilar, Madrid.

The present Executive Council is composed of fifty members,
each country affiliated with the Federation being represented by a
number of members varying from one as the minimum to five as
the maximum.

The present representatives of the United States, five in num-
ber, were elected by the National Dental Association at its meeting
held in the Coliseum Building, September 2. They are William
Carr, New York; B. Holly Smith, Baltimore; Edward C. Kirk,
Philadelphia; A. W. Harlan, New York; Burton Lee Thorpe, St.
Louis.

The next meeting of the Federation will be held in Switzerland
in 1905, the date and the city to be announced in the near future.

RULES AND REGULATIONS OF THE INTERNATIONAL DENTAL FEDERA-
TION, AS APPROVED BY THE FOURTH INTERNATIONAL DENTAL
CONGRESS, AT ST. LOUIS, MO.

Preamble.

(a) The International Dental Federation is an association or
universal union of national dental societies and those affiliated
therewith.

(b) The official title adopted is " Fédération Dentaire Internationale," abridged " F. D. I."

(c) The International Dental Federation is a permanent international body existing in the interim between international dental
congresses.

(d) It is governed by an Executive Council, composed of delegates representing different countries (receiving appointment from
the preceding congress). This Council organizes various Commissions that it deems will be beneficial to the advancement of dental
science in any of its phases; it is at the same time an advisory
committee on international affairs.

(e) The F. D. I. will hold a general meeting preceding the
opening of each international dental congress.

(f) The Executive Council and the various Commissions will
hold annual meetings, the time and place to be selected at the close
of each meeting.

(g) *Authority creating the F. D. I.:* Resolutions passed by the
Third International Dental Congress (Paris, France), August 14,
1900,—viz.:

" *Resolution 11.* There shall be organized an International
Dental Federation.

" *Resolution 12.* The national committees appointed to this
Congress will continue in office and will constitute the International
Dental Federation."

Rules and Regulations.

ARTICLE I.—The International Dental Federation was organized by the national committees present at the Third International
Dental Congress, at Paris, in 1900, and was created in conformity
with Resolutions 11 and 12 passed by the general meeting on the
closing day of the aforesaid Congress, August 14, 1900.

ART. II.—The objects of the Federation are as follows:

(a) The acceptance or rejection of invitations made by various countries to hold a regular International Dental Congress, and to fix the date and place where such congress shall be held.

(b) To maintain and strengthen the ties that bind the National Societies to each other.

(c) The organization of such International Commissions as it may deem necessary to create.

(d) In a general way, to promote the organization of bodies that will contribute to the advancement of odontological science throughout the world.

ART. III.—The International Dental Federation consists of—

(a) All the national committees gathered in Paris in 1900, or their successors.

(b) Associations or societies giving their adhesion to international dental congresses, and accepting these Rules and Regulations or sending their concurrence in them.

(c) Societies, or groups of societies, which may officially signify their acquiescence in these Rules and Regulations, and which are acceptable to the Executive Council.

ART. IV.—National dental associations or societies, or, in the absence of such, persons desiring to become identified with the F. D. I., should send their acceptance of the present Rules and Regulations. Such applications will be acted upon by the Executive Council, who will accept them as members of the Federation.

ART. V.—The general meeting of the F. D. I. will take place before the opening of each International Dental Congress. It will be composed of delegates from national or other societies. Extraordinary meetings may be called for special reasons by the Executive Council.

ART. VI.—The Executive Council may admit as members of the Federation—

(1) Members regularly appointed by societies.

(2) Honorary members.

(3) Persons in good professional standing who have been members of international dental congresses, and who shall subscribe to these Rules and Regulations.

ART. VII.—The programme for these meetings will be prepared by the Executive Council. It will deal with matters emanating from national or other societies, or with questions proposed by the

Council. Notices will be sent at least one month before these meetings to all affiliated societies, national or local.

Art. VIII.—The right of voting pertains to the regularly appointed delegates. Upon the request of representatives of at least two national dental associations, the vote may be taken by the said regularly appointed delegates in the mode of one vote for each country.

Art. IX.—The annual meetings of the Executive Council, and of the various commissions, are governed by the preceding Rules and Regulations.

Art. X.—The F. D. I. is composed of an Executive Council, as follows:

(1) Fifty original members, chosen by the Congress,—that is to say, for each country as a minimum one member, with a maximum of five members.

(2) In case of vacancy, by resignation, death, or other cause, the Council will ask the respective national dental association to fill the place of the missing member.

(3) The powers of the Executive Council will expire upon the opening of each International Dental Congress.

(4) The Council will hand over to a special committee appointed by the Congress all of its documents and records, at the time of opening of the Congress, the said committee receipting for the same.

(5) The treasurer of the F. D. I. will hold office until his successor is appointed.

Art. XI.—The Council is governed by nine officers, as follows:

(1) A president.

(2) Three vice-presidents.

(3) A secretary-general.

(4) Three assistant secretaries.

(5) A treasurer.

The officers of the Council are *ex officio* members of all commissions, and will direct them until they are properly organized.

Art. XII.—The duty of the Executive Council is—

(a) To supervise the execution of the rules of the Federation.

(b) To fix the place and date of annual meetings, and of International Dental Congresses.

(c) To organize various International Commissions.

(d) To supervise the carrying out of decisions made by the F. D. I.

(e) To examine propositions and resolutions offered by national committees, associations, or other societies.

The Council will keep all affiliated bodies informed of their work through the Bulletin of the Executive Council, which will be published in at least four languages,—viz., French, German, English, and Spanish.

ART. XIII.—The Council has already named several special Commissions, as follows:·

(1) A Commission on Education.

(2) A Commission on Hygiene and Public Dental Service.

(3) A Commission on International Dental Press.

And it will organize a Commission on Professional Jurisprudence, Deontology, and Nomenclature.

ART. XIV.—The sources of income of the F. D. I. are as follows:

(1) By dues from the members,—to wit: Members of the Executive Council (per year), $10.00; members of Commissions (per year), $5.00; honorary members and all others (per year), $5.00.

(2) Appropriations by Congresses.

(3) Subscriptions, gifts from governments or municipalities, from national associations, and from individuals.

ART. XV.—In case of deficit, the expenses of the F. D. I. shall be provided for by equal assessment on all societies having membership. Any excess above the receipts will be turned over to the next Dental Congress. The Council will give a detailed statement of receipts and expenditures to every Congress.

ART. XVI.—The Executive Council will send to the Congress during its sessions a list of those members best qualified to carry on the international work of the F. D. I.

ART. XVII.—

(1) International Dental Congresses shall be organized by a committee, composed of dentists, who shall be chosen as follows:

One-third of its membership shall be appointed by the Executive Council of the F. D. I.; the other two-thirds shall be appointed by the inviting dental bodies. The committee so composed shall constitute the Committee of Organization, all the members of which shall have the same powers.

(2) At the first meeting of the Committee of Organization they shall organize and select the following officers of the com-

mittee: One president; two vice-presidents; one secretary-general; one treasurer.

(3) The Executive Council of the F. D. I. has full power to decide all questions in dispute arising in the Committee of Organization.

ART. XVIII.—These Rules are operative during the periods between regular Congresses. They are subject to revision by the succeeding Congress.

FOURTH INTERNATIONAL DENTAL CONGRESS, ST. LOUIS, MO., AUGUST 29 TO SEPTEMBER 3, 1904.

Opening Session—Monday, August 29, 1904.

THE first general session was called to order at 11 A.M. Monday, August 29, by Hon. Howard J. Rogers, Director of Congresses of the Universal Exposition.

Rev. H. H. Gregg, St. Louis, invoked divine blessings on the deliberations of the Congress.

Hon. Howard J. Rogers, in opening the Congress, and welcoming the members on behalf of the Universal Exposition, spoke as follows:

MEMBERS OF THE FOURTH INTERNATIONAL DENTAL CONGRESS, LADIES, AND GENTLEMEN,—It gives me great pleasure to welcome you to this city to-day. To the members of the Fourth International Dental Congress; to the members of the National Dental Association; to the foreign delegates who are accredited by their respective governments; to the members of the profession, whether in this country or abroad, the Exposition extends a most cordial welcome, because we are glad to have you with us.

The profession of dentistry has made enormous strides during the past ten years, and our States are busily engaged at the present time in passing laws which shall govern the entrance to the study of this profession, and which shall improve the curriculum and govern the entrance to the profession itself. We expect, therefore, that from your sessions this week much of good and much of profit will accrue to this and the various States connected with your profession, and we expect from a legislative stand-point to receive valuable advice in framing proper laws for the development of dentistry. We hope, however, from an exposition stand-point, that you will find time during your deliberations to visit us at the great Exposition in the western part of the city, which should appeal to you sympathetically because it has been promoted upon educational lines. Our appeal to the government for funds, to foreign governments for co-operation, to the States of the Union for support, has been based upon this plea of education,—of course, meant in its broadest sense,—the education which comes to the people from observing arts and architecture, from exhibits which we have grouped together with due regard to their interrelation and interdependence, whereby the raw material is taken and under the eyes transposed into the finished article ready for the markets of the world. These exhibits have all been prepared with great expense and care, and we hope that you will avail yourselves of the opportunities there presented. If you are seeking for mental de-velopment this week, you will find it, I am sure, in the fifteen large buildings, crowded with the best things from all parts of the world, and from the many State and country exhibits surrounding them. If you are in search of physical development, you will find it, I am sure, while roaming over the twelve hundred acres comprised in the Exposition grounds. If you are seeking for relaxation and rest, we have to commend you to that apparatus of amusement, the Pike. All this we extend to you.

A very material part of the development of this Exposition has been a series of congresses and conventions. We have had some-thing like two hundred conventions held under the Exposition auspices. To these we have given every opportunity and attention to make it a satisfactory meeting-place. We have scheduled twenty international congresses connected with the different sciences and professions, and these will culminate in the latter part of next month in the great Congress of Arts and Sciences which can be designated as a symposium of the scientific work of the world.

The Fourth International Dental Congress is the third in number of this great series of international congresses, and per-haps the greatest of any preceding it. In the organization of these various congresses it has been our policy to work through the national association of this country allied with that specialty, believing that it was best to do so because it would bring the people interested in that science or in that profession closely in touch with its development, and furthermore because we believed that the best interests of the Exposition and of the profession concerned would be promoted simultaneously. For that reason we have worked in your own case through the National Dental Association, and made the committee appointed by that Association our Committee of Organization, and we have given them every support, believing that they represented the best element of the profession in all parts of the country, or else they would not have been certified to by the National Association.

No one who has not had experience in the development and promotion of a great international congress can have any idea of the amount of work, the amount of time, and the amount of sacrifice necessary to bring it to a consummation. I venture to say that if every member of the Committee of Organization could have known two years ago what they know to-day of what was required of them in work, money, and effort, they would all have been very reluctant to accept the commission. It means a great deal of hard work and much criticism. Every committee of organization, however, must have two things fixed before them in order to bring about a successful congress. They must have a programme which in strength and timeliness of subject-matters should be of special interest to its profession. It must also bring together an audience capable of appreciating that programme. These two objects must be sought, and I would be remiss of my duty and profligate of my opportunities if I did not take this occasion on the part of the Exposition to render thanks to the Committee of Organization for the magnificent work they have done since they were appointed. To the chairman, who has looked particularly after the funds and the many and varied details of organization, all of which have been conducted with consummate executive ability; to the secretary, who has had a correspondence which runs into reams and reams of paper; to every member of the Committee of Organization, who has done well and to the best of his ability the particular duty ascribed to him,—again on the part of the Exposition I express our appreciation of their work.

We come now, gentlemen, to the permanent organization of the Fourth International Dental Congress. Following the procedure which has obtained in all of the other international congresses held here in our city under our auspices, some time ago we instructed the Committee of Organization to make a permanent roster of officers to preside over this convention, believing that by so doing we were contributing to the stability of the Congress, to the contentment of individuals, and to the permanence of the programme, and that we were working for the best interests of the Congress. We have found, however, that there is a strong opinion among the members of this convention—whose opinion we most highly respect —that the report of the nominating committee of the Committee of Organization should be submitted to your honorable body for ratification (applause), and at the special request of the chairman of the Committee of Organization, Dr. Burkhart, and at the request, passed in due form, of the committee, we will now rescind that former order, and present to this convention the nominations individually, so that there may be an expression of opinion as to the gentlemen who shall preside over you during the Congress.

The question therefore is, What action shall be taken upon the original report of the nominating committee, certified to us in due form by the Committee of Organization, nominating Dr. H. J. Burkhart for President of the Fourth International Dental Congress?

Dr. B. Holly Smith, Baltimore, Md.—Mr. Director, it is more than pleasant for those who have been interested in the organization of this Congress to have your public commendation of the work of the Organization Committee.

Townsend, in a little book entitled " The Art of Speech," quotes from an unknown writer the following: " The ball of discord has been thrown in our midst, and unless it be nipped in the bud it will burst into a conflagration that will deluge the world." Mr. Director, I cite this quotation because it is my personal desire that you should not regard these evidences of contention as a serious matter. It may be that some simple men in this audience may have a ball or two in their pockets, but this ball, if it exist, is not of a kind with which to start a fire, nor, if there should be some little balls of feeling, is there any probability that they will deluge the world and interfere with the work of this Congress. I have personally known some of the members of this committee for a number of years, the chairman especially, before he became a practitioner of dentistry. I have known him to be an honorable, upright, conscientious, energetic man in all of his professional work, and I feel that this Congress will do itself credit, and do the graceful thing in honoring him who has borne the brunt of the work of organizing this Congress; and I therefore move you, Mr. Director, that the action of the nominating committee in nominating him for the presidency of this Congress be confirmed, and that Dr. H. J. Burkhart be elected President. (Applause.)

Dr. R. H. Hofheinz, Rochester, N. Y.—Mr. Director, as a member of the Committee of Organization, of which you have spoken so flatteringly and appreciatively, I take great pleasure in seconding the motion of Dr. Smith that the action of the nominating committee be confirmed, and that Dr. Burkhart be elected the President of the Fourth International Dental Congress.

Mr. Rogers.—The question before the house is, Shall the action of the nominating committee for the presidency of this Congress, as recommended by the Committee of Organization, be ratified?

The motion was carried, and Mr. Rogers declared the action of the nominating committee in nominating Dr. Burkhart for President ratified and adopted.

Dr. C. N. Johnson, Chicago.—Mr. Director, I should like to move that this motion be made unanimous.

Mr. Rogers put the motion, and the election of Dr. Burkhart for President was made unanimous.

Dr. Burkhart was escorted to the platform, and Mr. Rogers, introduced him as follows: " Gentlemen of the convention, I have the honor to introduce to you your presiding officer, Dr. H. J. Burkhart." (Applause.)

Dr. Burkhart.—Gentlemen of the Fourth International Dental Congress, I thank you deeply for this expression of confidence, and for confirming the action of the nominating committee and the work which that committee has tried to do conscientiously and for the best interests of this Congress.

The next order of business will be the election of the Secretary-General.

Dr. James Truman, Philadelphia, Pa.—Mr. President, I wish to nominate for the office of Secretary-General Dr. Edward C. Kirk, of Philadelphia. (Applause.) I take great pleasure in saying that Dr. Kirk has from the very inception of this movement done a large portion of the work connected with it. By day and by night that gentleman has worked faithfully up to the present moment, and he resigned from the Secretary's work simply because be found that the committee had decided to elect the officers of the Congress permanently, and because of the fact that his word, which had been sent broadcast over the world, was pledged to the

principle that the Congress would elect its own officers. He had
said that the Congress would and should elect its own officers, and
therefore he would not allow his name to be used when the time for
electing officers came. Now, the question before you is whether
you will elect this man, who has done so much for this Congress,
or elect some one else. I have no objection to that some one else,
but I do object to allowing an individual who has accomplished so
much to be overlooked by the Congress. I do not care personally
who the officers of this Congress are; that is not my object—my
desire is for the advancement of the dental profession scientifically;
but I want you to understand that when a man has done all that
Dr. Kirk has done for this Congress, it is our right and our duty
to elect him, and I therefore nominate him for Secretary-General
of the Fourth International Dental Congress. (Applause.)

Dr. E. T. Darby, Philadelphia, Pa.—Mr. President, it gives me
great pleasure to second the nomination which has been made for
Dr. Kirk as the Secretary-General of the Fourth International
Dental Congress. (Applause.)

Dr. G. V. I. Brown, Milwaukee, Wis.—Mr. President, the
motion is out of order. The method of procedure begun by Mr.
Rogers was that each of these nominations be submitted to the
Congress for ratification or non-ratification of the action of the
Committee of Organization.

Dr. William Conrad, St. Louis, Mo.—As a member of the committee which nominated the officers for the Fourth International
Dental Congress I would state that we nominated Dr. Burkhart
for President, Dr. Kirk for Secretary-General, and Dr. Finley
for Treasurer. Dr. Kirk resigned his position after being elected,
and Dr. A. W. Harlan was elected to take his place. I move, Mr.
President, that this Congress indorse the action of the nominating
committee in nominating Dr. A. W. Harlan for Secretary-General.

The motion was seconded by Dr. J. Y. Crawford, Nashville,
Tenn.

Dr. Conrad's motion was lost.

Dr. Truman.—Mr. President, I now renew my nomination of
Dr. E. C. Kirk for Secretary-General of the Congress.

Dr. William Conrad, St. Louis.—I nominate Dr. A. W. Harlan
for Secretary-General of the Fourth International Congress.

A rising vote was taken on the two nominees, and resulted in
the election of Dr. Kirk.

Dr. E. C. Kirk was escorted to the stage, and was presented to the audience by the President.

Dr. E. C. Kirk.—My friends, I have neither the strength nor nervous energy to at this moment say more than that I· thank you from the bottom of my heart for two things: First, for all· that this means of personal regard and confidence; and second, that it represents, I believe, the allegiance to the principle which has been so gracefully conceded by the Committee of Organization,—namely, the right of every man to express his views upon this question. (Applause.)

The President.—The next order of business is the ratification of the action of the nominating committee in nominating Dr. M. F. Finley for Treasurer of the Congress.

Dr. William Conrad, St. Louis, Mo.—Mr. President, I move that the nomination of Dr. Finley for Treasurer be ratified by this body.

The motion was put before the house, and Dr. Finley was duly elected Treasurer of the Fourth International Dental Congress.

Dr. Finley was escorted to the platform and introduced by the President as follows: " Gentlemen of the Fourth International Dental Congress, I have great pleasure in presenting to you the gentleman who presides over the funds of this Congress." (Applause.)

Dr. Finley.—Mr. President and gentlemen, I would like to be able to thank you as gracefully as has Dr. Kirk, and if you will accept his words for mine, I will thank you.

The President next introduced Dr. C. S. Butler, Buffalo, N. Y., chairman of the Finance Committee, who thanked the members for their hearty co-operation in carrying out the work of his committee.

The President then invited all of the honorary presidents and vice-presidents in the audience to come upon the platform.

The President.—Gentlemen and ladies of the convention, I have pleasure in presenting to you my long-time friend and colleague, Dr. C. N. Johnson, of Chicago.

Dr. Johnson.—Mr. President and gentlemen of the Congress, this is entirely a surprise to me, but I do want to thank most heartily your presiding officer for giving me the pleasure of looking you in the face, and begging you to go to work from this time forward with the one object of making this the best meeting ever held in the history of dentistry. If perchance there has been any feeling developed, let us crush it out and as one man let us all work together to do the best we can for the profession of dentistry.

The President.—The governor of Missouri was invited to make an address of welcome on this occasion, but was unable to be here, and in his absence you will listen to a letter from him, which will be read by the Secretary-General.

Dr. Kirk, the Secretary-General, then read the following communication from Governor Dockery:

St. Louis, Mo., August 28, 1904.

" To Dr. B. L. Thorpe:

My dear Sir,—I profoundly regret my inability to be present to-morrow and welcome the delegates to the Fourth International Dental Congress. It would have been a real pleasure for me, in behalf of the people of Missouri, to have extended a cordial greeting to this large body of representative and intelligent citizens. Please present to the Congress my regrets that official duties prevent my attendance, and also convey my best wishes for a pleasant and instructive occasion.

" Your friend,

" A. M. Dockery."

The President.—Ladies and gentlemen, I have the honor of presenting to you the honored president of the National Dental Association, Dr. C. C. Chittenden, of Madison, Wis., who will now address you.

Dr. Chittenden.—Mr. President, ladies, and gentlemen, great undertakings can only be brought to a successful issue by a careful, well-planned course of procedure and development, controlled by an intelligent comprehension of the objects sought to be attained. Time, patience, and unswerving courage and fidelity—regardless of all personal sacrifice—must be freely thrown into the balance by those who undertake to create and set in motion the machinery required to successfully bring together representative men from all the civilized nations of the earth for the uplifting of a common cause.

Two years ago the National Dental Association, which body I have the honor to officially represent to-day, received an invitation from the officials of the Louisiana Purchase Exposition to create and put in operation an International Dental Congress, to be held in St. Louis. That invitation was accepted, and a commission of fifteen was appointed to the arduous undertaking. The work was taken up by that commission, and despite the thousand difficulties and obstacles that beset the way,—some of them apparently impregnable as Gibraltar itself,—the result of its labors stands before us to-day in the form of a noble, completed, symmetrical achievement, —the Fourth International Dental Congress.

Too much cannot be said in appreciation of the untiring labor and self-sacrifice through which this result has been brought about. On behalf of the National Dental Association I here publicly thank the commission of fifteen collectively and individually for their faithful performance of the duties set them.

This Congress, whose opening we are met to celebrate, could not have been made possible but for the never-failing guidance, counsel, and (when needed) authoritative direction of a master mind in the person of the Director of Congresses, Mr. Howard J. Rogers, to whom each one of us here owes a deep debt of gratitude.

The deep interest created in this enterprise throughout the countries of the world is clearly evidenced by the presence here to-day of eminent, illustrious representatives and large delegations of dentists from practically every civilized nation of the earth. On behalf of the National Dental Association I extend to these professional brothers gathered under this roof from the very ends of the earth, seeking the development of scientific light and knowledge in their chosen calling,—to all these I extend the hand-clasp of greeting and warmest words of welcome.

Under the skilled business management of the Finance Committee there is every reason to expect that this Congress will present a happy contrast, as to its final solvency, to most such undertakings. An ample equipment for each of the sections has been assured.

Finally, to all who have in any way contributed to the success of this great enterprise I here offer the sincere thanks of the National Dental Association. (Applause.)

The President.—The address of welcome on behalf of the State of Missouri will be delivered by the gentleman to whom I believe belongs the credit of discovering this Congress. I take great pleasure in introducing to you Dr. Burton Lee Thorpe, of St. Louis, Mo. (Applause.)

ADDRESS OF WELCOME ON BEHALF OF THE STATE OF MISSOURI.

MR. PRESIDENT, AND MEMBERS OF THE FOURTH INTERNATIONAL DENTAL CONGRESS,—Proud to be an American citizen, prouder still to be an American dentist, and to have aided in a humble way in making it possible that this great meeting is held, this is the happiest opportunity of my professional career,—to be delegated the very delightful duty of bidding you a most cordial and sincere welcome on behalf of the profession of the State of Missouri and the city of St. Louis.

Recognizing that each of you delegates coming from foreign countries and the States, Territories, and provinces of North America represent the best interests of the profession of your various localities, and that each of you has contributed either to the science, art, or literature of dentistry, I am frank to confess that the profession of Missouri feels highly honored to greet and welcome such a distinguished body of representative men and women of the dental profession.

It is fitting, indeed, that during the great Universal Exposition now in progress at the western portals of our city, that is held in commemoration of that historic event when Napoleon Bonaparte, with a stroke of the pen, signed away and gave to Thomas Jefferson and the American people an empire of which imperial Missouri is the most important State,—it is fitting, I say, at this time that there be held, as one of a series of many important educational and scientific congresses, the Fourth International Dental Congress.

It is the spirit of the Exposition to show the achievement of human progress, so aptly illustrated by Mr. Chang You Tong, the talented interpreter of China of this Congress, in the following sentiment:

> " Well blessed with man's success, Columbia fêtes
> In festal hall the nations and her States;
> From every clime her honored guests have come,
> From far Cathay and Europe's Christendom,
> From silver-mantled regions of the poles,
> From golden shores where sparkling river rolls;
> Her States, like jewels in a coronet,
> Around the hall her loving hands have set.
> The wine of friendship bubbles in the glass,
> From hand to hand the fragrant roses pass;
> The song of thanks is swelled by every tongue,
> The nation's hymn is sung by old and young.
> Rejoice, Columbia! Lead the gallant van,
> And show the world the worth of man as man:
> Be thou the champion of the human race,
> And break the chains which manhood may disgrace.
> The nations, young and old, to thee resign
> The sacred sceptre and a task divine."

It is also the spirit of this Congress to welcome our professional *confrères* from every civilized country, and to unite with them in comparing the wonderful strides the humane and beneficent profession of dentistry has made by enmassing the investigators, teachers, journalists, and active progressive practitioners of dental surgery, the recognized leaders in art, science, and technique, to demonstrate both clinically and theoretically the latest and best in odontological science.

We are gratified that in the master minds of two American dental pioneers originated the three most potent factors in dental education,—the organization of the first dental college, the first dental journal, and the first dental society that brought our calling out of chaos, and made it blossom from a trade into a profession. We know that yesterday's achievements are not forgotten in the onward movement of to-day, when all nations in reverential homage do honor to the memory of the progenitors of dental science,— Horace H. Hayden and Chapin A. Harris.

We are not unmindful, however, of the achievements of the stanch pioneers of Europe, to whom we also must give ample credit for their contributions to our profession.

One hundred years ago, when St. Louis was a frontier trading-post on the banks of yonder river, records say that the first regular dental practitioner was Dr. Paul, a Frenchman of New Orleans, who located here in 1809, soon to be followed by other pioneers, such as Isaiah Forbes, B. B. Brown, Edward Hale, Sr., A. M. Leslie, Isaac Comstock, Aaron Blake, J. S. Clark, H. E. Peebles, C. W. Spaulding, Henry Barron, Homer Judd, C. W. Rivers, Henry S. Chase, William H. Eames, Edgar Park, William N. Morrison, and lastly our distinguished Henry J. McKellops, whose names will ever illumine the pages of Missouri dental history.

This coterie of men stood for progress, and were foremost in city, State, and national dental affairs, and I thank God that the better element of their successors are also imbued with the same progressive spirit, which is proved by their loyalty and liberality in making this Congress a success. On behalf of these self-sacrificing, broad-minded, liberal-spirited dentists of St. Louis and Missouri, I welcome you!

We welcome all nations. We welcome you of Spain, whose generous Queen Isabella long ago equipped the fleet that brought Columbus on his voyage of discovery to our shores. Our hearts

also go out to you for the courteous and chivalrous treatment tendered our sailors while the captives of your gallant Admiral Cer-
vera at Santiago.

To you, sons of England, the mother of America: We bid you
welcome! Once we were your unruly child; you tried to chastise
us, but we had outgrown our swaddling-clothes—you failed; but
now the British lion and the American eagle are bosom companions.
We heartily appreciate the recognition England has granted that
distinguished scientist, our fellow-countryman, J. Leon Williams.

To Sweden, who gave us Ericsson, and to Norway, who gave us
so many of your sturdy sons and fair daughters who have by their
industry made parts of America blossom as a garden: We bid you
welcome!

To France, who in the dark days of the American Revolution
sent us the gallant Marquis de Lafayette and Count Rochambeau
and their thousands of fellow-patriots who did so much to aid us
to gain our independence, we are especially indebted. With these
generals of army and navy came two men who have left their
imprint indelibly stamped on American dentistry,—Joseph Fran-
çoise Lemaire and James Gardette, distinguished as skilled operators, contributors to dental literature, and the pioneers in introducing dental surgery in America: We welcome you! Our national
emblem, symbolic of free thought and free speech, is the Stars and
Stripes. I believe if the American people were asked to add to it,
in recognition of the brotherly love between France and America
they would unanimously choose the *fleur-de-lis.*

To Germany, whose countrymen have done so much in developing America and have made such excellent citizens: We bid you
welcome! and we thank you for the fraternal recognition you
have given those two distinguished American practitioners who are
the foremost in the world in their specialties,—W. D. Miller and
N. S. Jenkins.

Lord Bacon says, "Every man owes a debt to his profession,"
and we feel that you who speak in different tongues, who have
crossed the seas to attend this Congress, have at least in part
liquidated your indebtedness to the profession.

To all nations: to all members of the Fourth International
Dental Congress: We bow our heads in salute to you; we bid you
welcome from the bottom of our hearts! Our homes are open to
you, our hands are at your service. We recognize the fact that

you represent the intellect and flower of dentistry of the world, and the profession of Missouri and of St. Louis are flattered to have you here. It is our hope that you may reap untold benefit from this historic meeting, and when you return to your respective homes, may you carry pleasant memories of our people, State, and city; and when your life's work is ended, may you each realize the reward that Kipling so beautifully pictures as the heaven of the honest workingman as epitomized by the painter:

" When earth's last picture is painted and the tubes are twisted and dried,
When the brightest colors have faded, and the youngest critic has died,
We shall rest, and faith! we shall need it—lie down for an æon or two,
Till the Master of all good workmen shall put us to work anew.
And those who were good shall be happy. They shall sit in a golden chair;
They shall splash at ten-league canvas with brushes of comet's hair;
They shall find real saints to draw from,—Magdalene, Peter, and Paul;
They shall work for an age at a sitting, and never be tired at all!
And only the Master shall praise us, and only the Master shall blame;
And no one shall work for money, and no one shall work for fame;
But each for the joy of working, and each in his separate star,
Shall draw the Thing-as-he-sees-it, for the God of Things-as-they-are!"

The President.—I now have pleasure in presenting to you the vice-president for America of the International Dental Federation, who will welcome the foreign delegates to the Fourth International Dental Congress.

Dr. A. W. Harlan, of New York, delivered the following address:

ADDRESS OF WELCOME TO THE FOREIGN DELEGATES.

MR. PRESIDENT, LADIES, AND GENTLEMEN, AND MEMBERS OF THE CONGRESS FROM FOREIGN COUNTRIES,—I am indeed fortunate to be able this day to greet you as the official mouth-piece of the Committee of Organization of this Congress. It looked for a long time as though the Fédération Dentaire Internationale and the committee could not come together, but to-day all differences are settled, and we appear before you as a united profession.

The World's Dental Congresses have become fixed institutions in the same way that other congresses have been evolved. The profession needed congresses. The world would be benefited in consequence of their evolution, and we have them. They are a part of our armament, just as physiology and chemistry are a part of the education of the dentist.

The members of our profession in the United States having chosen me to extend to every one present from a foreign shore the right hand of fellowship, I give you a cordial fraternal welcome in this noble hall and in the presence of this multitude of our own people.

This is the second time in the history of our profession that an international dental congress has been convened in the United States,—1893 and 1904. The origin of dental congresses, as you well know, was in the land of Ambroise Paré, Roux, Fauchard, Jourdain, Lefoulon, Robin, Magitot, Paul Dubois, Lecaudey, and Godon. It is our hope and wish that every one here this day will feel that he is thrice welcome to participate in the programme of the week, and that all will feel that time and distance will count as nothing when they sum up the benefits derived from what they see and hear.

On behalf of the officers and the management of the Congress, and the united dental profession, I again bid you all a hearty welcome.

(To be continued.)

Editorial.

THE FOURTH INTERNATIONAL DENTAL CONGRESS.

THE Fourth International Dental Congress has passed into history, and those who took an active part in it have equally moved onward to their several destinations. It now remains for the dental periodicals of the world to give their readers, not able to be present, the general impressions of this great gathering of dentists.

This self-imposed task seems to be a difficult one. It was very evident to the writer during the sessions of this Congress, that no single mind could do exact justice to this meeting. Each one present studied it from his own point of observation, and this, doubtless, led in many instances to false impressions of the Congress as a whole.

The meeting convened at the "Coliseum" on Monday, the 29th of August, 1904. The auditorium of this building would comfortably seat two thousand five hundred persons, and when the time arrived for calling the meeting to order it was fully two-thirds full.

It had been evident for several days prior to the organization of the Congress that a political storm was in progress, and this assumed very unpleasant proportions as the time of the meeting approached. The cause of this was the old and ever discreditable American fight for offices. We use the word American with a full understanding of its meaning. It is believed that in no other country could this happen to the same extent; and while human nature is very much the same everywhere, in no other land is the desire for office so intense as in this country. The reason for this is quite apparent to the student of racial proclivities, but space and time will not permit a thorough consideration of this part of the subject. It is sufficient to say that this contention crystallized itself on two positions, —those of President and Secretary-General. The origin of this controversy dates back to the appointment of the Committee of Fifteen by the National Dental Association and the appointment of the Committee of Nine by the "Fédération Dentaire Internationale" at Stockholm. The story is too long and too unprofitable to be repeated here. The result was that the first session of the Congress witnessed the culmination of this strife for office that must have astonished the foreign delegates.

The meeting was opened by Howard J. Rogers, Director of Congresses, in an able address of welcome. He, at the close of this, acted as temporary president to effect a permanent organization. The nominations for President were Dr. H. J. Burkhart, of Batavia, N. Y., and Dr. C. N. Johnson, of Chicago, the former having been president of the Committee of Organization. For Secretary-General the nominations were Dr. E. C. Kirk, of Philadelphia, secretary of the Committee, and Dr. A. W. Harlan, of New York City. For days previous to this meeting, this contest had been fought over behind closed doors, with the result that at the opening there was a general suppressed excitement and much uncertainty felt as to the final result. The vote for both offices was taken by each member standing until the vote was counted. The result for President was in favor of Dr. Burkhart by a large majority. The position of Secretary-General was decided by a practically unanimous vote for Dr. E. C. Kirk. The introduction of foreign delegates then followed, with short speeches from each. This occupied the first session, and the sections began their work in the afternoon.

In the opinion of the writer, the Congress was not opened with the dignity belonging to a great international organization. Had the permanent officers been selected months ago it would have permitted the successful aspirant for the office of President to have prepared a fitting address. This, of course, could not be done under the method adopted, resulting in a very informal opening, and to some very unsatisfactory.

No attempt will be made in this article to report the proceedings. As before stated, the story can only be told through the reports from Sections and the published volumes.

If the success of a congress is based on numbers—eighteen hundred being registered—and papers presented, this must be regarded as fulfilling all requirements. The world was well represented,— Europe, China, Japan, Philippines, Australia, New Zealand, America, and the islands of the oceans,—England alone not being represented by native Britons. Subjects of Great Britain were active in the Congress, but the mother country was not represented by any of her prominent workers. We presume this is capable of explanation, but it was an unpleasant feature in the complexion of the Congress.

The value of the papers can be judged only by careful reading after publication, for it is surmised that not one in attendance was entirely satisfied with the reading under conditions present. The writer had access to a limited number, and, if an opinion can be based on these, it may be safe to say that the final report will be of very great value.

The clinics were very extensive and the chairman and his assistants deserve great credit for the work accomplished. They exceeded anything of the kind ever attempted in this country. Their value the writer must leave to others to determine. The time was so much occupied in other directions, that but little could be spared for these or the exhibits. Both of these evidently were of more intrinsic value to the members than the sections, for the former were at all times crowded while the latter were almost entirely neglected.

Was the Congress a success? This question will, it is presumed, be asked over and over again, and the answer each time will be one of uncertainty. With a very few it will be regarded as having met all expectations, but with the large majority it was a serious disappointment, if not practically a failure. To the latter class the writer belongs, and it is due that large body that the reasons for this opinion should be given. That the Congress failed to meet the highest anticipations of its members is not, by any means, remarkable, for this, probably, may be said of all aggregations of men; neither can the Committee of Organization be censured for any shortcomings, for it simply followed precedent in its energetic and laborious work, but that this meeting was very unsatisfactory was the almost universal verdict.

The reason for this was primarily due to the fact that the Congress was divided into sections. This may be necessary in great gatherings, similar to the National Medical Association of this country, from the impossibility of accommodating the diversity of interests in any one building, and to some extent this is true of congresses of international character in dentistry, but experience has demonstrated that at no general meeting was it shown that all the papers possible to read could not have been read and discussed there. This was quite fully demonstrated when almost the entire membership occupied the auditorium to listen to Professor W. D. Miller's paper. The section work was well tested at the Columbian Dental Congress, and proved very unsatisfactory there, and why it should have been adopted again at this Congress remains for future explanation. The result was disastrous. In but few sections, from personal observation, was there more than ten or fifteen present, and oftentimes not that number, and in some the attendance was limited to the officers of the section. One chairman of an important section informed the writer that he was obliged to have most of his papers read by title, as he had no audience to listen to them. This is a humiliating confession, but it is better to give the exact truth now, that future congresses may profit by this unfortunate experience.

The reason for this indifference is not far to seek. The great Exposition attracted many; others found more instruction, as they did interest, in the exhibits, and still others found the social intercourse in the halls a very great pleasure; but above and beyond all these reasons, there was the main fact that some one invited this International Dental Congress to meet in a building that was in itself sufficient to stamp failure upon this and every other congress of the series, providing, as in this, they must branch out from the main auditorium to the widely scattered rooms below and above. This building, as it now stands, is a blot upon the character of American civilization, and the expressions of indignation in regard to this were loud and prolonged, but at the same time equally useless. The local committee had tried to clean it, but all efforts in this direction were futile. This building is recognized in St. Louis as having passed its day of usefulness, and it is proposed to have it demolished after the Exposition has been closed. It remains an unsolved problem why the Exposition managers should have selected this building for the various congresses. Its deplorable condition must have been well known, and the certainty that this would reflect upon American character and American civilization should have been seriously considered. Those who attended some of the congresses of the Columbian Exposition of 1893 could not fail to draw comparisons very unfavorable to the situation in St. Louis in 1904. The acoustic properties of the building throughout were so bad that even in the smaller rooms with lofty ceilings the members were in a constant strain to hear the papers and discussions. The result was that this, combined with the aforesaid uncleanly condition, broke up the sections. Had all the meetings been held in the main auditorium, it would have been better, but even here the conditions described were so unsatisfactory that many left the meetings, finding it impossible to hear, and others remained under protest rather than give the appearance of neglecting the work of the Congress.

The social features consisted of a reception at the Missouri Building, Exposition grounds. This the writer was unable to attend. The Grand Banquet was given at the Jefferson Hotel, at which some three hundred, including the writer, took part. A pleasant feature of this, and one worthy of future imitation, was the presence of ladies, the guests of the Congress. It was two A.M. before the long list of speakers, representing all civilized countries, had concluded the post-prandial work.

It is with profound regret that it is impossible to review the work of this Congress with any feelings of satisfaction. It failed, in the opinion of the writer, to represent the dentistry of America as he understands it, and it failed to give expression to that broader international dentistry of which we hear so much and know, intimately, so little. The undignified course pursued at the opening seemed to tinge the whole Congress, and if the residents of foreign countries return to their several homes with unfavorable opinions, it will be due to some who were unable to rise to the standard that the world demands of a professional cultured gentleman.

This article cannot be closed without entering a decided protest against the method adopted of having a door-tender to keep out all persons who failed to wear a button, the sign of membership. This senseless order resulted in several wordy conflicts with members, anything but creditable. Dental congresses are, in the estimation of the writer, educational bodies, or should be so, and the young men in the profession, or undergraduates, should be freely invited to take a listener's part. Not many of these can afford the ten dollars necessary to become a member. It seemed as though the committee, in ordering this, carried this Congress back to the middle of the last century when " No Admittance" was figuratively over every office door. This was not the least of the mistakes made in this Congress, and it certainly was one of the most unpleasant. The science worthy to be called by that name should be free to all able to understand.

It is with profound regret and with a sense of humiliation that nothing better can be said of the visible result of this Congress. We in this country had looked forward to it as a means of extending the professional view throughout the world, thus making our lives broader through a closer union with the dentists of modern civilization. In some instances this was secured, but upon the whole the true cosmopolitan spirit was not advanced, neither were we, to any great extent, aided by foreigners in the discussions. In the papers this was different, many of the most valuable being from the hands of foreign writers. It was, however, essentially an English-speaking congress, the international feature being almost entirely lost.

It is not probable that another International Dental Congress will be held in the very near future, but if such should be in contemplation, it is to be hoped that those who manage it will have learned to avoid the unfortunate errors committed by the various committees that managed the International Dental Congress at St. Louis, 1904.

Domestic Correspondence.

NATIONAL ASSOCIATION OF DENTAL FACULTIES.

I DO not know that I have any right to give expression in oppo-sition to the amount of fuss that has emanated from many of the colleges of late on account of the change of time from three to four years. It certainly looks strange to an outsider, one who is without partisan feeling for any of the colleges, and one who can see without the use of a field-glass just what the end will be if harmony is not restored. The colleges who have, and those who intend to, cut loose from the Association of Dental Faculties should be placed on a black list, and at no time during their existence should they be allowed to return to the fold. Their existence will be more than short. Students cannot and will not enter a college whose diploma is not recognized by the Association of Dental Facul-ties. Our dental laws in the majority of the States demand diplomas from colleges that are members of the Association. The falling off of students from these colleges means the closing of doors. To those colleges that have remained loyal will come the students who seek the higher dental education and a diploma which gives a standing and carries a professional dignity on the face of it. While we will be compelled to admit that the falling off in the attendance will be large and the loss to some of the colleges con-siderable, yet what the colleges lose the profession gains. For it will gain men who come well grounded in the English language, men who will have the interests of the profession at heart, and men who will work to place the standard as high as it is possible to reach. It means the closing of the dental parlors, protecting the laity and the profession.

The colleges should welcome the day when the weak and puny ones elect to go. The world demands the survival of the fittest. We need strong colleges and honest men to handle them. Men who can be turned by a key of gold are not fit to stand in a lecture-hall. If men of that stamp are allowed to fill the chairs, they will surely contaminate the student and open the gates of empiricism. We would not permit a minister of the gospel to preach other than holy writ from the pulpit. Then why allow our dental colleges to permit men to stand before a body of students and inculcate into them principals other than pertains directly to dentistry, not so much by word of mouth as by actions, and actions often speak volumes. To me dentistry is a holy calling. Do we not enter the homes of our patients as no other can except the family physician? Were we libertines and charlatans, would we be given the respect due our calling? As we conduct ourselves so are we judged. Then let us stand for higher education, moral principles, and ethical conduct at all times and in all places.

J. E. STOREY.

MORENCI, ARIZ.

Miscellany.

REPAIRING FRACTURED CASTS.—A valuable method of repairing fractured plaster casts may be found in the use of celluloid dissolved in camphor and ether to a creamy consistence. A good quality of celuloid should be selected, and to it should be added a mixture of equal parts of ether and spirits of camphor. This combination dissolves celluloid rapidly, and should be added to the material until a solution of a cream consistence is obtained. The preparation should be kept tightly corked to avoid its evaporation.

When it becomes desirable to repair broken casts, the fragments to be attached should be well dried and both surfaces should be freed from broken particles. The surfaces should be coated with the celluloid solution, and after being pressed firmly, should be allowed to dry.—S. M. WEEKS.

TO PREVENT SORENESS OF THE LIPS AFTER OPERATING.—White perfumed vaseline will be found a most excellent preventative of sore lips from long and repeated applications of the rubber dam. Although many ladies object to its use on account of the general impression that it stimulates the growth of hair, I find upon ex-

plaining the good results from its use, the avoidance of the so-
called cold sore, they will gladly submit to its application. Two
covered porcelain jars with the pure white vaseline are kept in
the operating-case, the contents of one for use as an application
around the mouth, the contents of the other for strips and disks.
By cleaning the porcelain jars every day, and placing in them a
small quantity of the pure clean vaseline, they are ready for use,
and if need be, the inspection of the most particular patient. It
is the exception that the most fastidious lady, when handed the
porcelain jar and the explanation is made for its use, will not
apply it immediately, and later bless you for having suggested
it. Undoubtedly the saliva saturating the skin and held there by
the rubber plays an important part in addition to our pulling and
stretching the mouth, in producing these disagreeable sores. In
long operations, especially in molars and bicuspids, a second and
third application sometimes is indicated, which can be made by
loosening the dam from the holder, drying the corner of the mouth
thoroughly with a napkin, then reapplying the vaseline. If applied to the lips when they are dry or cracked, it softens them
to such an extent that much of the discomfort of an operation is
avoided.—W. T. CHAMBERS, Denver, Col.

KEEP A RECORD OF YOUR TREATMENTS.—The various dental
ledgers will probably meet the requirements necessary to record
all permanent work, but a small book kept in a convenient place
near the operator's chair will be found useful for recording the
daily treatments. The busy dentist can not retain in his mind the
condition of each tooth he treats temporarily, and the result is that
he must practically diagnose every case when it is presented, no
matter how often he has treated the tooth before. The examination
form will at once show him which teeth require his attention, but it
will not give him any aid in determining the condition of the teeth
at the last sitting. Very often a dentist will remember the condition of an individual case, and it is right that he should. It will
not always be necessary for the careful practitioner to rely solely
upon records, but a record will show him the condition of the tooth
at the last sitting, and he can instantly determine what course to
pursue. It will take less time to record the treatment and prognosis than to make even a brief diagnosis when the patient calls

for treatment. This method will also serve as a reference for the operator to determine the correct fees he should receive for each tooth. After the work is completed he can refer the patient to his record and charge a reasonable fee, which might otherwise seem exorbitant.—*Review.*

METHOD OF TIPPING BRIDGE TEETH.—Prepare the tooth by grinding as is ordinarily done and burnish pure gold backing to position on the tooth, allowing the backing to project beyond the labial or buccal surface of the facing at the occlusal end. Hold the occlusal end of the tooth, with backing in position, against a flat surface having a right angle corner, such as a drawer in the bracket table, the labial surface of the facing being held even with the upper surface of the drawer. The projecting gold can now be turned down till it rests on the upper flat surface. Burnish the gold well against the facing and contour the tip if necessary. The case is now invested and 22-carat plate is flowed over the occlusal surface and tip as heavy as desired. After the crown is soldered grind away the gold that overlaps the edge in front, and this will produce a solid 22-carat tip. The same method can be adopted for bicuspids and molars in bridge-work. Flow 22-carat plate over the whole surface of the backing, making it heavy enough to protect the facing. Make lingual cusps, articulate, and attach with solder. —F. S. MILLER, Warsaw, Wis.

TREATMENT OF CONTRACTURE OF JOINTS WITH RONTGEN RAYS. —Moser reports the excellent results obtained in two cases by radiation. Almost all the joints of the first patient were ankylosed, and there was palpable friction during movement,—probably the results of gout. A skiagram was taken of one knee and the patient complained that she had had pains in all her joints thereafter. Moser noticed that the knee that had been exposed seemed less swollen than before, and he applied the Röntgen rays as a therapeutic measure for a minute to each knee. The patient reported four days later that there had been marked improvement since, not only of the exposed joints, but of all the others. The improvement progressively continued until the patient is now able to dress herself and do up her hair, previously impossible, and take a half-hour walk.—*Centralblatt Chirurgie*, Leipsic.

Current News.

INTERNATIONAL DENTAL CONGRESS—REPORT OF COMMITTEE ON PRIZE ESSAYS.

To the International Dental Congress:

The committee to whom was given the consideration of papers competing for the prize offered by the Committee of Organization begs leave to make its report to the Congress assembled at St. Louis.

Your committee decided upon the following rules for its government in considering papers presented:

1. The subject-matter must be new and original.

2. The paper must not be overloaded with quotations.

3. It must, in every respect, be in accord with the character and dignity of the Congress.

Ten papers have been presented and carefully considered. Several of these are so nearly up to the standard adopted that your committee has found some difficulty in reaching a united conclusion. It has, therefore, been regarded as proper and just, in deciding upon the paper worthy of the prize, to mention several equally worthy of " Honorable Mention."

The paper entitled " A Study of Certain Questions relating to the Pathology of the Teeth," prepared by Professor W. D. Miller, of Berlin, is, in the opinion of your committee, entitled to the highest honor that this Congress can bestow.

The prize, therefore, is conferred upon his work.

The paper entitled " The Pathology of Lime Salts in Nutrition," by Dr. Med. C. Röse, of Dresden, Germany, is regarded by your committee as one of the most thorough and valuable papers ever prepared upon this subject. It presents years of patient work, but unfortunately does not and, as yet, cannot go beyond clinical observation.

Your committee, therefore, report for " Honorable Mention" in the order of merit, the following:

1. "The Pathology of Lime Salts in Nutrition," Dr. Med. C. Röse, Dresden, Germany.

2. "Constitutional Causes of Tooth-Decay, Erosion, Abrasion, and Discoloration," Dr. Eugene S. Talbot, Chicago, Ill.

3. "Anatomic Changes in the Head, Face, Jaws, and Teeth in the Evolution of Man," Dr. Eugene S. Talbot, Chicago, Ill.

4. "The Development of the Teeth of the *Sus Domesticus*," Zahnarzt Max Hirsch, Halle, Germany.

The balance of the papers, valuable for section work, have been transferred to the proper custodians.

Two papers were sent in for examination, but both too late to compete for the prize. One by Dr. Michaels, of Paris, not in the hands of the committee, and title unknown, and one entitled: (1) "Investigations concerning the Corrosibility of Aluminum," and (2) "Applicability of Aluminum to Dentistry," a very full paper upon this subject, by Hof-Zahnarzt W. Pfaff, Dresden, Germany.

(Signed) WILBUR F. LITCH,

L. M. COWARDIN,

JAMES TRUMAN, *Chairman.*

ST. LOUIS, Mo., August 29, 1904.

NATIONAL ASSOCIATION OF DENTAL EXAMINERS— REPORT OF COMMITTEE ON COLLEGES.

IT will be remembered that the relations between the National Association of Dental Faculties and our Association which had obtained for some time during the past were left intact at the close of the meeting of this Association at Asheville last year. It will be unnecessary to more than briefly refer to the things that have transpired in the National Association of Dental Faculties since that meeting. Suffice it to say that that body has been wrestling with itself as to whether it would, or even could, keep faith with the public and with this Association in the carrying out of the requirements of course for graduation which it had definitely set up in

822 Current News.

1901 and put into actual operation beginning with the school year 1903–04.

It transpires that at least a majority of that Association, by official action, has seen fit, for reasons they consider paramount, to seriously modify their course requirements for graduation in a way and to a degree that your committee, as well as the profession at large, cannot interpret in any other way than as a most deplorable retrogression. It would appear, from what has thus occurred, that the National Association of Dental Faculties has clearly demonstrated that, no matter in how good faith it entered upon the establishment of the new standard in 1903–04, it was utterly powerless of its own unaided strength to permanently establish and maintain it.

After a careful earnest canvass of the whole situation by correspondence and interview with many of the leading dental educators of this country, as well as with many leading and influential practitioners of experience and observation, and also backed by some of the best legal advice procurable, as to what was the duty of this deliberative body, composed as it is of the various State boards, endowed under their various laws with the judicial and discriminative power and duty of establishing and maintaining reasonable dental educational standards and requirements, your committee is fully convinced that the time is ripe for this Association to declare in no uncertain tones what we hold to be most essential and necessary qualifications of a prospective dental college student in order to enable him to assimilate and appropriate the great fund of scientific knowledge offered him in any of our properly conducted dental schools.

Your committee would therefore recommend that this Association establish at once, to go into operation not later than the opening of the school year of 1905–06, the educational requirement for admission to the dental college course of graduation from an accredited high school or its full equivalent, all examination of credentials and equivalents to be placed in the hands of an acceptable appointee of the State Superintendent of Public Instruction where not otherwise provided for by law.

In view of the present disturbed and unsettled conditions existing in dental educational circles, and with a belief in the wisdom of avoiding all unnecessary disturbance of standards at this time, your committee would further recommend that no change be made at this time in the present requirements of this Association of not less than twenty-eight calander months of college attendance for graduation.

CHARLES C. CHITTENDEN, *Chairman,*
H. J. BURKHART,
J. A. HALL,
Committee on Colleges of the N. A. D. E.

Unanimously adopted by the National Association of Dental Examiners at St. Louis, Mo., August 27, 1904.

NEW JERSEY STATE BOARD OF REGISTRATION AND EXAMINATION.

THE New Jersey State Board of Registration and Examination in dentistry will hold their semiannual meeting in the Theoretical branches, in the Assembly chamber at the State-House, Trenton, N. J., on the 18th, 19th, and 20th of October, 1904. Practical prosthetic work to be done in the office of Dr. A. Irwin, 425 Cooper Street, Camden, N. J., and practical operative work to be done in the office of Dr. C. S. Stockton, 7 Central Avenue, Newark, N. J. Work to be done on dates assigned by the Examiner in those branches.

All applications must be in the hands of the secretary by the 15th of October.

CHARLES A. MEEKER, D.D.S.
29 FULTON STREET, NEWARK, N. J.

NORTHERN INDIANA DENTAL SOCIETY.

THE sixteenth annual meeting of the Northern Indiana Dental Society will be held October 18 and 19, at Huntington, Ind.

It is expected that we will have the largest attendance of any meeting ever held in this section of the country, and you cannot afford to miss hearing such essayists as Drs. G. V. Black, Hart J. Goslee, F. E. Roach, George E. Hunt, William T. Reeves, E. X.

Jones, J. Q. Byram, G. E. Johnson, F. R. Henshaw, F. M. Bozer,
Lavinia B. McCollum, C. G. Keehn, and many others that have
consented to appear on the programme, besides a very attractive list
of clinics demonstrating all of the newest and most valuable things
in practice.

All the leading manufacturers have signified their intention of
making an exhibit of their products.

Every up-to-date dentist will be present. Are you coming?

Special social features for Tuesday evening.

Remember the date.

Otto U. King,
Secretary.

ARKANSAS STATE BOARD OF DENTAL EXAMINERS.

The next meeting of the Arkansas State Board of Dental Examiners will be held December 2 and 3, 1904, in Little Rock, Ark.,
for the examination of all applicants. Those having applied for
examination will report to the secretary Friday morning, December 2, 1904, with rubber dam, gold, plastic filling-material, and
instruments, to demonstrate their skill in operative dentistry. Any
one who wishes may bring a patient; as far as possible patients
will be furnished. The board reserves the right to select the cavity
to be filled.

The examination will cover all branches of the dental profession.

No temporary certificate will be issued to any one. Examination
fee, $5.00. For further information write the secretary.

Dr. A. T. McMillin,
Secretary.

THE

International Dental Journal.

Vol. XXV.   November, 1904.   No. 11.

Original Communications.[1]

NEOPLASM (EPITHELIOMA) OF THE PULP.[2]

BY V. A. LATHAM, M.D., D.D.S., F.R.M.S., ROGERS PARK, ILL.

THE great importance of this subject from a clinical as well as a purely pathologic point of view must be my excuse for presenting this rather incomplete study. It is with diffidence that I put the case on record, for in looking through the literature at my command I have so far been unable to locate any other like condition. If we exclude the hypertrophies which have been described under the heading of "Polypus of the Pulp or Tooth," then I am led to the supposition that this may be the first case recorded of an exceedingly rare condition. In reviewing the literature, Ziegler[3] speaks of "tumors of dental tissue formed in later life, and described by dental pathologists as odontinoids."[4] Accordingly as they consist of enamel, dentine, cement, or a combination of these, they are classified as enameloid, enamelodentinoid, dentinoid, den-

---

[1] The editor and publishers are not responsible for the views of authors of papers published in this department, nor for any claim to novelty, or otherwise, that may be made by them. No papers will be received for this department that have appeared in any other journal published in the country.

[2] Read at the fifty-fifth annual session of the American Medical Association, in the Section on Stomatology, Atlantic City, June 7 to 10, 1904.

[3] Ziegler, Special Pathological Anatomy, section ix. p. 593, 1897.

[4] Ullrich, Ueber feste Neubildungen in der Zahnhöhle, 1852.

31   825

tino-osteoid, or osteoid.[1] They are all small, often to be recognized only by the aid of the magnifying lens. They are flat, round, pear-shaped, or warty in appearance. The first three-named varieties grow from odontoblasts, and arise from the pulp of the crown and from that of the root, generally in connection with caries, under metallic fillings, or as a result of periostitis, mechanical injuries, abnormal retention of teeth, or senile degeneration. The osteoid form grows from the pulp and from the periosteum, and is developed from osteoblasts. "Sarcoma, fibroma, and myxoma are in rare cases developed from the pulp as the tooth is being formed. Such growths, and particularly the sarcomata and fibromata, are, however, much more commonly derived from the periosteum of the dental socket or alveolar process, from the bone marrow or from the gum itself" (Ziegler).

Falkson[2] has described cases of cystadenoma arising from the rudimentary tooth papillæ and taking the form of a multilocular cyst, produced by cystic degeneration of the dental follicles. The growth encloses newly formed gland-like tubules and acini.

P. Bruns[3] and others have recorded certain rare instances of dental carcinoma, in which some of the epithelial cells of the tumor take on the appearance of enamel germs and produce enamel.[4] Unfortunately, the term "sarcoma" has been used when a simple hypertrophy or polypus of the pulp has been meant, and this has been passed down from Wedl[5] and Salter[6] to Black.[7]

Bödecker[8] states that the only known tumor of the pulp is malignant myeloma, as first described by C. Wedl. Bödecker adds

---

[1] Schlenker, Zahn- und Mundpflege, St. Gallen, 1883; Untersch. über das Wesen der Zahn-verderbniss, St. Gallen, 1882; Pulpen Odontinoide, Hdbuch d. Zahnheilkunde; Verknöcherung. der Zahnnerven, 1885; Vierteljahrsschrift f. 3, Wien, 1892.

[2] Falkson, Development of Rudimentary Teeth and Cysts of the Jaw, V. A. 76, 1879.

[3] Bruns, P., and Chibert, Adamantine Epithelioma. A. de méd. exp., 1894, with references.

[4] Mallassez, Epithelial Detritus round the Roots of Teeth in Adults. A. de Physiologie, v., 1885. Massin, Congenital Epithelioma originating from the Enamel, V. A. 136, 1894.

[5] Wedl, Pathologie der Zähne, 1870. Transl.

[6] Salter, Dental Surgery and Pathology, 1874.

[7] Black, American System of Dentistry, p. 915.

[8] Bödecker, Anatomy and Pathology of the Teeth, 1894.

one other example, but unfortunately nothing was known concern-- ing the history of the pulps affected.

In both cases, as seen by microscopic examination, they were the so-called round sarcoma, or, as Bödecker prefers to call them, lymphomyeloma. The term myeloma is used synonymously with sarcoma, some authorities objecting to sarcoma on account of its derivation from the word " sarkos" (Greek, flesh), whereas myeloma means what these tumors in reality are, medullary tumors. When combined with epithelial as well as connective tissues, we must not forget that they are termed " medullary carcinoma," and in some cases may lead to a wrong diagnosis.

Dr. Juan M. Alberdi,[1] Madrid, says, under affections of the dental pulp, " The organic affections consist in tumors, which reside in this organ. The tumors are hypertrophied productions, brought about by the simple hypergenesis of the normal elements of the tissue." The tumors are always the consequence of some lesion, especially penetrating caries, with exposure of the pulp. They are smooth, of a grayish color, and sometimes of considerable size, covered by a pellicle, which is only a thickening of that which covers the normal pulp. The treatment consists in removal of the pulp.

Dr. A. Pont[2] (de Lyon) mentions a case of tumor of the dental pulp without caries, which is not a tumor, pathologically speaking, but a polypus, or primary hypertrophied pulp with secondary in-flammation, without power to form secondary dentine, but which has absorbed the ivory dentine, which properly belongs to the tumor division, as seen so often in the osteosarcomata, and might incline one to place it in this group. " To what it was due is not clear, as it could not have been a chronic or hypertrophic pulpitis, there being no history of pain or caries. It might have been an aneurism of the pulp, but absence of hemorrhage excludes that, hence we will call it an hypertrophy of pulp, with total absorption of the dentine without caries."

When we review the histology and gross anatomy of the pulp, and note its close relation with the connective-tissue origin, we

---

[1] Alberdi, Dental Cosmos, p. 916, 1902, Third International Dental Congress.

[2] Pont, A., L'Odontologie, September 15, 1902; Dental Cosmos, November, 1902, Transl.; Ash's Quarterly Circular, December, 1902; Second report, with microscopic findings, in L'Odontologie, May 30, 1903.

easily see its liability to almost every known disease. Its peculiar formation enables it to supply the nutritive needs of the tooth with the vascular and nervous endowments, in which it is particularly rich.

The study of pulp diseases is best made by obtaining the affected teeth immediately after they are extracted. Great care is necessary that an observer be not led by his preconceptions. Just opinions are arrived at only after a thorough examination, and by comparison with many other similar cases. Diseased conditions of the pulp are to be studied in the pathologic associations of inflammation, trauma, and new formations.

Albrecht, in his monograph on " Diseases of the Pulp," follows these divisions: (*a*) disease of nerve; (*b*) disease of blood-vessels; (*c*) disease of secretion. To-day this will avail nothing, as it is founded on no anatomic pathologic observation, and only confuses by the intermixture of terms which is bound to exist.

When we consider the position occupied by the teeth at the entrance of the alimentary tract, the change of temperature, varieties of food, continual changes in blood-pressure as a peripheral area, and (in my mind one of the most important conditions to explain pathologic changes in their structure) liability to faulty development, fissures, cracks through acidity, abrasion, erosion, caries, and almost sure entrance of bacteria, as well as the relation and condition of surrounding structures as gingivitis, and the close effect of constitutional and systemic conditions of health, is it any wonder we have hyperæmia, which may readily be followed by more or less pulpitis, the quick follower of any irritation? Not always does it happen, however, that pain does follow pulp exposure of the peripheral tubuli; even when the inner aspect of the tubes is seen in a hyperæmic state, the pulp is often found in a fair state of resistance. The conductors of irritation, the odontoblasts, are common in their relationship to tubules and central organs; the filling up of these tubes and shrinkage of these cells break up the line of conduction, and this constitutes self-protection; then secondary deposits occur, and less pain usually follows. If the condition progresses, we may have a pulp exposure, with all the signs and symptoms of pulpitis. Pain is not necessarily an associate of the inflammation.

When a pulpitis has been of long continuance the pain seldom is found restricted to the tooth, but is apt to diffuse over all the trigeminal tract. Sympathetic neuralgias are not the sequences alone of pulpitis, one of the commonest causes being erosion just under the gingival margin.

Baume [1] considers pulpitis is rare in children, and only occurs when caries has attacked the organs before absorption begins.

There are many sequelæ of inflammation which bear on the etiology of neoplasms: 1. Chronic pulpitis, which may even be the primary condition. 2. Suppuration. 3. Hypertrophy. 4. Gangrene. 5. Periodontitis. 6. New formations. In chronic pulpitis we have little to distinguish between such as are inflamed or not, death of the pulp following very rapidly in some cases. There is no vital resistance, but an unresisting, decomposing, greasy mass, which easily explains the loss of pain during death of the pulp.

Suppuration.—This is indicated by a sense of fulness, uneasiness, and weight, and sometimes pulsation or boring pain, which may be of slight degree in some cases, but may be accompanied by œdema in and about the face in others. This is one of the commonest forms of termination of chronic pulpitis. Scanty watery pus, or pus of an acrid nature, is often met with where we have some constitutional disease, or where disease of the overlying parts has preceded or caused suppuration. When pus is sealed in 'a cavity for any length of time, without external agencies, we find it very much thicker, pasty, and with a vile odor of putrescence; microscopically it is very rich in fat.

Gangrene may rapidly follow suppuration, the nutritional cells becoming pus. The conditions due to congestion have been followed, and gangrene succeeds the high tension point of hyperæmia, the breaking up of the cell walls, passage and transformation of the cells, the coloring of the tooth, and the tissues melting down surely, if slowly, until all are destroyed; fat drops running in all directions, and even covering all the nerves and vessels, ánd cnding in a dark-colored, greasy, putrid mass,—sphacelus, or tooth discoloration. Dry gangrene is meant when evaporation of the circulatory secretions of the tooth has occurred.

Hypertrophy.—Inflammation may also cause a numerical increase in its constituents (hyperplasia), as well as hypertrophy, and form an enlarged mass so often and erroneously called a tumor. True, the increase in the new growth is allied to the histologic

---

[1] Dr. R. Baume, Lehrbuch der Zahnheilkunde.

structure in its cell elements and becomes a polypus resembling gum tissue, only projecting from the *interior* of the pulp-chamber. Microscopically, we see connective tissue, the vascularity being a characteristic feature. The nerve element being wanting, sensibility is often lacking—*unempfindlich.* Growth is rapid and often recurring readily, resembling malignant growths.

Salter speaks of a "sensitive sprouting of the pulp," differing very little from the above, except that it is clearer and softer and its vitality implies a more abundant nerve supply. It is often relieved only by extraction of the tooth.

Römer [1] has reported an examination of thirty patients with polypus, and gives three ·layers of granulation tissue: 1. Outer layer of pus cells. 2. Wider zone of endothelial cells,· and of capillaries with the appearance of gland strata. 3. Strong tissue, with enlarged blood-vessels and containing many round cells.

When the teeth are extracted they are placed in ten per cent. formalin and decalcified in thirty-three and one-third per cent. solution of formic acid. They are cut in half with a razor and the part wanted embedded in celloidin and stained by any dye, as alum-hæmatoxylin, and picrofuchsin (Van Giessen), or by Weigert's method.

In the head of the polyp ño nerve-fibres were seen, but in pulp-chambers and root-canals were nerve bundles, varying according to the degeneration found, which consisted usually of fibroid elements seen best in teeth whose pulps have been exposed by fracturing the tooth in faulty extraction. In the case under consideration there was little to note as being unusual.

The patient, an elderly woman, aged fifty-six, stout build, neurotic type, with signs of bronchial irritation and asthma (two sisters having died of cancer), called to see me regarding a partial plate. After examination, I advised that the few remaining teeth be extracted, as she gave a history of continued neuralgia around the face and head. The teeth were scattered in the mouth, and only the right upper first premolar and cuspid seemed peculiar, the former having a queer reddish color, no carious spots or other evidences of decay. The mouth was very cleanly kept; slight irritation of the gingivæ around the teeth and a feeling of un-

---

[1] Rümer, Ueber Pulpa Polypen der Zähne. Corresp. Blätt. f. Zahnärzte, C. Ash, Berlin, January, 1892.

easiness about the premolar. On percussing, I found that the nerve was not dead, but evidently congested. On extraction, hemorrhage was free and the tooth seemed to give way reluctantly, with a feeling of pulling from the apical attachment (hyperplasia cementum). I dropped it at once in warm saline solution, and then extracted the cuspid, which was an oddly shaped tooth, of a queer greenish-white tinge, so noticeable that the patient many times said people asked what was the matter with it. The cuspid was exceedingly difficult to remove, and on its coming out a drachm of yellowish clear fluid oozed from the alveolus. The apex of the root was covered with a thickened layer of peridental tissue, and I wondered if it was an abscess sac that had ruptured; the foramen showed a whitish thread hanging as the pulp, and I saw no evidences of suppuration, but some hypercementosis. So I preserved it in salt solution. The socket I carefully cleansed with peroxide of hydrogen; there was no effervescence to speak of, except when bleeding. Then I probed the cavity, and finally curetted it as thoroughly as I could, applied tincture of iodine, and then ninety-five per cent. carbolic acid, and plugged with gauze and wool. This I did for nearly a week, and then allowed the cavity to close. It healed steadily on the slow and gradual withdrawal day by day of the gauze tampon. The patient so far (after three years) has had no recurrence nor trouble, and seems much more comfortable, using no upper plate yet, as she prefers to wait.

The teeth were removed from the saline solution and carefully opened, one longitudinally, and the cuspid transversely about halfway, and the root longitudinally under normal fluid, till appearances were noted, and then it was changed to Zenker's solution. The cuspid had a fairly solid pulp, whitish-green. It looked like a fibroid, and was springy to the touch like a myxoma. I made microsections, and reproduce some photomicrographs from them. Taking the pulp at different levels, we find it complex and offering an unusual appearance.

Several points are worthy of note (Figs. 1 and 2) : 1. Evidence of granulation tissue and pulpitis. 2. Slight sclerosis or fibrosis. 3. Slight hyaline degeneration in this area. 4. Small vessels surrounded by fibrous thickening. 5. Many polynuclear leucocytes were scattered throughout, in some places massing together like a round-celled infiltration and mixed in with bands of fibrous trabeculæ. (Figs. 2, 3, and 4.) 6. Near the outer edge were more deeply stained cells and better formed fibrous tissue, which gave a more homogeneous appearance to the cells, and at one side was a dark bluish irregular body, a calcospherite or pulp-stone, longer than it was wide, and with a poorly stained area around it. (Fig. 1.)   At one edge of the specimen was an almost glistening hyaline mass of cells, inflammatory, and with some cells, much larger than others and multinucleated, lining the fibrous stroma spaces, almost like scirrhus cancer. (Figs. 5 and 6.)   Some of these cells were massed in cluster-nests, showing signs of considerable pressure; some cells staining a pale hyaline pinkish color, with the nuclei taking a darker stain, like cartilaginous cells, others appearing horny and taking no stain.   A number of dyes were used, prominently hematoxylin and eosin, Van Giessen, and Ranvier's picrocarmine and logwood, picrofuchsin and nigrosin, safranin, Unna's polychrome-methyl blue.

A method that will be found very useful for gum tissue, polypi, and epithelial structures is one modified and suggested by W. R. Smith, M.B.: Stain the section on the slide with hematoxylin and alum carmine, wash with water and put on the slide; dehydrate with absolute alcohol, stain a few seconds with a saturated solution of saffranin in aniline oil water, of which most is removed with blotting-paper, run over the section absolute alcohol for a few seconds, and immediately drop on clove oil; mount in Canada balsam in xylol or chloroform.   Great care is required in the washing out; it must only be partial.   Too little alcohol in the washing leaves the stain in the normal tissues, and does not differentiate the cell-nests from these or from other epithelial structures. Too much alcohol removes the whole of the stain from all pathologic and normal tissues.   If sections are cut fresh, it is much harder to stain with hematoxylin and to dehydrate.   For fresh sections, soak a few minutes in four per cent. formalin or methyl alcohol and then use alum carmine and wash thoroughly in water, and dehydrate.   The carmine stains faster if gently warmed.   In studying these specimens we must clearly note:

1. Whether normal non-pathologic growths of epithelium in the form of processes are growing inward from an epithelial surface,—*e.g.,* gum, epidermis, mucous membrane, pulp, or glandular organ which can resemble an epithelial pearl when cut in some ways.

2. Pathologic processes, papillary prominences, epithelial col-

FIG. 1.

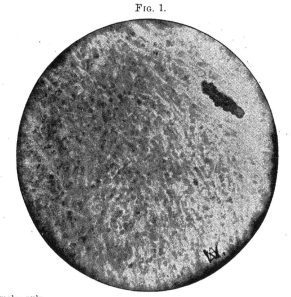

T. S. premolar pulp. × 143. Taken from a central area. Pulp-stone, fibrous tissue, with cells showing cloudy swelling, fat.

FIG. 2.

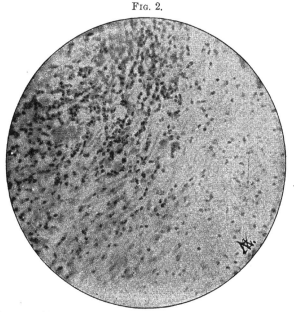

T. S. pulp. × 148. Showing polynuclear leucocytes. Early fibrous tissue with connective tissue corpuscles.

FIG. 3.

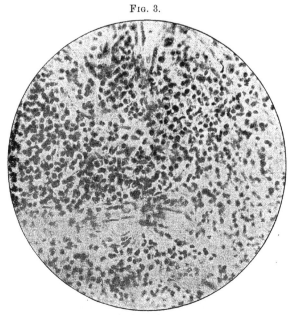

T. S. pulp. × 250. Showing cell infiltration, proliferation of blood-vessels—fibrous tissue
—more advanced than Fig. 2.

FIG. 4.

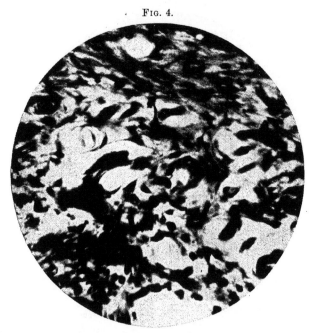

Pulp. × 400. Connective tissue. Spindle cells. Thickening of inner coats of vessel.

FIG. 5.

/ Artery.

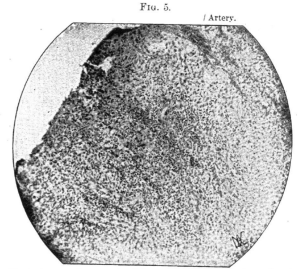

T· S. cuspid pulp from another area of periphery. Showing inflammatory cells, arteries, and the margin free from odontoblasts. × 50.

FIG. 6.

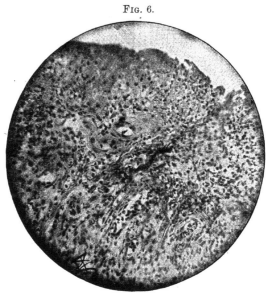

T. S. cuspid pulp. × 143. Showing horny or hyaline areas, here and there large cells and early masses with fibrous tissue resembling a scirrhus growth.

Fig. 7.
Vessel with cancer cell.

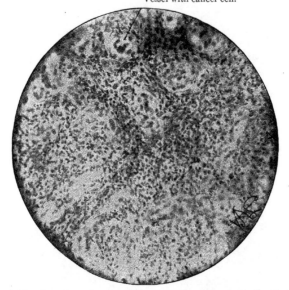

T. S. peripheral surface of pulp. × 143. Showing early whorls of cells, large and small. A binucleated cell to the left, on the outer edge a vessel with a carcinoma cell in the wall.

umns of homogeneous masses of epithelial cells with ovoid nuclei (papillary prominences of Lebert), which may be found in the surrounding tissue, and simulate cell-nests. Neither of these correspond with Billroth's classical description of cell-nests. What distinguishes these masses in their earliest known form? (Figs. 7 and 8.)

They appear at first sight like spherical or oval cysts from one one-hundredth to one five-hundredth of an inch in diameter, walled in by irregular fibrous tissue, and containing granular matter, nuclei, or cells within them. They may be in cluster or cylindrical; their nuclei are shrivelled or not visible; contents often granular.

The termination in horny material is an extreme form of specialization, and such is not the destiny of all cell-nests. Indeed, the study of these extreme forms is much desired, for observers have thus been misled as to the true nature of the structure and mode of growth of cell-nests in general.[1] (Fig. 13.) In all probability epithelial cell-nests start from one cell, by division and subdivision, except in such a disease with large pearls, as seen by Hamilton.[2]

In Figures 7 and 8 we find a single cell with two nuclei standing out; around it various-sized cells are massed, forming an early cluster, and surrounded by one outer layer of cells; in places, only a single cell and small cohorts of a few cells each. In some places we find here and there a thickened capillary or arteriole, showing well-marked cells lining the endothelium (Fig. 7); here and there a large cell and nucleus, or an alveolus filled with a cluster of cells, almost forming an island. (Fig. 10.)

We find masses like those just described mixed in with the small-celled infiltration of Virchow, indicating active proliferation and irritation, with the intermediate areas breaking down or staining only poorly, but with here and there well-marked nucleated cells. Lying near these masses we see some typical cell-nests with granular detritus among them, singly and in groups. How these cell-nests grow is yet to be understood. Paget[3] is in favor of the

---

[1] Woodhead's Pathology, second edition, 1885, p. 481; third edition, 1892, p. 174.

[2] Text-book of Pathology, 1889, part 1, p. 406.

[3] Paget, Lectures on Surgical Pathology, third edition, 1870, p. 720.

theory of the growth being from one central cell, and Snow,[1] who, with others, gives us a theory of surrounding pressure, says " a small area of cells always appears as the original point of the globe, never a single cell." (Figs. 9, 10, 12.)

That this specimen is a carcinoma, epithelioma, is very evident. It certainly cannot be classed, like Wedl's and Bödecker's cases, as a lymphomyeloma or round-celled sarcoma, for it certainly possesses epithelial nests, fibrous trabeculæ, and stroma, lined with large cells; granulation cells of the polynuclear type, degeneration, and a reaction to dyes that marks the carcinoma group. (Figs. 6, 7, 11, 12, 13.)

In polypus of the pulp the parenchymatous connective tissue is the seat of the proliferation described as sarcoma of the pulp, in which the parenchyma is gradually destroyed, and indicated by the absence of nerves and the altered character of the blood-vessels. As the sarcoma is located on the outside of the remains of the pulp, it serves in a measure to protect the latter.[2]

The study of the odontoblasts is a very vexatious one, as on account of their close relation to the dentine it is difficult to procure good sections without decalcifying the hard tissues, or preparing a tooth by the Koch-Weil process, which loses much valuable material; and the disarrangement of the pulp, unless this is done, renders it valueless.

In removing the pulp from its chamber the layer of odontoblasts clings tenaciously to the dentinal walls, either partly or as a whole, and hence we can easily understand how little progress has been made in this study. Black[3] states that this layer of cells seems to remain unchanged in acute inflammation until combined with suppuration. This seems, judging from my own work, to be hardly the case, for the cells are seen in every state of disease, and many times are not present, showing plainly the odontoblast cells act very similarly to the ciliated cells in bronchitis, and the falling off before the pulp is very much affected shows how easily any irritant affects the deep pulpal ends of the cells, and so causes atrophy and degeneration. (Figs. 4 and 5.) Hopewell-Smith[4]

---

[1] Snow, Cancer and Cancer Processes, London, p. 65.
[2] Wedl, Pathologie der Zähne, 1870. Transl.
[3] Black, American System of Dentistry, p. 915.
[4] A. Hopewell-Smith, The Histology and Pathological Histology of the Teeth, 1903.

F<small>IG</small>. 8.

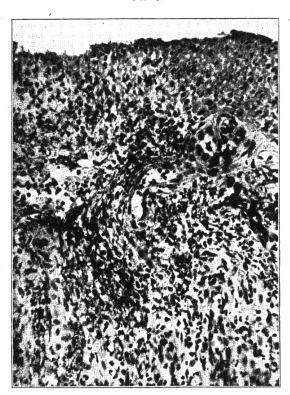

Pulp. ✕ 240. Note the large cells in places of the inflammatory tissue around vascular areas.

FIG. 9.

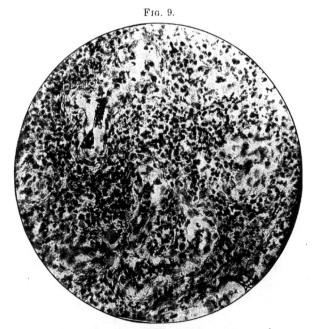

T. S. pulp nearer to the centre. × 225. Showing the inflammatory condition and the scattered cancer cells.

FIG 10.

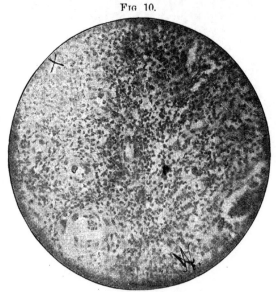

T. S. pulp following Figs. 7 and 9. × 143. Showing medullary type of growth. Multinucleated cells.

FIG. 11.

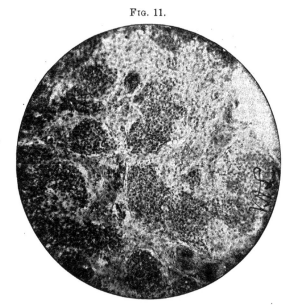

T. S. pulp continued from Section 10.   Medullary masses all through with a typical epithelial arrangement in the lower area.   Fragmentation.   × 137.

FIG. 12.

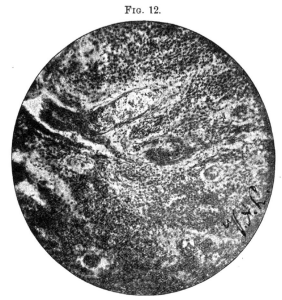

T. S. pulp.   × 137.   Showing the change from the closely massed areas to the epitheliomatous cell nests and the pressure points surrounded by fibrous tissue—detritus.

FIG. 13.

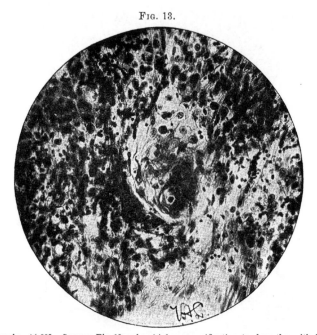

T. S. pulp. × 225. Same as Fig. 12, only a higher magnification to show the epithelioma, with layers of cells. Nucleated characters plainly seen. Yeast infection.

also shows illustrations which correspond to my own slides of inflamed odontoblasts, showing in some a numerical hyperplasia. It would be an interesting study to make careful sections of pulps *in situ* and extracted from teeth excised in cases of neoplasms of the jaw, as myeloid sarcoma, epithelial growths, fibroma, epulis, etc., and so note if the pulp shows any metastatic deposits or any other pathologic conditions. I have a few specimens so made which exhibit many problems for elucidation, and especially as regards their origin.

In the specimen here presented it may be asked how and from what did this growth originate. The teeth were, to all appearance, sound; even with an aplanatic lens nothing could be seen but the change in color, which gave me the idea of a dead tooth, and the percussion note was negative. The sensitiveness and neuralgic pain pointed out pulp and peridental irritation. Stanley Colyer [1] shows a "burrowing epithelioma from the periodontal membrane" which illustrates my section of neoplasm of the pulp very well, but he found the pulp dead and suppurating. His theory as to origin would certainly be questioned by many of the workers in carcinoma to-day. (Figs. 11 and 13.)

If we accept the theory that "like cells produce like," then how did odontoblasts produce epithelial cells, if the former originate from the stomodeal mesoblast,—*i.e.,* from the periphery of the dentinal or pulp organ? If odontoblasts could be proved as arising from the epiblast or hypoblast, many difficulties would be removed. Their nerve-endings and their close relationship to the cells at the terminations of the optic and auditory or sensory nerves, not only as regards the physiology, but the morphology and pathology, their functions being allied somewhat to the glandular organs, as in the stomach and intestine,—namely, secretion, excretion, and manufacture of chemical problems for metabolism,—and the situation and better development of odontoblasts at the coronal cervical part show that we have here a close relationship of epiblast and hypoblast structures. This points to the nerve-impressions passing through the tubules, and shows a closer relationship to the nervous system than is usually given.

In looking over the question of treatment we must note the

---

[1] Stanley Colyer, Transactions Odontological Society of Great Britain, June, 1901, pp. 231, 242.

use of the cautery, escharotics, and iodine. In this instance the best and only treatment was extraction, and if it had not been for the usual plan of study by breaking open the teeth and making sections, the great danger the patient ran would never have been recognized, and the chance of continual watching afterwards, as well as the curetting which was done, would have been lost. It is well known that arsenic has been accredited with causing epithelioma, and J. Hutchinson[1] considers that many of the cases of multiple cutaneous sarcomata may be fairly attributed to the use of iodine and its salts. When we note the frequency with which iodine is used in dentistry, externally and internally, that many patent medicines contain it, and consider its use in the arts, photography especially, and in the preparation of antiseptic gauzes, we can find another point for study. The frequent stimulation used by dentists for pericemental and periodontal irritation should cause an increase in hypertrophy, gingivitis, and the papilloma and epulis forms of growth, to say nothing of the epitheliomata; but I think it can be shown we have less neoplasms in the oral cavity now than formerly, due, possibly, to better hygiene and methods of operating.

CONCLUSIONS.

The points of interest are:

1. The freedom from urgent symptoms beyond neuralgia.

2. The great rarity of neoplasms of the pulp.

3. Lack of literature and careful pathologic and histologic study.

4. The want of further and more complete examination of the tooth-structures, in relation to the pathology of neoplasms of the jaw.

5. The question of metastases in the pulp from periodontal tumors.

6. The value of microscopic study should be urged in dental schools, as an aid to differential diagnosis and treatment.

7. The changes which may attend the killing of pulps by irritants and care to thoroughly cleanse the pulp-canals.

8. To emphasize the better treatment and value of closing up fistulous openings in the gingivæ for fear of further infection, and

---

[1] Archives of Surgery.

irritation of the peridental membrane, which may cause the growth of neoplasms.

9. That all dead teeth should be discovered early and treated thoroughly with the best of surgical skill.

10. The frequency with which hypercementosis is found at the radical point of the dead tooth.

11. The embryonic origin of the various structures of the pulp.

12. That great care should be used when examining the dental structures in elderly people, and all causes of irritation removed.

13. From what did this epithelioma originate, since it is a primary growth, enamel or odontoblasts—most probably the nerve elements? [1]

DISCUSSION ON PAPERS BY DRS. ANDREWS, TALBOT, AND LATHAM.

Dr. M. L. Rhein, New York City.—The deductions which Dr. Andrews has made I do not think are logical or warranted by what he has presented to our Section in the last few years. I have never taken the position attributed to me of believing that pulps were merely for formative purpose, and that in adult life they would be better out than in. I do radically disagree with the argument laid down by Professor Andrews that we are too prone to remove diseased pulps, and I believe Dr. Latham's conclusions show the error of conservative treatment of diseased pulps. One of the unfortunate things that meets the practising dentist is the impossibility of making microscopic examination of pulps in a pathologic condition. We can only draw inferences and conclusions. There has come into practice in my locality in the last few years a pulp-capping imported from Germany, known as "iodoformagin." I have a large collection of radiographs taken from one to three years after this medium has been used, and in every instance macroscopic examination has shown an apparent degeneration of pulp-tissue. It has been impossible to make microscopic examinations. In some cases the entire contents of the pulp-canal have apparently been consolidated, so that, so far as a circulating medium, or pulp proper, it has disappeared up to within a close border of the end

---

[1] Other references which may be consulted are: Latham, Résumé of the Histology of the Pulp, Journal American Medical Association, July 12, 1902; New York Medical Journal, May 10, 1902; also American System of Dentistry, vol. i. p. 883.

of the root. It is for this purpose that I have been for years a strong advocate of the aseptic removal of every portion of the contents, not only of the pulp-chamber, but the canals where this is liable to occur, or where it is feared. The criticism made by Professor Andrews in his paper as to the results of removing the pulp and the subsequent deterioration of the cementum and pericementum tissue is one that I naturally disagree with, and the basis of that disagreement is the observation of following this practice for over twenty years. I do say that there is a vast difference in the manner and methods of removing pulp-tissue and of taking care of those tissues afterwards. The trouble is that the majority of the profession are not willing to give the time required to thoroughly remove every portion of the contents of the pulp. There is another procedure necessary after every portion of the pulp contents has been removed surgically; the introduction of proper therapeutic agents will remove so much of those fibrils that enter the canalicular portion of the dentine as to leave that tooth absolutely free from any danger of breaking down and infection. These agents should be followed by scientific sterilization of the canals. Finally, the hermetical sealing of those canals is one of the means which will keep the roots in healthy condition. Where this healthy condition does not continue, it is, in the majority of cases, due to faulty operation. There is no excuse for a darkened tooth-substance after the removal of tooth-tissue.

Dr. E. A. Bogue, New York.—Dr. Rhein has called attention to my misunderstanding of his position. I am glad to have him set right the question of removing a living pulp. He has just acknowledged what I wished to have him,—that a living pulp cannot always be removed instrumentally. This morning he said that he had been misinterpreted and made to say that he considered the pulp of no value after adult life had been reached, and it might better be removed than not. That was not my understanding, but I understand him to publish this statement, that after adult life is reached he regards the pulp, being a formative organ of the tooth, as of little further value. I agree with him in regard to preserving a pulp exposed by decay. I have never seen any capping or treatment of any kind effectual in restoring health, or a condition that would lead to restored health, in these pulps, once exposed. Dr. Rhein told me on one occasion that he had removed a living pulp from a right lower molar. I have that tooth in my possession to-day. It and I do not agree with them. I surely do not mean to remove the pulp. When brought to me, it had considerable of the pulp in it, showing that his skill was not sufficient to get it out; nor could any one else have done it.

Dr. E. C. Briggs, Boston.—I take the ground which I have taken before, which is that after adult life the pulp is more often a menace to the tooth than a help. That does not mean that every tooth should have the pulp killed. I think that after the able papers by Drs. Latham and Talbot we are appalled at the ills the flesh is heir to, and it makes one more convinced than ever that the pulp had better be out of the way. The surgical removal of the pulp is the thing that these men do not seem to consider. We know Dr. Andrews's ability and power of research, which I bow to with great respect; yet his deductions are not necessarily correct, and I do not agree with them. I surely do not mean to remove the pulp with acids and arsenic and such things that will destroy the tooth, but if the pulp is removed surgically it does not destroy the tooth any more than removing the appendix destroys the whole alimentary canal; so that I indorse what Dr. Rhein says in respect to removing the pulp with rather more emphasis than perhaps he puts on it.

Dr. N. S. Hoff, Ann Arbor.—Would you have removed this pulp that Dr. Latham reports, simply because of the symptoms?

Dr. Briggs.—I think I would. It is one of my preliminary treatments in interstitial gingivitis or pyorrhœa alveolaris. I knew enough of the evils which are the result of this condition of the pulp before Dr. Latham and Dr. Talbot referred to the subject. I knew of the exostosis and the reverse action of the odontoblasts in removing calcareous matter from the root, and I knew of the pulp-stones, and now all these other conditions only emphasize, to my mind, the importance of the surgical removal of pulp when there is any irritation.

Dr. M. L. Rhein.—Dr. Briggs has stated my position, and I stand exactly on what I have published. Dr. Bogue has misunderstood what I have published. All that has ever been brought before this Section has shown us how difficult it is to find the pulps in adult life in a normal physiologic condition. As I understand Dr. Bogue, he advocates in the multiple-rooted teeth the use of arsenic in preference to removal under anæsthesia by cocaine. I differ entirely with him. I think he has held up the case which he cites a number of times, and very erroneously. The posterior root of this lower molar had coalesced with the anterior canals, and there was a slight amount of this deposit between the two roots. This is the description of the tooth given me by Dr. Taggart, of Burlington, Vt. After the pulp was surgically removed from the posterior canal and both anterior canals of these teeth were in such a condition that it was impossible to find a trace of any pulp-tissue, the canals were subjected to a most vigorous treatment by sodium and potassium, which practically destroyed any vitality that remained in this coalescent site. The subsequent history of this case proves absolutely the correctness of my position. It does not follow that arsenic would have acted any better. On the contrary, I have histories of cases in which arsenic has failed to do its work, and where cocaine enabled me to remove surgically the pulp from the canals of multiple-rooted teeth where it was impossible to proceed after numerous arsenical applications had been made. Where arsenic would have been of any further value in a case of coalescence of these two roots I fail to see.

Dr. A. W. Harlan, New York City.—It seems to me the summing up of Dr. Andrews's paper is the desirability of retaining the pulp in a tooth for other than formative purposes. Dr. Andrews's position on the retention of the vitality of the pulp when not diseased is probably correct. When a pulp becomes exposed there are certain changes that take place within a certain period which render that pulp as a normal organ valueless, and it might just as well be destroyed. Referring to the paper of Dr. Latham, I think perhaps the extraction of that tooth was correct, but I challenge the statement that there is no method of knowing whether the pulp has died, because we have ample means at present, although somewhat imperfect, of determining whether the pulp is alive.

Dr. V. A. Latham.—I said that our means of diagnosing dead teeth was not as yet very perfect or absolute.

Dr. A. W. Harlan.—So far as determining the vitality or non-vitality of the pulp is concerned, I should contend that with heat, cold, or electricity we can determine that absolutely. I was interested in Dr. Talbot's statement that abnormalities of the teeth occur from non-use. In the publication of Oakley Coles, more than thirty years ago, there are shown a number of abnormalities of the pulp. It is absolutely certain that when a tooth is not in use it deteriorates either by elongation or by the growths on the external surface of the root, or that it gets out of position and the tissues around the root become so inflamed and irritated that it becomes a useless member. It is further absólutely determined that in the rapid eruption of the teeth certain changes of the pulp take place. The chewing of tobacco and the holding of pipes in place also cause changes in the pulp. When the pulp is diseased we have a formation which may be in the shape of a cyst, and within that cyst we may have a deposit of calcareous matter which is a pseudo-form of tartar. There are growths around the ends of the teeth after the pulps die that may cause serious disturbance of the general system, so great as to result fatally. I would, therefore, conclude that when the pulp becomes exposed it should be destroyed, no matter whether it is surgically removed or poisoned; destroy it so that you will get every vestige of it out. The root of the tooth should be filled and there should be a sufficient amount of contact with the opposing jaw to keep the tooth in use.

Dr. J. L. Williams, Boston.—Pulps that are nearly exposed and not diseased I have proved in years of practice can be saved and means taken to protect them; but, after a pulp has become inflamed I have learned not to expect its total recovery. It may be kept comfortable, but I suppose its nutritive quality is lost, and I often question whether it is worth while to tamper with it. Some years ago I saw a case in which the pulp was exposed, but not wounded. I tried a process of treatment, which I was the first to introduce and systematize. I made the softest possible antiseptic covering for it; I looked at it at the end of a month and again treated it. At the end of about a year I opened it. It looked perfectly clear, and in passing my instrument over the transparent secondary dentine there was no sensation. It was then filled. In two years the tooth decayed on the other side. There was some sensation on excavating the new cavity, showing that we should discriminate between an exposed pulp and a diseased pulp. I do not believe that when a pulp has its growth it does not contribute to the continued welfare of the tooth. When it can be made healthy it should be saved for the benefit of the tooth.

Dr. E. C. Briggs.—We should bring out clearly that the idea brought forward is not that one is to go around slaughtering pulps of teeth, but that, if things are in any way wrong concerning the teeth, the chances are that there is more menace from the presence of the pulp than without it. In answer to Dr. Bogue, I do not like to have the principle destroyed by his questioning one's ability to remove the pulp. I do not pretend that I can do these things, but I think the chances are that I or some other one will find a perfect way of doing this work. We are doing now a great many things that could not be done ten years ago. The underlying principle is not affected.

Dr. E. A. Bogue.—Dr. Dawbarn, in a paper on malignant growths, speaks of an operation of his own devising,—viz., excision of a portion of both external carotids after ligation; and in speaking of that he has two or three times wondered why we as dentists did not more often observe the incipient beginnings of cancer. He says that sarcoma and carcinoma are acted on quite differently by his operation. In sarcoma he has had no instance up to the present in which he has felt that his operation has been a failure. In carcinoma he regards the operation as helpful only for a short time. That brought to mind Dr. Latham's case, which would show that it was through the circulation that carcinoma took its way, while sarcoma may more particularly be called a local condition. I hope we may have a further report concerning Dr. Latham's case.

Dr. Talbot.—There has been for several years a symposium on the dental pulp, and the results have been more than satisfactory. Dr. Andrews's paper is far-reaching, and I fear the importance of the paper is not understood. It has been discussed from the degeneration stand-point, but the fact has been lost sight of that the pulp at any period of life has its influence on tooth-structure. The paper is most valuable, because it leads to the point of the necessity of the vitality of the tooth. If it be necessary, as Dr. Andrews shows, it must follow that diseases of the human body have a great influence on tooth-structure. It must be admitted that there is a difference between supposition that certain conditions of the pulp exist, or that they have been found and actually demonstrated. Supposing a condition exists in the human body; to state it is one thing, to demonstrate it another. I wish all these papers on the pulp could be published in book form. It would be a most remarkable collection of papers.

Dr. Latham.—I came before this Section asking for a diagnosis, for advice, and also for bibliography. My main object was to bring my contribution before the Section for discussion as to the origin of the growth. I have held this case in hand for some three years, and only recently thought of publishing it. I have had experts in

Germany and in England looking up bibliography for me, with no success. The papers are not published in a way easy to be found, especially since the *Dental Cosmos* stopped its bibliography, and I would suggest greater care in choosing titles. I ask from what tissue did this epithelioma arise, if the pulp is a mesoblastic structure?

A REPORT ON ORTHODONTIA.[1]

BY LAWRENCE W. BAKER, D.M.D., BOSTON, MASS.

At the request of our president, Dr. Stanley, I have prepared, for you to-night a report on the subject of Orthodontia. This. report will consist of the explanation of some lantern-slides illustrating a series of cases that I have treated by means of the expansion arch appliance, perhaps better known to you as the Angle appliance.

Owing to the full programme, I shall endeavor to be as brief as possible.

The first slide that I am to have thrown upon the screen (Fig. 1) represents a type of normal occlusion which is familiar to you all. The more of this work I do the more I see to study and admire in this wonderful piece of nature's work, and I trust that by again bringing this picture to your attention you may also profit by it. It is the model that I have attempted to approach in the treatment of the various cases that we are to consider. I only wish that this picture could be permanently placed upon the screen, so that it could be compared with each and every case we are to discuss; for I fully realize that in order to obtain permanent results in this work the establishment of normal occlusion is essential.

It is essential simply for this one reason—that when the teeth are in a state of normal occlusion there is produced an *equilibrium of the occlusal forces* which can be obtained in no other possible arrangement of the occlusal planes. We should study, plan, and work to obtain this balance, for with it the teeth are placed in their most *retentive positions,* and there is the least possible chance of the

---

[1] Read before the Harvard Odontological Society, April 28, 1904.

arches returning to their malformed condition when once the tissue about the teeth becomes normal.

Perhaps by classifying these cases into several groups I may be able to explain them more clearly. I have adopted the Angle classification which has done so much for the advancement of this science by giving us a definite basis to work upon.

The first two cases have this one feature in common,—that the first molars occlude normally mesio-distally, placing them in the first group. Cases III., IV., and V. are characterized by a distal displacement of the first molar; therefore they belong to the second group. In Case VI. the occlusion has been so mutilated by extraction that I have been forced to put it in an out-of-class group.

Since this classification is based upon the normal mesio-distal relations of the first molars, let us consider our model and see what their normal relations are. We find that the lower first molar is one occlusal plane in advance of the upper one, allowing the point of the upper antro-buccal cusp to fall into the buccal fissure of the lower first molar, as shown by the lines marked upon these landmarks.

CASE I.—Fig. 2 shows us two side views of a case before treatment. The relations of our molar landmarks are normal, placing this case in the first class, according to our Angle classification. The reason for attempting correction of this case is evidently to improve the facial and dental expression.

Fig. 3 shows the results of the attempt at copying our model, normal occlusion. This change has given us a marked improvement in appearance and in utility, and has also greatly minimized the danger from dental caries, all resulting from the fact that the balance of the occlusal forces has been established.

CASE II.—Fig. 4 illustrates similar views of a case having this one occlusal characteristic in common with the preceding,—the molar landmarks are normal mesio-distally, although the cases differ widely in other respects.

Fig. 5 shows the results obtained. I think you will all readily appreciate that the occlusal balance was reached, when I tell you that, after correction, I depended largely upon the occlusal force for retention. This normal locking of the teeth not only held what I had gained, but greatly improved upon my work.

CASE III.—Fig. 6. We notice at once that the character of this

Fig. 1.

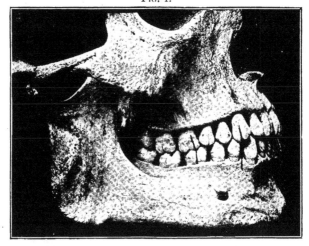

Fig. 2.

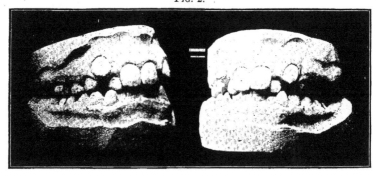

Fig. 3.

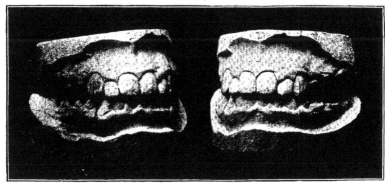

FIG. 4.

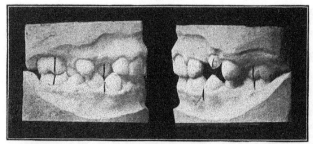

FIG. 5.

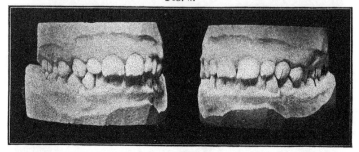

FIG. 6.

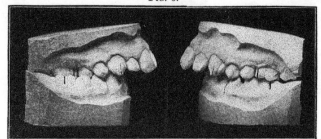

FIG. 7.

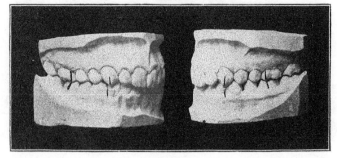

case is entirely different from that of the two preceding ones. It belongs to a different class,—to Group II.,—because of the distal displacement of the lower arch.

Formerly this deformity was supposed to be confined to a protrusion of the upper arch alone, but since the importance of the relations at normal occlusion to this work was realized, it has been noted that this deformity is caused by a distal displacement of the lower arch, as well as to a slight protrusion of the upper incisors. The deformity of one arch unfortunately exaggerates that of the other, producing a marked facial disfigurement, which can be easily imagined by studying the models before treatment. Fig. 7 shows the results obtained. The protrusion of the upper incisors has been reduced, and at the same time the receding lower jaw has been brought forward to its intended position, producing a great improvement in the balance of the facial lines; which goes to show that the relations between facial and dental harmony are closely associated. This result was obtained by the use of the inter-maxillary elastics, first used with marked success by my father, Dr. H. A. Baker.

CASE IV.—This I consider the most interesting case that I am to present this evening. It is one of those rare cases of distal occlusion in which the bite was jumped entirely unaided. To understand the changes that took place, close attention must be paid to the illustrations and description.

The apparent deformity is confined to the anterior part of the superior arch (see Fig. 9), but on consulting our occlusal landmarks in Fig. 8 it is seen that the lower arch is in distal occlusion, which places this case in the same general class with the preceding one. However, in that case the incisors *protruded,* while in this case they *retrude,* which fact places them in different subclasses of this second division.

Fig. 9 shows the occlusal aspect of the two arches before treatment. Note the crowded condition of the upper incisors, while the lower arch is perfectly regular.

Fig. 10 presents the same view of the corrected models. The only change noted is the correction of the upper arch, the lower arch remaining unaltered; in fact, no force whatever was applied to it during the progress of the work.

The next figure, 11, shows the effect of this change upon the occlusion. See that the receding lower arch has come forward to its correct position; the contraction of the anterior part of the upper arch having been the cause of its distal displacement. When the upper arch was made normal the lower arch simply slid forward to its proper place,—another case in which we see that as soon as nature was given a chance she re-established the occlusal balance.

CASE V.—It is with great hesitancy that I present this case, for two reasons: in the first place, I fear that you will doubt that there could be, due to the teeth, such a malformation of the jaws; and again, because I am unable to give you the finished result, the case being still under treatment.

Fig. 12 shows that the lower arch is not only in distal occlusion, but is doubly so; that is, instead of being one plane distal, it is distal two planes, causing a marked facial deformity.

By way of history, I should like to state that when the child came to me the lower sixth-year molars were beyond saving. At the proper time I had the bits of roots removed, allowing the twelfth-year molars to come forward, with the result that you see here.

In undertaking this case I should have hesitated at the responsibility had I not known something of the possibilities of the intermaxillary elastics.

The next illustration, Fig. 13, shows the study models as the case is. To get the exact relations of the two jaws I had the patient bite in wax and placed the models together accordingly. I am of the opinion that later, when the occlusion settles, a permanent benefit will result.

In this case many would have considered extraction in the upper arch necessary. I believe that by keeping the upper arch intact and bringing this receding lower jaw forward the facial lines will be placed in much better balance; for instead of weakening the lower part of the face, by moulding it to the weak receding lower jaw, it was strengthened by bringing the chin forward to harmonize with the general facial contour.

CASE VI.—Figs. 14 and 15. After considering the preceding case the one at hand will appear very simple. It is one of those cases in which there has been such wholesale extraction that I considered it impossible to obtain the normal state of affairs, so worked to get the best abnormal occlusion I could. For this reason we might consider it an " out-of-class" case, and I have placed it at the end of the report.

It is similar to most cases in which the arches have been mutilated by extraction, in that the deformity was progressive. In fact,

Fig. 9.

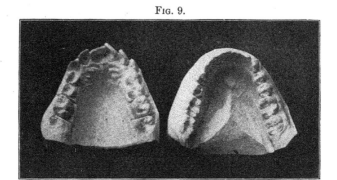

Fig. 10.

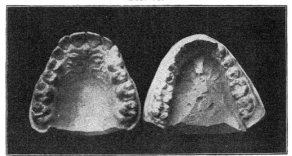

Fig. 11.

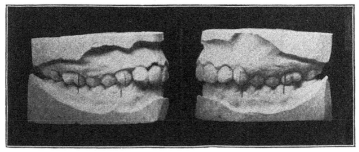

FIG. 12.

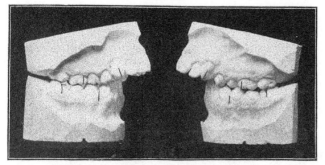

FIG. 13.

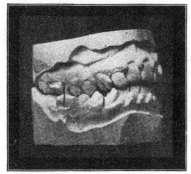

FIG. 14.

FIG. 15.

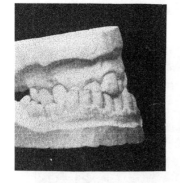
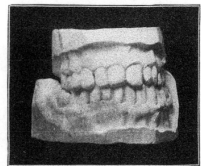

recently conditions had changed for the worse so rapidly that an increasing facial deformity was resulting, as might be expected from studying the models before treatment. The patient being a middle-aged woman, I could not anticipate an ideal result.

In bringing the retruding superior teeth over the lower ones spaces were necessarily formed. This condition was overcome by carrying the poorly spaced teeth towards the median line, converting the spaces into one large one between the cuspid and bicuspid and supplying this space with what might be termed a retaining bridge.

From the cases that we have briefly considered some may get the idea that I am an extremist regarding the non-extraction of teeth in the practice of Orthodontia. While my observations are that the use of the forceps has caused more harm than good, still we do find cases which have been previously mutilated by extraction, where an occlusal balance is impossible, and in which by resorting to judicious extraction, to balance planes previously lost, we may improve conditions by getting the best abnormal occlusion possible. Or, again, we find a limited number of cases where the lost planes can be successfully restored artificially.

In cases where the teeth are all present many mouths are ruined by the carrying out of the erroneous idea that extraction simplifies matters, whereas, as a rule, the case is usually made more difficult to correct and to retain.

MULTIPLE FRACTURE OF THE LOWER JAW COMPLICATED BY DOUBLE FRACTURE OF THE UPPER JAW.[1]

BY THOMAS L. GILMER, M.D., D.D.S., CHICAGO.

THE following case, with treatment, is considered of sufficient interest to present for your consideration:

From St. Luke's Hospital record of May, 1902, is taken the following:

---

[1] Read at the annual session of the American Medical Association, Section on Stomatology, Atlantic City, June 7 to 10, 1904.

"*Patient.*—G. C. was brought to accident ward about one A.M., May 12, 1902, in police ambulance, presenting the following lesions:

"1. Fracture of lower jaw multiple: (*a*) just to left of symphysis between two left incisors, compound in mouth; (*b*) on right side between bicuspid and first molar; (*c*) at angle of jaw right side, simple; whole lower jaw was flattened antero-posteriorly and dropped somewhat toward sternum.

"2. Fracture of upper jaw: (*a*) palate and alveolar processes broken from attachments and freely movable; (*b*) both alveolar processes broken loose from palate; (*c*) hard palate seemed fractured—antero-posteriorly throughout nearly the whole length—near the middle line. (Later examination did not positively confirm this.)

"3. Loss of teeth. Upper jaw: (*a*) four incisors; (*b*) both canines. Lower jaw: (*a*) left central incisor.

"4. Anterior portion of upper alveolar process detached from bone above and space so formed communicated freely with right nostril and probably with right antrum of Highmore.

"5. Extensive laceration of lower lip.

"6. Incised wound of chin.

"7. Hemorrhage from right ear not manifested until twelve hours after accident.

"8. Hemorrhage into soft parts about both eyes and into conjunctivæ.

"9. Hemorrhage subcutaneous about both ears.

"*Cause of Injury and Emergency Treatment.*—Fall from second-story window on a stone pavement. History of intoxication obtained from room-mate and confirmed by breath. Was in a heavy stupor, not unconscious, rather restless, and was continually spitting blood. Lower lip and wound of chin sutured with silkworm gut, about three sutures in each, in accident ward. Hemorrhage from nose and mouth was free and showed no tendency to stop. Both nostrils packed with iodoform gauze about three A.M. Hemorrhage only partly checked, and about five A.M. space leading up to nose, above the fractured alveolar process, was tightly packed with iodoform gauze. Hemorrhage then ceased after sufficient loss of blood to be appreciated constitutionally. Patient became more wideawake towards morning and has remained conscious and rational. Was seen by Dr. Gilmer about two P.M., who wired, provisionally,. the two teeth at sides of fracture near symphysis. Wet cold compresses were applied over face, and mouth and nose were thoroughly irrigated. t. i. d. with saturated boric solution, two ounces; oil cassia, one drop. Ear cleaned, filled with boric powder, and drained.

"Rectal temperature, 100.4; pulse, 86; respiration, 20."

Examination.—After a careful examination of the patient I found that the nature of the fracture and injuries of the jaws were more extensive than history of the internes indicated. I found the man in a semicomatose condition, blood oozing from the right ear, and also a conjunctival ecchymosis. His condition was so serious that I concluded absolute quiet more important for a few days than the setting of the bones of the jaws and face; indeed, I was quite positive that he could not recover. All of the injured parts were maintained in as nearly an aseptic condition as possible, the bowels kept open, and he was kept quiet. On the fifth day he had improved to such an extent that I felt it was safe to proceed with the treatment of the fractures.

A corrected diagnosis showed that there were five fractures of the lower jaw. On the left side, one at the angle, another on the line of the first bicuspid. On the right side there was a break at the neck of the condyle, one at the angle, and one at the cuspid tooth. The upper jaw was broken in half, through the median line, and the two halves were broken from their attachment above. All of the incisors and both cuspids on the upper jaw were knocked out and lost; the other teeth on this jaw were in place. On the lower jaw, strangely, only one tooth, an incisor, was missing. Those on a line with the fracture in the body of the bone were loosened.

Treatment.—In such a case no one method of treatment is applicable, therefore I decided on a combination of wiring and splinting, hoping by this means to at least partially restore the contour of the face and get a reasonably good occlusion of the teeth. Looking to this end, assisted by Dr. Arthur D. Black, an impression was made of the upper jaw and teeth in very soft modelling composition, the two lateral halves of the jaw having been temporarily restored to their normal position. On a cast from this impression a modified Kingsley splint was formed of vulcanite, square brass tubes being vulcanized in the splint on each side to receive the side arms. On the lower part of this splint wire staples were secured to receive the wires which were to be attached to the lower teeth (Fig. 1).

Holes were now drilled through the bone on either side of the anterior fracture on the lower jaw and the fragments caused by this break securely wired to each other by heavy silver wire. This gave stability to a considerable portion of the body of the bone. German silver wires were now placed around the necks of the firmly set teeth on the lower jaw and secured by twisting. The splint was adjusted to the upper teeth and the two halves of the upper jaw were drawn forward and pressed upward in their normal relation with the bones above it and secured in place by laces extending from the side arms, to which they were attached to eyelets in a skull cap (Fig. 2). The wires on the lower teeth were now secured to the staples on the lower part of the splint, the lower jaw being drawn forward by this attachment to its normal position and the teeth held in apposition with the splint, the lower surface of which was shaped to correspond with what I believe to represent the normal occlusion.

Results.—The result was far more satisfactory than could reasonably have been anticipated, and is fairly well shown in Fig. 3, made from a photograph taken immediately after the removal of the appliances. The occlusion of the teeth was so nearly correct that a trifle grinding made it approximately perfect. To prevent the laces slipping on the metal arms extending out from the mouth, pieces of adhesive plaster were attached to them. Through these holes were punched to receive the laces (Fig. 2).

The progress of the case was uneventful, the temperature never rising above 100.6. Primary union was secured in each fracture, and the patient was discharged one month and three days after the application of the splint and the wiring of the bone and teeth.

DISCUSSION.

Dr. G. V. I. Brown, Milwaukee.—I suppose it is only those who have been through the trials of excessive fractures and who are familiar with the conditions under which such cases come to the stomatologist and oral surgeon for treatment who can appreciate the very great difficulties that Dr. Gilmer has so successfully overcome in this case. Any one of the five fractures that was reported in this one jaw would have been sufficient difficulty in itself, but to take a multiple fracture with surrounding tissue having its in-

FIG. 1.

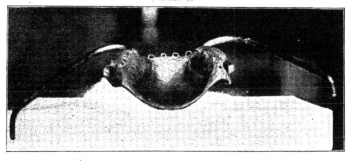

FIG. 2.

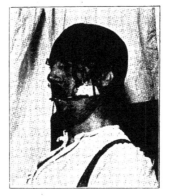

FIG. 3.

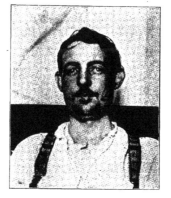

tegrity almost entirely destroyed by the traumatism makes the appearance of the patient as shown in the final result something almost beyond expectation. Commonly, the teaching with regard to the treatment of fractures is that it is necessary to apply the splint almost immediately. I note that Dr. Gilmer found it necessary to allow several days to elapse, and I think that that is the part of wisdom. Not only was it so in this case, but I believe it to be true in many other fractures of less degree. I have found it extremely useful to construct a temporary splint of modelling compound. I always carry this modelling compound in my surgical bag, and for use in an emergency it is extremely valuable. It can be softened in hot water and placed before there has been opportunity for swelling, soreness, or other complication to arise. When these conditions have subsided and the patient is in condition to control with comparative comfort, a better splint can be constructed, but even without the construction of another splint, modelling compound can be made to serve the purpose.

REPORT OF A CASE OF VINCENT'S ANGINA AND STOMATITIS.[1]

BY G. C. CRANDALL, B.S., M.D., ST. LOUIS.

THIS infection of the throat and mouth, as described by those who have reported cases, is characterized by a membranous, ulcerative process, quite painful, but with slight systemic reaction—the lesions, especially of the mouth, usually healing slowly; the secretion, pseudo-membrane, and tissue beneath containing a fusiform bacillus associated, as a rule, with a spirillum.

As comparatively few cases of Vincent's angina have been reported in this country, the following case will be of interest:

History.—Patient, male, single, twenty-three years old, medical student, family history good, always having been well except for an attack of measles and of typhoid fever some years ago. No

---

[1] Read at the annual session of the American Medical Association, Section on Stomatology, Atlantic City, June 7 to 10, 1904.

venereal disease. He had never suffered from sore throat nor sore mouth of any kind, and his teeth were unusually good.

The first indication of the disease which he observed appeared one morning at breakfast, when he noticed that swallowing hot coffee caused some pain in the region of the left tonsil. Looking at his throat he found it somewhat congested on the left side. During the following day it became gradually worse, so that the mere act of deglutition was very painful, much more, however, when swallowing anything hot; the tonsil, soft palate, and uvula becoming more congested. The second day a small diphtheritic spot was observed on the upper anterior border of the left tonsil, and the pain increased somewhat.

The spot was about one-fourth inch in diameter, and did not enlarge much during the six days it was present. It was covered by a grayish-white, friable pseudo-membrane, which could be easily removed, leaving a slightly depressed bleeding surface, over which membrane would again form in a few hours.

The fourth day of the disease he had a dentist clean his teeth, and the following day the disease appeared along the margin of the gums and between the teeth, the gums rapidly receding from the teeth, and the infection extended in places over the gums to the buccal surface, especially about the last molar teeth. Wherever the infection extended it had the appearance of the primary spot on the tonsil,—ulceration, accumulation of pseudo-membrane, congestion of surrounding mucous membrane, bleeding of the ulcerative surface when disturbed, and pain. The bleeding of the gums was very annoying, and with the pain prevented him from eating anything which it was necessary to masticate. With the extension of the infection to the gums, the breath became very foul, due to decomposing blood and membrane about and between the teeth. This unpleasant symptom continued to some extent until the disease entirely disappeared.

During the early part of the attack there was a slight increase in salivary secretion, but of no consequence. There was some swelling of the lymphatic glands near the angle of the jaw on the side where the infection first appeared; later there was slight swelling and tenderness of the lymphatics of the submaxillary region after the gums were invaded.

Throughout the course of the attack there were only slight constitutional symptoms; temperature was raised one-half to one

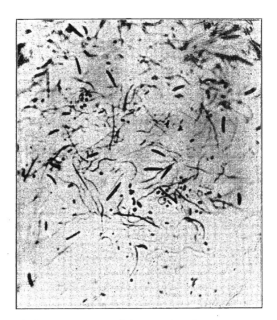

Photomicrograph of bacilli and spirilli of Vincent, with other organisms, as seen in smear taken from gums, stained with carbol-fuchsin. × 1000.

degree during first few days, after which it was normal. The patient became somewhat debilitated because of his inability to take the usual amount of food, but continued attending his college work without missing a day. He drank liquids, and ate only bland soft food neither hot nor cold.

Treatment.—On the third day the patient began treatment, applying a ten per cent. silver solution without apparent effect. On the fourth day the spot of the tonsil was touched with pure carbolic acid, followed by a gargle which consisted of 1 to 1000 bichloride in two per cent. carbolic solution. This relieved the throat at once, but had little effect on the infection of the gums, which later was relieved by chlorate of potash in solution, and better in the form of tablets, which the patient dissolved in the mouth frequently, expectorating the saliva. The tablets were used to the end of the attack. The throat symptoms cleared up in a week, but the lesions about the gums resisted treatment much longer, showing a tendency to recur, apparently because of the infection between and about the teeth which was so inaccessible to the local remedies used. While the throat was well in a week, the gums showed traces of the disease for six weeks.

Bacteriology.—A smear was made from the tonsil on the fourth day, first drying the spot with cotton to remove the mucus from the surface. This showed the bacillus of Vincent and a spirillum, the latter appearing identical with the *Spirochæta dentium* (Cohn), which is common in the mouth. Both organisms were abundant, with very few other germs present. Smears taken from the margin of the gums showed both organisms, but with numerous other organisms from the decomposing material about the teeth.

The organisms stained readily with carbolic fuchsin, also with gentian violet, and with Loeffler's methylene blue. The bacillus took the stains, as a rule, much better than the spirillum, although the latter took the gentian violet fairly well.

Efforts to make cultures of the organisms on the common media, gelatin agar, and blood serum were all negative.

The bacilli were distinctly fusiform, averaging large, but varying in length from eight to twelve microns, and in thickness from one-half to one micron. The spirilli were thirty-six to forty microns long, and of quite uniform thickness, about one-third micron (see illustration).

The organisms were found abundant during the first few days of the disease; later only a few could be found.

In this case the disease was at first confined to the throat, but was quickly and thoroughly inoculated into the gums by the irritation incident to cleaning the teeth.

The dentist was not aware of the infectious process in the throat; however, this case illustrates the necessity of caution on the part of the dentist in so simple a procedure as cleaning the teeth when any acute infectious process exists about the throat or mouth; at most, then, only the teeth and not the gums should be disturbed; every precaution should be taken to avoid irritation of the mucous membrane, since the slightest abrasion is inoculated with the infected secretion.

When we have an acute infectious process of the throat or mouth which has a tendency to spread, it would be well to confine the diet of the patient to bland liquids and soft food requiring no mastication, thus avoiding, so far as possible, all irritation of the mucous membrane.

So far as known, no other cases developed, although the patient was associating with other students constantly, avoiding, however, using any common drinking-cup.

Briefly reviewing the literature, we find that in 1896 Vincent[1] reported a form of ulcerative angina due to these organisms. In 1897 Bernheim[2] reported a series of thirty cases which conform in general to this disease, although he did not feel certain that the fusiform bacilli and spirilli found were the cause. Vincent[3] again, in 1898, reported fourteen cases. In 1901 Nicolet[4] and Morotte described the morphology of the organism. Mayer[5] in 1902 reported a typical case, with clinical data. In 1903[6] Fisher reported two typical cases, with description of organisms and illustrations. Hess[7] in 1903 reported two forms of the disease,—the croupous form, due to the fusiform bacilli, and the diphtheritic form, in which both the bacilli and the spirilli are present. In 1903 Anchi[8]

[1] Annales de l'Institute Pasteur, 1896.
[2] Deutsche med. Woch., 1897.
[3] Bull. de la Soc. des Hôpitaux, March, 1898.
[4] Revue de Médecin, April 10, 1901.
[5] Jour. Am. Med. Sci., 1902, p. 187.
[6] Ibid., 1903, p. 438.
[7] Deutsche med. Woch., vol. xxix., No. 42.
[8] Gaz. Hebd. d. Sci. Méd. de Bordeaux, 1903, vol. xxiv. p. 555.

called attention to the possibility of considerable tissue destruction incident to the disease. In 1903 Tarruella[1] discussed the clinical and bacteriologic features of what he terms the ulcerative-necrotic angina of Vincent. In 1903 Conrad[2] reviewed the literature to date quite thoroughly and gave some clinical reports.

Most of the observers emphasize the tendency of the disease to run a protracted course, especially when the gums are affected.

The differential diagnosis will come, as a rule, within three diseases,—syphilis, diphtheria, and Vincent's angina,—which can usually be readily cleared up by the history of the attack and a microscopic examination of the secretion from the ulcerated surface.

DISCUSSION.

Dr. Vida A. Latham, Rogers Park, Chicago.—I had the good fortune to see this specimen, which, I understand, is only the third ever reported in America. From a dental or stomatologic point of view it is of value, showing that dentists must recognize this disease. I had one case some time ago, but it was never recorded, as I was not sure at the time what it was. The patient's lips became almost black from the disease, and in consequence it was called gangrenous stomatitis. There was considerable pain and great nervous prostration. The only way of identifying the disease is by the microscopic examination.

Dr. E. C. Briggs, Boston.—I think I must have had a similar case, but no microscopic examination was made. When I first saw the case I thought it must be syphilis. There was excessive ulceration of the mucous membrane with severe pain. The patient was a man of character and courage, and I did not feel that he was exaggerating when he told me how intolerable his days and nights were. At another time I shall have a microscopic examination made for diagnosis. The case cleared up after a while, during which time I treated him vigorously.

Dr. Latham.—I would suggest in these cases the use of orthoform tablets for pain on deglutition.

[1] Rev. de Med. y Cirug. Barcel., 1903, vol. xvii. p. 180.
[2] Arch. f. Laryngol. u. Rhinol., Berlin, 1903, vol. xiv. 525.

Reviews of Dental Literature.

MEDICAL EDUCATION IN THE UNITED STATES.—The present issue of the *Journal* is the fourth annual educational number, and contains statistics regarding medical education in the United States, covering the year ending June 30, 1904. The information contained in this statistical study was obtained largely from the colleges directly, and has been certified to by some one in authority in each school, so that we have every reason to believe that all the data are as correct as can be obtained. It has been no easy task to gather all this information, and any errors that may have crept into the work are only such as are likely to occur when information is gathered from many sources. Only one college in the United States (not including the Manila and San Juan schools) flatly refused to give any information, but the data which might have been obtained would not have changed the totals appreciably. We take this opportunity of extending our thanks to all those who aided us in gathering these statistics.

A perusal of our study will show that medical education, so far as students and colleges are concerned, has not changed materially during the past year, although a slight improvement is noticeable in the advances made in the length of the college term. This improvement is, on the whole, very gratifying, inasmuch as it shows the disposition of all the schools to better medical education. In the statistics contained in this number, we have embodied some new features which, we are convinced, will be of interest to medical educators.

Number of Medical Students.—The number of medical students in the United States for the year ending June 30, 1904, was 26,138, a decrease of 1477 below the year 1903. Of this number, 23,662 were in attendance at the regular schools; 1105 at the homœopathic; 1014 at the eclectic, and 357 at the physiomedical and nondescript schools. There was a decrease in the attendance of the regular schools of 1268 below last year, and a decrease of 1216 below the year previous,—1902. In the homœopathic schools there was a decrease of 393 below that of 1903, and a decrease of 512 below 1902. The eclectic schools have been increasing steadily since

1900. In 1904, 1014 students attended the eclectic schools, an increase of 166 over the attendance of the year previous,—1903. The physiomedical and nondescript schools show an increase in attendance of 18 over the previous year, the attendance in 1903–04 being 357. This increase, however, occurred in the nondescript schools and not in the physiomedical.

TABLE OF MEDICAL COLLEGE ATTENDANCE.

Year.	Reg.	Homœo.	Eclec.	Physiomed. and Nondes.	Total.
1880	9,776	1220	830	...	11,826
1890	13,521	1164	719	...	15,404
1900	22,710	1909	552	...	25,171
1901	23,846	1683	664	224	26,417
1902	24,878	1617	765	241	27,501
1903	24,930	1498	848	339	27,615
1904	23,662	1105	1014	357	26,138

Number of Graduates.—The total number of graduates for the year ending June 30, 1904, was 5747, an increase of 49 over the preceding year. The increase in 1903 over 1902 was 699, so that the increase during the present year was much less than that of the year previous. Of course, there are nine more colleges this year than there were last year, but three of the nine were not in session, and the others, with the exception of one, taught only a portion of the medical course. Although the graduates have increased slightly, the matriculants have decreased considerably, and we must assume that the decrease has occurred largely in the Freshmen classes, partly because of the increase in entrance requirements, partly because of the increase in fees and general expense of the medical course, and, perhaps, because of the prosperity in the business world in general, which usually lowers the attendance in the professional schools. In some colleges there was a decided falling off in the Freshmen class, while in others there was a very slight increase. The falling off was noticeable, particularly, in those schools that raised their entrance requirements. The decrease in the number of graduates in the homœopathic schools— 49—represents the lowest number of graduates since 1902. The eclectic schools show a decrease of 3 in the number of graduates below last year, and the other school a decrease of 1. In the regular schools, on the other hand, there has been an increase of 102 over 1903.

TABLE OF MEDICAL COLLEGE GRADUATES.

Year.	Reg.	Homœo.	Eclec.	Physiomed. and Nondes.	Total.
1880	2673	380	188	..	3241
1890	3853	380	221	..	4454
1900	4715	413	86	..	5214
1901	4879	387	148	30	5444
1902	4498	336	138	27	4999
1903	5088	420	149	41	5698
1904	5190	371	146	40	5747

Number of Colleges.—Our report last year showed that there were at that time one hundred and fifty-seven medical colleges, three of which did not grant the degree of M.D., but taught only the first two years of the medical curriculum. Since then one college has passed out of existence, and ten new ones have been formed, making a total of one hundred and sixty-six colleges at the present time. Of these one hundred and thirty-three are regular, nineteen homœopathic, ten eclectic, three physiomedical, and one institution which teaches all the " pathies" and " isms," including osteopathy. Of the regular colleges, two are not yet active, and seven do not grant any degree. Of the latter number, six teach only the first two years of the medical course, and one only the first year. Two of the regular colleges are located in our island possessions; one is the Medical Department of the University of Porto Rico at San Juan, and the other the Medical Department of the San Tomaso University of Manila, P. I.

COLLEGES IN STATES AND CITIES.

ALABAMA—2.
Birmingham 1
Mobile 1

ARKANSAS—1.
Little Rock 1

CALIFORNIA—8.
San Francisco 5
Oakland 1
Los Angeles 2

COLORADO—3.
Denver 2
Boulder 1

CONNECTICUT—1.
New Haven 1

DISTRICT OF COLUMBIA—3.
Washington 3

GEORGIA—3.
Augusta 1
Atlanta 2

ILLINOIS—16.
Chicago 15
Galesburg 1

INDIANA—6.
Indianapolis 4
Fort Wayne 1
Bloomington 1

IOWA—5.

Iowa City 2
Des Moines 1
Sioux City 1
Keokuk 1

KANSAS—3.

Lawrence 1
Topeka 1
Kansas City 1

KENTUCKY—7.

Louisville .... ı

LOUISIANA—2.

New Orleans 2

MAINE—1.

Portland .... ı

MARYLAND—8.

Baltimore 8

MASSACHUSETTS—4.

Boston 4

MICHIGAN—6.

Ann Arbor 2
Detroit 3
Grand Rapids 1

MINNESOTA—3.

Minneapolis 3

MISSISSIPPI—1.

Oxford .... ı

MISSOURI—15.

St. Louis 6
Kansas City 6
Columbia 1
St. Joseph 2

NEBRASKA—3.

Omaha 2
Lincoln 1

NEW HAMPSHIRE—1.

Hanover 1

NEW YORK—11.

New York City 8
Albany 1
Buffalo 1
Syracuse 1

NORTH CAROLINA—4.

Raleigh 2
Davidson 1
Wake Forest 1

OHIO—10.

Cincinnati 4
Cleveland 3
Columbus 2
Toledo 1

OKLAHOMA—1.

Norman .... ı

OREGON—2.

Salem 1
Portland 1

PENNSYLVANIA—7.

Philadelphia 6
Pittsburg 1

PHILIPPINE ISLANDS—1.

Manila .... ı

PORTO RICO—1.

San Juan .... ı

SOUTH CAROLINA—1.

Charleston .... ı

TENNESSEE—11.

Nashville 4
Knoxville 2
Chattanooga 2
Memphis 1
Jackson 1
Sewanee 1

TEXAS—8.		VIRGINIA—3.	
Galveston	1	Charlottesville	1
Fort Worth	1	Richmond	2
Dallas	5	**WEST VIRGINIA—1.**	
Texarkana	1	Morgantown	1
VERMONT—1.		**WISCONSIN—2.**	
Burlington	1	Milwaukee	2

Three colleges are exclusively for women; sixty for men; one hundred and three are co-educational; four hold only night sessions, and two both day and night sessions. There are seven schools to which only colored people are admitted. Four schools operate under the continuous course system, the year being divided into quarters, the student being allowed to attend only a specified number of quarters or semesters in each calendar year. Sixty-six regular schools, four homœopathic, and one eclectic college have a university connection or affiliation. The baccalaureate and medical degrees are granted at the end of six years' study by six colleges, and at the end of seven years by one college.

Seventy regular colleges are members of the Association of American Medical Colleges, twelve belong to the Southern Medical College Association, eighteen of the homœopathic schools are recognized as in good standing by the American Institute of Homœopathy, and eight of the eclectic colleges are members of the National Confederation of Eclectic Medical Colleges. Many of the colleges not in these associations abide by their entrance requirements.

A study of the following comparative table of medical colleges is of interest. The regular schools have increased in number since 1903, while the other medical colleges number as many as last year. It must be remembered, however, that last year only three schools gave instruction in the first two years' work of the medical curriculum, whereas this year seven schools were engaged in doing this preparatory work. Each of these preparatory schools are integral parts of recognized universities, and this work, therefore, is accepted as a full credit by other medical colleges. By subtracting these seven colleges, and also the two schools in Porto Rico and Manila, from the number of regular medical schools, it gives us an actual increase of only two colleges which grant the degree of M.D., or a total of one hundred and fifty-six.

Year.	Reg.	Homœo.	Eclec.	Physiomed. and Nondes.	Total.
1880	72	12	6	..	90
1890	93	14	9		116
1900	121	22	8	..	151
1901	124	21	10	4	159
1902	121	20	10	4	155
1903	121	19	10	4	154
1904	133	19	10	4	166

Length of Terms.—A study of the length of terms, in months, of the various medical colleges discloses some very interesting facts. Of the one hundred and sixty-three schools from which we were able to obtain the necessary information, 40.3 per cent. have a course of at least eight months' duration. Only 16.3 per cent. have a course of less than seven months' duration. The figures are as follows:

TABLE OF COLLEGE TERMS.

Term.	Schools.	Per cent.
6 months	27	16.3
7 months	44	27.0
7½ months	22	13.5
8 months	34	20.8
8½ months	13	7.9
9 months	19	11.6
10 months *	4	2.4

* Night Schools.

Nearly all the shorter term schools are located in the South, where medical educators feel that the conditions are such as to prohibit a longer term. Most of the non-sectarian schools have seven months' terms. A very small percentage of the regular colleges have less than a seven months' term. Many of the colleges which last year had seven months' terms have adopted the eight and nine months' terms for the coming year. It is probable that another year will see the passing of the six months' school. Of course, the term "months" is elastic, inasmuch as seven months means anywhere from twenty-six to twenty-eight weeks; eight months, thirty to thirty-two weeks; and nine months, thirty-three to thirty-six weeks. It would be far better to regulate the length of each annual course by specifying a definite number of teaching days or number of hours spent in college.

Women in Medicine.—It is of interest that, in spite of the apparent passing away of colleges for women, the number of women medical students and graduates has been increasing steadily. During the past year only two of the three colleges for women were in session, but ninety-seven colleges are co-educational, which may account for the increase in women students. During the past year 1129 women were engaged in the study of medicine—4.3 per cent. of the total number of medical students—and 244 graduated,—four per cent. of the total number of graduates. Of the total number of matriculants, only 183 were in attendance at the two woman's colleges, and 46 graduated from them.—Editorial, *Jour. Amer. Med. Assn.*

THE TEACHING OF MATERIA MEDICA IN MEDICAL SCHOOLS. Abstract of a paper by Torald Sollman, M.D.[1]

DESIRABILITY OF RESTRICTING THE COURSE OF MATERIA MEDICA.

" I must confess, if I had my way I should abolish materia medica[2] altogether. . . . Not one trace of a knowledge of drugs has remained in my memory from that time to this; and really, as a matter of common sense, I cannot understand the arguments for obliging a medical man to know all about drugs, and where they come from. Why not make him belong to the Iron and Steel Institute, and learn something about cutlery, because he uses knives?

" I entertain a very strong conviction that any one who adds to medical education one iota or tittle beyond what is absolutely necessary is guilty of a very grave offence."—HUXLEY, " On Medical Education," 1870.

Every one will agree with this last sentence. In most medical schools the required class attendance exceeds thirty hours per week, leaving the student a very insufficient time for home study. This condition tends naturally to become worse, for the domain of medical knowledge is constantly extending, and the teaching must follow these extensions. It is, therefore, imperative to lighten the curriculum as much as possible by curtailing such studies as are no longer essential.

A case in point is presented by the relation of pharmacology, materia medica, and therapeutics. The study of the action of drugs

---

[1] Professor of Pharmacology and Materia Medica, Western Reserve University, Cleveland, Ohio.

[2] It will, I hope, be understood that I do not include therapeutics under this head.

by laboratory methods is a new branch and one which requires considerable time, which must be taken from some other subjects. It is very true that a knowledge of pharmacology facilitates the study of therapeutics so greatly that a part of the time formerly devoted to therapeutics can be assigned to pharmacology without injury. The saving thus effected is not, however, sufficient. What further time is' needed can be profitably drawn from materia medica (including pharmacy) if the course in these branches is wisely reorganized. This can be readily done, especially if they are taught in the same department as pharmacology, as they should be, in my opinion.

No one can doubt that the action of drugs is of vastly greater importance to the medical practitioner than their natural history. The latter can only be of essential importance when the physician is located remote from a pharmacist, a condition which is rather rare in this country. Nothing prevents those who expect to be so situated from taking a special, optional course, and such should be offered by the college, if it is needed. Were there no other demand on the students' time, an exhaustive course of materia medica might be profitable to all other students, but there can be no question that the other demands are more important. Indeed, I incline to the belief that the above advice of Huxley has not been sufficiently heeded by many schools, doubtless because it is somewhat too radical.

WHAT PARTS OF MATERIA MEDICA SHOULD BE RETAINED?

How far, then, may the study of materia medica be safely curtailed? What is essential? What may be made optional and what omitted entirely? There is surely room for much honest difference of opinion in this connection. I venture to give my views, as they may serve as a basis for reflection.

I believe that the students should be given, by way of introduction, some general ideas about the classes of chemical and structural constituents of drugs. Sufficient botany should have been learned in school, and zoölogy is quite superfluous. The systems of weights and measures should be made thoroughly familiar. In regard to pharmacy, the student should learn the different classes of pharmaceutic preparations, their common characteristics and special uses, and he should be given (by demonstration) a broad conception of how they are prepared. A little practice in simple dispensing is very desirable. All these data will be invaluable in understanding the materia medica of special drugs.

As regards the latter, only those should be discussed at all which have a real, living therapeutic or toxicologic importance. Of the former the student should be required to know, in the first place, those data which are needed in prescribing: The correct Latin name (faulty orthography indicates a faulty education, in materia medica as elsewhere), the methods of administration, the most useful preparations, *and these only!* [1] Their dose, solubility, incompatibility, and in a few cases, their composition; constituents should be taught only in so far as important therapeutically or by incompatibility.

Furthermore, I believe that there should be required considerable familiarity with the appearance and other physical characters of the important drugs and their principal preparations, so that the more common poisons may be identified or excluded. This seems to me very important, and I believe that I lay rather more stress on it than is commonly done. The knowledge so obtained is also very valuable, in that it often enables the physician to adapt the medicine to the peculiarities of the patient, and sometimes to prevent the results of an error on the part of a druggist. I require this acquaintance rather oftener in the case of preparations than of crude drugs. I need hardly add that a good deal of discrimination must be exercised in selecting the drugs to be studied. The study must, of course, be made directly from the specimen.

It will be seen that the principal abridgment which I advocate in the teaching of materia medica concerns the number of drugs and preparations to be studied, neglecting all those—and they are quite numerous—which are unimportant.[2] A further saving is obtained by limiting pharmacy, and by paying no attention to habitat, natural order, method of collection, etc. These are quite useless for practical purposes, and those students who are interested

---

[1] There is some excuse for the Pharmacopœia retaining obsolete drugs and preparations, because these are sometimes used in certain localities or by the laity, but there is no reason for burdening medical students with them. It is to be wished that all State boards would discourage such questions as, " Give *all* the preparations of ——."

[2] This refers only to materia medica. It is often desirable to say a few words about the action of these unimportant drugs in the lectures on pharmacology.

in them can easily find the information. The natural orders are sometimes useful in explaining relationships, but these can be touched on in pharmacology. In this way, and by arranging the course as indicated below, the class-work in materia medica and pharmacy may be reduced to something like forty-five hours. Besides this required work, I believe that a more thorough study of the chemistry of drugs and of pharmacy is very useful, not so much by the direct knowledge which they give, but because the handling of drugs which they require gives a greater familiarity. This advantage is not sufficient, to my mind, to make them compulsory, but they may be offered as elective or optional work.

ARRANGEMENT OF THE INSTRUCTION.

The dryness of materia medica is almost proverbial, and it is, indeed, difficult to render interesting a study which consists so largely of memorizing. This difficulty is enhanced by constituting the subject into a separate course, as is so often done, and especially by letting this course precede that of pharmacology or therapeutics. What interest can there be for the student in memorizing certain tabulated information which he does not fully understand, about a drug which, too often, he has never seen, and about the uses of which he has no clear idea? What opportunities I have had of observing have only confirmed my objections to this plan. I believe that only the preliminary subjects of pharmacy, etc., should be taught separately, and that the materia medica of the individual drugs should be studied immediately *after* their action and uses. It is my practice to give the student his first experience with drugs by letting him use them in the laboratory, as this is the most efficient way of arousing his interest and showing him the importance of the drug. When he has in this way obtained an objective knowledge of the effects of most drugs and has become curious to have them explained, their action is studied systematically in class, and after each lecture the students are supplied with the specimens of drugs, with instructions to describe them, again objectively, in their note-books. Around this nucleus the other information is grouped. In this way the interesting parts of the study carry the more mechanical parts, so that these are less felt. It will be noticed that lectures are not emphasized in this scheme. If there is any study in which formal lectures are misplaced this is certainly materia medica. The subject is taught with us almost purely by laboratory work and recitations.—*Jour. Amer. Med. Assn.*

Reports of Society Meetings.

ACADEMY OF STOMATOLOGY.

A REGULAR monthly meeting of the Philadelphia Academy of Stomatology was held at its rooms, 1731 Chestnut Street, on the evening of Tuesday, June 28, 1904, the President, Dr. I. N. Broomell, in the chair. The evening was occupied with the consideration of incidents of practice.

Dr. M. Schamberg.—There is a case which should be reported by Dr. Fogg. He brought to my office about a week ago a patient who had a rather peculiar condition upon the root of a central incisor tooth. He noticed a swelling upon the gum overlying the root of that tooth, and upon testing it found it to be vital and decided that the condition must be a pericemental abscess. He was very anxious to find some cause for the trouble, and a radiograph was taken, which showed a large area of tooth destruction. This destruction indicated resorption. The tooth was kept under observation for quite a while. Yesterday the doctor told me that, in addition to this tooth, quite a number of the other teeth exhibited this irregular resorption, to such an extent, indeed, that the tooth-crown was lost. It is the only case of the kind I have ever seen, and it is of such an unusual type that I thought it might be interesting for the Academy to hear of the case. I would be very glad to know whether any have met with a similar condition.

Dr. E. T. Darby.—Were they all vital teeth?

Dr. Schamberg.—They were in the main vital. In some of the lower teeth the pulps were dead.

Dr. James Truman.—How old was the patient?

Dr. Schamberg.—The patient was about thirty-two or thirty-five years old.

Dr. H. R. D. Swing.—Was there any pyorrhœa?

Dr. Schamberg.—There was no pyorrhœa, but there was a certain amount of recession. The tooth was vital up to the time of its removal.

Dr. I. N. Broomell.—Had the alveolar bone filled in the space?

Dr. Schamberg.—No; the alveolar process in most cases was

resorbed over the site of the root resorption, due more to infection which reached the part in consequence of the food débris entering the spaces. Almost every surface of the molar teeth affected showed resorption.

REPORT OF A CASE.

Dr. A. N. Gaylord.—I had an interesting case some time ago of a gentleman upward of sixty, who called upon me and said that two and a half years previously he had a badly inflamed jaw and face and was unable to open his mouth. He was fed through a tube. He went to a physician, who stated that he had a malignant growth and suggested that he go to a specialist. The specialist concurred in the opinion and sent him to a surgeon for operation. The tissues were laid open, the bone scraped, and the man told that he would recover. From that time the man had a sinus discharging on the border of the jaw. Fortunately he had a heavy growth of whiskers, which covered it, but he was obliged to carry absorbent cotton to keep it in a respectable condition. The history was the familiar one of alveolar abscess, although there was nothing on the inside of the mouth to indicate one. There was no sign of an embedded root, although I suspected one, and suggested that the man have a skiagraph taken. The first one taken of the entire jaw showed a faint outline of a root. That was not satisfactory, and I had a second one taken, using a film on the side of the border of the jaw, and that showed a root plainly. I made an application of cocaine and cut down upon it, but it was too firmly embedded to be removed by the forceps. I used a surgical burr, took the root out, and passed a probe from the opening on the outside of the face through the tissues and found that it came out through an opening in the bone. This was washed out with antiseptics. There was no discharge the next day, and on the second day the opening on the face had closed up. I opened it again, fearing that it had closed too quickly, but from the third day the wound has remained closed and there has been no discharge. I saw the patient this afternoon. The inside of the mouth presents an entirely healthy appearance and the wound is entirely healed. For this credit is due to the X-ray diagnosis.

Dr. E. T. Darby.—Dr. Gaylord's narrative of that case reminds me of one I had a few years ago, which I mention to show that we may be sometimes mistaken about the vitality or non-vitality of a tooth. Some years ago a gentleman was brought to me by his dentist, and the facts of the case were these: The man was a fine healthy specimen of about thirty-five or more. He had had a discharge upon the jaw opposite the bicuspid or molar tooth for a year or more. He had consulted his family physician, who told him that his blood was diseased, and had given him remedies. He was obliged to wear a black patch for the discharging sinus. He was travelling one day in one of the New England States, and a gentleman sitting behind him leaned forward and said, " My friend, that comes from a tooth." He said, " You are mistaken; my physician in Philadelphia tells me it is from the condition of my blood." The reply was, " Well, I am a surgeon. I simply say that comes from a tooth." The gentleman was a little indignant, but when he came to Philadelphia he consulted Dr. Agnew, who said, " I think he told you the truth," and referred him to me. The gentleman brought his dentist with him for a consultation. The dentist began by saying, " I know, doctor, this does not come from his teeth; I have examined them over and over and over again." I looked into the patient's mouth and opened the right lower second bicuspid. I passed in a probe, and pus welled up. The dentist had been for thirty years in practice and had never seen one of these cases. I advised extraction, which was done, and three days later I met the gentleman, who said there had not been a particle of pus since.

I mention this to show that a man with thirty years of experience had never happened to see an abscess discharging at the angle of the jaw from a lower molar or bicuspid tooth, and when he had it before him he did not recognize it. One can hardly conceive of that happening. The surgeon in that instance was brighter than the dentist. In Dr. Gaylord's case the dentist was brighter than the surgeon.

Dr. P. B. McCullough.—Four or five years ago I mentioned a case which is in accord with the present discussion. It is already recorded in the transactions of the Academy. I was asked by a veterinary surgeon to examine the mouth of a dog with an abscess discharging below the line of the lower jaw. Such cases were so common in dentistry that I suspected an abscess. I examined all the teeth, but could find no decayed tooth. I felt that the only way to diagnose the condition was to allow the probe to be a guide as it passed through the fistulous tract. The abscess was in the neighborhood of the first or second lower molar. I called the attention of the veterinary surgeon to this, and he recommended extraction. I assumed that he should know more about the anatomy of the tooth of the dog. The tooth was extracted and found to be devitalized.

I would like to mention some experiments made with plaster. There is soon to be published in the INTERNATIONAL DENTAL JOURNAL a *résumé* of these experiments in practical work. There has been much written about the difficulty of working with plaster because of its different stages of expansion. The Academy will remember that work of this kind dates far back into dentistry. Recently Dr. Spencer announced that he had a plaster which was non-expanding. I have made no experiments with his product, and therefore do not know of its value. I have, however, discovered a plaster which is absolutely non-expanding. I mention in this article to be published how my attention was first called to it and the circumstances that led up to the discovery of the trick that makes the non-expanding plaster. The method consists of the proper treatment of lime-water. The water must be boiled. Unslaked lime is added and the clear liquid is drained off. If a fraction of salt is added the plaster will expand. If boiled water is used alone the plaster will expand. There was no difference in the degree of expansion from all the combinations I tried. I have soaked the plaster in water several days after it was mixed and then vulcanized it into the tube, but without any change. I also made another test with gum-arabic water, without boiling, and in this case there was no expansion. This is not of much value for the reason that the gum-arabic is so readily soluble in water that I felt that in vulcanizing it might soften.

Dr. James Truman.—I think the report of Dr. McCullough is very important. I would like him to explain his use of the glass tube with the plaster made with lime-water boiled.

Dr. McCullough.—I will say, briefly, that the first test that I made was with lime-water that had been boiled for domestic use. In making some further tests I noticed that the first test was made with boiled water, the second, without boiling. I then went through a series of experiments. All of the tubes cracked within twelve minutes, except the one with the plaster which had been mixed with the boiled lime-water. This is interesting from the stand-point of the chemist. I do not know that the chemistry of plaster is known. I remember being taught that it was a problem that was not understood. I am inclined to think that it can be understood, but why boiled lime-water should affect plaster as it does I do not know. It occurred to me as possible that the water being deoxygenated by boiling would account for it, but the fact that I tested boiled water without the lime shows the error of this.   The water was sterile without the addition of lime.   With gum-arabic water the plaster did not expand, yet that water was not boiled.

Dr. Schamberg.—Dr. McCullough's report is very interesting, and the discovery should be of much value.   One thing occurred to me when he spoke of water losing its oxygen through boiling.   When I was in Porto Rico we boiled the water for drinking, and we found it very flat.   With an ordinary bicycle tube which we placed in the water we forced the air through it.   In that way it took up a certain amount of oxygen.   It occurred to me that Dr. McCullough might try that method with his experiments to find out whether boiled water so treated would influence the expansion of the plaster.

Dr. Gaylord's remarks interested me particularly, because I have recently had three cases where a fistulous tract was established upon the line or beneath the lower jaw, and due to abscessed teeth.   In many instances that have come to my attention prior to this time I have noticed that it was largely due to the advice of the medical practitioners, and occasionally the dentist is at fault.   This is not surprising when we consider how hard it is to test a tooth for vitality.   When an obscure case comes into my office I always use the rubber dam and test each tooth separately by the use of the ethyl chloride spray.   I have been at times much humiliated, after advising dentists that certain teeth were not vital, to find that they were vital.   I have concluded that often there is a loss of sensation in tooth-pulps without loss of vitality.   The sensory nerves may have lost their function, but there is a certain amount of circulation in the pulp, and the pulp is vital.   We can conceive of such a thing being possible when we realize that we may have a palsied arm and yet have circulation in that arm.   So in several cases where I thought I was at the bottom of some troublesome neuralgia and the tooth has been opened, the dentist has found a vital pulp.   I have, therefore, hesitated much more about advising the drilling into teeth when they give no sensation upon the application of the cold test.   I believe it is a good thing to try the transillumination method.   When there has been doubt as to whether there was a small apical inflammation, I have followed up these tests with the X-ray, and in many instances have noticed the most incipient abscess where we might scarcely expect to find a drop of pus.   We are all familiar with the immense amount of cellulitis involving the face when there has been less than a drop of pus at the apical space.

Dr. McCullough.—Dr. Schamberg's reference to the pulp having physiological function without sensation recalls to me a case of a woman for whom I had to drill into the labial face of a cuspid tooth for arsenical application. I knew that if she had the slightest pain she would tell me. I drilled into that tooth until I reached the pulp, and yet there was no blood and she felt no pain whatsoever. The tooth was without cavity or decay. As soon as I struck the pulp-cavity I got blood.

In another case I moved the entire upper set of teeth in a girl when she was quite young. The extent to which the central incisors had to be moved to articulate was so great that it took two years to move them. They were very slowly moved a certain distance during the winter months, and then retained with a fixed appliance. In the summer there was no change made. In the winter the teeth were again moved. Several years afterwards the girl complained that her teeth were turning yellow. I asked several men if they thought they were devitalized. The interesting point is that these teeth for a period of four years after completion of the operation showed no change.

Dr. James Truman.—I can appreciate very fully the difficulty of diagnosing a devitalized pulp. Ethyl chloride is one of the best things for the purpose, but I think it is often fallacious; so is ice. I am well aware of Dr. Jack's rather exhaustive formula, but I have not been as successful as he has in that direction. I have had as much satisfaction with the galvanic current as with any other method. I often wonder that it is not more generally used. It seems to me more exact than the cold test. My experience, however, is not sufficiently large to prove that as a fact; in my hands it has worked well.

OTTO E. INGLIS,
Editor Academy of Stomatology.

FOURTH INTERNATIONAL DENTAL CONGRESS, ST. LOUIS, MO., AUGUST 29 TO SEPTEMBER 3, 1904.

Opening Session—Monday, August 29, 1904.

(Continued from page 810.)

Dr. A. W. Harlan, of New York, called upon by the President to introduce the foreign delegates to the Congress, made a few appropriate remarks in presenting Dr. Otto Zsigmondy, Vienna, the official representative of Austria, who spoke as follows:

Mr. President, Ladies, and Gentlemen,—I thank you from the bottom of my heart for this very kind and enthusiastic reception. In Austria, as in other countries, a remarkable change has taken place, in the sense that dentistry is now fully recognized by the government as being of the utmost importance to public hygiene. As a proof of the increasing interest our authorities are taking in dental matters, I should state that, not content to gather information about international dental congresses from the official reports, they deemed it fit to appoint an official delegate to this Congress. The desire often expressed by the Austrian dental societies may now be considered almost realized.

I wish to be permitted to mention another improvement which is likewise the result of our efforts. Special dental courses have been organized for army surgeons in which they can obtain not only the special training desirable, but at the same time they attend gratuitously to the teeth of the soldiers of the Vienna garrison.

To these statements I have only to add my sincerest thanks for the privilege of having been permitted to address to you these words, and to express a confident hope that the results of this great and memorable Congress will bear further good fruit for my country also. (Applause.)

Dr. Rudolph Weiser, of Vienna, Austria, delegate from the Central Union of Austrian Stomatologists and the Association of Dentists of Prague, was next introduced and spoke as follows:

Mr. President, Ladies, and Gentlemen,—If the wonderland America is in general a voyage-aim for the cultivated classes of society, a dental congress in the United States will exert upon us as professionals an attractive power to a most exceptional extent.

The Americans have always been ahead in converting theoretical results into practical applications of benefit to mankind. Consequently, and by natural logic, they ought to distinguish themselves in dentistry, and indeed they may be considered pioneers in this branch of knowledge.

I should now like to inform you that we Austrians have a still greater incentive to study your institutions thoroughly and to enter into friendly personal contact with you because the universities in our country are just about to place education in this branch of surgery upon a new and sound basis.

I have the honor to express to you, in the name of the Central Union of Austrian Stomatologists and of the Association of the Czech Dentists of Prague, the most cordial thanks for your kind invitation and warm reception. As the delegate of the aforenamed dental associations I feel happy to transmit you the sincerest wish that the results of your enterprise may be of real benefit to the nations of the world. (Applause.)

Dr. Harlan next introduced Dr. Alfred Burne, the representative of Australia, who spoke as follows:

MR. PRESIDENT, LADIES, AND GENTLEMEN,—I trust I shall be pardoned this morning if I take for my cue a line from the ghost in Hamlet, "Brief let me be." I feel that there are so many to follow me that I do not desire to take your time. From the state of Victoria, New South Wales, I desire to extend to the Congress congratulations and good wishes for a very successful meeting. I feel that we who have come such long distances to this Congress are like the wise men who followed the star of Bethlehem. We are looking to the Fourth International Dental Congress, seeking the light that we need, and which I think we shall find. Gentlemen, I thank you. (Applause.)

Dr. J. M. Magee, of St. Johns, N. B., Canada, was next introduced and spoke as follows:

MR. PRESIDENT, LADIES, AND GENTLEMEN,—I came here simply as a dentist, and it was with the greatest distress that I learned I would be called upon to speak for the great country to the north. I am very sorry that I cannot respond on behalf of the profession in Canada as befits the occasion, but the representative who could worthily represent it is unfortunately absent, and I was unexpectedly called upon to take his place. I am very proud to be honored on this occasion by being permitted to speak to you, and, as my predecessor from the antipodes expressed it, I thank you. (Applause.)

Dr. E. Sauvez, of Paris, was next introduced. He said, Mr. President, in the name of the government of the French Republic, of which I have been commissioned delegate together with my eminent *confrère* and friend Dr. Godon, I have the honor of saluting the aurora of the Fourth International Dental Congress.

I will also present you the good wishes for the success of this meeting on behalf of the Directeur de l'Assistance Publique of Paris, who has delegated us for the purpose; and finally, as president of the French committee on publicity and propaganda and of the national federation of France, I want to offer you the assurances of our sentiments of confraternity and sincere admiration for the constant efforts which American dentists have been making for so many years for the purpose of elevating the status of our profession.

The École Dentaire, Paris, which represents the most important institution for dental education and the most vital one in our country, takes the greatest interest in your work, in your journals, in your schools, because you have travelled towards the ideal with gigantic strides. Sixty-five years ago the first dental school in the world was created in Baltimore. To-day about sixty-five schools are being operated upon United States territory. It must be clear to every one that a country capable of creating on an average a school per year must necessarily be the one in which the status of the profession is the highest.

We are particularly happy to bring to you our token of admiration in this beautiful city of St. Louis, the heart of the United States, where so many names remind us of France, the first one to give to the modern centuries, through the cession of Louisiana, the example of a colony voluntarily ceded by the parent country, and when we look at the prosperity of your beautiful country, and at the splendor and importance of your Exposition, we cannot refrain from thinking of the just statements made by Livingston, the ambassador of the United States, at the time of the signing of the Louisiana Purchase. He then prophesied the future in such a precise way that you have not hesitated to inscribe part of it upon the monument commemorating the event.

Dr. W. D. Miller, Berlin, the representative from Germany, was greeted with loud applause.

Dr. Harlan.—It is not necessary, it seems, that I should introduce Professor Miller, our distinguished representative from Germany and the guardian of American dentistry in Europe.

Dr. Miller.—Mr. President, ladies, and gentlemen, I do not need to say that I thank you very heartily for this courteous show of friendship on your part, and that I reciprocate it most fully.

I come to you as the representative of the National Dental Association of Germany, of the National Association of Dental Societies, and of the National Association of Dental Faculties of Germany. These three bodies embrace, I may say, practically all the prominent dentists of the country, and they have asked me to convey to you an expression of cordial good-will and sympathy. They wish me to assure you also of their great appreciation of the grand work done in America by the dental profession, and of their hope and confidence that this meeting will, like all other dental meetings held on American soil, contribute much to the advancement of our profession. (Applause.)

Dr. Harlan.—I have pleasure in introducing to you the representative of the government of Holland, Dr. John E. Grevers, who was a member of the International Medical Congress held in Washington in 1887, and of the World's Columbian Congress of 1893 in Chicago.

Dr. John E. Grevers, Amsterdam, Holland.—Mr. President, ladies, and gentlemen, I thank you very heartily for your kind reception, and I thank you for the opportunity you have given me of coming before you as the representative of a very small country —a country, however, which is full of love and interest for everything pertaining to dentistry. My gracious little Queen Wilhelmina has kindly delegated me to represent her government at this Congress; and this act marks the beginning of a great period for Holland, as the government is becoming more and more interested in matters relating to dentistry. Dentistry in our country has for many years been regulated by law, but not to the best interests of dentistry, I am sorry to say. I think I can now prophesy that the present ministry will do much towards bettering the conditions for those desiring to enter upon the study of our specialty.

I have also come to bring you greetings from two dental societies, the Odontological Society of Holland and the Union Society of Dentists. Both have delegated me to represent them, and to bring to you their heartfelt greetings, and the hope that the outcome of this Congress will be beneficial to dental science through-out the world. Again I thank you for your very kind reception. (Applause.)

Dr. Vincenzo Guerini, of Naples, the representative of Italy, was introduced by Dr. Harlan, and spoke as follows:

MR. PRESIDENT, LADIES, AND GENTLEMEN,—As the represent-ative of the Odontological Society of Italy and of the Neapolitan Medical Association, I have the honor of bringing to you a fra-ternal greeting from the Italian dentists.

A strong current of sympathy, originating from great histor-ical events that are known to all of us, unites and will ever unite Italy to America. Every new manifestation of progress, every fresh success of yours, has our sincere applause; and my colleagues in Italy hope that this great dental Congress may add new glory to the many accomplishments which your nation can already boast.

It is the source of great happiness to me to find myself for the first time in the United States, in this great centre from which the light of civilization and of progress radiates so abundantly over the whole world; and this day, when I have the honor of standing in the midst of so eminent an assemblage of talent, con-stituted for the most part of the elect of the dental profession in America, will ever be one of my dearest remembrances.

In conclusion, gentlemen and ladies, I will express my fervent desire that the brilliant results of this great international congress may constitute a new and solemn affirmation of the autonomy of dental science, which Americans have the merit of being the first to recognize, and which is the indispensable condition of rapid progress in dentistry.

May this Congress strengthen still more the bond that unites all of the dentists of the world into one body, rendering it more easy for the dental profession to achieve fresh triumphs in the field of scientific and practical dentistry for the welfare of humanity. (Applause.)

Dr. José J. Rojo, Mexico City, Mexico.—Mr. President, ladies, and gentlemen, I thank you for your kind reception. It is with great pleasure that I have the honor of addressing you as delegate from the National Mexican Dental College and from the Mexican Dental Society. Permit me to express our feelings of appreciation and special sympathy with the organizers of and co-operators in this great historical event, the Fourth International Dental Congress. Besides this, in the name of the dental profession of the republic of Mexico, I want to express our best wishes for a successful meeting, and many beneficent results to our profession. (Applause.)

Dr. Jaime D. Losada, of Madrid, one of the representatives from Spain, spoke as follows:

MR. PRESIDENT, LADIES, AND GENTLEMEN,—I feel a deep sense of emotion on this occasion, as it is for me a great honor and pleasure to address you in the name of Spain. My government takes the greatest interest in all matters relating to dental science, and as a further proof of this interest has sent, besides myself, as governmental delegates, two of the greatest dental men we have in Spain, Drs. Florestan Aguilar and Dr. Luis Subirana, and it is through their courtesy and also in their names that I address you.

I have to thank you most heartily for the kind way in which we have been welcomed by the city of St. Louis and by the Fourth International Dental Congress. We are full of admiration for your magnificent exhibition, one of the greatest wonders the world has ever seen. This sentiment of admiration is still greater to us, coming as we do from countries which have existed almost since the prehistoric periods, as we realize that your wonderful land has accomplished in a few years—thanks to the progressive genius of the American people—that for which other countries have consumed centuries.

I am happy to say that dentistry is one of the up-to-date sciences in Spain. Our teaching of this branch compares very favorably with that of any other country, and our requirements are very high. My *confrères* in Spain are most progressive, and, of course, as in every part of the world, American systems are in vogue. Many of the young dentists from my country, knowing that America is the true spring of modern dental science and the mother of dental education, come to your land, regardless of sacrifices, with the object of improving their knowledge, and then return to the mother country usually with the American D.D.S. appended to their names.

Again I thank you for your cordial welcome, and my only regret is that I am not familiar enough with your language to be able to express well enough the sentiments of admiration and friendship from my professional brethren in Spain. (Applause.)

Dr. L. C. Bryan, of Basel, the representative of Switzerland, spoke as follows:

MR. PRESIDENT, LADIES, AND GENTLEMEN,—Considering the late hour, the small spot which I represent on the map of the world, and the large number of speakers to be heard from, I will only extend to you the cordial greetings of the profession of Switzerland, and say that it is our great desire that the next dental congress may be held in our hospitable country, the playground of the world. I thank you very much. (Applause.)

Dr. Harlan.—Among those who have been appointed as official delegates to this Congress you have standing before you Dr. J. Y. Crawford, of Nashville, Tennessee, delegate of the United States government. (Applause.)

Dr. J. Y. Crawford, Nashville, Tenn.—Mr. President, dental diplomats of the world, ladies, and gentlemen, in all the experiences of my life I have never felt more profoundly my responsibility than in the duty which I am now trying to perform. I extend to you, the representatives of the nations of the earth, on behalf of the government of the United States, our greetings, and welcome you most heartily on this auspicious occasion. The people of America, and particularly the departments of our government, whether it be the executive, legislative, or judicial, are in sympathy with the idea of gathering together at stated intervals congresses representing the various interests of the world, and we come with our congratulations, most earnestly invoking such interest and solicitude in the discussions of odontological questions at this time as will bring great benefits to the world, and result not only in the improvement of the masticating apparatus of the human family, but tend to relieve suffering humanity and add to the comfort of the population of the world. We are created upon the fundamental principle of equal rights to all, and special privileges to none. We therefore enter most heartily into the business of this Congress for the improvement and betterment of the condition of mankind. By the authority of the great government located at Washington, resting upon the will of the people of this great nation, we extend our most hearty congratulations. Mr. President, as the humble representative of the government of the United States, I pledge you to do all that we can for the advancement of the interests of this Congress and the profession of dentistry the world over. (Applause.)

Dr. Edwin P. Tignor, representative of the Army Dental Corps, was next introduced, and spoke as follows:

MR. PRESIDENT, LADIES, AND GENTLEMEN,—It gives me great pleasure to be able to be present at this great meeting. It was a great surprise to me, and a very agreeable one, to receive the order directing me to proceed here in order to represent the Army Dental Corps, and I thank you very much for the privilege of being allowed to speak to you to-day.

Dr. Harlan next introduced Dr. J. M. Whitney, of Honolulu, the representative of the Hawaiian Islands, who spoke as follows:

MR. PRESIDENT, LADIES, AND GENTLEMEN,—As I was sitting greatly enjoying the proceedings, my friend Dr. Kirk touched me on the shoulder and said, " We must hear from the baby of our republic," to which I replied, " No, you had better excuse me," but Dr. Harlan says no excuses are acceptable here. I am here not as representing the baby country, because we had an organization in Hawaii long before California was known to most of us. I was privileged to stand before you at the Second International Dental Congress, at that time as a foreigner, but now I am proud to stand before you as one of you. You are one with us and we are one with you, and I thank you for this honor. (Applause.)

Dr. Harlan.—Ladies and gentlemen, it affords me particular pleasure to be able to now present to you my old associate and collaborator in the preparation of the proceedings of the World's Columbian Dental Congress of 1893, Dr. Louis Ottofy, the representative of the Philippine Islands. (Applause.)

Dr. Ottofy.—Mr. President, ladies, and gentlemen, it is with the greatest of pleasure that I join my distinguished predecessors upon this floor in expressing to you my sincere thanks for your most cordial welcome. I assure you that I highly appreciate the opportunity and privilege of being present to witness the erection of another milestone in the history of the progress of dentistry, a progress which may not inaptly be likened unto the progress of our great nation—a nation which during the last few years has extended her civilizing hand across the seas to a people emerging from the darkness of semi-ignorance into the bright rays of intelligence. Some idea of this influence may be formed when I mention the fact that, while I come from a territory over which wave the Stars and Stripes, I have travelled a greater distance to come here, excepting one gentleman from Java, I believe, than any other member of this Congress.

While here with you, it shall be my sacred duty to learn all I possibly can of the advance made by our profession, and to carry the fruits of your thought and labor back to the Philippines. On behalf of the dental profession of the Philippine Islands, which I have the honor to represent, I again thank you heartily for your cordial welcome. (Applause.)

Dr. Salvador Pratto was introduced by Dr. Harlan, and spoke as follows:

LADIES AND GENTLEMEN,—As delegate of the Odontological Society of Uruguay I desire to express to you our most cordial sentiments of confraternity and esteem.

You no doubt know that there is a little country in the southern extremity of this hemisphere, a small country in area, but large in brains and activity, and its organization in educational lines places it at the head of the South American intellectual movement. In my country, as in all other South American republics, we carefully follow the progress achieved by dentistry in this country, without any delay save that implied by the distance which separates the two countries.

I feel a deep sense of gratification, realizing that I shall be the medium of conveying to the Odontological Society of Uruguay an account of your deliberations and a description of your operative ability and of your discoveries in the field of practical dentistry.

I am a sincere admirer of the genius of America's sons, whom I regard as the first to establish permanently the separate profession of dentistry upon an autonomous basis—thus cultivating the fruits of a plant which germinated in France, and which is now being diffused throughout the universe for the welfare of suffering humanity.

I wish to express my earnest desire for the success of this gathering, and I furthermore wish to say that I feel proud and happy to be a member of the foreign delegation.

Dr. Harlan.—In every country with a population of five hundred thousand or over will be found installed somewhere a representative of America practising dentistry. I have pleasure in presenting to you Dr. J. W. Noble, of Hong Kong, China.

Dr. Noble.—Ladies and gentlemen, it gives me great pleasure to appear before you this morning, and to have the opportunity to thank you for the cordial reception you have given to the members from foreign countries—with whom I feel I am included this morning—as well as to myself. I regret very much that all those practising dentistry in my part of the world cannot be with me here to-day to see the progress taking place in our profession in science and art. They are missing that which we are gaining, and we can only sympathize with those who are absent from us during the present week. (Applause.)

Dr. Benjamin Vidaurre, representative from Nicaragua, was next introduced, and spoke as follows:

MR. PRESIDENT, LADIES, AND GENTLEMEN,—The government of Nicaragua, whose duly accredited representative I am proud to be, sends greetings to the Fourth International Dental Congress. Please accept from my profession and myself sincere thanks in the name of my country for the courtesies that have been extended to me. I am glad to say that my government has always shown not only a desire, but an eagerness, to assist in any scientific work or lend aid in any way that will further the ends of progress. Our president, on being invited, did not hesitate to send a representative of the government to the Congress, and while that representative may not shed much light upon the deliberations of this body, he will endeavor to take back with him part at least of the great treasures which will emanate from this Congress. Again I thank you most heartily for the cordial reception tendered me. (Applause.)

Dr. Joaquin Yela, Jr., official delegate of the government and dental faculty of the republic of Guatemala, Central America, was presented, and spoke as follows:

MR. CHAIRMAN, FELLOW DELEGATES, LADIES, AND GENTLE-MEN,—If I were to speak now in my own native tongue, very few of you, I am sure, would understand me; although, from my speaking in my broken English the number of sufferers may be greater. Relying then, on your own well-known patience and goodness, I will try to make myself understood in the beautiful language of Shakespeare and Longfellow.

For many reasons I could have wished that it had fallen to the lot of a delegate of greater distinction and experience than myself to respond to your very kind invitation to speak, but I do recognize that in letting your choice fall upon me you have acted, not out of regard to the special delegate, but out of compliment to the country whose government and dental faculty I have the honor, however unworthy, to represent at this Congress; a country which is linked to the United States of America by so many ties both of a commercial nature and of sincere friendship.

I observe wth great pleasure that there are to be discussions and conferences on many and very important dental topics which it will be for us to report to our respective governments and faculties.

It only remains for me now, Mr. Chairman and fellow-delegates, to express once more my very cordial thankfulness for the benevolent reception accorded me here, and to present as well the same sentiment of thankfulness to the people of this beautiful city of St. Louis, assuring you all that I am the interpreter of the feelings of the government, faculty, and people whom I have the honor of representing in this highly distinguished assembly. (Applause.)

Dr. Ragnwald Hendricsen, of Christiania, the representative from Norway, was presented, and spoke as follows:

MR. PRESIDENT AND MEMBERS OF THE FOURTH INTERNATIONAL DENTAL CONGRESS,—On behalf of the dental profession of Norway and the Christiania Dental Society, it is with the greatest pleasure that I greet you. Norway is the farthest northern country represented here, and although cool of climate we are warm of heart, and our profession as a whole and individually are profound admirers of American dental science. We all try to follow your methods and are eager to know more and more, and therefore have sent and are sending to your colleges many students.

The cordial, friendly spirit which you have shown to all of us foreigners will always be a delightful remembrance, and I wish to express the most sincere thanks both from myself and my Norwegian brethren.

The official representative of the Norwegian government, Mr. Anderson, has not arrived, and I could not refrain from expressing a few words on behalf of my nation. (Applause.)

Dr. N. S. Jenkins, of Dresden, Germany, was presented to the Congress, and spoke as follows:

MR. PRESIDENT, LADIES, AND GENTLEMEN,—With all my heart I wish to bring to you the greetings of the body of colleagues practising their profession under the American degree in the empire of Germany. They send to you their most cordial and fraternal greetings, and beg you to believe that they are heart and soul with you in every effort towards uplifting and carrying forward the ever-increasing influence of the great profession to which we all belong. (Applause.)

The President.—Ladies and gentlemen, members of the Fourth International Dental Congress, the next order of business is the address by the President of the Fourth International Dental Congress, and as an evidence that I never really intended to preside over this body, until the election had been finally ratified on this floor, I am here to-day at this wedding-feast without a wedding-gown,—namely, the " President's address." My remarks therefore shall be brief.

At the threshold of this great gathering of the profession from all parts of the world, I bring you the greeting of the Hon. Theodore Roosevelt, President of the United States, for a most pleasant, profitable, and successful Congress. I desire also to acknowledge the courtesy and interest of his Excellency the governor of Missouri.

To the official delegates representing foreign governments, and the representatives of dental societies in other countries, assembled here to-day, I extend a most cordial and hearty greeting, and beg to express the hope that their stay among us may be most agreeable and pleasant. It is a matter of sincere congratulation to welcome this splendid representation from abroad, and to be able on behalf of the profession in America to felicitate them upon their achievements in the advancement of professional interests in the various countries from which they are accredited.

We in America are pleased to note the great interest which our brethren from abroad evince in this Congress, not only by their presence, but more particularly by their contributions to the excellent programme which has been prepared for this meeting. We welcome them with open hearts, and cordially reciprocate the warm sentiments which they have ever expressed to representatives of the profession from America on occasions like the present.

It is indeed a pleasure to commend the enterprise, enthusiasm, and liberality displayed by State and local societies and colleges in America, in their very generous contributions to assist in defraying the necessary expenditures in preparing for this Congress.

The Organization Committee also desires to acknowledge at this time their indebtedness to the Hon. Howard J. Rogers, Director of Congresses, for the ready and willing support which he has at all times rendered, and for his unfailing interest and solicitude in everything having for its object the complete success of the Congress.

To the members of the profession in America assembled here to-day I bring the greeting of the authorities of the Louisiana Purchase Exposition, and that of the officers and committees in charge of the preparations for this great meeting. In point of numbers this is the largest dental congress ever held, which must be a source of great satisfaction to all our people. The programme, from a literary and a scientific stand-point, has never been equalled. No such array of talent has ever before been brought together, and I am sure that the results achieved at this meeting will make an epoch in dentistry that will for many years be referred to as one of the most brilliant in the annals of the profession.

Many questions will come up for discussion, the correct solution of which will require earnest and thoughtful deliberation, and I urge upon you the necessity of cultivating a broad and liberal spirit in the consideration of the great problems with which you are confronted.

This is not the time nor the place to burden you with references to matters of history or to treat in an academic way the great questions of the hour.

You are conversant with the early history of dentistry, the lack of sympathy and support by the medical profession, the great obstacles to proper professional recognition; the difficulties encountered by the early practitioners; the wonderful achievements with crude facilities for practice, and withal the splendid and brilliant results obtained by the great men who have shed undying lustre upon the profession which they honored and served so well. The past is secure; so let us approach the duties of the hour, with the same spirit of self-sacrifice and love for the profession that animated the fathers of dentistry.

I trust that every member of the Congress will do his utmost to promote harmonious action throughout the various committees and sections, so that all shall work together for the complete success of the Congress and the glory of dentistry. (Applause.)

The President.—We are signally honored by having with us to-day the president of the International Dental Federation, a distinguished gentleman who is well known to all of you for his sterling qualities, and for the great ability he has shown not only as a practitioner of dentistry, but as an executive officer, and I now have the honor of presenting to you our distinguished *confrère* from France, Dr. Charles Godon, of Paris, who will address you. (Applause.)

Dr. Godon.—Mr. President, ladies, and gentlemen, at this, the first meeting of the Fourth International Dental Congress, I should have liked to speak in the name of France, being one of the official delegates of the French government and of the National Federation, to recall to you all the ties of sympathy which unite our two republics. The fraternal relations existing since the time when you achieved your independence under Washington, with Lafayette and Rochambeau, are also of a professional nature, because of our common ancestors, Gardette and Lemaire, who brought over to America the French dentistry of the eighteenth century; and they are finally assured at the present time because of our common ideals of liberty, equality, and fraternity.

I left to my friend and co-delegate, Dr. Sauvez, the honor of speaking in the name of France, because I have to-day another duty, that is to speak at this opening meeting in the name of an association which is above nationalites, since it is a universal association of national dental societies, a permanent international body existing in the interim of international dental congresses; in the name of this great association which you all know now as the great advisory council on dental international relationships.

The F. D. I. has taken a part in the work of this Congress which for a while was surrounded by many difficulties. But now these are all over, and I bring you in the name of the F. D. I. a fraternal greeting. We can but congratulate you upon this first result, and now we turn over to you our powers and all documents relating to the work accomplished since 1900.

The following statement, which is approved by all the members of the executive council of the F. D. I., will give you an idea of the work which has been performed.

To conclude, let me tell you of my satisfaction in seeing that the F. D. I. has found in your great land this hearty hospitality, characteristic of the American dental profession, for which I thank you sincerely. It is with the greatest confidence that I place its destiny in your hands, quite sure that it will continue to grow and to develop, as does everything here pertaining to the progress of science and to the good of humanity.

The President.—If there is no objection this report will be accepted and referred to the Committee on Resolutions.

The Secretary-General, Dr. Kirk, read the following cablegram from Dr. John S. Burnett, of Salto, Uruguay:

"DR. H. J. BURKHART, *President Fourth International Dental Congress,* *St. Louis:*
"Success to the Congress. I am mentally with you.
"JOHN BURNETT."

The next order of business being the report of the Committee on Prize Essays, the President called upon Dr. Truman to present the report of that committee.

Dr. James Truman, chairman of the Committee on Prize Essays, then read the report.

[This report was published in the October number.]

On motion, the report of the Committee on Prize Essays was accepted and adopted.

The Secretary-General then read a communication from the Dental College of Sheffield, England, as follows:

"UNIVERSITY COLLEGE, SHEFFIELD, DENTAL DEPARTMENT.
"At a meeting of the dental practitioners held in Sheffield, on Tuesday, July 19, 1904, it was unanimously decided to send their congratulations and fraternal greetings to the members in meeting assembled at the St. Louis Dental Congress.

"Also: The members of the Sheffield and District Association of Licentiates of Dental Surgery have pleasure in sending their heartiest good wishes to the members of the Congress at St. Louis.

"The members of the above society have delight in announcing that their honorary secretary, Mr. H. James Morris, L.D.S. (Eng.), will attend the Congress and in person express their hearty good wishes for a happy and successful meeting.
"GEO. HENRY LODGE, *President,*
"CHARLES STOKES,
"FRANK MORDAUNT,
"*Council.*
"H. JAMES MORRIS,
"*Treasurer-Secretary.*"

A letter from Mr. W. H. Williamson, president of the British Dental Association, to Dr. M. H. Cryer, as follows, was received too late to be read, having been delayed in transmission:

"Kindly express to the officials of the Congress my great regret at my inability to be present, and at the same time convey the best wishes of the British Dental Association for the success of your great gathering.

"I shall send a cable on the opening day in case this should not reach you in time.

"Yours sincerely,

"W. H. WILLIAMSON."

The President.—If there be no objection, the Secretary-General is instructed to reply to all telegrams and letters to the Congress.

There being no other business before the Congress, the President declared the meeting adjourned until Tuesday morning at ten o'clock.

(To be continued.)

Editorial.

THE SOCIAL STANDING OF DENTISTS.

ONE of our contemporaries is spending much time, mental effort, and printer's ink in discussing the social side of dentistry. This may be very important to a certain class of mind, but the writer fails to understand why this should disturb the gray matter in any well-considered intellect.

Society, and the world, is made up of a heterogeneous mass of humanity, all the product of evolution, and with an ever-present tendency to a reversion to the intellectual standard of lower forms; in other words, the barbaric element is never entirely eliminated from the human mind, notwithstanding the general uplift through higher civilizing influences. Hence the various ratings we find in the social world. In one class it is ancestors. This has its highest development in the Chinese, where it assumes the garb of a religion. In this country it builds on the "Heralds' College" in England, and in Philadelphia it must bear the stamp of age, and that age must have begun with the cave-dwellers along the banks of the Delaware. In New York City and its environs, not to have been a descendant of the renowned Knickerbockers is not to be worthy of much consideration. Then there is another class who sail with their yachts, run automobiles at the risk of their necks, and try to kill time in a hundred different ways to get even with their income. This class ordinarily requires a clean certificate that the money possessed should have passed through at least two generations to be clean of the smut and soil of labor, the foundation of their millions. This is the barbaric side of society, and its idol is gold and its heaven, if it has any, is paved with gold and precious stones. These sum up its earthly and spiritual desires.

There is another class that regards all social intercourse, worthy the name, to be based on intellectual culture, and the certificate for entrance into this high estate must be clearly defined. Naturally the devotees of this cult are not inclined to mingle with either of the previous classes, neither of which may furnish a clear title to those mansions of a higher, but perhaps narrower, life.

There is still another class, composed, it may be, of many minds entitled to enter the sacred precincts of one or all of the previously named, but prefer to occupy, to them, a broader platform capable of holding all willing and able to aspire to its demands. Its motto is, an intelligent aspiration for the highest. This may be the ambition of the mechanic, the man behind the hoe, the laborer in the trench, the shoemaker on his bench, the man at the anvil, each and all ambitious to become perfected in the world's work.

It is no new cry for some dentists to mourn that they are unable to secure entrance to society, as they understand and appreciate its value. The writer knew one who seemed to feel that he was somehow and in some way deprived of his just rights for the reason that society would not recognize him on account, as he believed, of his occupation.

The world is more and more dividing itself into classes. The lines are quite well defined in the older civilizations, and no one there specially grieves that he is interdicted from passing over the border. This latter phase is as it should be. It is impossible to avoid these separate spheres of activity, or non-activity, for mind naturally falls in with congenial mind, and it is certainly true that these affinities are governed by a natural law controlling the relations of all worlds, physical and spiritual.

The individual who wishes to be other than he is, to receive recognition because of a large bank balance, or to be accepted into the circle of ancestor worship, or in the cultured body that ignores the labor of the hands as unworthy to be compared with that of the brain, lives in a region where the fool dreams.

Dentistry occupies a peculiar position in the social life of the world. It is a mixed profession. It labors with its hands as well as with its brains. It has in the past been largely recruited from the ranks of the semi-educated. The after-experiences have resulted, with many, in an educated body worthy to mingle in any of the refined circles of the world. The number of this class is necessarily limited, but the "curse of labor," if it be a curse, still clings to these as individuals and the body they represent. The set who worship ancestors will have nothing to do with them. The worshippers of the golden idol will thrust them aside. They say, in substance, "The man who cleans teeth and handles instruments is unworthy to sit at my table." This is all very amusing, and yet very natural, but why the man or woman who loves the work that dentistry offers should complain, or feel grieved when debarred entrance to clubs or societies, is an incomprehensible problem to the writer.

That which is needed more than aught else in the dentistry of the period is not recognition by any set of men or women, but a mental poise that aspires to a higher standard of self and professional respect. The great demand of the best thinkers should be that dentists should cultivate a dignified deportment, and aim for the best life possible in our profession, leaving nothing unattempted, however much may be unattained, that will make for the best. There is amply sufficient room in dentistry and in its social life to satisfy the most aspiring mind. Let it form its own clubs, and not wait, hat in hand, while the ballots of the Golden Idol Club reject the applicant. He ought to be rejected. He is trying to enter doors barred against him. It is difficult to see any difference between the man demanding admission to a club and one knocking at the doors of a private mansion insisting that he be placed on the visiting list.

A friend of the writer's in large practice in Europe once said to him, "I never speak to my patients on the street." This was a man who fully recognized his true position. He made no demands, yet no one received greater consideration from all classes, high and low, than he, or was more beloved by all.

The element that makes for social advancement is true self-respect, and with this is correlated character, the last naturally following the first. The man in dentistry is, or should be, a man devoted to science, and science means knowledge. This being developed in the man, he is ever growing towards the highest. Nothing

33

can take this away, death will not destroy it, but over the border it will ever remain the great force, the true wealth of the spirit.

To the writer, therefore, this humiliating aspiration for recognition not only to be in society, so called, but in medical circles, by a certain class of dentists, should be frowned upon as an unworthy thought. It is unmanly and degrading to professional character. Our work is, beyond question, one of the most important to the health and comfort of the race of any of the callings devoted directly, or indirectly, to the aid of humanity. No arguments are here needed to impress this upon dentists, for they all fully appreciate the fact. If the great mission of this profession is thoroughly understood, then live by and for it, and pass by on the other side the sneers of the unthinking. Emphasize this faith by true dignity, and above all remain true to the work to which your life is dedicated, mingling with your own, and your own will never refuse admission into its inner sanctuary. Thus in congenial intercourse the days will pass serenely, and the products of that life will be for the increasing advancement of the profession of your choice, and your own self-respect will grow with years and experience.

Bibliography.

A Text-Book of Dental Pathology and Therapeutics for Students and Practitioners. By Henry H. Burchard, M.D., D.D.S., late Special Lecturer on Dental Pathology and Therapeutics in the Philadelphia Dental College. Revised by Otto E. Inglis, D.D.S., Professor of Dental Pathology and Therapeutics in the Philadelphia Dental College. Second Edition. Illustrated with five hundred and forty-five Engravings and a Colored Plate. Lea Brothers & Co., Philadelphia and New York, 1904.

It is six years since (1898) the long-to-be-lamented Burchard wrote the preface to the first edition of this book. No attempt has been made since to reproduce it under proper editorial revision until the present time. The difficulties attending this were well understood by those conversant with the book as originally prepared. It was well understood that much of it would necessarily have to be rewritten. Professor Inglis undertook this serious task, and has completed it in a volume of six hundred and thirty-nine pages, against five hundred and eighty-five in the first edition. This, however, does not indicate the difference in pages between the two volumes, as forty-three pages have been eliminated by omitting the section on Pharmacology in the first edition.

The editor has followed Dr. Burchard in the arrangement of chapters, but has so thoroughly revised the text that the book must be reviewed, in its second edition, as an original production, the editor standing sponsor for all that has been written in both editions. There can be but one opinion, it is presumed, as to the faithfulness of the editor to his own convictions while, at the same time, retaining an almost sacred devotion to the man who originally planned and wrote the book. That he has succeeded in everything, as some may have desired, is not to be expected, but that he has brought the work up to present standards must be conceded. Whatever criticisms the reviewer may feel called upon to make after a careful perusal of its contents are simply the difference of individuals and methods of teaching, and may not be regarded as directly detracting from the value of the book as a whole.

The chapter on Inflammation is an improvement on that by Burchard, but it does not seem to the reviewer to be a full statement of this very important foundation subject. The reviewer recognizes the value and necessity for condensation in a book of this character, but condensation can be secured without omitting essentials, and these seem to have been to some extent excluded. The history of the work of histologists that led up to the final rediscovery of Conheim, from Döllinger (1819), through Williams, Waller, Von Recklinghausen, Beale, and others, would not have occupied much room, and would have been not only an instructive lesson to students, but would have given credit justly due to these pioneers in histological discovery. Further, the chapter fails to do justice to the classical terms of Redness, Heat, Swelling, Pain, and Impaired Function. These all cover very important facts, and are as important to-day in modern study of abnormal conditions as they were at any former period.

Necrosis of the jaw is very inadequately treated from the standpoint of the reviewer. The dentist should regard this as one of the important pathological problems to be met and conquered, and it will not do to relegate it entirely to the oral surgeon. Hence, while it may at the last fall into the hands of the specialist, its preliminary treatment should be, as a rule, in those of the dentist. Aside from this, the ever-present danger of producing serious lesions through modern methods of force in operating, and resulting in necrotic conditions, seems to make more extended explanation absolutely necessary. No allusion is made to these traumatic disturbances or to the means of avoiding or treating them.

A typographical error occurs on page 141, where Gyse's name is spelled Geise.

The chapter on Dentition is fairly well treated. The editor adopts Constant's suggestion as to the causes producing eruption of the teeth. It is, of course, a matter of theory and not one of proof, hence it is hardly worth while to devote much attention to it, but the illustration of the truth of Constant's theory does not seem very conclusive, for he says, " A simple accident demonstrated this to the editor. While excavating with a large bur the softened dentine about a decayed pulp-chamber, the cementum was widely removed from the pericemental tissue beneath, which latter fortunately remained unbroken. It immediately protruded into the perforation." This the editor regards as the result of internal pressure. It is questionable whether this furnishes proof of a pressure sufficient to force a tooth towards the gum, producing resorption of that and the enveloping process.

The editor is at times profuse in his credits, and at others, as already stated, he seems to have failed to do justice. This is marked wherever it becomes necessary to make use of the reviewer's name and work. On page 201, in writing on " Pathological Second Dentition," he explains that " The lower second molars may cause some irritation owing to an insufficient development of the jaw at the angle, leaving an inadequate accommodation for the crown. At about nine years of age the second molar occupies the angle of the jaw in much the same position as shown in Fig. 101 for the third molar. If held back, a pathological condition equivalent to that occurring in the temporary teeth may result. . . . Truman has prevented a threatened second attack of this sort by deep incisions in the gum over the site of the crown." This is all very imperfectly stated, which is all the more strange, as the editor quotes the facts from an article written by the reviewer in 1899 and read before the National Dental Association. The entire subject-matter, from the time the second molar of the mandible passed from the ramus to assume the direct vertical, was based on original investigation by the reviewer some twenty years previous to that time, and these observations had been so fully confirmed by experience that he had felt justified in calling attention to it as an unobserved pathological problem in second dentition. If any one had noticed this and its resultant nervous reflexes, it had not been observed in the reviewer's reading.

The subject of impacted third molars is generally satisfactory. The editor follows Cryer mainly both in illustration and general ideas. Much might be said of value to the student, but is not mentioned here, especially as to the possible pathological conditions following malposition, where the third molar of the lower jaw abuts against the second molar in an inclined position, inviting caries and final exposure of the pulp.

On page 256 the editor is in error in stating that it was first suggested by " Truman that erosion is due to an altered secretion of the mucus-forming glands of the lip which lie in close relation to them. Truman found these to secrete an acid at night, while during the day the secretion might be alkaline." It may be added to this that Truman found nothing of the kind, but what he did find, after an extended investigation as to the cause of erosion and abrasion, was that at night, when the alkaline saliva practically ceased to flow from the salivary glands, the fermentative process was exceedingly active, with the result that tests at night and early in the morning gave invariably an acid reaction. The lip being held directly upon the anterior teeth during this period acted as an agent to retain the acid fluids in contact with the enamel, and the mucous membranes of the cheeks did the same service for the buccal surfaces of the posterior teeth. Kirk was the one who demonstrated that the mucus glands of the lip gave an acid reaction during the day. His tests were not carried into the night, but it was presumed that there was a continuous action during the twenty-four hours more pronounced during the periods of rest at night.

The chapter on " Stains of the Enamel and Dentine" is satisfactory although brief, but the treatment will not be of much use to the average student. There is great need of more practical detail on this very important branch of operative procedures.

The history of dental caries as given under that chapter is lacking in much that would have been of value. While Miller completed the labor of investigation of dental caries, his work supplemented that of a long line of investigators, but the editor begins his history of the micro-organic theory with Leber and Rottenstein, whereas it should have gone back to Erdl, Ficinus, and Klencke. Writers of books are apt to forget that they are making a repository of history, and that this requires careful compilation of facts, that future writers may not be led into error.

The following very curious statement, to be found on page 327, seems to require notice. He states that " Dentine cannot become inflamed, as leucocytes cannot enter the tubules; nevertheless the irritability of the fibrillæ, like that of other protoplasm, may be heightened." It is altogether a novel idea that leucocytes by entering the tubuli could arouse inflammation. Have blood-vessels ever been discovered permeating dentine? and are the leucocytes the originators of inflamed areas, or, are they simply the final products, through an abnormal condition in the circulation? This certainly should be corrected in future editions, as it fails to properly explain the subject.

" Hypersensitive Dentine and Therapeutics" is well treated from the therapeutical side of the question, but is not equally as well considered from the histological. To mention hypersensitive dentine carries the thought at once back to Tomes, but his name is not mentioned in connection with the discovery of the fibrillæ that bear his name.

This neglect in giving proper credit is manifest in the use of silver nitrate on children's teeth. This properly belongs to the late Dr. Stebbins, and its importance in controlling caries in deciduous teeth should have decided the editor in giving a very full report of his procedures and the results obtained.

The following paragraph is very far from the position held by some, at least, of the leading histological observers of to-day. The editor states, on page 355, " That the caries fungi may be present in the mouth and be harmless, unless conditions favor the formation of gelatinous plaques upon the teeth, as has been shown by Black and Williams.

" These facts demonstrate that the sole requirement in the prevention of caries is the prevention of the formation of gelatinous plaques upon spots favoring their retention.

" It has been shown by Williams that caries is a reasonably slow process; therefore, the removal of plaques at frequent intervals is sufficient for the prevention of caries."

It is doubtful whether Williams or Black would go as far as

this statement presumes to carry them. The editor might profitably have quoted Miller, who has demonstrated very conclusively that the so-called gelatinous plaques have little or nothing to do with the production of caries.

On results of secondary dentine the editor asserts that this tissue unquestionably brings about a degeneration in the pulp " which may become a cause of neuralgia." This statement requires further confirmation. It has been the observation of the reviewer that secondary dentine rarely or never results in neuralgia or other pathological conditions.

The editor still adheres to the use of aconite and iodine painted upon the gum in pericementitis. Aconite, as thus used, is of more than doubtful value, as its effect is to paralyze the sensory nerves of the part to which it is applied, and therefore produces results exactly the reverse of what is desired in a counterirritant.

The editor separates " interstitial gingivitis," as named by Talbot, from pyorrhœa alveolaris, making it a distinct disease. This is not as Talbot intended, for he distinctly renamed pyorrhœa alveolaris by this term, and it is difficult to understand how any pathologic distinctions can be made between these two as described by the editor.

In the treatment of this disease aromatic sulphuric acid is recommended. This is a very poor substitute for the commercial.

Leucoplakia is not mentioned in the book. This is a very important disease for dentists to become familiar with and be able to treat, or, at least, to advise a patient thus afflicted. This neglect of an important topic is to be regretted, as the dentist should be the first to call the patient's attention to this, as it is generally unnoticed. Intelligent advice in the earlier stages may save a surgical operation rendered necessary in severe cases.

The reviewer has felt it a duty to call attention to a few of the minor defects in this otherwise valuable production, but these do not militate against the book as a whole. It is regarded as covering the majority of the subjects included under the name of Dental Pathology with marked ability. It is, at present, the only work that can be recommended to dental students with a feeling that they can use it with profit to themselves as a text-book. It should be placed on the list of text-books in all dental colleges, and equally upon the shelves of the practitioner's library.

The book is sent out in the usual excellent style of Lea Brothers & Co.

ESSENTIALS OF MATERIA MEDICA, THERAPEUTICS, AND PRESCRIPTION WRITING. By Henry Morris, M.D., Fellow of the College of Physicians of Philadelphia, etc. Sixth Edition, thoroughly revised by W. A. Bastedo, Ph.G., M.D., Tutor in Materia Medica in Columbia University. W. B. Saunders & Co., Philadelphia, New York, and London, 1904.

This small volume, while classed among the compends, richly deserves a higher place than is usually given works of this character. The original author of this book very clearly understood the value of a compend, for in the Preface to the first edition he says, " The Author hopes that, if properly used, this book will be of service to the student and young practitioner, but he is sure, from his experience as a teacher, that neither this or any other ' Compend' will suffice to form the groundwork of what is really the study of a lifetime." While this is true, a good compend is of great value to the student, probably more in this study than some others, for the acquisition of a knowledge of drugs, with the general student of medicine and dentistry, must largely depend on memory. The more thorough work must come later.

This book, in its sixth edition, covers most of the more recently introduced drugs; consequently it has a value for the dental operator, as well as to the student, as a convenient and reliable book of reference. For those who desire a more exhaustive treatment resort must be had to the larger works devoted to this subject.

Domestic Correspondence.

THE PRESENT SITUATION OF THE D.D.S.

THREE RIVERS, CANADA, October 13, 1904.

To THE EDITOR:

SIR,—Enclosed please find statement requested of me by several college men. It will serve the best interests of all concerned to publish same at an early date. The exhibits referred to I shall gladly furnish also.

There should be prompt and pronounced action by the colleges and it might be wise to invite me to the meeting and allow me to enter into the council.

Very respectfully,

J. H. WORMAN.

The German government has been instructed by their consuls that any three persons may obtain a charter and found a college or professional school, that their founders may be wholly unqualified, morally or intellectually, to conduct such an institution, and that there is *no supervision on the part of the State* to insure the reputable conduct of manager, preceptor, or student, and that therefore the American Academic honors are questionable ones. I refer especially to the reports of Consuls Bopp and Wever. (See Exhibits A to E.)

They have also reported that political influences prevail in the schools and in the State boards, and that while the dental schools now belonging to the National Association of Dental Faculties may be regarded as " reputable," there is after all no guarantee that they will remain so, for " changes are in America always to be looked for." (See Exhibit   .)

Erich Richter, who at one time carried great influence in the German courts as an Expert, although now retired, still uses every opportunity to call in question the character of our institutions, and for the purpose of saving the Huxmanites from their just deserts has even belittled my standing as a consul, leaving the impression on German judges that I am only a political creature and in nowise comparable with a general consular officer. Richter has testified under oath that Huxman's G. A. D. S. of Chicago was reputable in 1890–93, and recognized by the Illinois Board of Dental Examiners, although the minutes of the board do not permit any such statement. (See Exhibit   .) Richter may have been given a hearing in the Imperial foreign office, and his statements should have been contradicted everywhere.

Professor Dr. Miller, of whom the Americans are justly proud, aimed some years ago to give the Germans a better comprehension of American dental surgery, but did, unwittingly no doubt, more harm than good. Although he recognized the worth of the National Association of Dental Faculties, he weakened their standing by the statement that the smaller schools do not observe their obligations like the stronger ones, and by the imputation that only in a few colleges were the conditions for admission comparable to the preparation in Germany. The German minds cannot grasp the situation so indefinitely stated, and false impressions now prevail. He also repeated the unfortunate statement printed in the report of the United States Commissioner of Education in 1899–1900 regarding the many aliases of our swindling colleges, so that a German unfamiliar with the facts must conclude that we have hundreds of swindling institutions, scholastic and professional, although the facts are that we never had a score of them, and that at the present hour none exist; at least, none are operating successfully.

Professor Miller bestowed much praise on me, and, therefore, this criticism on his course must seem ungrateful to those who do not realize that I seek first, last, and always, simply the suppression of an unlawful traffic in American academic honors and the just treatment of American interests; that I would go to any length to suppress the impostor and traducer, and would not hesitate to combat any attempt to belittle our good name, even though it might for the moment work greatly to our disadvantage. It is our duty to uproot the evil done in our name abroad and bring to justice all who have imposed on foreign governments; thus, and thus only, may we hope to prove ourselves worthy of confidence and our institutions of recognition.

There is a kindly feeling for America in the educated and beaurocratic ranks of Germany, and we could easily obtain an international standing for the dental profession if the States of the Union would legislate on the lines of New York, or the Philippines.

By the law of reciprocity, when once adopted everywhere at home, we would provide further means to effect through diplomatic channels the fullest acknowledgment for our schools, not as private foundations for personal gain, but as institutions conducted *pro bono publica,* bearing the stamp of State authority, also a quasi recognition from the national government.

The various states of Germany have issued edicts for regulating the use of titles in their states and territories as the central government of Germany, that is to say, the imperial German government cannot interfere in church and school matters, the autonomous rights prevailing in the individual states.

Much variability has existed, therefore, in Germany as to the use of foreign academic titles and the values of foreign academic degrees. In some states the edicts, while apparently establishing the manner in which holders of such foreign academic honors might obtain permission for their use of the respective authority of the state, that is to say, of the minister of the interior and cultus, seem to have been merely intended to do away with former usage without the direct declaration against any foreign titles, for in recent years all petitions outside of Bavaria by the holders of American academic degrees have been unfavorably replied to.

The unfavorable decisions are, however, largely due to the fact stated above,—viz., that the German governments have come to look upon our academic and professional schools as affording no guarantee as to the worth of the academic honors conferred by them.

The German courts have also differed widely in their decisions regarding the rights of the holders of American academic honors who are desirous of using their titles in public life, and, as the title plays a most important part in European professional life, any abrogation of the practitioner's rights in this connection means a considerable curtailment of his income, if not the ruin of the practitioner.

Wherever the courts have been duly informed by me of the *bona fide* of our reputable institutions, the courts have ruled favorably, despite the fact that the prosecution was instituted by the state's attorney upon the direct allegations, or, still worse, instigations, of German practitioners.

As late as last August an appeal taken in the kingdom of Bavaria by a graduate of the Maryland Dental College from the ruling of a district court, where local prejudices had resulted in an unfavorable verdict, the higher court ruled the practitioner holding an American reputable degree entitled to its use, and I believe that with proper counsel and truthful representations an appeal to the still higher courts would result no less favorably.

The statement originally given out by Richter, and widely circulated and published in the professional and general press, that the imperial supreme court of Germany had rendered a decision against the use of the American academic title, the "Doctor of Dental Surgery," is groundless, as the ruling was on the title "Doctor Chirurgiæ Dentariæ," the supreme court holding that the American institutions having *private* foundation could not confer titles in other than the language of the land, and that Latin titles should emanate only from institutions of the State with concurrences of the same.

My efforts aim to effect a twofold result,—viz.:

1. An harmonious legislation in the States of our Union making the licenses exchangeable and the diploma a conferment of the school and profession (*i.e.,* the Board of Examiners).

2. An international comity in the profession according to the American State licenses and academic honors of a recognized (reputable) college the same recognition abroad that we accord to their university honors and state approbations.

"OCCLUSION" AND "ARTICULATION."

THE words "occlusion" and "articulation," so frequently quoted in dental literature, are often, we believe, erroneously referred to. The term occlusion, for instance, is not uncommonly made to imply the several and distinct relations of the teeth as witnessed in the act of mastication; whereas, in my conception, this term can refer to only one movement,—viz., to the closing of the jaws. Occlusion, therefore, refers to the normal relations of the inclined occlusal planes of the teeth when the jaws are closed (Angle). Articulation, on the other hand, is a name applied collectively to the relations of the lower teeth to the upper as exhibited in the several movements performed by the mandible during mastication.

JULIO ENDELMAN.

Obituary.

DR. GEORGE H. CHANCE.

THE announcement of the death of Dr. Chance, of Portland, Ore., will create a feeling of serious loss to the dental profession throughout the country, but this will be more pronounced upon the Pacific coast where his long and active service has made his name familiar to all in dental practice. He has demonstrated in his life and work the very best of that type of the pioneer dentists of the western coast, a type honored throughout the United States for the high standard maintained in education and practice.

The personal intercourse of the writer with Dr. Chance was necessarily limited, but it was sufficient to mark him as a man genial in disposition, lovable in character, and earnest always for the best in his profession.

One by one the old standard-bearers are passing to the eternal beyond. This demands at our hands a more serious devotion to the work they left uncompleted. We must emulate, and surpass if possible, their unselfish devotion to a great trust. They went up to the altar of sacrifice and carried there the best fruits of their lives. Let us aim to follow in their footsteps.

Dr. Chance worked to almost the last hour of active life. He was taken sick while attending the California State Society. Up to the time of this visit he had been in active practice. His sufferings from that hour were severe. An operation enabled his friends to remove him to his home, where he lingered for over two months.

Dr. Chance was born in England seventy-four years ago, and came to this country about the year 1850. The gold regions of California drew him to the Pacific coast, and about 1860 he settled in Salem and lived there until 1874 when he removed to Portland, where he lived until the time of his death.

Dr. Chance's last visit East, it is believed, was in attendance at the National meetings held at Niagara Falls a few years since. He accompanied the National Association of Faculties upon a trip to Toronto, and those who were with him on that trip will not soon forget the pleasure he gave by his conversation and thorough enjoyment manifested in association with his professional co-workers. How thoroughly he enjoyed life is manifest by this quotation from his little book entitled " Sunshine Thoughts for Gloomy Hours."

" Is it not better for us to take a broader and therefore a clearer view of this life than most of us do, and soar for awhile above the clouds and thus get a little more sunshine into our souls. On our journey to what we all hope will prove to be the larger and the better life, we pass this way but once; let us keep our eyes for the bright spots in the landscape, for the fruits, the birds, and the flowers, and avoid, in all possible ways, the poisonous swamps of pessimism."

As a dentist Dr. Chance enjoyed a large practice. He was an active official in the Taylor Street Methodist Episcopal Church. He was also a thirty-third degree Mason.

He leaves a widow and the following children: Mrs. F. A. Kenny, Alameda, Cal.; Miss S. E. Chance, Miss W. E. Chance, Miss Alna B. Chance, Charles H. Chance, and Dr. Arthur W. Chance.

The funeral took place September 5, 1904.

DR. STEPHEN G. STEVENS.

I WRITE to notify you of the death of Dr. Stephen G. Stevens, of Boston. He was born in Brooks, Maine, in 1844. He served in the Civil War as a member of Company D, New York Frontier Cavalry; commenced the practice of dentistry in Lynn, Mass.; graduated at the Boston Dental College in 1877; bought the practice of the late Dr. R. L. Robbins and removed to Boston, where he has practised dentistry at 2 Commonwealth Avenue. Dr. Stevens was an honored member of the dental profession and was a very skilful operator. He was a trustee of the Boston Dental College; was ex-president of most of the dental societies in his city and State, and at the time of his death was a member of the Boston Society of Dental Improvement, the American Academy of Dental Science, the Northwestern Dental Society, and the Alumni Association of the Boston and Tufts Dental College. I thought perhaps you would wish to notice Dr. Stevens's death in the JOURNAL.

R. R. ANDREWS.

CAMBRIDGE, September 22, 1904.

DR. J. H. BENTON.

DR. J. H. BENTON, of Newbern, died suddenly at Black Mountain Station, Thursday, September 15, 1904. His remains passed here *en route* for Kinston Saturday morning. Burial service and interment took·place Saturday afternoon. He was placed to rest in the family burial lot beside a son and daughter that had preceded him.

Dr. Benton had been in feeble health for several months, and had recently gone to the mountain section to recuperate, but gradually grew worse, and the end came suddenly.

He anticipated the approach of death with composure and had no fears to disturb and harass a peaceful state of mind. He died as he lived,—true in the faith of the love and mercy of a blessed Redeemer, and at peace with all men. Tidings of his death came as a shock to many, and has brought sorrow and sadness to the hearts of a bereaved wife and many loving kindred and friends.

Dr. Benton was truly a good and true man in the fullest acceptation of the term, and discharged well and faithfully the varied duties of life. He was a man of sound judgment, and always acted in strict accord with his honest convictions of what was right, and lived more for others than for self. He was a devoted, loving husband and father, and as a friend there was none truer; and he was ever benevolent, kind, and helpful to the poor and needy. To appreciate his character rightly and to realize fully the beauty of the many noble traits and virtues with which he was so richly endowed, was to know him well. Those who knew him best loved him most.

He had been a successful practitioner of medicine in his native county—Sampson—for more than twenty-five years, and for ten years past had made Newbern his home and had enjoyed a lucrative dental practice, and was held in the highest esteem by all who knew him professionally and personally. He occupied a prominent position as a dentist in the State and in the State Dental Society, and it will be difficult to fill his place. He served well while he lived, and is at rest.

Peace be with him.

B. F. ARRINGTON.

Current News.

SOUTHERN BRANCH OF THE NATIONAL DENTAL ASSOCIATION.

THE eighth annual meeting of the Southern Branch of the National Dental Association will be held February 21 to 23, 1905, at Memphis, Tenn.

J. A. GORMAN,
Corresponding Secretary.

ASHEVILLE, N. C.

SOUTH DAKOTA STATE BOARD OF DENTAL EXAMINERS.

THE South Dakota State Board of Dental Examiners will hold its next regular session for the examination of candidates at Sioux Falls, S. D., Tuesday, December 6, beginning at 1.30 P.M. All candidates will be required to bring operating-instruments, prepared to do all kinds of clinical operative work, also a bridge of not less than four teeth, including one Richmond and one gold shell crown invested ready to solder. All candidates must positively send in their application to G. W. Collins, secretary, Vermilion, S. D., not later than December 2.

G. W. COLLINS,
Secretary.

THE

International Dental Journal.

VOL. XXV.   DECEMBER, 1904.   No. 12.

Original Communications.[1]

RADIOTHERAPY IN SOME MALIGNANT CONDITIONS OF THE MOUTH.[2]

BY MILTON FRANKLIN, M.D., NEW YORK.

THE now almost universally accepted theory of the action of the X-ray upon the human organism supposes that in all tissue exposed there is effected a high degree of stimulation, which, when continued for a time disproportionate to the resistance of the affected tissue, assumes the proportions of an inflammation, of gradually increasing severity, finally ending in sloughing and necrosis.

Whether the tissue be normal or pathological, whether the result be beneficial or destructive, the action of the ray is the same, and can be said to differ only in degree. Assertions that there exist a distinct curative and burning action are erroneous.

A consideration of the phenomena which occur in an area that has been exposed to the action of the rays will elicit the fact that they strikingly resemble in character and sequence those of typical

---

[1] The editor and publishers are not responsible for the views of authors of papers published in this department, nor for any claim to novelty, or otherwise, that may be made by them. No papers will be received for this department that have appeared in any other journal published in the country.

[2] Read before The New York Institute of Stomatology, June 3, 1904.

classic inflammation. There is the same congestive hyperæmia, followed by the slowing of the blood-current, diapedesis, and vascular exudation, with their accompanying alteration in the vascular walls. There is the increased flow of leucocytes to the part and the infiltration of the tissues by them. These changes are followed in turn by the other well-known changes of inflammation, and may extend through the stages of fibrinous exudation or even to the formation of pus followed by necrosis with sloughing. The causes of inflammation are various, such as traumatism, the action of strong chemicals, heat, electricity, and the X-ray. Each of the different causative agents gives rise to a somewhat different train of phenomena, and while the course of inflammation is in the main the same in each, the different causes may be generally recognized from the resulting inflammation. So also in the case of the X-ray, there are certain peculiarities which render the character of the inflammation slightly different from the rest.

This difference, as far as can be deduced from facts thus far known, consists in that the action commences generally only after a varying period of latent inactivity, that the effect seems entirely due to action upon the nerve terminals, and that the resolution of the scar so closely resembles that of healthy tissue that it is unlike any class of scar heretofore observed, both in absence of tissue loss and of tendency to hypertrophy.

Besides this action in causing inflammation through direct stimulation, there is the almost paradoxical coincident inhibitory effect upon lower forms of cell life. This action has been so certainly established that I shall not attempt to detail the experiments which have led to a knowledge of the fact.

In the main these effects are common to the X-ray, the ultra-violet ray as applied by Finsen, and to the emanations of radium. In the case of the X-ray the destructive action is dominant; in the case of the ultra-violet ray there seems at the present time to be strong reason to suppose that the germicidal factor plays no inconsiderable part, while the ability to cause the growth of almost normal new tissue in the area formerly occupied by the diseased tissue is quite remarkable, excelling even that of the X-ray. In the case of radium there has been so little evidence up to the present time that is likely to prove of any therapeutic value, that I shall not consume the time or space necessary to discuss it. At the same time it may be well to point out that on account of the small size of the tubes, combined with their independent activity, apart from any connection with an outside source of electricity, they might prove of interest in conditions of the mouth if they are ultimately found to possess any value in medical science.

In considering which method to use when dealing with a malignant condition, much judgment should be exercised. The disadvantages and limitations of operative methods should be carefully compared with those of the X-ray, and the method chosen which, in the case under consideration, offers the greatest number of advantages and the fewest disadvantages.

In the treatment of diseased tissues with the X-ray, it should be remembered that all tissues are affected in the same way, the action being the same upon healthy as upon morbid tissue. The different effects are attributable, in the main, to the lower vitality of the latter. The changes that are gone through follow each other with comparatively greater rapidity in the less resisting tissue, while the normal tissue is but mildly stimulated. Thus the stage of sloughing and cell proliferation may be reached in the tumor, while in the adjacent healthy tissue, equally exposed, there may be only mild irritation, or, at the most, burn of the first degree. At the same time the retarding action upon lower forms of cell life should be taken into consideration as probably inhibiting the growth of the neoplasm.

The advantages of surgical measures over the X-ray may be briefly summed up as follows:

1. Celerity. The whole diseased tissue as well as the threatened tissue may be removed at once, while in the case of the ray, weeks, months, and in some few cases a year, or even more, has been necessary.

2. Conservation of the patient's strength. By removing from the body, at one operation, the whole malignant growth, a great drain upon the patient is avoided, together with the constant danger of metastasis.

3. The removal of the growth from the body by an outside route instead of causing it to be eliminated by the body organs, with the consequent accompanying autointoxication from the presence of the degenerated noxious tissue products. The strain upon the eliminating organs and the danger of metastasis, which it is now generally accepted is increased by the action of the ray, is avoided.

The considerations in favor of the ray method are briefly as follows:

1. Avoidance of surgical shock and anæsthetic complications.

2. Better ability to differentiate, and assurance that only the diseased tissue will be destroyed.

3. Better appearance of the resulting scar, which in the majority of cases so far resembles the normal tissue as to almost entirely escape detection.

Considerations of locality will in a measure determine which of the two methods is to be preferred in some cases, it being remembered that the ray cannot be focussed, and that the tissue surrounding the area to be treated should be protected as far as possible from the action of the ray.

In deep-seated conditions the ray as a curative agent cannot be too strongly condemned. The necessity of traversing healthy tissue by the inflammatory rays subjects them to the great danger of burn, with the accompanying inflammatory changes. Besides this the delicate nature of the lining membranes of the bodily viscera renders them liable to so great irritation as to endanger life. Besides this there is no authentic case of cure of deep cancer at present extant.

The determination of which method is to be used in any instance should be based upon a consideration of the features of the case in connection with the characters of the methods available.

In general terms cases in which the X-ray is to be recommended are those in which (1) the condition is essentially superficial; (2) where the loss of any great amount of tissue would be serious; (3) where there is little likelihood of other organs being involved through metastasis; (4) where cosmetic considerations outweigh all others; (5) where time is a negligible quantity and does not add danger; and (6) where the case is for any reason inoperable. In general all other cases are preferably treated by operative methods.

I make mention here of only those conditions of the mouth in which, in my opinion, there is nothing to be gained by employing the radiotherapeutic in preference to the operative method. There are numerous other cases where either some difference of·opinion exists, or the ray is generally accepted as inapplicable.

Epithelioma of the mouth, when situated on the edge of the lip, is frequently better treated with the ray than by other methods.

Here the loss of tissue should if possible be avoided. The condition is among the most amenable to treatment by the ray, and the superficial character renders it the more so. In cases where there is much involvement of the submaxillary glands, while it is the experience of some practitioners that the size of the glands decreases simultaneously with that of the lesion, it is better practice to extirpate the whole of the threatened and diseased tissue and then apply the ray for the purpose of preventing recurrence. Where the epithelioma involves the tongue, it is preferable to use the rays where conditions do not specifically contraindicate. Here any loss of tissue is followed by grave consequences, and the results in cases that have been treated by the rays have been such as to render the method of unquestionable value. In cancer of the larynx or pharynx, notwithstanding some reputed cures, it is certain that there is little to be gained by using the ray. Because of the impossibility of applying the rays direct, but only through the tissues of the neck, it is doubtful if any benefit can be obtained without seriously impairing the tissues traversed. The ray may be used after the operation to lessen the likelihood of recurrence. This is in no way inconsistent with anything that has been said regarding the danger of raying deep-lying structures, as it is necessary to apply the rays only a few times to obtain reasonable assurance.

In noma the results of raying have, on the whole, been of negative character. Here the utmost despatch is needed in ridding the mouth of the offending mass, as any delay is apt to result in irreparable loss of tissue or even of life.

Catarrhal and croupous stomatitis, though not malignant diseases, are worthy of mention here because of the striking manner in which they respond to the ultra-violet treatment of Finsen. In the former condition the degeneration of the epithelium and the formation of pus cease after a few treatments, and the substitution of a new membrane follows speedily. In the croupous condition the false membrane melts away under the action of the light, and is followed by no perceptible scar. Where there has been tendency to necrosis, there appears a cicatrix after the cessation of the morbid process, which closely resembles the normal tissues.

Tubercular stomatitis is readily influenced by the ultra-violet ray, and as there is rarely any communication of the process to other parts of the body, there is little danger in a prolonged treatment. It is therefore preferable to proceed by phototherapeutic methods instead of resorting to operation. The X-ray also exercises a marked benefit upon these cases, but on account of the danger of burning the face, the ultra-violet rays are to be preferred.

Papillomata are best treated by the X-ray when they are of small extent, and by operation when large. The ray is recommended, as the results are obtained in small tumors before the lining membrane of the mouth is affected, and in these cases this method is simpler than operation.

Angiomata respond very readily to the action of the X-ray, the internal walls of the vessels undergoing a change resulting in early occlusion, followed by atrophy and final disappearance of the whole mass. The elaborate measures necessary to prevent excessive bleeding in all operations render them less to be desired in these conditions.

To conclude: it may be stated that in the present condition of the science the radiotherapeutic method may be used on some few cases in preference to all others; in some cases where the operative method, *cæteris paribus*, would be preferred, but in which on account of existing complications cannot be performed; and in nearly all cases, after operation, to minimize the possibility of recurrence.

Regarding the value of the ray in post-operative cases, for the purpose of minimizing to the fullest extent the likelihood of recurrence, it may be stated that herein lies the most satisfactory feature of the whole method. Scarcely any difference of opinion exists at all among surgeons who have made a practice of having their cases undergo a course of X-ray exposures after operation, as to the influence in preventing recurrence.

MALIGNANT GROWTHS IN THE MOUTH.[1]

BY R. H. M. DAWBARN, M.D., NEW YORK.

GENTLEMEN,—The chief forms of malignancy directly of interest to stomatologists are, the bony tumors of the jaws, malignant epulis, cancer or sarcoma of the tonsils or pharynx, cancer of the tongue and of the lip.

In order to compress my paper within modest limits I shall only refer to such points in diagnosis as have a very practical bearing for you. As to tumors of the jaws, the case narrated by Dr. Howe demonstrates the ease with which a growth filling the antrum can be overlooked. I show you to-night the jaw and antrum tumor of this patient sent me by Dr. Howe about seven years ago upon a shrewd suspicion. It proved spindle-celled sarcoma, was excised, and remains cured. The use of a stout needle in this case, held in a firm holder, at once revealed decalcification of the bone. This you can verify for yourselves upon this specimen. The electric-light test also showed the antrum filled on that side. Another case, sent me last December by Dr. W. C. Dears, ex-president of the First District Dental Society, presented nothing but a very trifling swelling of the bony roof of the mouth; but the needle test showed, where there should have been almost stony hardness, a softened area, about as firm as articular cartilage and shading gradually into the surrounding dense bone. This area was considerably larger than a silver dollar and irregular in outline. I operated upon her at the Polyclinic Hospital in December, 1903, removing by drill and rongeur the softened area, also about one centimetre of dense bone beyond, for safety, and of course the same extent of periosteum and mucous membrane. I could then have passed both thumbs into the nose through the gap so left. Professor Jeffries, pathologist at this school, pronounced the pieces of softened bone sent him typical carcinomatous.

At first, after healing, this lady wore a temporary plate, for obvious reasons; but by continuous maintenance of unhealed edges, thus inviting growth by granulation, I have almost closed the gap. It is now not larger than the head of a pin. She is courteous

---

[1] Read before The New York Institute of Stomatology, June 3, 1904.

enough to be present to-night for your examination. So far as I can ascertain, early decalcification, permitting successful use of the needle test, is the rule rather than the exception; but it has not heretofore been recognized that such is the case. I have proved it in a considerable number of instances now; but one each of sarcoma and carcinoma of the upper jaw suffice to-night to remind you of it.

As to cancer of the tongue, unquestionably neglect of decaying teeth, sharp-edged and persistently irritating the tongue against their lingual surface, constitutes the chief predisposing cause. The cancer begins almost always at the edge of the tongue, continually chafed by such a tooth; and here, as in epulis,, or, indeed, any other soft growth, it is wise for the dentist to inject a few drops of, say, one per cent. solution of cocaine, and then with curved scissors and forceps remove a small piece for the opinion of an expert in pathology. Then you will know what to expect, as to prognosis, after your surgeon has operated; and this report will also be his guide as to how extensive must be his excision.

Turning to treatment, we may put it rather concisely by saying that as yet there is no known means of a medical nature which is curative of malignancy; although arsenic pushed as far as is safe, by hypodermic, unquestionably slows and even checks the growth for a time of certain forms of sarcoma.

Prompt and wide excision remains our only safeguard, and by early diagnosis you have it in your power to save many lives through wise advice not to delay operation. But if the tumor be too extensive when first seen, or if it be so placed as to make excision anatomically hopeless, then our resources are either radium, X-rays, or Finsen light, naming them in order of speedy efficacy; or in just one instance, certain fusiform-celled sarcomata, the Coley antitoxin treatment; and finally my own plan of attempted starvation by depriving the tumor of its nourishment.

Regarding the use of radium and X-rays, doubtless Dr. Franklin will speak fully; but it is the opinion of surgeons that where excision is possible it is unwise to delay. There have been some really brilliant cures by these means; but, on the other hand, I have seen several cases go from bad to worse, and beyond hope of excision, during the delay of several weeks or longer with X-ray treatment. We cannot yet say why one case is helped and another is not. Apparently radium or X-rays are more hopeful in sarcoma than in carcinoma; but even in the latter I have noted a marvellous relief from the agonizing pain of cancer of the bodies of the vertebræ by placing a small radium tube of great power for an hour in contact with the back. Fully twenty-six hours of freedom from suffering followed; and this could not have been merely psychical, for the patients did not even know that anything unusual was to be tried.

'Our wisest plan, in cases still operable, is to excise; and after the wound has healed, to begin X-ray or radium treatment several times a week for a month or more, hoping in this way to prevent recurrence. Of late I have been following this plan quite regularly; and so do most other surgeons, I think; and not alone about the mouth, but after removal of the uterus or breast for cancer, or, indeed, wherever it may chance to have been.

But if the tumor cannot be excised, and if the other two plans indicated have failed, what then? Are we at the end of our rope? In the region supplied by the external carotid we are not; and it means much to a patient to know this, and thereby to substitute for the certainty of death once more the uncertainty of life!

When first I began experimenting in this unknown field, just nine years ago, I feared that attempted starvation of malignancy would result also in starving the nose, tongue, or other normal parts. Fortunately, this is untrue; and we now know that normal flesh is able to survive with surprisingly little blood—much less than is necessary in order to permit so very vascular a thing as a cancer to continue growing. Also, it was demonstrated that no good would result from merely tying the external carotid on one or even on both sides. Nothing short of complete excision of both these arteries was effective—doing it for safety at two different periods of time.

At present the writer has excised the external carotids in nearly sixty instances. The operation is quite surprisingly safe. If the patient is not badly cachectic, and if the surgeon is not so unwise as to attempt removal of the growth at the same sitting, there ought to be not over five per cent. of mortality. And simple ligation of both external carotids should have hardly any mortality at all.

What are the results?

In carcinoma, which spreads, as we all remember, not through the blood-vessels, but through its lymphatic channels, the results have been disappointing. Even here, however, we can expect with some confidence a considerable degree of shrinkage, but lasting

only a few weeks or months,—up to a year in one case, who otherwise would certainly have died within a month. But in sarcoma
there is reason for a more cheerful view; and, remembering that
this malignant tumor spreads by its blood-vessels rather than its
lymphatics, one could guess, *a priori*, that sarcoma would be better
controlled by the starvation of blood than would carcinoma.

In Butlin, " On Malignant Disease," round-celled subperiosteal
sarcoma of the jaws is considered hopeless, whatever we do; and
yet in my Gross prize book are recorded two cases of this nature
which have remained shrunken for much longer than the Volkmann
period of three years, after which we may with some degree of certainty claim a permament cure, and which still remain quiescent.
The tumor did not, of course, disappear, but it became much
smaller, harder, and inactive. In several other instances of sarcoma
there has been only a temporary checking; but this is generally
longer than we have learned to expect in carcinoma. We must
recollect that if a growth is so situated that it can get blood from
the *internal* carotid or its branches,—about the orbit, for example,
—the prognosis is necessarily bad. Of course, we cannot tie off
the internal carotid too, for this would be useless unless done on
both sides, and that would kill the patient promptly from anæmia
of the brain. (Roughly, the internal carotid may be said to supply
brain and eye; the external carotid all parts of the upper neck,
and of the head except as just stated.)

Here in New York about a dozen members of the New York
Surgical Society have tried my plan, and sent me their results, all
of which have been published. In every instance of recovery from
the operation itself cancer—*i.e.*, carcinoma—has been the form of
malignancy; and, as it happens, in no case sarcoma as yet. This
is unfortunate; and in fairness to this plan it is evident that it
should be given a trial in sarcoma.

I trust it is plain to this society that this operation is not recommended by me for trial except as a last resource—after other
things fail; and since a coffin is the only alternative, surely it is
worthy of trial. In many instances patients are eager if only for a
few weeks' longer life; perhaps for business reasons, to straighten
out their affairs; and this at the very least we can give them.
Again, in a case inoperable through size, and yet not extremely so,
it is quite likely that we may be able, because of a few weeks' shrinkage, so to reduce the mass that it can safely be subjected to thorough

work by the knife. I have within the past fortnight received from Professor J. Chalmers Da Costa, of Philadelphia, the account, sent me for publication, of a case of this very sort, refused as impossible of excision by two other prominent surgeons, but made easily operable by the starvation plan; so that after a few weeks' shrinkage Dr. Da Costa safely cut out the now shrunken tumor.

These points, then, we can surely claim for this method of the *dernier ressort,* and, in addition, in sarcoma, in some cases a real and permanent cure, in the sense that the shrunken mass has remained shrunken for years, and, so far as I know, permanently. The case sent the writer by Dr. Howe is such an instance, definitely cured; only there we could excise the tumor as well as the carotids.

In two cases in my book, of especial interest to you, as involving the lower jaw, one detail of the operation I must particularly mention and recommend. This is, upon completing the excision of the external carotid, to do a short, blunt dissection in the front of the wound high up, thus exposing the inner surface of the ramus and the inferior dental nerve and artery as they are about to enter the canal. The artery and also its mylohyoid or main branch, at this point easily seen, are tied. Thus we deprive the bone of a free anastomosis, for the inferior dental, coming from the internal maxillary, anastomoses freely through orbital branches with the ophthalmic from the internal or deep carotid. In cases of lower-jaw malignancy starvation, where this ligation is omitted, we can well see how the excision of the external carotid alone would prove almost valueless. This step does not add more than a few minutes to the length of the operation. Finally, in each of these cases an inch or more of the inferior dental nerve was excised; for, in case the growth in the mandible should start up again at some future time, at least we have made sure by this means that there will be little or no suffering. Of course, it is essential that this be done upon both sides of the neck, just as with the work upon the arteries; otherwise little is gained.

In conclusion we may claim the following advantages from the starvation plan in the external carotid area, in cases wisely selected.

1. In some instances of sarcoma it saves life by permanent shrinkage of a tumor too large to excise, or so placed that this is impossible.

2. In all instances surviving the carotid excisions there is a

prolongation of life not otherwise possible of accomplishment; even in carcinoma this is true. This may in unfavorable cases be only a few months' gain, but patients are grateful even for this time in which the better to arrange their affairs.

3. Every operator has agreed that one striking effect is the lessening of pain, which is a prompt result of the anæmia produced.

4. In some instances the shrinkage permits the removal of a tumor not possible of excision because of its size and vascularity at first.

PERICEMENTAL ABSCESS.[1]

BY D. D. SMITH, D.D.S., M.D., PHILADELPHIA.

THE affection here denominated pericemental abscess was first noticed by the author about 1890, and first described by him in a paper read at the Tri-union Meeting of the Virginia State, Maryland State, and District of Columbia Dental Societies, held at Old Point Comfort, Va., May, 1897. Prior to this all abscesses associated with the teeth and alveolus were styled alveolar abscess; the only exception to this being the occasional use of the meaningless term " blind abscess."

It was not until quite a number of these peculiar tumoric growths found on the roots of teeth—especially between the roots of molars—had been observed and noted that their distinguishing characteristics were made a subject of special interrogation and study.

ATTENTION FIRST ARRESTED.

While treating the putrescent root-canals of a superior left bicuspid, in the year 1890, two hitherto unobserved diagnostic conditions came prominently into notice. It was evident that the tooth was associated with an abscess, yet the most persistent efforts to relieve it by treatment through the root were wholly without results; at the same time the previously cleansed and disinfected canals of the tooth remained entirely devoid of infection. Repeated dressings and medication during a period of three weeks failed to

---

[1] Read before the Philadelphia County Medical Society, September 23, 1904.

develop any odor or to make any impression whatever for the better. At the end of four weeks the tooth was extracted, when the cause of the trouble and the negative results in treatment became apparent. Lodged in an irregular depression of the root, formed by a slight sharp bend, about one-quarter of an inch from the apex, was a glandular, fibrous tumor of the size of an ordinary pea, covered with globules of pus. The base of this tumor, or abscess, was relatively large and strongly attached to the pericemental membrane. It was entirely independent of the pulp or canals, having no communication with them whatever, either at the basal attachment or at the apex. I remember well, that in reciting this feature of the case at the meeting referred to, several who took part in the discussion refused to believe that such conditions could exist.

THE DAWNING OF RECOGNITION.

In the dawning of my observation of these pathological conditions, the recognition of them was so confused and imperfect—for in the beginning only chronic cases were apprehended—that it required several years to differentiate them from the ordinary alveolar abscess.

THE REVELATIONS OF AN ACUTE CASE.

The observation and conduct of an *acute* case, in the spring of 1895, developed the missing diagnostic links, opened the way to a more perfect understanding of the etiology of the trouble, and suggested the nosology we have adopted.

This case is of peculiar interest, and is here cited in the hope that it may serve to fix the special pathognomonic features of the disorder. It was in connection with a second left upper molar, a tooth of typical formation, in the mouth of a young M.D.—a mouth marked, because of virulent infection on all surfaces of the teeth.

BEGINNING OF AN ACUTE CASE.

The patient presented rather hesitatingly, complaining of an uneasy sensation only, which he hardly classed as pain, but which he located without hesitation in the offending tooth. Examination disclosed no diagnostic symptoms except a very slight loosening of the tooth and a barely distinguishable response to tapping and pressure. There being no evidence of periosteal irritation, and the pulp being alive, I was disposed to regard the complaint as having origin more in the imagination than in a real pathological state. Following an application of tincture of iodine to the gum over the affected·tooth, the case was dismissed with the suggestion that the pain was probably due to some unusual or misdirected pressure in biting.

APPREHENSION A DIAGNOSTIC SYMPTOM.

The next day the patient returned, with the local symptoms equally obscure; there was little evidence of inflammation, no swelling, no decided pain on pressure. The most prominent feature of the case at this stage was the feeling of apprehension, the decided conviction of the patient that there was something wrong with that particular tooth.

The case was a regular daily visitant for about eight days. During the first five days no strongly marked diagnostic features developed, but it excited interest and. not a little anxiety. The treatment consisted of external applications only, the quieting effect of which seemed to be most evanescent. Neither heat nor cold applied directly to the tooth and gums gave rise to any unusual sensations of pain or relief. There was no appreciable swelling, no marked periostitis or other evidence of the inflammation save the pain; this had become continuous, and was definitely located *in the tooth.*

On the fifth day a diagnosis of acute pericemental abscess was made. The tooth had become looser and perhaps more painful; it responded more acutely to tapping and pressure, but the pulp was deemed to be alive. To assure myself that it was not implicated in the trouble, I decided upon devitalization.

(IN PARENTHESIS.)

And here parenthetically I desire to put on record a protest against much that has been written in disparagement of arsenic for the devitalization of pulps, and present the one proper method for using this valuable agent.

ARSENIC AS A DEVITALIZER.

Although wholly contrary to accepted teachings and practice, the *arsenical paste*—white arsenic, morphia acetas āā, creosote

q. s.—should *never* be placed in contact with pulp tissue; this application should always be made to intervening vital dentine.

The cavity in the tooth in which the application is to be made should be so shaped and arranged that the arsenic shall be securely confined in contact with vital, sensitive dentine only. There should be no possibility of its escape to other mouth tissues, either through the confining filling or around the margins of the cavity. If the cavity of decay cannot be made to securely confine the arsenic,— and very frequently it cannot,—or if it is desired to destroy the pulp in a sound tooth, a special cavity or large drill-pit should always be made *in another part* of the tooth, one in which the arsenic can be perfectly confined. The application may be made in a cavity remote from the pulp with perfect assurance, provided it is secured there in contact with sensitive dentine (temporary gutta-percha stopping is the best confining medium).

WHY PAIN AND SYSTEMIC SYMPTOMS RESULT FROM THE USE OF ARSENIC AS A DEVITALIZER.

It is placing the arsenic upon living pulp-tissue that induces the pain, and it is the escaping of the arsenic from the cavity to the pericementum and gums, through or around the confining filling, that has been and is the cause of all supervening troubles—gum inflammations, alveolar absorption, and necrosis—which result from the use of this agent.

Manipulation in accordance with the method suggested will insure painless and perfect devitalization in any tooth in from twenty-four to seventy-two hours, and that with no possible systemic injury, neither inflammatory manifestations in any contiguous tissues.

THE NARRATIVE RESUMED.

Drilling through a small crown filling into the dentine, the tooth-bone was found in an exalted state of sensibility. Assured of my diagnosis, I determined, if possible, to reach the seat of the abscess and evacuate the pus in the hope of effecting a cure. An arsenical application was accordingly made to the dentine, which so perfectly destroyed the pulp that its removal was effected within thirty-six hours. This operation produced no disturbance, neither was there any incident following it. The removal of the pulp and dressing of the roots had no appreciable influence on the abscess symptoms; the soreness of the tooth, the continuous (not throbbing) pain, and the mental disturbance—a feeling of apprehension—continued unabated. I next drilled entirely through the crown, reaching the alveolus at the point which extends down between the roots. This operation was very disappointing in that it failed to evacuate any pus or to develop any odor. The third day after the opening was made upon the alveolus there appeared unmistakable signs of infection in the left antrum. Unwilling to risk further treatment, the offending molar was extracted, when the cause of all this trouble became apparent. Just above the opening which had been made with the drill, and closely adherent to the inner side of the distal buccal root, was the peculiar but well-developed lobular sac of the abscess, with small globules of pus disseminated over its surface. The night following the removal of the tooth there was a copious discharge from the antrum through the left nostril. An opening was at once made through the alveolus into the antrum and treatment instituted through it. The antral cavity was syringed twice daily with phénol sodique, diluted about one-half with water, and at the end of two weeks the case was discharged entirely well.

WHY THIS CASE POSSESSES GENERAL INTEREST.

This acute case should possess general interest for the profession, not alone because it presents the distinguishing peculiarities and diagnostic symptoms of this affection, but more because it discloses the serious nature of the malady and points to some of its usual but unrecognized complications.

A COMMON AND SERIOUS MALADY.

It is manifest that the pathological condition we are discussing is not only far more common than has hitherto been supposed, but that the infection resulting from it is the occasion of many grave systemic diseases as yet unsuspected. It is a condition which may be readily diagnosed when in a state of activity, but when chronic and apparently inert, it is difficult to recognize. In the guise of innocent inactivity it gives rise to perpetual infection, and frequently arouses most serious systemic maladies, conditions far more to be dreaded than its most aggravated local expressions.

Fig. 1.

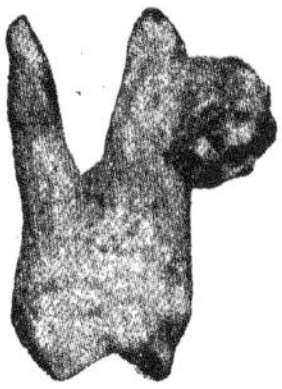

Fig. 2.

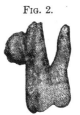

Pericemental abscess.

Fig. 3.

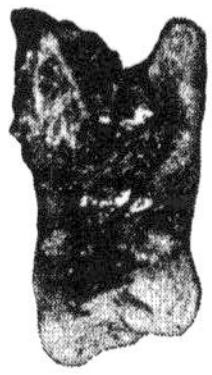

Fig. 4.

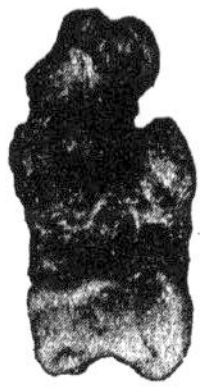

Fig. 5.

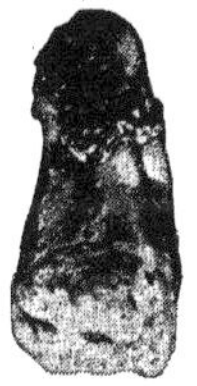

During the ten years which have followed the treatment of the case cited I have seen and treated a goodly number of these abscesses, both acute and chronic, but never with encouragement or pronounced success. One of the former occurred in my own mouth in connection with a maltreated, split molar, which eventuated in an obstinate ·double antral infection. Another—chronic—illustrated in this article (Fig. 3), was the occasion of a grave head trouble—a burning pain under the scalp, attended with exhaustion and despondency. These conditions were immediately relieved by extracting the tooth. Fig. 4 was the cause of the ·development of a severe double antrum infection. Fig. 5 was the occasion of a marked condition of malaise, attended with mental depression and hallucinations. In the two latter cases, extraction of the offending teeth afforded immediate and pronounced relief; the antrum trouble progressed rapidly to complete cure, and the malaise and mental depression to complete systemic restoration.

In but two instances, where pericemental abscess has been surely diagnosed, has there been any prolonged effort to retain and preserve the teeth. In these cases—both teeth superior molars—the abscesses have extensive basal attachment, which supplants and occupies the territory on the inner surface of the roots at their junction with the crown. These abscesses are quiescent, and have no perceptible pus discharge; while the teeth are somewhat loose, they are in use in mastication, and occasion no complaint. In both instances the teeth were experimentally retained: there is absolutely no hope of bettering their condition by treatment, either through surgical removal or lymphatic absorption.

TESTIMONY FROM DR. FORMAD.

The histological researches of the late Dr. Formad, of the Medical Department of the University of Pennsylvania, as revealed in a private letter under date January 20, 1898, fully confirm the status ascribed to this pathological condition as a new discovery; they also stamp its nosology as correct, and reveal why it may, and does, occur indiscriminately on teeth with and without vital pulps. Caused, as it is, by an irritant on the outer surface of the pericemental membrane, it is wholly unaffected by any known method of treatment, either through the root, by external application, or by surgical interference.

DIAGNOSTIC SYMPTOMS.

The diagnostic symptoms of pericemental abscess are distinct and plain when once recognized. In acute cases the first manifestation is pain; not severe, but continuous, and located by the patient in the offending tooth. Nervous apprehension on the part of the patient is, I believe, always incident to it. The trouble is liable to be confounded with periodontitis, but is readily distin-guished from it. In acute pericemental abscess there are no marked inflammatory symptoms in the alveolar and gum tissue; no swelling, no acute pain in response to tapping or pressure, no marked distinction between hot and cold applications, and no relief afforded by any local medication. The loosening of the tooth, slight in the beginning, becomes more and more marked as the case progresses. It will thus be noted that while this affection has been, and is, liable to be confounded with periodontitis, all the diagnostic symptoms (except the pain and the response to pressure) in the former are exactly the opposite to those in the latter.

Chronic pericemental abscess is distinguished by absence of pain and all other active inflammatory symptoms. Occasionally there is some hypertrophy of the gum tissue, but no marked swelling, nor soreness of the tooth on pressure. The tooth itself can generally be used in mastication without special discomfort. The escaping pus is discharged at the edge of the alveolus—between the alveolus and the gum. The point of egress may be distinguished by a peculiar lip, or mouth-like opening, marked by a circumscribed turgescent condition of the gum tissue; a condition wholly unlike the fistulous opening of an alveolar abscess.

TEETH SPECIALLY LIABLE TO PERICEMENTAL ABSCESS.

Any tooth having a pericemental membrane, and a conformation to accumulate infection, may be the subject of pericemental abscess. Molars with large, bell-shaped crowns and constricted necks, because of their shape and location in the mouth, are more especially liable to it.

WHAT IT RESULTS FROM.

The conditions preceding its development are neither systemic inclination through aberrant nutrition, nor a circulation floating a so-called gouty poison. It is not a result of infection from putrescent pulp-tissue, nor from the prolific gaseous emanations resulting from nitrogenous decomposition within the tooth. Infection from such sources finds expression on the *inner* surface of the pericementum about the apical foramen, and eventuates in the ordinary alveolar abscess. The nucleus of this inflammation, and the resultant tumoric abscess, is in touch with some stagnant, septic irritant upon the tooth or teeth, the external surface of the pericemental membrane alone being involved.

PUS DISCHARGE SMALL.

The amount of pus disengaged from these abscesses is relatively small. It is not confined within a sac or limiting membrane, as is generally the case with an ordinary alveolar abscess, but it is sparingly distributed over the irregular surface and within the folds of the tumor-like body which forms the abscess.

HOW A PERICEMENTAL ABSCESS DISCHARGES.

The pus from a pericemental abscess never forces an outlet through the alveolus and gums in the form of a fistulous opening, neither does it come into the pulp-canals through the apical foramen. It escapes at the edge of the alveolus, at the free margins of the gums,—commonly between root bifurcations,—or it may be found oozing around one particular root of a molar; frequently it is the palatine root of a superior molar or the distal root of a lower molar. Turgidity of the gum tissue at the point of egress marks the exact location of the abscess. No pus whatever can be obtained from a pericemental abscess in its earlier or acute stage. Even in chronic states the discharge is seldom profuse in connection with a single-rooted tooth. In a goodly number of cases, where the abscess had assumed a hopelessly chronic form, I have found pus in large quantities and very offensive, in a few instances in connection with lower bicuspids, but more especially around lower molars. The incessant inflammatory action induced by this abscess not only increases its own substance, but it loosens the tooth, and through necrotic absorption forms, enlarges, and deepens cavities and pits in the alveolus which become cesspools of pus prolific in infection.

The nerve-centres, from my observation, are the special points attacked by the pyæmic toxins from this abscess. Depression of spirits, loss of appetite, enfeebled digestion, malaise, headache, tonsillar and pharyngeal inflammations, are the direct outcome. They also become the exciting cause of many far more serious troubles, both acute and chronic; among these we have found neurasthenic, gastric, gastro-intestinal, rheumatic, and renal complications, including diabetes and albuminuria. From all these maladies we have not only afforded relief but effected cures by relieving septic mouth conditions, complicated with pericemental abscess.

POTENCY OF MOUTH CONDITIONS ORIGINATING SYSTEMIC INFECTION
  JUST IN THE DAWNING OF RECOGNITION BY MEDICINE AND DEN-
  TISTRY.

Since the publication of the article on " Systemic Infection due to Natural Teeth Conditions," in January, 1903, there have appeared two papers of marked significance, by medical men,—one by Dr. Robert T. Morris, of New York City, entitled " Infections of the Lymph-glands of the Mouth and Throat," and the other, " Buccal Antisepsis," by Dr. E. Dunogier, Bordeaux, France. The former makes this significant and commendable remark: " We are finding at my clinic very many more infections proceeding from the teeth than are found in some other clinics," and then goes on to say, " One class of infections, very dangerous ones, have been frequently overlooked by dentists: these are infections following the removal of abscessed teeth. Patients die and the cases are not reported; they come in to be treated for pneumonia. There are patients dying this minute in this city from the result of having abscessed teeth extracted while in course of acute infection."

Dr. Dunogier speaks of " dangerous systemic results accompanying purulent conditions about the oral cavity," and recites the case of a " young man aged twenty-one, a sufferer from albuminuria for over six years," who was cured through, what seems to me, very indifferent attention to the teeth and mouth, which had previously been wholly neglected. To prove positively " whether the mouth-infection had been directly concerned in the causation of albuminuria, the patient was directed to abandon temporarily all dental care. This was followed five days afterwards by the reappearance of the albumin, and thus," is is stated, " the original diagnosis was definitely established." Another case of a diabetic is noted by Dr. Dunogier with similar treatment and like favorable results.

When the day shall dawn when medicine and dentistry shall fully recognize the human mouth as the field of most prolific and dangerous infection and truly differentiate its pathologic conditions, the prevention of disease, the relief of suffering, and the lengthening of the average of human life will be accelerated a hundred-fold.

If it is true, as Dr. Morris says, that in dentistry and surgery " we find whatever we are looking for," how important that we keep our eyes fixed on actual conditions. Actual conditions do not reveal that the extraction of a tooth with an ordinary alveolar abscess was ever the precursor of pneumonia. Pericemental abscess, with its pyogenic infection and enfeebling results, has undoubtedly been a predisposing factor in many cases of pneumonia. How important that medicine and dentistry distinguish between the two conditions!

Mouth conditions would appear very different to both professions if they could be viewed in the light in which they really exist. We do not need the hypothetical conditions of " thrombi" and " embolic infection," said to be induced by equally hypothetical " crushing of cancellous bone-structure in tooth extraction," for the induction of systemic infection. Infection is found as a natural exudate along the whole linear gum margin about the teeth; it is found upon the twenty to thirty square inches of tooth surface in every mouth, between and under the teeth, and in crypts and pockets about roots. It is found in nasal passages, upon the tongue, on tonsils and pharynx. There is infection in the breath, in salivary and mucous sediment, in decaying food remains, and in mouth débris of every kind. Add to these *normal* infectious states the many serious pathological mouth conditions,—decay in the teeth, putrescent pulp-tissue, the retrograde metamorphosis of devitalized teeth, alveolar abscess, alveolar pyorrhœa, and, more than all, the infection we are considering, pericemental abscess,— and we have a combination of infection in the human mouth which should startle the community and rouse to highest intensity the interest of medicine and dentistry alike.

The question may arise, Is pericemental abscess a state of pyorrhœa? My answer is emphatically in the negative. Pericemental abscess and alveolar pyorrhœa are often associated in the same mouth, and they may have similar origin, but they are separate and distinct affections. Pericemental abscess develops from a point of irritation on the external surface of the pericementum, usually some inaccessible depression in which the infection lodges and is confined. It is generally found between the roots of double- or multi-rooted teeth, or it may be at the end of a tooth having fused roots. Alveolar pyorrhœa is more commonly found in connection with single-rooted teeth; when associated with molars, the infection is between, rarely, if ever, under them.

Pericemental abscess is a characteristic tumoric growth, generally between the roots of teeth; alveolar pyorrhœa is an inflammation beginning in the pericementum at the free margin of the gums; in its progress it destroys cemental and alveolar tissue, uncovers portions of the roots of teeth, develops pus, and imparts a characteristic odor to the breath. This inflammation leaves in its train not degenerate, serofibrous *growths,* but broken-down tissue remains, calcic sedimentary matter, and other débris which destroys permanently all vital relations between the uncovered portions of the affected roots and the alveolus..

Pericemental abscess, virulently infectious, is incurable, except through loss of the tooth.

Alveolar pyorrhœa, often equally infectious, is wholly amenable to rational surgical treatment.

Reviews of Dental Literature.

BONE-CYSTS: A CONSIDERATION OF THE BENIGN AND ADA-MANTINE DENTIGEROUS CYSTS OF THE JAW AND BENIGN CYSTS OF THE LONG PIPE BONES.[1] By Joseph C. Bloodgood, Baltimore.

Recent accumulated experience, in the ultimate results after amputation for sarcoma of the long pipe bones, and complete resection for sarcoma of the upper and lower jaw, has demonstrated that local recurrence is unusual, but death from internal metastasis is common in a certain number of cases. When these cases are studied pathologically it is found that the patients who have remained well suffered from special types of sarcoma essentially different from the tumors removed from the patients who ultimately succumbed to internal metastasis. In other words, we were not accomplishing

---

[1] Read at the fifty-fifth annual session of the American Medical Association, in the Section on Pathology and Physiology. We are under obligations to the *Journal of the American Medical Association* for the loan of cuts illustrating this article.

a cure in the latter group of cases even after amputation at the highest joint, because internal metastasis takes place early and is present at the time the patient seeks surgical treatment, and we were subjecting the first group of patients to an unnecessarily extensive operation.

In 1899 [1] I discussed the literature and the experience of the surgical clinic at the Johns Hopkins Hospital in regard to the different relative malignancy in sarcoma of bone, and that in certain varieties much less extensive operations would accomplish a cure with as great a certainty as amputation at the highest joint.

Experience has demonstrated that in some cases curetting is sufficient; for example, the benign bone-cysts of the long pipe bones, dentigerous cysts of the jaw, and medullary giant-cell sarcoma. The latter was advocated many years ago by Koenig. In other cases resection, the extent of which is indicated by the local infiltration of the disease. For example, the various forms of epulides of the upper and lower jaw; the periosteal and medullary giant-cell sarcoma; the periosteal fibrosarcoma and osteosarcoma; the myxochondrosarcoma and a special tumor of the jaw,—the cystic adamantine epithelioma. Such local resections as against amputations have been advocated by von Mikulicz, Weisinger, Morton, Karewski, Hinds.[2]

Amputation is indicated in these varieties of sarcoma only when the necessary resection would result in a useless limb. Infiltration of muscle is not a positive indication for amputation. In this group of cases amputation at the highest joint, except due to the position of the tumor, is never indicated.

In April, 1901, in a discussion before the Philadelphia Academy of Surgery,[3] I advocated this more conservative procedure. Since then the further experience of Dr. Halsted's clinic and my own and the reading of the literature have accumulated additional facts justifying the more conservative operation in this group of sarcoma of bone, of relatively low malignancy.[4]

In December, 1902, I removed with the curette a large medullary giant-cell sarcoma filling and expanding the upper third of the

---

[1] Progressive Medicine, December, 1899, p. 234.

[2] Ibid., pp. 38–42.

[3] Annals of Surgery, 1901, vol. xxxiv. p. 94.

[4] Progressive Medicine, 1902, pp. 151–186.

tibia.[1] This patient has no evidence of recurrence and a limb with unimpaired function.

The experience of the surgical clinic in tumors of the jaw and long pipe bones can be expressed in a few words.

In Group 1 the patients have remained well since operation, the time varying from six months to twelve years. There has been a slight operative mortality, and a few cases in which, on account of the size and position of the tumor, the disease was considered inoperable.

Benign Cysts of Long Pipe Bones.—Three cases; one died after operation (Fig. 2); two cases are well.

Benign Dentigerous Cysts.—Ten cases (upper jaw, four; lower jaw, four; ethmoid, two cases). Inoperable, no cases. Death after operation, two cases (Figs. 5 and 6). In these two instances a complete resection was performed. Well, eight cases. In these eight cases the operation consisted in partial removal of the bony wall, curetting and packing.

Adamantine Epithelioma.—Twelve cases; inoperable, one case (Fig. 8). Death after operation, one case (Fig. 9). Well, ten cases. In one instance there was a second operation for local recurrence; this patient has remained well eight years since the second operation.

PERIOSTEAL SARCOMA.

Epulis.—Twenty-three cases; upper jaw, thirteen; lower jaw, ten. One patient died of pneumonia; in this case, an extensive giant-cell tumor of the lower jaw, it was necessary to do tracheotomy and perform a complete resection of the jaw. Well, twenty-two cases. In all of these cases the operation consisted of removal of the tumor with the alveolar border of the jaw. In only one case was there a local recurrence, and this patient has remained well since the second operation.

Spindle-Cell Fibrosarcoma or Myxosarcoma.—Eight cases; antrum, three, all well; lower jaw, three, two well, one died of pneumonia after complete resection; orbit and antrum, two cases; one, a young child, died after an extensive operation; the other, also a child, has remained well since the less extensive operation, two years.

Osteosarcoma.—(I employ the term osteosarcoma only in those periosteal tumors in which new bone formation predominates.) Eight cases; lower jaw, four, two well, two refused operation; upper jaw, two, both well; long pipe bones (humerus and fibula), two, both well.

Giant-Cell Sarcoma.—Those situated on the jaw and called epulis have already been considered. It is a rare tumor of the long pipe bones. We have observed three cases: Ulna, one case, resection, well twelve years. Tibia, upper third, two cases, both well; in both the tumor was recurrent;

---

[1] Johns Hopkins Hospital Bulletin, May, 1903.

FIG. 1.

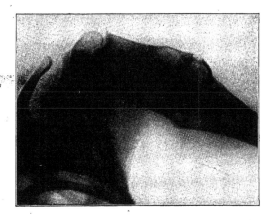

Characteristic shadow thrown by any medullary tumor which in its growth produces a shell
of bone. A pathologic fracture is also seen.

FIG. 2.

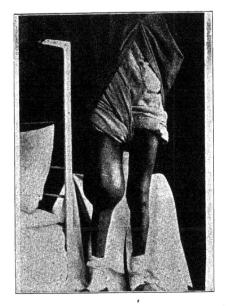

Bone-cyst of lower end of femur of four years' duration.

FIG. 3.

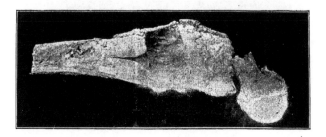

Bone-cyst of upper portion of femur. Dr. Halsted's case.

FIG. 4.

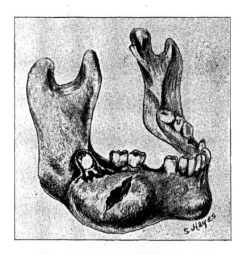

Sketch of reconstructed lower jaw in a case of dentigerous cyst. The expansion of the body, chiefly on the outer side, is well shown and the recess containing the non-erupted wisdom-tooth.

in one the tumor was excised without destroying the continuity of the tibia, in the other the limb was amputated at the thigh.

MEDULLARY SARCOMA.

Giant-Cell Tumors (Myeloma).—Eight cases, all well; lower jaw, one; long pipe bones, seven.

Myxochondrosarcoma.—Three cases; one involving the sacrum, inoperable; one involving the upper third of the humerus, well; one of the femur, death two years after operation from tuberculosis of the lungs.

Seventy-eight bone tumors in this group are either benign or of relatively low malignancy. Sixty-nine cases are well, two inoperable; two refused operation; seven died after operation. In six of these cases the tumor involved the upper or lower jaw. In these six cases, I believe, a less extensive operation could have been performed which would have reduced the dangers of the operation, but not the probabilities of an ultimate cure.

Group 2 includes patients who have not been cured, either because the condition was inoperable when they presented themselves at the clinic, or because of death from internal metastasis after operation.

PERIOSTEAL TUMORS.

Spindle- and Round-Cell Sarcoma.—Six cases; lower jaw, two; long bones, four.

Perithelial Angiosarcoma.—Long bones, two cases.

MEDULLARY TUMORS.

Spindle- and Round-Cell Sarcoma.—Long bones, four cases.

Perithelial Angiosarcoma.—Long bones, two cases.

In these fourteen cases a complete operation was performed. In the twelve cases of the long pipe bones a high amputation; in the two jaw cases, an extensive resection. In every case death has taken place, usually within a year after the first symptom of the tumor. In only one case was the duration of life longer than two years.

Sarcoma of the Upper Jaw involving the Antrum.—Clinical diagnosis: Six cases, all inoperable.

Carcinoma of Upper Jaw.—Twenty-one cases; inoperable, sixteen; one death of pneumonia; remainder not cured.

We have, therefore, observed forty-one cases of tumors involving bone of a relatively high malignancy, none of which has been cured, as compared with seventy-eight of a relatively low malignancy, of which sixty-nine are well.

These facts demonstrate the hopelessness of the more malignant varieties of bone tumors.

Surgeons who take the view advocated in this paper must educate themselves to recognize clinically, or through the Röntgen negative, or at the exploratory incision, the different varieties of sarcoma of bone, and govern the extent of the operative procedure by the relative malignancy and extent of the tumor.

In this paper I shall discuss only the benign bone-cysts of the long pipe bones, the dentigerous cysts of the jaw, and the cystic adamantine epithelioma.

BENIGN BONE-CYSTS.

The benign bone-cysts of the long pipe bones are rare tumors. Up to the present time we have observed but three cases in the surgical clinic.

CASE I.—Bone-cyst of the humerus. White girl, aged seven, tumor one year, pathologic fracture. Operation, curetting and drainage, June, 1904, ten months, well.[1] I saw this patient in August, 1903. The parents gave the following history:

History.—The apparently healthy child one year ago fractured the upper third of the humerus of the right arm after a slight fall. The fracture was treated by their family physician and united. After the dressing was removed a swelling was observed which has never disappeared. If the swelling had been present before the fracture, it had not attracted the attention of the parents or the physician who treated the fracture. For a year there were absolutely no symptoms except swelling. Three days ago, after a very slight fall, the child refused to use the arm because of pain, and for this reason was brought to the surgical clinic. ·

Examination.—On examination there was a fairly uniform expansion of the upper third of the humerus, easily seen, greatest towards the surgical neck. On palpation the soft parts were normal, but one could feel the normal shaft of the humerus expanding into a thin shell of bone. The surface of this shell of bone was not smooth like the normal shaft, but irregular. In a few places one could elicit definite parchment crepitation, first described by Dupuytren, or what I have called " ping-pong ball" crepitation. The arm was very tender.

Clinically, a diagnosis of bone-cyst was suggested, because so far in my experience every sarcoma of the more malignant type in children at this age had caused death by internal metastasis within a year.

The only medullary tumors of the long pipe bones which, in their growth, expand the bone and produce a definite shell, are the bone-cysts, the myxochondrosarcoma and the giant-cell sarcoma. Of the latter two we had no observations in the clinic, in patients

---

[1] Progressive Medicine, December, 1903, p. 191.

Fig. 5.

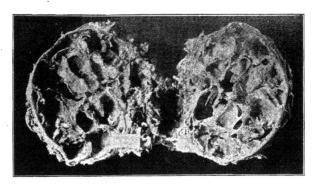

Photograph of the alcohol specimen of an excised lower jaw, in which the dentigerous cysts are multiple.

Fig. 6.

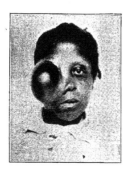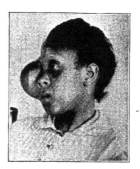

This illustrates the huge size which a dentigerous cyst of the upper jaw may reach.

FIG. 7.

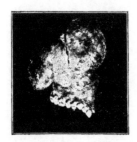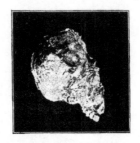

Photograph of the alcohol specimen of Fig. 6 after removal.

FIG. 8.

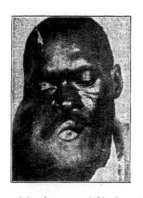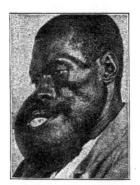

Colored man, aged fifty-four; tumor of twenty years' duration.

at this age, and so far I have been able to find none in the literature. The Röntgen negative is illustrated in Fig. 1.

Operation.—At the exploratory operation the tissues were normal
until the periosteum was separated. The bone beneath was irregular and
varied in thickness from 1 to 4 mm. On removing a piece of the shell
of bone a cavity was exposed filled with blood; there was no connective
tissue lining, and no evidence of cartilage, but as only sufficient bone was
removed to allow curetting of the cavity, one cannot exclude the possibility that cartilage was present in some part of the wall. After curetting,
the cavity was partially packed with gauze, the remainder allowed to fill
with blood-clot. Eight weeks after operation an X-ray picture demonstrated
that the cavity was almost completely filled with new bone.

The origin of these bone-cysts has been demonstrated by Virchow, Zeronie, Schlange, Koenig and others to be due to liquefac-
tion of misplaced islands of epiphyseal cartilage, and in the majority of cases cartilage has been found in some parts of the wall.[1] In
the two other cases observed in Dr. Halsted's clinic cartilage was
demonstrated in the wall of the cyst.

CASE II.—Colored woman, aged thirty-seven. Expansion of the lower
end of the right femur, four years.

History.—The swelling shown in Fig. 2 reached its greatest height
about one year after the onset, and during the last three years there has
been little or no increase in size. This patient refused amputation. Five
years and eight months later she returned to the clinic.

Examination.—The tumor had increased in size, but had not changed
its characteristics. The shell of bone was rough, similar to Case I., but
thicker, and one could not elicit parchment crepitation. The X-ray showed
a shadow somewhat similar to Case I. The diagnosis lay between a bone-
cyst and a myxochondroma. The long duration and the preservation of
the shell of bone excluded a malignant bone tumor.

Operation.—The findings at the operation by Dr. Follis, the resident
surgeon, were similar to the case just discussed, except that cartilage was
present within the shell of bone in many parts of the wall.

CASE III.—The age, clinical history, appearance, and X-ray shadow
were almost identical in this patient with Case I., except that the first
pathologic fracture had been five years instead of one year before the
patient came under observation. The expansion of the upper two-thirds
of the femur in this case was produced in the upper portion by cartilage,
in the central portion by a cyst filled with blood, and in the lower portion
by a fibromyxomatous connective tissue which extended down the medullary
cavity of the femur some distance below the point of its expansion (Fig. 3).

---

[1] Progressive Medicine, December, 1899, p. 236.

Dr. Halsted exhibited this patient and the specimen at a recent meeting of the Johns Hopkins Hospital Medical Society. Later a detailed report, with the interesting histologic findings, will appear. The extensive formation of fibromyxomatous connective tissue histologically like ostitis fibrosa, described by von Recklinghausen, is, I think, a unique finding in both cysts.

Koch [1] gives the most complete *résumé* on the subject of bone-cysts, collecting from the literature, in addition to his one observation, twenty-two cases.

Heineke [2] has recently published the first case of multiple bone-cysts in which X-ray negatives were made. He is inclined to the conclusion that the cystic degeneration is part of a general osteomalacia. I have recently learned that Dr. Goldthwaite, in Boston, has under observation, confirmed by X-ray studies, a similar case of multiple bone-cysts, in which there is no doubt clinically as to the presence of osteomalacia.

The etiology of these multiple cysts is apparently entirely different from the single cyst, but in every case numerous X-rays should be taken to exclude multiple cysts. Codman,[3] in Boston, reports a very interesting tumor in the digital phalanx which undoubtedly represents the cartilage stage of the beningn bone-cyst.

The benign cyst of the long pipe bones cannot always be recognized clinically, nor does the X-ray negative differentiate it from medullary giant-cell sarcoma or the myxochondrosarcoma. As a rule, these three tumors can be distinguished from the more malignant and rapidly growing medullary sarcoma. However, if there is any doubt, one should never proceed with an amputation without excluding these tumors of less malignancy by an exploratory incision.

BENIGN DENTIGEROUS CYSTS.

Ten cases. Upper jaw, four cases; lower jaw, four cases; ethmoid, two cases. The age of the patients varied from six to thirty years; four were under fifteen years of age, six between twenty and thirty. The duration of the tumor varied from three months to thirteen years. Whether the tumor is situated in the

---

[1] Archiv f. klin. Chir., 1902, vol. lxviii. p. 976.

[2] Beiträge z. klin. Chir., 1903, vol. xl. p. 481.

[3] Boston Med. and Surg. Journal, vol. cl., No. 8, p. 211, February 25, 1904.

FIG. 9.

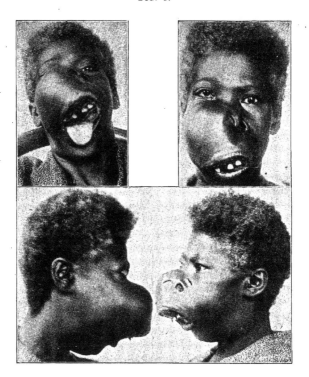

Dentigerous cyst of upper jaw. Death followed complete excision.

FIG. 10.

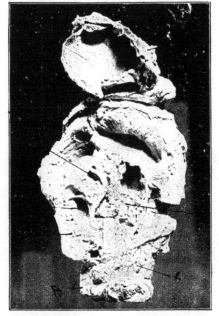

Photograph of resected lower jaw.

FIG. 11.

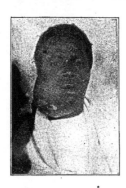 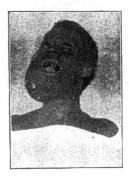

Patient from whom tumor shown in Fig. 10 was removed.

upper or lower jaw, it is of slow growth and usually painless. There is a slow expansion of the jaw, and on palpation one can feel a smooth, thin shell of bone. Usually there is parchment crepitation. At the exploratory incision the periosteum is normal. The outer shell of bone is smooth; lining the bone there is a thin, vascular connective tissue membrane. The contents of the cyst is usually a blood-stained serum.

Microscopically, one finds frequently cholesterin crystals, blood-corpuscles, and degenerated cells, which suggest epithelium. Histologically, however, I have never been able to demonstrate an epithelial lining.

Usually the cyst is single; now and then there are thin partitions. In a few cases the cysts are multiple. Complete resection is unnecessary. Partial resection with curetting and drainage will accomplish a cure. In three of our cases a non-erupted tooth was found in a recess of the cyst. These dentigerous cysts are apparently due to the distention of the connective tissue capsule of a non-erupted tooth.

CASE IV.—Fig. 4. The patient was a white boy, aged fifteen.

History.—The swelling of the body of the lower jaw was of three months' duration. Because of the painless and uniform expansion, the distinct shell of bone, and parchment crepitation, I made the diagnosis of a dentigerous cyst.

Operation.—The exploratory incision revealed the pathologic findings already described. The outer expansion was cut away with the chisel without destroying the continuity of the lower jaw. The connective tissue membrane and tooth were removed. The bone cavity was then curetted, allowed to fill with a blood-clot, and the skin incision closed. The wound healed *per primam.*

Result.—June, 1904, six years after operation, there is a slight depression in the jaw at the site of the scar, but no other deformity.

CASE V.—Fig. 5. The patient was a white girl, eight years of age, the tumor of some years' duration.

Operation.—Complete resection was done. The child's hæmoglobin was but fifty-two per cent. at the time of the operation, and although there was no loss of blood the patient died of shock. The tumor was a very large one and extended from the zygoma almost to the symphysis of the jaw. I believe incision and curetting would have been sufficient in this case.

CASE VI.—Fig. 6. The patient was a colored girl, nineteen years of age, the tumor of thirteen years' duration. Complete resection was performed (Fig. 7). The patient died at the end of the third week from abscess of the lung.

In the remaining five cases of dentigerous cysts, two of the upper jaw and three of the lower, the operation was similar to that followed in Case IV. The patients recovered and have remained well for from two to eight years since operation.

The two cases of cysts of the ethmoid bone presented themselves clinically with a tumor projecting from the angle between the nose and the supraorbital ridge, producing slight exophthalmos. On palpation the tumor was smooth and presented a thin shell bone giving parchment crepitation. In both, partial excision with curetting and drainage was performed. The patients have remained well, one four years and the other eighteen months since operation.

ADAMANTINE EPITHELIOMA.

Of these there were twelve cases. In four the tumor projected from the alveolar border of the jaw (three lower, one upper). The tumor was covered with normal mucous membrane and did not invade the bone. In eight cases the epithelial tumor was situated within the body of the jaw (one upper and seven lower), and in its growth produced an irregular expansion very similar to a dentigerous cyst. The age of onset varied from eighteen to sixty-one years. The majority of cases were twenty and thirty-five years of age; the duration of the tumor from seven months to twenty-nine years, the majority from six to twenty years. In one case the condition was considered inoperable (Fig. 8). In the remaining eleven cases a complete resection of the diseased area was made. Nine cases have remained well for from one to twelve years. In one instance there was a local recurrence, but this patient has remained well eight years since the second operation. One patient (Fig. 9) died after complete excision of a huge tumor involving both upper jaws.

This epithelial tumor is apparently of a very low grade of malignancy. In none of our cases was there metastasis to the glands of the neck. The tumor can be differentiated from the more malignant neoplasms of the jaw by its very slow growth. The adamantine epithelioma involving the alveolar border cannot always be differentiated clinically from the connective tissue epulis. The epulis is more apt to be associated with ulceration of the mucous membrane.

When the adamantine epithelioma originates in the body of the jaw and produces expansion, with the formation of a thin shell of

FIG. 12·

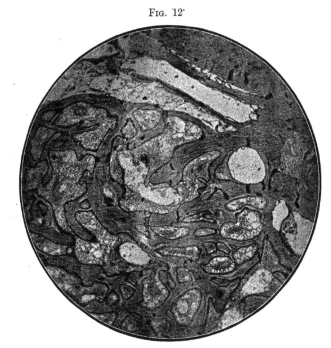

Microphotograph of a section of an adamantine epithelioma, involving chiefly the alveolar border of the lower jaw. In this section the basal columnar cell and its various morphologic changes towards the centre of the alveolus are well shown. (Sent me by Dr. Steensland.)

Fig. 13.

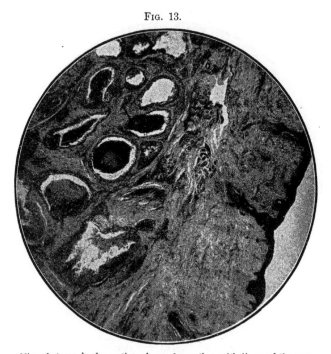

Microphotograph of a section of an adamantine epithelioma of the gum.

bone, it cannot be differentiated from a benign dentigerous cyst until the exploratory incision is made. Then, when the shell of bone is incised, we do not find a cavity, but a white, finely granular tumor containing connective tissue trabeculæ, and usually many small and large cystic cavities. The gross appearance is well illustrated in Fig. 10. This patient (Fig. 11) was a colored man, forty-two years of age, tumor of eight years' duration. The patient has remained well three years since operation.

The microscopic appearance is well illustrated in Fig. 12.

CASE VII.—Fig. 13. The patient was a white woman, aged fifty-two.

History.—Four years ago, when forty-eight years of age, she observed a tumor like a gumboil on the outer side of the alveolar border of the left lower jaw, opposite the canine and first molar teeth. At the end of two years, when it had reached the size of a hickory-nut, it was removed. A local recurrence took place within six months.

Examination.—The recurrent tumor is the size of an egg and involves the alveolar border of the left lower jaw from symphysis to within one centimetre of the angle. The tumor is present on both sides of the alveolar border. It is distinctly circumscribed. The mucous membrane at one point has ulcerated, exposing a small cyst.

Operation.—The tumor was removed by turning back flaps of mucous membrane which were not adherent to the tumor. Then the tumor and the alveolar border of the jaw were removed in one piece. The patient has remained well since the operation, a period of ten years.

Appearance of Tumor.—The fresh appearance was quite typical: white, friable, granular alveoli of various sizes and cysts in a definite fibrous stroma.

Under the microscope (see Fig. 13) one sees the normal mucous membrane of the gum, then a zone of connective tissue, beneath which is the circumscribed tumor. The tumor is composed of branching epithelial alveoli in a connective tissue stroma. Some of the alveoli are cysts lined by the typical basal adamantine epithelium. Other alveoli are solid, with cells showing the various morphologic changes of the adamantine epithelium.

DISCUSSION.

Dr. F. J. Hall, Kansas City, Mo.—It would be of interest to know what distinction, if any, Dr. Bloodgood makes between the cystic bone tumors of the long bones; in particular, two varieties of pathologic bone condition: one is the myeloma and the other is the traumatic myositis ossificans. Several cases of both these conditions have occurred in my own territory, and three of the cases of myeloma—so-called central sarcoma of the bone—have been

he New York Institute of Stomatology.

. I do not think there is any relation between
its observed in myositis ossificans and the cysts
nes.
question of the origin of the giant cells, recent
uld indicate that the periosteal or medullary gia
robably an angioma or an angiosarcoma, and

subject is by Friedlänger.[1] Further investigati

ical Association.

Reports of Society Meetings.

YORK INSTITUTE OF STOMATOLOGY

operated on, and none has recurred. Three cases also of myositis ossificans have occurred wherein the central portions of the tumors were occupied by these cysts, and I should like to know if Dr. Bloodgood has had any experience with these other two varieties of conditions, and what relation they bear to the conditions which he has described.

Dr. Joseph C. Bloodgood, Baltimore.—I am inclined to think that what you mean by myeloma is a giant-cell tumor.

Dr. Hall.—Yes, sir.

Dr. Joseph C. Bloodgood.—Dr. Hall, in his question·in regard to myeloma, undoubtedly means the medullary giant-cell sarcoma. This tumor is one of a relatively low grade of malignancy. We have observed about ten cases; all have remained well since operation. I have reported them in the Johns Hopkins Hospital Bulletin for May, 1903. In regard to the question as to the origin of the blood-cysts in the condition called myositis ossificans, they are probably due to hemorrhage. Recently there has appeared in the literature a number of interesting articles and reports of cases on this subject. These I have reviewed in *Progressive Medicine* for December, 1903. With or without a history of trauma an indurated mass associated with some pain and tenderness is observed by the patient in one of the large muscles, most frequently the thigh. The tumor rapidly becomes bony in hardness. In some cases the X-ray demonstrates a zone of normal tissue between the shaft of the bone and the osteoid tissue in the muscle. In other cases the two bony shadows are in contact. This has given rise to two views as to the etiology of the new bone formation in the connective tissue between the muscle bundles. A number of authorities conclude that the bone is a product of detached pieces of periosteum, others that it rises from the connective tissue cells between the muscle bundles. Clinically the condition is not difficult to recognize, especially with the aid of the X-ray. However, when the new shadow rests directly on the shaft of the neighboring bone it will be difficult to differentiate the ossifying myositis from a condition called traumatic exostosis or ossifying periostitis. Blood-cysts have been observed only in the ossifying myositis. Extensive operations are not necessary. One should remove as much of the new bone production as possible without destroying function. Slight local recurrences of the bone formation are to be expected. Fortunately the amount is never great, gives little or no discomfort, and second operations are rarely necessary. I do not think there is any relation between the hemorrhagic cysts observed in myositis ossificans and the cysts of the long pipe bones.

As to the question of the origin of the giant cells, recent investigation would indicate that the periosteal or medullary giant-cell tumor is probably an angioma or an angiosarcoma, and that the giant cells are due to budding of the endothelial cells of the vessels in these very vascular tumors. The most interesting publication on this subject is by Friedlänger.[1] Further investigation, however, should be made of this most interesting tumor.—*Journal American Medical Association.*

Reports of Society Meetings.

THE NEW YORK INSTITUTE OF STOMATOLOGY.

A MEETING of the Institute was held at the Chelsea, No. 222 West Twenty-third Street, New York, on Friday evening, June 3, 1904, the President, Dr. A. H. Brockway, in the chair.

The minutes of the last meeting were read and approved.

COMMUNICATIONS ON THEORY AND PRACTICE.

Dr. C. O. Kimball presented a set of Dr. D. D. Smith's scalers upon which he had made some slight alterations that in his hands he had found to improve their utility. He had found them excellent for cleansing teeth.

Dr. J. Morgan Howe.—I have for some time wanted to express my appreciation and thanks to our fellow-member, Dr. Strang, for introducing the method of mixing amalgam and cement which he has recommended. I have found such mixture of the two materials to be so valuable that I think those who have not tried it would do well to do so. The use of a rather slow-setting amalgam and a quick-setting cement works best, in my estimation. The filling being mixed and introduced, in five or six minutes the filling can be shaped and margins made flush; then lightly rubbing the

---

[1] Archiv f. klin. Chir., vol. lxvii. p. 202.

surface with a burnisher will cause the particles of amalgam to coalesce, giving practically an amalgam surface. This method will prevent the filling from wearing rough, at least in a great degree.

Dr. S. E. Davenport.—Will Dr. Howe kindly tell us for what class of cases he thinks this combination is best adapted?

Dr. Howe.—The filling is adapted for those cases where adhesion to the walls of the cavity is desirable, the cement giving the filling the adhesive qualities, while the amalgam protects the cement and gives durability. Cavities that run under the margin of the gum, filled with it, have made a good record in mouths where cement alone would quickly waste away and gutta-percha had proved to be practically worthless.

All conditions unfavorable to the retention of the filling because of the shape of the cavity or the weakness of the walls are indications for this mixture of amalgam and cement.

Dr. F. Milton Smith.—I would be willing to part with almost anything else in the way of a filling-material rather than with this combination. I believe that almost any one will make a failure in the use of this filling-material if he does not use the utmost care, following the little details of preparation according to Dr. Strang's directions. I had in my office to-day a patient for whom I inserted one of my first fillings of this kind, a posterior cavity in an upper first molar. It was something over five years ago, and the tooth is practically perfectly preserved. I am sure that in that time it would have been filled four or five times with either cement or amalgam. I have had almost uniform success, although I have had cases where the combination has worn away quite rapidly. This, however, I have ascribed to some fault of my own in the mixing.

The President.—I have used this combination in many cases with great satisfaction. Dr. Strang does not claim that he originated this method, but gives the credit, I believe, to Dr. Tillotson. Our Dr. C. B. Parker, I remember, read a paper describing it several years ago.

Dr. Smith.—Regarding the proper proportions for this mixture, the amount of cement powder is one-half as much as the amount of filings in bulk. The filings are amalgamated first and placed in a mortar with the oxide of zinc and the two ground to almost an impalpable powder. It is then placed on the slab and mixed with the liquid of the cement, the mass then being kneaded with the fingers for a little while. A matrix should always be used for approximal cavities, and the filling inserted with pressure. Then a thorough burnishing over the surface makes a filling that will last.

Dr. C. O. Kimball.—Might I modify Dr. Smith's excellent method? I too am very much indebted to Dr. Strang, and have used this method continually. I do not altogether like the "rule-of-thumb" method followed by Dr. Smith. I have the powders taken out separately and placed in two heaps. I prefer a rather slow-setting cement, and find the Dirigo very satisfactory for this purpose. The amalgam is mixed dry, rubbing it up in a mortar, not touching it with the hands at all. The powder is then placed in the mortar and thoroughly incorporated with the amalgam. It is then placed on the slab and mixed with the phosphoric acid, then not rubbed in the hand but with the spatula until the right stiffness is obtained, which can be judged by the feeling of the spatula. It is not rolled in the hand, but taken up by the spatula and put directly into the cavity, where it is thoroughly and rapidly moulded into the required contour. I think it is well, as far as possible, to avoid all contact with the hand, and above all the tooth must be kept perfectly and absolutely dry from the beginning to the end of the operation. A little fresh amalgam may be burnished over the surface after the proper shape has been given to the filling. If carefully done it will make a filling that will stand in a wonderful way.

Dr. Fossume.—I wish to present for your inspection a set of instruments made of ivory for burnishing inlay matrices. These instruments will not iron or stretch the matrix, and thereby overcome, to a great extent, the rigidity and pulling away of the metal.

I also pass around some aseptic dental-bracket covers that Johnson & Johnson are putting on the market. They are made in three sizes, for the Allen, Holms, and Harvard tables, and are put up in boxes containing from one hundred to five hundred covers. The idea is to get an aseptic cover at a small cost, so that they can be changed after each patient. These covers will be supplied, I believe, at seventy-five cents a hundred.

Dr. J. Morgan Howe.—Mr. President and gentlemen, the subject of malignant growths in the mouth has interested me for a number of years, not because I know anything about it, but because a good many cases have come under my observation. I have been willing to speak upon the subject this evening in order to urge upon dentists the desirability of their giving attention to the subject, that they may early recognize any suspicious indications. I have seen several cases where the patient was passed from dentist to physician and back to the dentist again, the physician supposing the trouble to originate from the root of a tooth and the dentist not being certain whether it was a tooth or not, the patient being encouraged to await developments, action being postponed until— in one case—fatal results followed. I got the patient into the hands of a surgeon,—the late Dr. Garretson,—and he was operated upon the very same day that I saw him first, but the tumor recurred. I would not urge upon dentists the study of malignant growths with any other object than to have their suspicions aroused when they should be. I have in mind a patient who, when I suggested that a section for examination be made of a tumor, stated that this had already been done and the tumor pronounced benign, the patient giving the name of a dentist whom I knew to have given some attention to microscopy and histology. My examination of the case was some months later. I would not advise dentists to set themselves up as pathologists, but to make such a study of malignant growths as to be able to give patients good advice. It not infrequently happens that patients are needlessly alarmed about some little thing that need not be suspected of malignancy, and the dentist is fortunate who can dissipate such fears.

We are very fortunate in having with us to-night a gentleman who can tell you a great deal about this subject. I will say, in this connection, that I have been very much interested in reading Dr. Dawbarn's book, for which he received the Gross prize. The book contains a description of diseased growths in a good many parts of the body and not a few about the mouth. It is one of the books that is well worth the attention of dentists.

Of course it is understood that in speaking of this subject I merely call attention to it from a dentist's point of view. We expect the information from the gentlemen who are to follow.

(For Dr. Dawbarn's paper on "Malignant Growths in the Mouth," see page 911; for Dr. Franklin's paper on "Radiotherapy in some Malignant Conditions of the Mouth," see page 905.)

Dr. Dawbarn.—In the main I have nothing to differ from Dr. Franklin's very interesting paper, except in one respect. If I understood him correctly, in cancer of the tongue he would advise using the X-ray instead of the knife. I have known of two

.instances of cancer in this locality where the patient lost his life in just this manner. There is no exception to the rule that the proper thing to do is to use the knife at once. The doctor refers to the great danger of the application of the X-ray to deep-seated conditions. In this connection the value of the X-ray in locating gall-stones is of great value. Also in fractures of the thigh-bone or in fracture of any of the bones it aids materially in properly reducing the fracture.

Dr. Davenport.—I hope, Mr. President, you will extend our cordial thanks to these gentlemen for what they have done for us this evening. Dr. Dawbarn being one of us, perhaps we may take his efforts in our behalf more as a matter of course, though we should not be less appreciative of his many services to this society. From what we have learned of Dr. Franklin to-night I am sure we all hope he will be a frequent visitor.

Dr. Kimball.—In seconding Dr. Davenport's suggestion, I wish to state that while we cannot very well discuss this subject, the society certainly owes a debt to these gentlemen for giving us this information so clearly and forcibly.

Dr. Franklin.—Regarding the point upon which Dr. Dawbarn differs from me, I really do not believe that he differs from me, or that I differ from him, so much as he thinks. While it has been my custom to X-ray cases of the tongue first, at the very first sign of lack of response or of further involvement I turn the case over to the surgeon. A reason why the ray has been used so much in cases that should have been operated upon is to be found in the fact that there exists in the hearts of most women an extreme dread of surgical interference. Cases have come to me in which I have actually begged the patient to place herself in the hands of a surgeon, and insisted that every day the growth was X-rayed the danger was increasing. In many cases they have been obdurate. In many cases they have gone to others who have held out more hope. I know of two cases that have died because they would not allow themselves to be operated upon.

The President.—Before entertaining a motion to adjourn, I wish to tender to Dr. Dawbarn and Dr. Franklin the thanks of the society for their instructive and interesting papers.

Adjourned.

FRED. L. BOGUE, M.D., D.D.S.,
Editor The New York Institute of Stomatology.

Editorial.

ESSENTIALS IN DENTAL EDUCATION.

WHAT is to be understood by this use of words? Does this mental training in any sense differ from any other education in the final results? Is not all education, however effected, but a cultivation of the brain-cells and, in addition thereto, reflex power, represented in thought? These are questions of great importance, yet we are met with the assertion that education, to be of value, must be acquired through certain methods of training, an inheritance from mediæval periods, and that professional culture has no place in the mental standards of the twentieth century.

To the writer this view is radically wrong and unworthy the great accomplishments of this utilitarian age.

It is a problem remaining unsettled with many, whether it is possible to make a thinker—a philosopher—unless the education is based exclusively upon what are known as the humanities. This is the natural outcome of the standard of learning established centuries ago, and may find its best example in the study given to Confucius and his works by the recognized scholars of China. It is not the purpose, however, of this article to discuss this much-mooted question, and it is only alluded to here as a basis for related thought.

Dental education as understood fifty years ago was simply the acquirement of a trade. It consisted in its last analysis in the manufacture of artificial masticating substitutes and the stopping or filling cavities in teeth to prevent further destruction by caries. The man who labored in the laboratory found his work a succession of repetitions, doing to-morrow what he did the day previously, and the man over the chair had no other expectations or higher ambitions, each branch aiming at greater perfection as experience necessarily gave manipulative skill. There was but a limited sphere here for thought. The tendency was to a life of repetitions, and repetitions had the usual result of narrow thinking. There was no room for the broader life common to the older professions. The work was regarded as useful and necessary, but the men who followed it were held not to be worthy the consideration due professional men, and their claim to be such was derided, and socially they became, in a certain sense, outcasts and their claims to the doctor title was regarded as an assumption.

The fathers in dentistry were not satisfied with this anomalous position, and the effort was made to increase the curriculum to something more nearly that of medicine. The slow development of this through over sixty years has been fruitful through its slow progress in the evolution of acquirement that at this period marks it as equal to the mother profession in broader conceptions and more accurate modes of thinking and practice. The man in dentistry to-day aspires to a mental power that will enable him to hold communion with the more profound thinkers of his own and past ages. He is no longer satisfied with the nomenclature of his profession. He has cast aside the word mechanics, as related to artificial substitutes, and now labors under the prosthetic name. He is beginning to feel that the word dentist does not comport with the dignity of his calling, and recognizes that stomatology more nearly answers to his higher thought. The man who regulated teeth in the earlier periods is now an orthodontist, and the continuous-gum worker has been transformed into a practitioner in ceramics. This is encouraging. The superficial thinker may laugh and regard it as bordering on shallow conceit, but to the thoughtful mind it gives a positive evidence of a growing taste for the artistic in thought as well as in practice, for its indications, while limited, point unerringly to a higher standard through the evolution of ideas.

The curriculum of forty years ago, in the few dental colleges then existing, consisted of operative dentistry, didactic and practical; mechanical dentistry the same; a minimum of anatomy through lectures; lectures on chemistry with no practice in the laboratory; materia medica from the stand-point of the medical practitioner; the therapeutics limited to few drugs, and those used empirically; dental pathology was scarcely recognized as a distinct study, and, above all, there was no standard of entrance. To-day the diploma of a four years' high school, or its equivalent, is demanded by the higher schools. This, as a preliminary, presupposes higher thinking and a dissatisfaction with the drudgery regarded as essential in the older methods of work. The man of to-day is finding his place, not so much in what is called the mere mechanics of his profession, but in the elaborating of its more artistic features that have in the past been mainly neglected.

He is brought in contact in his first year with the sculptor, modeller. He must rise to the conception of the beauty of form of the human mouth and all that it contains. He must think as he works over his chemical problems in the laboratory. He must grasp the limitations of his human intellect as he searches for the ultimate in his histological work. He will gather new inspiration as he studies the life history of the minute forms of activity in his bacteriological examinations. He will over the cadaver speculate on the dynamic power of the muscles, activity of the nerves, and the strength of the frame, and he must watch the knife of the surgeon as he skilfully dissects out the tumor or calls to his aid the mechanism prepared by the stomatologist to assist nature while she restores normal powers to the fractured jaw. He listens to lectures and works, it may be, in the physiological and pathological laboratory,—in a word, he has become in the evolution of sixty years a thinker and a professional man.

This may not be true of all the dental colleges of the country, but it will be true in the not far distant future. The higher ideals are being grasped and slowly but surely are being made part of the curriculi of the schools, and before the curtain is rung down on the present century the thorough training outlined will be regarded as the essentials in dental education.

This brings the thoughtful individual to the consideration of the question, Have we, as dentists, lost or gained in this gradual evolution? It must be evident that there has been both a loss and a gain. We have lost to a large extent prosthetic ability. We have also lost in our manipulative skill in operative dentistry. This, we are aware, will be denied; but taking the country through, the percentage of skilled operators will not compare with those of thirty or forty years in the past. In a word, then, the mechanical side of dentistry is gradually giving way to a higher professional culture, and this, in the progressive development of time, must be relegated to a special class. It is difficult to view this possible change with any other feeling than that of profound regret. Prosthetic dentistry is, in the view of the writer, the second greatest boon given to humanity during the nineteenth century. It ranks, in his opinion, a close second to the discovery of anæsthesia. It ought not to be cast aside as unworthy the highest efforts of the thinker; indeed, it should be to him, more than aught else, the very foundation and support of that higher spiritual life manifest in the human brain. It has extended the life of the race, but while this is important, it has not the same value as is its service in keeping the digestive apparatus in order and through this normal activity holding the nerve forces in harmonious and in working condition, thus preserving mentality to the last days of life. If there is anything higher than this in any profession the writer is not aware of its existence.

The art of filling teeth as understood fifty years ago and at present will undoubtedly give place to something better, at least as far as material is concerned. This is not to be mourned. The dentist has been too long the slave of a master of his own creating, and the release from the drudgery will be a happy fulfilment, when it comes, of the hopes of many years.

The bright side of this picture is the release it will give the practitioner and a larger devotion to those studies that make for a more liberal view of life and its duties, and those things that count for the spiritual elevation of man. To-day the dental practitioner is a drudge, not the drudge of fifty years ago, but still bowed down over his daily work for daily bread. He fails to grasp the possibilities lying dormant in his profession. He reads but little and thinks less. His days are given over to labor and his nights to disturbed repose. He has no hours and no desire to devote to the cultivation of those amenities that go so far to make beautiful our civilization. It is time he was aroused from this lethargic state, and the question of the hour is, How may this be accomplished? Education, as already stated, has done much, will do more; but we need an education that will lead the dentists of the period out of the morass of mere money-getting into the more perfect soulful life of the thinker.

Are we viewing dental education from the stand-point of the real educators in dentistry? Are we not laying down uncertain laws that will land our profession again into the depths from which we have laboriously emerged? There seems to be in a certain class of mind a feeling of rejoicing that the dental colleges of this country halted progress in this direction and turned the wheels of our civilization backward. When that body assuming the name of the National Association of Dental Faculties met at St. Louis and adopted three years as the course of college training, it cared nothing for higher education. The slogan was sounded broadcast, " We will be financially ruined if this four years' course is continned." Gold, gold, gold, has been the cry of the besotted world in all ages, drowning the "still small voice crying in the wilderness" of confused thought. Come out of the temples dedicated to the brazen god and in the clearer atmosphere of a broader culture breathe a new inspiration and a more perfect life.

Recently one of our best writers, in discussing this subject of dental education in colleges, cried, in tones of agony, "Time! Time! Time! Always time, as though the length of a term was a true measure of the quality of the education imparted." Yes. Time we must have. There can be no real value in hurried work. The brain-cells need time for an impression. The superficial mark fades rapidly. There is such a thing as indigestion of the brain-forces. They become over-saturated and refuse to further act. The power to think is measurably lost. That some may be able to accomplish in two years that which requires four in others is no argument to prove that the two years' man will be the standard bearer in the future; indeed, in the experience of the writer this has been reversed in almost every instance. The man of two years has taken his intellectual pabulum too rapidly, with the result—mental indigestion.

The idea entertained that three years of nine months each is equal to four years of seven months is based on wrong conclusions and imperfect knowledge of the possibilities of dental education. Every one practically familiar with dental training is aware that the last two months of a nine months' course are the least profitable months, and relatively so of a shorter period. The human mind staggers under the continuous load and must have rest and time for recovery. For this the fourth year is imperatively necessary.

Some of the dental colleges tried bravely to resist the current that threatened to engulf them. That they failed is now an historical record, but their day of triumph will surely come. This will be when dentists cease to worship mammon. When they cling closely to their higher conceptions, treading under feet all baser motives. When they give their influence for a dental education that will draw out all that there is in a man. When they cultivate the best in literature and cast away that which drags down the profession. In a word, when they aim for the highest attainable.

The time may come when the man who studies will be graded according to his ambitions. The prosthetic worker may conclude his preparation in three years, the operative expert in four, and the stomatologist in five. Whether this will be the logical outcome of educational effort remains to be seen, but it is to be hoped that whatever course may be adopted it will be to the honor of dentistry and the broadening of the mental horizon of all who labor within its folds.

DR. OTTOLENGUI OBJECTS.

In a private letter to the editor, Dr. Ottolengui states that the editorial in the October number of the INTERNATIONAL DENTAL JOURNAL contains an erroneous statement in regard to the nominations for President of the Fourth International Dental Congress, held at St. Louis, August 29 to September 3. His statement is as follows :

" As I was personally associated with the party who advocated the election of Dr. Johnson, I beg leave respectfully to take exception to the way you have reported the matter in your editorial in the October number of the INTERNATIONAL DENTAL JOURNAL. You say that the nominations for President were Dr. H. J. Burkhart and Dr. C. N. Johnson; also that the vote for both officers was taken by each member standing until the vote was counted. Will you pardon my reminding you that as a matter of fact Dr. Johnson was never placed in nomination at all? indeed, by the most arbitrary sort of ruling we were not permitted to introduce his name."

It is true that the ticket headed by Dr. Johnson for President was not nominated in the usual formal manner, and the editorial statement was thus far in error, but the difference between a formal nomination and a general open understanding that the ticket was prepared to be voted for at the proper moment is about the difference between tweedledum and tweedledee. Dr. Ottolengui was not permitted the floor by Mr. Rogers, the temporary President. The writer regarded this then, and still regards it, as the most arbitrary decision it has ever been his experience to meet with, coming from a President claiming any knowledge of parliamentary law, and under other circumstances should have been very properly resisted. While this was true, and the nomination was not permitted to be made properly, there was not a person familiar with the English language present who was not aware of the nominations to be made, and it was equally well understood that had Dr. Burkhart failed of an election, Dr. Johnson's name would have been presented to the Congress. The part of the editorial in question, in which it was stated, " The vote for both officers was taken by each member standing," had allusion to the offices of President and Secretary, and not to the two nominations for President.

That the writer is correct in stating that it was universally understood that Dr. Johnson was to be placed in nomination,—indeed, was practically nominated,—the following quotation from a St. Louis daily paper is given in evidence. After giving a very true and detailed account of the difficulty that led up to this contest, the report proceeds:

" The opposition retaliated yesterday by putting an independent ticket in the field. For President their choice is Dr. C. N. Johnson, of Chicago, editor of the *Dental Review*. Dr. Kirk became their candidate for Secretary. The issue has been clearly drawn, and was the absorbing undercurrent topic at the dentists' meetings yesterday. Some of the members declare that they will not be drawn into the wrangle, and will not take sides, but all are watching the outcome expectantly. The foreign delegates are standing aside and permitting the Americans to have it out. When approached on the matter they give a nod of the head and show an air of amused interest."

The fact that Dr. Johnson followed the usual custom of moving the unanimous election of Dr. Burkhart was sufficient proof, if any were needed, that he, at least, felt he was practically in nomination.

Space is given somewhat reluctantly to this somewhat extended explanation, but it is deemed due to the parties interested that the matter should be corrected.

The writer at the time had but a very mild interest in this contention for office. From first to last it was an undignified exhibition of a morbid ambition for office, that created a bad impression upon all reasonable thinking persons present. The writer was personally favorable to both nominees. He regarded either as eminently qualified for the responsible position, but his preference had been in the direction of an international character who fully represented both America and Europe. Such a nomination, had it been made, would have given character and dignity to the Congress. This view, however, received no consideration, and the elected President was placed in the unenviable position of being the head of a great congress without an address suitable for the occasion. Had the appointment been made months previously, this could have been avoided. The matter is now, however, past history, to be read and pondered over for the benefit of future dental congresses. .

DR. J. E. GARRETSON, DENTIST OR SURGEON?

THE following paragraph taken from a paper on " The Danger of allowing Warts and Moles to remain," etc., by Dr. W. W. Keen, read before the American Medical Association, at Atlantic City, in June last, is one of those peculiar discriminations dealt in by some medical men whenever they have occasion to allude to the work of another member of the same profession, provided he happens to practise a specialty such as dentistry. " He is a dentist," and that of course settles his place in the domain of medicine. The quotation is as follows :

" *History.*—Mrs. F., aged about sixty, was first seen in consultation with Dr. Rhoads, February 7, 1894. Ever since she can remember she had a wart on the right ankle, just below the inner malleolus. In 1889, five years ago, this began to enlarge, and some time afterwards the late Dr. J. E. Garretson, a dentist, transfixed it with a pin and ligated it. It soon returned, and a year later was again pinned and ligated by her son, who was also a dentist. Recurrence again took place, and in July, 1893, the growth was again transfixed and ligated by Dr. Garretson. Ten months before the last operation the saphenous glands were observed to be enlarged. At the time of the last operation the saphenous tumor had grown to the size of a lady apple. A considerable amount of pigmentation also had appeared in the neighborhood of the original tumor, extending towards the toes."

The fact was that Dr. Garretson was a graduate of medicine, University of Pennsylvania, 1859, a professor of anatomy, a surgeon, and an author of world-wide celebrity. As far as the writer is aware, his practice of dentistry was limited, his tastes running in the direction of surgery, for the practice of which he was well qualified by education and experience.

The quotation seems to imply that the fact of the ligation

being performed on two separate occasions by two dentists, it was not done according to the high standard of the surgeon. Why was it necessary to mention the specialty at all? It will be some generations hence before the feeling, "He is only a dentist," is eradicated from the minds of medical practitioners, who dwell in the narrow confines of their own specialty and are apparently oblivious to the fact that the world of intelligence progresses steadily towards a higher standard of thought and practice.

Bibliography.

ESSIG AND KOENIG'S DENTAL METALLURGY. A Manual for the Use of Dental Students and Practitioners. By Charles J. Essig, M.D., D.D.S., formerly Professor of Mechanical Dentistry and Metallurgy in the Dental Department of the University of Pennsylvania, and Augustus Koenig, B.S., M.D., Demonstrator of Metallurgy in the Dental Department of the University of Pennsylvania, etc. New (fifth) edition, revised and enlarged. In one 12mo volume of three hundred and eighteen pages, with seventy-six engravings. Lea Brothers & Co., Philadelphia and New York, 1904.

This publication, originally prepared by Dr. Charles J. Essig, and now, in its fifth edition, revised by Augustus Koenig, B.S., M.D., still remains as the most satisfactory text-book on metallurgy.

When Professor Essig originally issued this book it was regarded as of more value to practitioners than to students, for the subject was indifferently taught in dental colleges; in fact, it was not thought of sufficient importance to have it introduced as a separate study. This book changed all this, for through its quiet influence courses in metallurgy have been established universally.

It requires no argument here to demonstrate the importance of this study to the dentist,—in fact, a knowledge of this to some extent, at least, is demanded of every practitioner, and he who failed to secure it at college will find it to his advantage to follow Essig and Koenig through this book.

Thirty-two new cuts have been added to this edition, which with those previously in place increase the illustrations to seventy-six.

The fact that this has been translated and used as a text-book in foreign colleges is a sufficient recommendation, and an assurance that under its present able editor it will remain as the standard publication on the subject.

NORMAL HISTOLOGY. By Edward K. Dunham, Ph.B., M.D., Professor of General Pathology, Bacteriology, and Hygiene in the University and Bellevue Hospital Medical College, New York. Third edition, revised and enlarged. Illustrated with two hundred and sixty engravings. Lea Brothers & Co., New York and Philadelphia, 1904.

The fact that a work on any subject has reached a third edition is sufficient evidence that it has met a demand. This book, however, carries its own credentials with it and must necessarily command attention, for it has been prepared by an experienced teacher in this direction.

The author begins the study of histology by " First, the conception of the cell as the active constituent of tissues; second, the general rule that the elementary tissues are composed of cells and intercellular substances, and that their differences depend upon the proportions or characters of those constituents; third, that the structural details of the different tissues are intimately correlated to their usefulness—*i.e.*, that function and structure are mutually dependent upon each other, being but two aspects of a single device or arrangement; and fourth, that the ability of tissues to perform active functions is, in the main, roughly proportional to the number or size of the cells entering into their structure."

With this as a basis of work the author has prepared an exceedingly valuable text-book on " Normal Histology" that cannot fail to have a distinct value to students of medicine and also to students of dentistry in their general histological work.

The author fails, however, as all medical authors do fail, to meet the needs of the dental student in his special work. It is strange that medical teachers when called to explain anything dental immediately make it a fit subject for indifferent treatment. The author devotes just one page and a quarter to " The Teeth," with three illustrations, two showing development and one the tissues diagrammatically. The author says, " Only a brief description of the structures entering into the formation of the fully developed tooth can be given here." It seems to the writer that the development of teeth from the histologist's stand-point is as important and interesting as any portion of the organism, and the various tissues composing the teeth are of quite as much importance in the human economy as bone, to which the author devotes six pages.

Dental students can secure this knowledge elsewhere, but in other respects the book can be cordially recommended for their study in connection with their practical work in the laboratory.

THE HISTORY OF A HISTORY. Souvenir. Fourth International Dental Congress, St. Louis, Mo., August 29 to September 3, 1904.

This is a very interesting little volume giving a brief history of the foundation of the present *Dental Cosmos* and that of the *Dental News Letter* of 1847, and also the history of the house of S. S. White Dental Manufacturing Company since it was founded by Dr. Samuel S. White in 1844, at the age of twenty-two.

To one familiar, as the writer is, with every stage of progress made by this great house, from the time when Dr. White opened his first place of business on Seventh and Race Streets, Philadelphia, to the present time, when it has branches all over the world, this souvenir claims special interest. To the pleasure of recalling facts is added the feeling of mournful regret as we look into the face of the founder and that of his brother James to feel that they are no longer part of the active life of this world. It is something of a compensation to know, however, that the house and our able contemporary, the *Dental Cosmos*, have gone steadily forward, each step taken indicating, indirectly it may be, but still indicating the growth of the dental profession, with which during all these years they have been so intimately connected.

The temptation is, when examining such a souvenir, to allow the mind to travel back to the past and to the men connected with this house and with dentistry, but space does not permit the reminiscent mood.

Excellent pictures are given of all connected with the house at the present, as well as those of the past. These add much to the interest. From President Lewes, General Manager Gilbert, down to the branch managers, each and all tell a story of progress. The congratulations of the INTERNATIONAL DENTAL JOURNAL are extended.

GENERAL CATALOGUE OF MEDICAL BOOKS. P. Blakiston's Son & Co., Philadelphia.

This is a very convenient pocket catalogue, giving title and price of the leading medical and dental books published. In this respect it seems to have been very carefully compiled, and with its interleaves will enable memoranda to be made for future reference. The question of price is one constantly made and not always readily answered. The firm of Blakiston have, therefore, given a really valuable compilation in small compass to the profession.

Current News.

BANQUET TO DR. C. T. STOCKWELL.

DR. CHESTER TWITCHELL STOCKWELL was the recipient last evening of such recognition of notable service as comes but rarely to a man while he is yet alive. Sixty-five friends of many professions, dentistry predominating, tendered him a complimentary banquet at the Massasoit House, of which the features, aside from the bountiful feast, were a preliminary reception and after-dinner speaking, which set forth in terms of fine eulogy the feeling of the company towards its honored guest.

The dinner was given in recognition of the great service done by Dr. Stockwell to dentistry as a science in bringing clearly before the world the germ theory of dental decay, which since his epoch-making paper has become everywhere recognized as the truth, upsetting and forever doing away with the old theory of acids as the cause of destruction. This paper preceded the notable experiments made by Dr. Miller, of Berlin, which demonstrated the truth of Dr. Stockwell's position. It was also in recognition of the many years of faithful and helpful work and counsel among the dentists of the Connecticut Valley. They have been talking for several years of giving him this dinner, and the further testimonial of books, and the convenient time had now come.

The early part of the evening was given over to a reception in the upper parlor of the hotel. At the right of Dr. Stockwell in the receiving party stood Joel H. Hendrick, and at the left Charles

Goodrich Whiting, both intimate friends of the doctor for many years. Other members of the party were Dr. Herbert Stockwell and Professor A. E. Dolbear, of Tufts College. After an hour spent in kindly greeting and reunion, the gathering repaired to the dining-room, where a substantial repast was enjoyed, enlivened by selections by the Home City Quartette and recitations by C. B. Richardson. The tables were arranged in the form of a U, and were radiant with chrysanthemums, contributed by Mrs. Stockwell and Dr. Stockwell's daughter. Autumn leaves and palms supplied further decorations.

The toastmaster for the speaking was Dr. Newton Morgan, of this city, at whose right sat Dr. Stockwell. As a prelude, Dr. George A. Maxwell, of Holyoke, read specimens of the letters of regret received from those of the one hundred and fifty invited guests who could not attend. All testified to the great esteem in which Dr. Stockwell was held throughout this and other countries. The first speaker was Dr. Andrew J. Flanagan, of this city.

Dr. A. J. Flanagan gave a clear history of the remarkable pioneer work which was done by Dr. Stockwell in assisting to establish the bacteriological theory of the decay of teeth. He called attention, in opening, to the great revolution in science and medicine during the past twenty-five years. Three immortal names stand as a synonym of what this revolution implies—Tyndall, Pasteur, and Koch. The germ theory of disease may be traced back with more or less distinctness for two hundred years before the days of Pasteur, but in a practical way the world is more largely indebted to Pasteur than any man who lived during the nineteenth century.

Professor A. E. Dolbear, of Tufts College, presented a view of Dr. Stockwell as one of the philosophers of science. The scientific students discovered and proclaimed facts, and then it was the work of the philosopher, in the broader view, to correlate these facts, and deduce from them their higher and spiritual significance. It is in this class, which many thinkers regard as the higher, that Dr. Stockwell is to be placed. From his close study of science he has drawn inspiration for faith in the ultimate excellence. Dr. Stockwell's philosophical writing, he said, was on a plane of its own because of his trust that the universe was built by one who knew how to do it, and his feeling that he did not need to worry about looking after it. All kinds of knowledge seemed welcome to him. He welcomed the truth, he believed that goodness would triumph. His work has been, then, the raising of mere fact to ideal planes, by deductions of a supreme purpose of good in all manifestations of life.

Charles Goodrich Whiting said that he should speak of the intimate qualities that had made Dr. Stockwell the man he was. His studies in science had developed a close affection for Nature, and it was from her mother-breasts of exhaustless nourishment that he had drawn his interior life. The brief remarks were closed by the familiar lines from Wordsworth's " Tintern Abbey," as expressing the character of Stockwell:

> For I have learned
> To look on Nature, not as in the hour
> Of thoughtless youth, but hearing oftentimes
> The still, sad music of humanity,
> Not harsh or grating, though of ample power
> To chasten and subdue. And I have felt
> A presence that disturbs me with the joy
> Of elevated thoughts; a sense sublime
> Of something far more deeply interfused,
> Whose dwelling is the light of setting suns,
> And the round ocean, and the living air,
> And the blue sky, and in the mind of man;
> A motion and a spirit, that impels
> All thinking things, all objects of all thought,
> And rolls through all things.
> Therefore am I still
> A lover of the meadows and the woods
> And mountains, and of all that we behold
> From this green earth,—of all the mighty world
> Of eye and ear,—both what they half create
> And what perceive; well pleased to recognize
> In Nature and the language of the sense
> The anchor of my purest thought, the nurse,
> The guide, the guardian of my heart; and soul
> Of all my moral being.

Dr. John Dowsley, of Boston, president of the Massachusetts Board of Registration, said in the course of his remarks that during the recent general convention in St. Louis Dr. Stockwell was inquired for more than any other man. Dr. Waldo E. Boardman, of Boston, president of the National Dental Association; Dr. Edgar O. Kinsman, of Cambridge, president of the Massachusetts

Current News.

Dental Society; Albion F. Bemis, of Clinton, Massachusetts State Senator; Dr. James McManus, of Hartford, president of the Northeastern Dental Society; and Dr. Maxfield, of Holyoke, were other speakers. Dr. Maxfield's words were in his happy vein, and as an appropriate climax for the evening's pleasure he presented Dr. Stockwell, in behalf of his friends of the dental profession, a beautiful bookcase containing the world's great thinkers' series,— Kant, Hegel, Plato, Aristotle, Spencer, Mill, and others, in large library octavo; a set of John Burroughs's works, a set of Thoreau, and others. When the programme had been completed, Dr. Morgan invited Dr. Stockwell to speak, if he should so desire.

Dr. Stockwell, evidently touched by the tributes and expressions of good will towards him, gave voice to his feelings in a short address. He said that the older he grew the more convinced he was that kindness and good will is the fundamental fact in human nature. The antagonism, the competition, the jealousies and afflictions of life sometimes lead us to feel that hate or, at least, indifference is the fundamental fact, but it is not so. These belong to the superficial side of life, they are temporary, transient, evanescent. As an example of this Dr. Stockwell related his experience, when, some thirty-five years ago, after he had begun his professional career in Des Moines, Iowa, his health failed. The generous and warm-hearted friendliness of the people of the town and the indorsement which they gave him on his leaving, of his record as a dentist and a citizen, he would never forget. It was no small consolation to reflect that if the shades of these older friends could be present and listen to the kind words of the evening, they might not, after all, regret their indorsement of him. In closing he thanked the company warmly for their kindness, and said, " I can think of no greater boon, as one approaches the evening hour of life, than to be assured that he shall live in the hearts of his fellows. That I conceive to be the most desirable mansion in our Father's house. With that boon to look forward to, I think I may say this is, if not the happiest, at least the most blessed hour of my life. With this inadequate expression of gratitude I bid you all good-night."

Singing of an appropriate arrangement of " Auld Lang Syne" was the closing feature.

The following were present at the dinner:

Senator Albion F. Bemis, of Clinton; R. M. Chase, of Bethel,

Vt.; Dr. H. E. Stockwell, of Stockbridge; Dr. Carl R. Lindstrom, of Lynn; Dr. Waldo E. Boardman, of Boston; Dr. Edward O. Kinsman, of Cambridge; Dr. J. N. Davenport, of Northampton; Dr. Civilion Fores, of Bridgeport, Conn.; Professor A. E. Dolbear, of Tufts College; Dr. A. G. Doane, of Northampton; Dr. Edward B. Griffith and Dr. Frederick Hindsley, of Bridgeport, Conn.; Dr. L. C. Taylor, of Hartford; Dr. F. D. Murlless, of Windsor Locks; Dr. R. H. Clark, of Northampton; Dr. C. S. Gates, of Amherst; Dr. P. T. Nichols, of Northampton; Dr. A. J. Nims, of Turners Falls; Dr. James McManus, of Hartford; Dr. F. Milton Smith, of New York; Dr. Clinton W. Strang, of Bridgeport, Conn.; Dr. George A. Maxfield, of Holyoke; Dr. John H. Dowsley, of Boston; Dr. E. E. Mitchell, of Haverhill; Dr. C. Frank Bliven, of Worcester, Mass.; Dr. Charles McManus, of Hartford; Dr. A. C. Fones, of Bridgeport, Conn.; Dr. Henry McManus, of Hartford, Conn.; Dr. A. J. Cutting, of Southington, Conn.; Dr. Frederic D. Murlless, Jr., of Hartford; Dr. Albert W. Crosby, of New London, Conn.; Dr. W. H. Rider; Dr. Edward B. Dickinson, of Amherst; Dr. P. W. Soule, of Monson; and Dr. J. Wesley Shaw, Dr. Cornelius S. Hurlbut, Samuel D. Sherwood, William F. Adams, A. M. Ross, Harold Ward, Dr. Andrew J. Flanagan, Samuel Bowles, Dr. Newton Morgan, Dr. C. T. Stockwell, Dr. C. Wesley Hale, H. B. Powers, Dr. H. C. Medicroft, Dr. R. A. Baldwin, Dr. James Martin, Dr. Walter W. Swazey, Dr. P. H. Derby, Dr. De Witt C. Shaw, Dr. P. J. Woodward, Dr. E. T. Sherman, Edward S. Hitchcock, Dr. D. Hurlbut Allis, Charles Goodrich Whiting, J. H. Hendrick, Charles H. Churchill, Dr. F. E. Hopkins, Francke W. Dickinson, all of this city.—*Springfield Daily Republican.*

INSTITUTE OF DENTAL PEDAGOGICS.

THE Institute of Dental Pedagogics will hold its annual meeting at Louisville, Ky., December 28, 29, and 30, 1904. This has come to be the most important gathering of the year, and no dental teacher or practitioner interested in dental education can afford to miss the session.

H. B. TILESTON, *President.*
W. E. WILLMOTT, *Secretary.*

HARTFORD DENTAL SOCIETY.

At the annual meeting of the Hartford Dental Society, held October 10, 1904, the following officers were elected for the ensuing year:

President, Dr. G. M. Griswold; Vice-President, Dr. C. E. Barrett; Secretary, Dr. A. E. Cary; Treasurer, Dr. E. R. Whitford; Librarian and Curator, Dr. Henry Dryhurst; Historian, Dr. Henry McManus.

Executive Committee.—Dr. E. H. Munger, Chairman, Dr. W. S. Youngblood, Dr. A. A. Hunt.

A. E. Cary,
Secretary.

THIRTY-SIXTH ANNIVERSARY MEETING OF THE FIRST DISTRICT DENTAL SOCIETY OF THE STATE OF NEW YORK.

The First District Dental Society will celebrate its thirty-sixth anniversary by two great meetings on the 12th and 13th of December. The essayists of these meetings will be Dr. G. V. Black, of Chicago, and Dr. E. K. Wedelstaedt, of St. Paul. Dr. Black will read an exhaustive *résumé* on the subject of " Extension for Prevention," illustrating his lecture with one hundred and twenty-five or more lantern-slide pictures. Dr. R. H. Hofheinz will open the discussion. On December 13 Dr. E. K. Wedelstaedt will read a paper on the " Packing of Gold in Approximo-Occlusal Cavities in Bicuspids and Molars," illustrating his method with the use of clay in large wooden models of teeth. The discussion of this paper will be opened by Dr. G. V. Black, and followed by Dr. R. Ottolengui and Dr. B. Holly Smith. This meeting will be held at the New York Academy of Medicine, 17 West Forty-third Street, at eight o'clock in the evening.

In addition to this meeting the Clinic Committee has arranged for a most interesting clinical exhibition to be held during the afternoons of these days, at the Grand Central Palace, Lexington Avenue and Forty-third Street. This programme comprises porcclain work, X-ray, different methods of packing gold, orthodontia, exhibits of different anatomical and histological specimens, etc.

Dr. Black will exhibit new instruments for testing the finger-power in the handling of operative instruments. Every facility will be afforded to enable the largest number to witness the demonstrations. The entire mornings of both days will be devoted to manufacturers' exhibits, which will be an interesting feature of the programme. All communications pertaining to clinics or exhibits should be addressed to the chairman of the Clinic Committee, Dr. S. L. Goldsmith, 129 East Sixty-ninth Street.

The following dental societies have been officially invited: The New York Institute of Stomatology, the New York Odontological Society, the New York Institute of Dental Techniques, the Second District Dental Society of the State of New York, the Central Dental Association of Northern New Jersey, the Hartford Dental Society, and the New Haven Dental Society.

A cordial invitation is extended to all members of the dental profession, and it is confidently expected that a large number of prominent dentists will be in attendance.

F. L. Fossume, *Chairman,*

A. M. Merritt,

A. G. Lansing,

Executive Committee.

OHIO STATE DENTAL SOCIETY—THIRTY-NINTH ANNUAL MEETING.

Following is the programme of the thirty-ninth annual meeting of the Ohio State Dental Society, to be held at the Great Southern Hotel, Columbus, Ohio, December 6, 7, and 8, 1904:

ESSAYS—TUESDAY.

" Personality," Bert E. Saunders, Elyria. Discussion, C. R. Butler, A. O. Ross.

" The Nerve Broach," W. I. Jones, Nelsonville. Discussion, H. J. Bosart, W. A. Holmes.

" Care of the Teeth of the Poor," W. T. Jackman, Cleveland. Discussion, C. I. Keely, W. G. Ebersole.

" The Dental Nurse," C. M. Wright, Cincinnati. Discussion, J. R. Callahan, H. F. Harvey.

960 *Current News.*

"The Advantages of the Pyrometer for Obtaining Exact Results in Baking Porcelain," Weston A. Price, Cleveland. Discussion, L. E. Custer, H. M. Semans.

"Removable and Fixed Bridge-Work," Fred A. Peeso, Philadelphia, Pa. Discussion, Geo. H. Wilson, W. O. Hulick.

"Selected," Edward K. Wedelstaedt, St. Paul, Minn. Discussion, O. N. Heise, L. L. Barber.

"Pathological Irregularities," M. H. Fletcher, Cincinnati. Discussion, C. A. Hawley, W. S. Locke.

"Development and Maldevelopment Incident to Infant Dentition" (stereopticon), S. D. Ruggles, Portsmouth. Discussion, H. A. Smith, E. H. Raffensperger.

CLINICS—WEDNESDAY.

1. A. C. Searl, Owatonna, Minn., "Gold Filling, Mesio-Occlusal Surface of Molar or Bicuspid."

2. Henry C. Raymond, Detroit, Mich., "Porcelain Inlay."

3. G. W. Wasser, Cleveland, "High-Fusing Porcelain Inlay."

4. Frank J. Smith, Columbus, "Porcelain Inlay, Brewster's Body."

5. Edward E. Hall, Columbus, "Ambler's Tin and Sibley's Felt Gold."

6. H. C. Brown, Columbus, "A Method of reducing Pain in Cavity Preparation."

7. Chas. K. Teter, Cleveland, "Extracting under Prolonged Anæsthesia with Nitrous Oxide and Oxygen."

8. L. O. Green, Chicago, Ill., "Extracting under Local Anæsthesia."

9. C. H. Thompson, Athens, "The Use of Distilled Water for the Painless Extraction of Teeth."

10. M. E. Fenton, Cleveland, "Ethyl Chloride in Dental Surgery."

11. C. V. Lanum, Washington C. H., "Immediate Regulating."

12. Fred A. Peeso, Philadelphia, Pa., "Removable and Fixed Bridge-Work."

13. W. O. Hulick, Cincinnati, "Carved Cusps for Gold Crowns and Bridges."

14. Edward B. Spalding, Detroit, Mich., "A Shell of Porcelain reproducing the Entire Natural Enamel and thoroughly

. protecting the dentine of a Living Tooth when made necessary by Erosion or other Cause."

15. Geo. E. Bratton, Manchester, " One Method of making the Gold Bicuspid and Molar Crown."

16. E. S. Fuller, Piqua, " Partial Gold and Rubber ·Plates."

17. Weston A. Price, Cleveland, " The Advantages of the Pyrometer."

18. W. H. Hayden, Youngstown, " The Whiteside Crown as a Bridge Dummy."

19. Geo. H. Wilson, Cleveland, " Expansion and Compressibility of Plaster."

20. Varney E. Barnes, Cleveland, " Adjustable Regulating Appliances."

21. W. L. Gares, Columbus, " Method of repairing and packing Partial Dentures." (*b*) " Method of setting Logan Crown."

22. W. I. Jones, Nelsonville, " One Way to set a Fractured Inferior Maxillary."

23. Clare Smith, Columbus, " Crown- and Bridge-Work, Removable Facings."

24. R. C. Brophy, Chicago, Ill., " Porcelain Work, using Gasoline and Gas Furnaces."

25· F. W. Stephan, Chicago, Ill., " Anatomical Articulator."

26. L. E. Custer, Dayton, " Demonstration of a New Electric Appliance."

CLINICS—THURSDAY.

1. A. C. Searl, Owatonna, Minn., " Gold Filling, Mesio-Occlusal Surface of Molar or Bicuspid."

2. Geo. H. Woodbury, Cleveland, " High-Fusing Porcelain Inlays."

3. Gillette Hayden, Columbus, " Treatment of Diseased Pulps."

4. G. S. Junkerman, Cincinnati, " Soft Foil *versus* Cruelty."

5. W. G. Hamm, Chillicothe, " Pressure Anæsthesia, Immediate Pulp Extirpation."

6. J. W. McDill, Cleveland, " Flexible Rubber Attachment for Partial Rubber Dentures."

7. Holston Bartilson, Columbus, " A Practical Bridge, using Steele's Detachable Facing."

8. Sidney A. Rauh, Cincinnati, " Use of Napkins in Operative Work."

9. S. M. Weaver, Cleveland, " Pressure Anæsthesia by Automatic High-Pressure Syringe."

10. Karl C. Brashear, Columbus, " Anæsthesia, using Somnoform."

11. Nelson D. Edmonds, Wilmington, " Hollow Gold Inlays, Dr. C. N. Thompson's Method."

12. Fred A. Peeso, Philadelphia, " Removable and Fixed Bridge-Work."

13. H. E. Jenkins, Ironton, " Porcelain Jacket Crown."

14. E. Ballard Lodge, Cleveland, " Stereoscopic Dental Skiagraphs."

15. A. P. Bell, Zanesville, " Richmond Crowns."

16. J. O. Hawkins, Wellston, " Some Original Ideas on swaging Plates and Crowns."

17. Alden Bush, Columbus, " Anatomical Models for teaching Cavity Preparation, Dental Anatomy, etc."

18. J. C. Newton, Cleveland, " Knapp Crown."

19. M. L. Leob, Cleveland, " Crown and Bridge, using Over-Top Facing."

20. Edward B. Spalding, Detroit, Mich., " A Shell of Porcelain reproducing the Entire Natural Enamel and thoroughly protecting the Dentine of a Living Tooth when made necessary by Erosion or other Cause."

21. F. M. Casto, Cleveland, " Construction of Plain Bands (Orthodontia)."

22. H. H. Phillips, Cincinnati, " The Justi Porcelain Crown."

23. J. R. Bell, Cleveland, " Matrices."

24. R. C. Brophy, Chicago, Ill., " Cast-Metal Dentures."

25. M. H. Fletcher, Cincinnati, " Pathological Irregularities."

26. C. G. Myers, Cleveland, " Obtunding Sensitive Dentine."

CALIFORNIA BOARD OF DENTAL EXAMINERS.

THE Board of Dental Examiners of California will hold an examination in San Francisco, commencing on Thursday, December 15, 1904.

F. G. BAIRD,
Secretary.

INDEX TO VOLUME XXV.

D

This book must be returned to
the Dental Library by the last
date stamped below.   It may
be renewed if there is no
reservation for it.

270-7-60

Lightning Source UK Ltd.
Milton Keynes UK
UKHW020432210219
337573UK00007B/1608/P